Designing Next-Generation Drug-Like Molecules for Medicinal Applications

Designing Next-Generation Drug-Like Molecules for Medicinal Applications

Guest Editors

Imtiaz Khan
Sumera Zaib

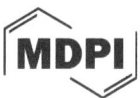

Basel • Beijing • Wuhan • Barcelona • Belgrade • Novi Sad • Cluj • Manchester

Guest Editors

Imtiaz Khan
Department of Chemistry
The University of Manchester
Manchester
United Kingdom

Sumera Zaib
Department of Basic and
Applied Chemistry
University of Central Punjab
Lahore
Pakistan

Editorial Office
MDPI AG
Grosspeteranlage 5
4052 Basel, Switzerland

This is a reprint of the Special Issue, published open access by the journal *Molecules* (ISSN 1420-3049), freely accessible at: www.mdpi.com/journal/molecules/special_issues/Drug_Like_Molecules.

For citation purposes, cite each article independently as indicated on the article page online and using the guide below:

Lastname, A.A.; Lastname, B.B. Article Title. *Journal Name* **Year**, *Volume Number*, Page Range.

ISBN 978-3-7258-3008-4 (Hbk)
ISBN 978-3-7258-3007-7 (PDF)
https://doi.org/10.3390/books978-3-7258-3007-7

© 2025 by the authors. Articles in this book are Open Access and distributed under the Creative Commons Attribution (CC BY) license. The book as a whole is distributed by MDPI under the terms and conditions of the Creative Commons Attribution-NonCommercial-NoDerivs (CC BY-NC-ND) license (https://creativecommons.org/licenses/by-nc-nd/4.0/).

Contents

About the Editors vii

Imtiaz Khan and Sumera Zaib
Designing Next-Generation Drug-like Molecules for Medicinal Applications
Reprinted from: *Molecules* **2023**, *28*, 1860, https://doi.org/10.3390/molecules28041860 1

Komal Sharma, Shams Aaghaz, Indresh Kumar Maurya, Shreya Singh, Shivaprakash M. Rudramurthy and Vinod Kumar et al.
Ring-Modified Histidine-Containing Cationic Short Peptides Exhibit Anticryptococcal Activity by Cellular Disruption
Reprinted from: *Molecules* **2022**, *28*, 87, https://doi.org/10.3390/molecules28010087 5

Mariangela Agamennone, Marialuigia Fantacuzzi, Simone Carradori, Anél Petzer, Jacobus P. Petzer and Andrea Angeli et al.
Coumarin-Based Dual Inhibitors of Human Carbonic Anhydrases and Monoamine Oxidases Featuring Amino Acyl and (*Pseudo*)-Dipeptidyl Appendages: In Vitro and Computational Studies
Reprinted from: *Molecules* **2022**, *27*, 7884, https://doi.org/10.3390/molecules27227884 25

Reda G. Yousef, Wagdy M. Eldehna, Alaa Elwan, Abdelaziz S. Abdelaziz, Ahmed B. M. Mehany and Ibraheem M. M. Gobaara et al.
Design, Synthesis, In Silico and In Vitro Studies of New Immunomodulatory Anticancer Nicotinamide Derivatives Targeting VEGFR-2
Reprinted from: *Molecules* **2022**, *27*, 4079, https://doi.org/10.3390/molecules27134079 49

Ibrahim H. Eissa, Mohamed S. Alesawy, Abdulrahman M. Saleh, Eslam B. Elkaeed, Bshra A. Alsfouk and Abdul-Aziz M. M. El-Attar et al.
Ligand and Structure-Based In Silico Determination of the Most Promising SARS-CoV-2 nsp16-nsp10 2′-*o*-Methyltransferase Complex Inhibitors among 3009 FDA Approved Drugs
Reprinted from: *Molecules* **2022**, *27*, 2287, https://doi.org/10.3390/molecules27072287 74

Niels V. Heise, Daniel Major, Sophie Hoenke, Marie Kozubek, Immo Serbian and René Csuk
Rhodamine 101 Conjugates of Triterpenoic Amides Are of Comparable Cytotoxicity as Their Rhodamine B Analogs
Reprinted from: *Molecules* **2022**, *27*, 2220, https://doi.org/10.3390/molecules27072220 99

Lubna Atta, Ruqaiya Khalil, Khalid Mohammed Khan, Moatter Zehra, Faiza Saleem and Mohammad Nur-e-Alam et al.
Virtual Screening, Synthesis and Biological Evaluation of *Streptococcus mutans* Mediated Biofilm Inhibitors
Reprinted from: *Molecules* **2022**, *27*, 1455, https://doi.org/10.3390/molecules27041455 116

Kashif Rafiq, Najeeb Ur Rehman, Sobia Ahsan Halim, Majid Khan, Ajmal Khan and Ahmed Al-Harrasi
Design, Synthesis and Molecular Docking Study of Novel 3-Phenyl-β-Alanine-Based Oxadiazole Analogues as Potent Carbonic Anhydrase II Inhibitors
Reprinted from: *Molecules* **2022**, *27*, 816, https://doi.org/10.3390/molecules27030816 127

Atsushi Yoshimori, Filip Miljković and Jürgen Bajorath
Approach for the Design of Covalent Protein Kinase Inhibitors via Focused Deep Generative Modeling
Reprinted from: *Molecules* **2022**, *27*, 570, https://doi.org/10.3390/molecules27020570 141

Mohammed I. El-Gamal, Seyed-Omar Zaraei, Moustafa M. Madkour and Hanan S. Anbar
Evaluation of Substituted Pyrazole-Based Kinase Inhibitors in One Decade (2011–2020): Current Status and Future Prospects
Reprinted from: *Molecules* **2022**, *27*, 330, https://doi.org/10.3390/molecules27010330 153

Md. Khalid Anwer, Essam A. Ali, Muzaffar Iqbal, Mohammed Muqtader Ahmed, Mohammed F. Aldawsari and Ahmed Al Saqr et al.
Development of Sustained Release Baricitinib Loaded Lipid-Polymer Hybrid Nanoparticles with Improved Oral Bioavailability
Reprinted from: *Molecules* **2021**, *27*, 168, https://doi.org/10.3390/molecules27010168 238

Md Yousof Ali, Susoma Jannat, Hyun-Ah Jung and Jae-Sue Choi
Structural Bases for Hesperetin Derivatives: Inhibition of Protein Tyrosine Phosphatase 1B, Kinetics Mechanism and Molecular Docking Study
Reprinted from: *Molecules* **2021**, *26*, 7433, https://doi.org/10.3390/molecules26247433 253

Mohammed I. El-Gamal, Nada H. Mewafi, Nada E. Abdelmotteleb, Minnatullah A. Emara, Hamadeh Tarazi and Rawan M. Sbenati et al.
A Review of HER4 (ErbB4) Kinase, Its Impact on Cancer, and Its Inhibitors
Reprinted from: *Molecules* **2021**, *26*, 7376, https://doi.org/10.3390/molecules26237376 269

Faisal Usman, Hamid Saeed Shah, Sumera Zaib, Sirikhwan Manee, Jahanzeb Mudassir and Ajmal Khan et al.
Fabrication and Biological Assessment of Antidiabetic α-Mangostin Loaded Nanosponges: In Vitro, In Vivo, and In Silico Studies
Reprinted from: *Molecules* **2021**, *26*, 6633, https://doi.org/10.3390/molecules26216633 300

Sumera Zaib, Rubina Munir, Muhammad Tayyab Younas, Naghmana Kausar, Aliya Ibrar and Sehar Aqsa et al.
Hybrid Quinoline-Thiosemicarbazone Therapeutics as a New Treatment Opportunity for Alzheimer's Disease-Synthesis, In Vitro Cholinesterase Inhibitory Potential and Computational Modeling Analysis
Reprinted from: *Molecules* **2021**, *26*, 6573, https://doi.org/10.3390/molecules26216573 314

Mahmoud M. Gamal El-Din, Mohammed I. El-Gamal, Young-Do Kwon, Su-Yeon Kim, Hee-Soo Han and Sang-Eun Park et al.
Evaluation of the Inhibitory Effects of Pyridylpyrazole Derivatives on LPS-Induced PGE_2 Productions and Nitric Oxide in Murine RAW 264.7 Macrophages
Reprinted from: *Molecules* **2021**, *26*, 6489, https://doi.org/10.3390/molecules26216489 337

Abdullah Mohammed Al-Majid, M. Ali, Mohammad Shahidul Islam, Saeed Alshahrani, Abdullah Saleh Alamary and Sammer Yousuf et al.
Stereoselective Synthesis of the Di-Spirooxindole Analogs Based Oxindole and Cyclohexanone Moieties as Potential Anticancer Agents
Reprinted from: *Molecules* **2021**, *26*, 6305, https://doi.org/10.3390/molecules26206305 345

Md Yousof Ali, Seongkyu Park and Munseog Chang
Phytochemistry, Ethnopharmacological Uses, Biological Activities, and Therapeutic Applications of *Cassia obtusifolia* L.: A Comprehensive Review
Reprinted from: *Molecules* **2021**, *26*, 6252, https://doi.org/10.3390/molecules26206252 365

About the Editors

Imtiaz Khan

Dr. Imtiaz Khan received his PhD degree in Chemistry from The University of Nottingham, United Kingdom. Later, he worked as a postdoctoral research associate at the same University. He then spent two years (2016-2018) as a Leverhulme Trust research fellow at Cardiff University before joining The University of Manchester, UK, in 2018. He has made significant contributions to the scientific and academic communities by publishing over 140 peer-reviewed articles and reviews with an impact factor of >670 that have been cited over 4800 times. He also received the Research Staff Strategy Group (RSSG) Excellence Award 2020/21 from the University of Manchester and Horizon Prize: Rita and John Cornforth Award 2023 from the Royal Society of Chemistry. His research interests include the development of novel synthetic methodologies for the efficient synthesis of biologically active heterocycles and integrated chemo- and biocatalysis.

Sumera Zaib

Dr. Sumera Zaib received her PhD degree in Biochemistry from Hazara University, Pakistan. During her PhD, she has visited University of Bonn, Germany, as a DAAD research fellow. Dr. Zaib has worked as a Postdoctoral Research Fellow for over 2 years at COMSATS University, Islamabad. Afterwards, she joined University of Central Punjab, Lahore, and is currently working as an Associate Professor and leading the department of Basic and Applied Chemistry. She has successfully produced 1 book, 3 international book chapters, 7 national patents, >180 publications in reputable international journals with an impact factor of >700 and a 33 h-index, and over 3500 citations. Dr. Zaib is also recipient of multiple research productivity awards by Pakistan Council of Science and Technology. She has also been awarded "The Best Researcher and Innovator Award 2021" by University of Central Punjab. Dr Zaib has supervised and co-supervised >90 BS, MS and PhD students. She has successfully secured several research grants of over 7 Million PKR from Pakistan Science Foundation, Higher Education Commission of Pakistan and BioSolveIT, Germany. Her research interests include protein chemistry and enzymology with special emphasis on clinical biochemistry and enzyme inhibition studies.

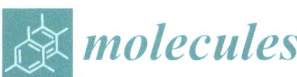

Editorial

Designing Next-Generation Drug-like Molecules for Medicinal Applications

Imtiaz Khan [1,*] and Sumera Zaib [2,*]

1. Department of Chemistry and Manchester, Institute of Biotechnology, The University of Manchester, 131 Princess Street, Manchester M1 7DN, UK
2. Department of Basic and Applied Chemistry, Faculty of Science and Technology, University of Central Punjab, Lahore 54590, Pakistan
* Correspondence: kimtiaz@hotmail.co.uk (I.K.); sumera.zaib@ucp.edu.pk (S.Z.)

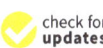

Citation: Khan, I.; Zaib, S. Designing Next-Generation Drug-like Molecules for Medicinal Applications. *Molecules* **2023**, *28*, 1860. https://doi.org/10.3390/molecules28041860

Received: 1 January 2023
Revised: 2 February 2023
Accepted: 3 February 2023
Published: 16 February 2023

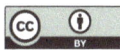

Copyright: © 2023 by the authors. Licensee MDPI, Basel, Switzerland. This article is an open access article distributed under the terms and conditions of the Creative Commons Attribution (CC BY) license (https://creativecommons.org/licenses/by/4.0/).

The development of new drugs/drug candidates for medical treatment remains an exciting but challenging process as only a limited number of synthetic compounds fit well into the discovery and development process after multiple experiments and screening for their preclinical properties. Over the years, this continuous demand has been fueled by the use of organic/synthetic chemistry protocols that deliver new molecules or improve the existing toolbox diversifying libraries of pharmacophores of medicinal interest. The application of new methodologies, particularly employing green and sustainable commercial feedstock chemicals for the discovery and development of biological therapeutics, opens up new avenues of research. In parallel, the discovery and development of new organic molecules have always proved effective in designing drugs, while overcoming critical challenges to the pharmaceutical industry and providing innovative solutions towards commercialized medicines.

This Special Issue aims to provide a far-reaching overview of the most recent developments in synthetic methodologies as well as medicinal chemistry applications of small molecule inhibitors. This Special Issue encompasses fourteen original research articles and three authoritative reviews covering exciting developments in the design strategies of new drugs/drug molecules, structure–activity relationships, in vitro and in silico analyses, and pharmacokinetic properties. These articles not only summarize the recent developments in different perspectives of drug development but also present a wealth of information and possible structural leads to explore new drug inhibitors against various targets of medicinal importance. Herein, we briefly summarize the contributions reported in this Special Issue.

Chang and co-workers summarized the phytochemistry, ethnopharmacological uses, biological activities, and therapeutic applications of *Cassia obtusifolia* L., a member of the Leguminosae family. The ethnomedicinal importance of *C. obtusifolia* indicates that the whole plant, roots, seeds, leaves, stem bark, pods, and fruits are used for the treatment of various health issues. The pharmacological features of the plant include- antimicrobial, anti-inflammatory, antidiabetic, antioxidant, anticancer, neuroprotective, hepatoprotective, immune-modulatory, larvicidal, anti-Alzheimer's, and anti-Parkinson's properties [1].

El-Gamal and co-workers reviewed the structure, location, ligands, and functions of HER4 kinase, which play a key role in the normal physiological functions of body systems such as cardiovascular, nervous, and endocrine systems. They have also summarized the relationship of HER4 with the development of various cancers such as colorectal, lung, gastric, prostate, bladder, ovarian, breast, pancreatic, brain, endometrial, melanoma, osteosarcoma, and hepatocellular carcinoma. They also presented a concise summary of selective HER4 inhibitors developed between 2016 and 2022. These classes include quinazoline, quinoline, imidazo-pyrimidine, pyrrolo-pyrimidine, and imidazo-thiazole compounds [2].

In the subsequent study, El-Gamal and co-workers reviewed the pyrazole-based kinase inhibitors developed between 2011 and 2020. Pyrazole is a well-known nitrogen-containing five-membered heterocycle with a proven track-record of a diverse pharmacological importance. Among many other biological functions, pyrazole derivatives have shown their potential as kinase inhibitors that play a crucial role in various cancers. The reported pyrazole-containing compounds have displayed inhibitory effects against various kinases, including Akt, ALK, Aurora, Bcr-Abl, CDK, Chk2, EGFR, ERK/MEK, FGFR, IRAK4, ITK, JAK, JNK, LRRK, Lsrk, MAPK14, PDK4, Pim, RAF, ROS1, Src, and VEGFR [3].

Barakat and co-workers developed a concise library of spirooxindole derivatives through a one-pot three-component approach. α,β-unsaturated ketones, substituted isatin, and (2S)-octahydro-1H-indole-2-carboxylic acid were coupled together in methanol under reflux conditions. The target compounds were obtained in high regio- and diastereoselectivity. The synthetic compounds were evaluated for their antiproliferative activity against four cancer cell lines, including prostate PC3, cervical HeLa, and triple-negative breast cancer (MCF-7 and MDA-MB231) using an MTT assay. Molecular docking analysis was also performed to rationalize the key binding interactions and results, which demonstrated that the active compounds accommodated well in the binding pocket of MDM2 [4].

Kim and co-workers reported a series of pyridylpyrazole derivatives and evaluated their potential to inhibit lipopolysaccharide (LPS)-induced prostaglandin E2 (PGE2) and the production of nitric oxide (NO) in RAW264.7 macrophages. A multistep synthetic route was established using commercial starting materials to obtain the target compounds. Some of the tested compounds exerted a stronger inhibitory effect on the production of PGE2 than over NO [5].

Khan and co-workers demonstrated a facile multistep synthetic approach to access quinoline-thiosemicarbazone derivatives. A molecular hybridization strategy was used to combine quinoline and thiosemicarbazone pharmacophores in one unit. The in vitro cholinesterase inhibitory assessment of the tested derivatives revealed that several compounds can act as potential drug candidates against Alzheimer's disease. Kinetics studies were performed, presenting the competitive mode of inhibition. Molecular docking analysis further revealed the conspicuous role of vital binding interactions in the active pocket of cholinesterases, whereas the ADMET profile suggested the safe and druggable properties of quinoline-thiosemicarbazone hybrids [6].

In another study, Khan and co-workers prepared α-mangostin (MGN)-loaded nanosponges using a quasi-emulsion solvent evaporation method and investigated their potential to treat type 2 diabetes mellitus. The nanosponges were characterized through FTIR spectroscopy, differential scanning calorimetry (DSC), and scanning electron microscopy (SEM). Various physicochemical properties, including the zeta potential, entrapment efficiency, hydrodynamic diameter, and drug-release properties were also tested. The in vitro α-glucosidase inhibition potential demonstrated appreciable results, which were reinforced with in vivo studies [7].

Choi and co-workers reported the anti-diabetic potential of naturally occurring hesperetin and their glycosylated derivatives using protein tyrosine phosphatase 1B (PTP1B). The acquired results were promising and PTP1B inhibition was found to be dependent on the nature, position, and number of sugar moieties in the flavonoid structure. Molecular docking analysis showed a significant binding interaction with key amino acid residues in the PTP1B allosteric site cavity [8].

Anwer and co-workers demonstrated the preparation of four different baricitinib (BTB)-loaded lipids (stearin)-polymer hybrid nanoparticles using a single-step nanoprecipitation method. The nanoparticles were characterized through various physicochemical parameters. The in vitro release and in vivo pharmacokinetic studies in rats revealed the enhanced bioavailability of BTB formulations [9].

A computational approach was designed and utilized by Bajorath and co-workers to explore covalent kinase inhibitors by combining fragment- and structure-based screening with deep generative modeling learning. The approach was exemplified with the design of Bruton's tyrosine kinase (BTK) inhibitors, which are employed as a major drug target for the treatment of inflammatory diseases and leukemia [10].

Al-Harrasi and co-workers designed and synthesized a small library of 1,3,4-oxadiazole compounds that contain a phenylalanine amino acid. The structures were fully established through various spectroscopic methods. The carbonic anhydrase inhibitory profile was examined and the acquired in vitro efficacy was remarkable, which was further validated with computational modeling analysis [11].

Ul-Haq and co-workers performed in silico screening (virtual screening) for the identification of small-molecule inhibitors of *Streptococcus mutans* glycosyltransferases. They have developed various pharmacophore models which were validated with multiple datasets. Several hits were identified, showing a high binding affinity, and hydrophobic and electrostatic interactions with vital amino acid residues. The identified hits exhibited remarkable antibiofilm activity [12].

Csuk and co-workers synthesized a selection of rhodamine B or rhodamine 101-conjugated pentacyclic triterpenoic amides. Piperazine or homopiperazine were successfully coupled with different acids. The cytotoxic activity of the synthetic derivatives was evaluated using SRB assays. The in vitro results demonstrated that the piperazinyl and homopiperazinyl amides are more cytotoxic than their parent acids or acetylated congeners. Moreover, rhodamine 101-conjugated homopiperazinyl amide showed good results against ovarian cancer cells [13].

Metwaly and co-workers applied an in silico approach for the identification of the best SARS-CoV-2 nsp16-nsp10 2'-*o*-methyltransferase (2'OMTase) inhibitor among several FDA-approved drugs. They have utilized molecular fingerprints, structure similarity analysis, molecular modeling, and MD simulations to identify and support the results [14].

In the search of new VEGFR-2 inhibitors, Eissa and co-workers designed and synthesized several nicotinamide compounds. Anti-proliferative activity results against human cancer cell lines (HCT-116 and HepG2) showed significant promise and excellent VEGFR-2 inhibitory activity. Furthermore, immunomodulatory effects against TNF-α and IL-6 were also examined. In silico molecular docking and dynamics simulation demonstrated the high affinity to the target resides and the ADMET profile indicated the acceptable drug-likeness properties [15].

Carradori and co-workers reported coumarin-based amino acyl and (pseudo)-dipeptidyl derivatives. The in vitro dual inhibitory potential against membrane-bound and cytosolic human carbonic anhydrases (hCAs) and monoamine oxidases (hMAOs) as anticancer agents was evaluated. The synthetic compounds exhibited a nanomolar inhibition efficacy. Computational studies shed light on the interesting features required for the inhibitory profiles as well as the isoform selectivity [16].

Jain and co-workers reported a series of ring-modified histidine-containing short cationic peptides. The anticryptococcal activity was evaluated and the acquired results revealed promising antifungal activities against *C. neoformans*. The SEM and TEM analyses indicated the involvement of the cell disruption mechanism [17].

In summary, the current Special Issue encompasses both synthetic and natural inhibitors of various drug targets. The synthetic classes include pyrazole, pyridylpyrazole, oxadiazole, amides, spirooxindole, quinoline-thiosemicarbazone, and coumarin derivatives. The conjugation of amino acids with other biologically active pharmacophores as well as the synthesis of short peptides for medicinal purposes have been achieved. The use of nanotechnology to address the burgeoning health complications have also been illustrated. Various drug delivery approaches highlighted the sustained drug release and enhanced bioavailability of nanoformulations. Moreover, in silico approaches were successfully exploited not only for the identification of potential inhibitors but also for the elucidation of a high affinity to the target residues, thus strengthening the in vitro assay results. Overall, the presented research in this Special Issue demonstrates a significant advancement towards achieving the next-generation drug-like molecules for medicinal applications.

Acknowledgments: We thank all the authors for their valuable contributions, all the peer reviewers for their valuable comments, criticisms, and suggestions.

Conflicts of Interest: The authors declare no conflict of interest.

References

1. Ali, M.Y.; Park, S.; Chang, M. Phytochemistry, Ethnopharmacological Uses, Biological Activities, and Therapeutic Applications of *Cassia obtusifolia* L.: A Comprehensive Review. *Molecules* **2021**, *26*, 6252. [CrossRef] [PubMed]
2. El-Gamal, M.I.; Mewafi, N.H.; Abdelmotteleb, N.E.; Emara, M.A.; Tarazi, H.; Sbenati, R.M.; Madkour, M.M.; Zaraei, S.-O.; Shahin, A.I.; Anbar, H.S. A Review of HER4 (ErbB4) Kinase, Its Impact on Cancer, and Its Inhibitors. *Molecules* **2021**, *26*, 7376. [CrossRef] [PubMed]
3. El-Gamal, M.I.; Zaraei, S.-O.; Madkour, M.M.; Anbar, H.S. Evaluation of Substituted Pyrazole-Based Kinase Inhibitors in One Decade (2011–2020): Current Status and Future Prospects. *Molecules* **2022**, *27*, 330. [CrossRef] [PubMed]
4. Al-Majid, A.M.; Ali, M.; Islam, M.S.; Alshahrani, S.; Alamary, A.S.; Yousuf, S.; Choudhary, M.I.; Barakat, A. Stereoselective Synthesis of the Di-Spirooxindole Analogs Based Oxindole and Cyclohexanone Moieties as Potential Anticancer Agents. *Molecules* **2021**, *26*, 6305. [CrossRef] [PubMed]
5. Gamal El-Din, M.M.; El-Gamal, M.I.; Kwon, Y.-D.; Kim, S.-Y.; Han, H.-S.; Park, S.-E.; Oh, C.-H.; Lee, K.-T.; Kim, H.-K. Evaluation of the Inhibitory Effects of Pyridylpyrazole Derivatives on LPS-Induced PGE2 Productions and Nitric Oxide in Murine RAW 264.7 Macrophages. *Molecules* **2021**, *26*, 6489. [CrossRef] [PubMed]
6. Zaib, S.; Munir, R.; Younas, M.T.; Kausar, N.; Ibrar, A.; Aqsa, S.; Shahid, N.; Asif, T.T.; Alsaab, H.O.; Khan, I. Hybrid Quinoline-Thiosemicarbazone Therapeutics as a New Treatment Opportunity for Alzheimer's Disease-Synthesis, In Vitro Cholinesterase Inhibitory Potential and Computational Modeling Analysis. *Molecules* **2021**, *26*, 6573. [CrossRef] [PubMed]
7. Usman, F.; Shah, H.S.; Zaib, S.; Manee, S.; Mudassir, J.; Khan, A.; Batiha, G.E.-S.; Abualnaja, K.M.; Alhashmialameer, D.; Khan, I. Fabrication and Biological Assessment of Antidiabetic α-Mangostin Loaded Nanosponges: In Vitro, In Vivo, and In Silico Studies. *Molecules* **2021**, *26*, 6633. [CrossRef] [PubMed]
8. Ali, M.Y.; Jannat, S.; Jung, H.-A.; Choi, J.-S. Structural Bases for Hesperetin Derivatives: Inhibition of Protein Tyrosine Phosphatase 1B, Kinetics Mechanism and Molecular Docking Study. *Molecules* **2021**, *26*, 7433. [CrossRef] [PubMed]
9. Anwer, M.K.; Ali, E.A.; Iqbal, M.; Ahmed, M.M.; Aldawsari, M.F.; Saqr, A.A.; Ansari, M.N.; Aboudzadeh, M.A. Development of Sustained Release Baricitinib Loaded Lipid-Polymer Hybrid Nanoparticles with Improved Oral Bioavailability. *Molecules* **2022**, *27*, 168. [CrossRef] [PubMed]
10. Yoshimori, A.; Miljković, F.; Bajorath, J. Approach for the Design of Covalent Protein Kinase Inhibitors via Focused Deep Generative Modeling. *Molecules* **2022**, *27*, 570. [CrossRef] [PubMed]
11. Rafiq, K.; Ur Rehman, N.; Halim, S.A.; Khan, M.; Khan, A.; Al-Harrasi, A. Design, Synthesis and Molecular Docking Study of Novel 3-Phenyl-Alanine-Based Oxadiazole Analogues as Potent Carbonic Anhydrase II Inhibitors. *Molecules* **2022**, *27*, 816. [CrossRef] [PubMed]
12. Atta, L.; Khalil, R.; Khan, K.M.; Zehra, M.; Saleem, F.; Nur-e-Alam, M.; Ul-Haq, Z. Virtual Screening, Synthesis and Biological Evaluation of *Streptococcus mutans* Mediated Biofilm Inhibitors. *Molecules* **2022**, *27*, 1455. [CrossRef] [PubMed]
13. Heise, N.V.; Major, D.; Hoenke, S.; Kozubek, M.; Serbian, I.; Csuk, R. Rhodamine 101 Conjugates of Triterpenoic Amides Are of Comparable Cytotoxicity as Their Rhodamine B Analogs. *Molecules* **2022**, *27*, 2220. [CrossRef] [PubMed]
14. Eissa, I.H.; Alesawy, M.S.; Saleh, A.M.; Elkaeed, E.B.; Alsfouk, B.A.; El-Attar, A.-A.M.M.; Metwaly, A.M. Ligand and Structure-Based In Silico Determination of the Most Promising SARS-CoV-2 nsp16-nsp10 2′-o-Methyltransferase Complex Inhibitors among 3009 FDA Approved Drugs. *Molecules* **2022**, *27*, 2287. [CrossRef] [PubMed]
15. Yousef, R.G.; Eldehna, W.M.; Elwan, A.; Abdelaziz, A.S.; Mehany, A.B.M.; Gobaara, I.M.M.; Alsfouk, B.A.; Elkaeed, E.B.; Metwaly, A.M.; Eissa, I.H. Design, Synthesis, In Silico and In Vitro Studies of New Immunomodulatory Anticancer Nicotinamide Derivatives Targeting VEGFR-2. *Molecules* **2022**, *27*, 4079. [CrossRef] [PubMed]
16. Agamennone, M.; Fantacuzzi, M.; Carradori, S.; Petzer, A.; Petzer, J.P.; Angeli, A.; Supuran, C.T.; Luisi, G. Coumarin-Based Dual Inhibitors of Human Carbonic Anhydrases and Monoamine Oxidases Featuring Amino Acyl and (Pseudo)-Dipeptidyl Appendages: In Vitro and Computational Studies. *Molecules* **2022**, *27*, 7884. [CrossRef] [PubMed]
17. Sharma, K.; Aaghaz, S.; Maurya, I.K.; Singh, S.; Rudramurthy, S.M.; Kumar, V.; Tikoo, K.; Jain, R. Ring-Modified Histidine-Containing Cationic Short Peptides Exhibit Anticryptococcal Activity by Cellular Disruption. *Molecules* **2023**, *28*, 87. [CrossRef] [PubMed]

Disclaimer/Publisher's Note: The statements, opinions and data contained in all publications are solely those of the individual author(s) and contributor(s) and not of MDPI and/or the editor(s). MDPI and/or the editor(s) disclaim responsibility for any injury to people or property resulting from any ideas, methods, instructions or products referred to in the content.

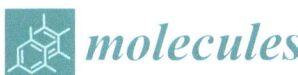

Article

Ring-Modified Histidine-Containing Cationic Short Peptides Exhibit Anticryptococcal Activity by Cellular Disruption

Komal Sharma [1], Shams Aaghaz [1], Indresh Kumar Maurya [2], Shreya Singh [3], Shivaprakash M. Rudramurthy [3], Vinod Kumar [4], Kulbhushan Tikoo [4] and Rahul Jain [1,*]

1. Department of Medicinal Chemistry, National Institute of Pharmaceutical Education and Research, Sector 67, S.A.S. Nagar 160 062, Punjab, India
2. Center of Infectious Diseases, National Institute of Pharmaceutical Education and Research, Sector 67, S.A.S. Nagar 160 062, Punjab, India
3. Department of Medical Microbiology, Post Graduate Institute of Medical Education and Research, Sector 12, Chandigarh 160 012, India
4. Department of Pharmacology and Toxicology, National Institute of Pharmaceutical Education and Research, Sector 67, S.A.S. Nagar 160 062, Punjab, India
* Correspondence: rahuljain@niper.ac.in

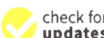

Citation: Sharma, K.; Aaghaz, S.; Maurya, I.K.; Singh, S.; Rudramurthy, S.M.; Kumar, V.; Tikoo, K.; Jain, R. Ring-Modified Histidine-Containing Cationic Short Peptides Exhibit Anticryptococcal Activity by Cellular Disruption. *Molecules* **2023**, *28*, 87. https://doi.org/10.3390/molecules28010087

Academic Editors: Imtiaz Khan, Sumera Zaib and Jean-Marc Sabatier

Received: 9 November 2022
Revised: 19 December 2022
Accepted: 19 December 2022
Published: 22 December 2022

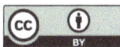

Copyright: © 2022 by the authors. Licensee MDPI, Basel, Switzerland. This article is an open access article distributed under the terms and conditions of the Creative Commons Attribution (CC BY) license (https://creativecommons.org/licenses/by/4.0/).

Abstract: Delineation of clinical complications secondary to fungal infections, such as cryptococcal meningitis, and the concurrent emergence of multidrug resistance in large population subsets necessitates the need for the development of new classes of antifungals. Herein, we report a series of ring-modified histidine-containing short cationic peptides exhibiting anticryptococcal activity via membrane lysis. The *N*-1 position of histidine was benzylated, followed by iodination at the C-5 position via electrophilic iodination, and the dipeptides were obtained after coupling with tryptophan. In vitro analysis revealed that peptides Trp-His[1-(3,5-di-*tert*-butylbenzyl)-5-iodo]-OMe (**10d**, IC_{50} = 2.20 μg/mL; MIC = 4.01 μg/mL) and Trp-His[1-(2-iodophenyl)-5-iodo]-OMe (**10o**, IC_{50} = 2.52 μg/mL; MIC = 4.59 μg/mL) exhibit promising antifungal activities against *C. neoformans*. When administered in combination with standard drug amphotericin B (Amp B), a significant synergism was observed, with 4- to 16-fold increase in the potencies of both peptides and Amp B. Electron microscopy analysis with SEM and TEM showed that the dipeptides primarily act via membrane disruption, leading to pore formation and causing cell lysis. After entering the cells, the peptides interact with the intracellular components as demonstrated by confocal laser scanning microscopy (CLSM).

Keywords: iodinated histidines; membrane active peptides; anticryptococcal activity; iodopeptides; pore formation; cell lysis; antifungal agents

1. Introduction

Multidrug resistance and a compromised immune system due to underlying diseases such as HIV, cancer and COVID-19 infection have rendered easily treatable fungal infections as life-threatening. Cryptococcal meningitis is one such condition, and caused 580,000 deaths in 2020, accounting for 19% of the AIDS-related deaths globally [1]. Various classes of drugs approved for the treatment of invasive fungal infections act on the fungal membrane (polyenes, azoles and echinocandins) and DNA (pyrimidines). For the treatment of cryptococcal meningitis, the first line of treatment includes induction, consolidation and maintenance therapy which primarily relies on the administration of amphotericin B, fluconazole and flucytosine in different combinations for varied time durations [2]. Moreover, various formulations of the most potent and commonly used drug amphotericin B have been developed over a period of time that have shown promising results as compared to the conventional therapy [3]. However, due to acute and chronic toxicities, such as nephrotoxicity associated with amphotericin B and flucytosine, neurotoxicity with fluconazole and various gastrointestinal complications, along with development of resistance in microbes due to extensive and reckless use of antifungal drugs, there is a need for the development of newer classes of antifungals [4]. Hence, various new chemical structural classes are being explored and different anticryptococcal agents are being developed. Some of them act via interactions with various components of the fungal cells such as inhibition of glycosyl phosphatidylinositol (fosmanogepix), fungal-selective calcineurin inhibitor (APX879) and fungal-selective Hsp90 inhibitor (resorcylate aminopyrazoles). However, anticryptococcal agents acting via membrane disruption and lysis are quite popular, for example peptides [5,6], benzothioureas, ibomycin and hydrazycins [7].

Antifungal peptides (AFPs) primarily act via membrane disruption; however, their mechanism may involve complex secondary actions, such as reactive oxygen species (ROS) generation, mitochondrial dysfunction, induction of apoptosis, cell cycle interruption and interaction with genetic material [8]. The membrane interacting properties of AFPs basically depend on a few structural characteristics of the peptide such as positive charge and hydrophobicity [9–13]. The choice of amino acids in a peptide sequence specifically determines its toxicity and pharmacokinetic profiles along with biological activities. Peptides with more hydrophobic residues may lead to hemolysis whereas hydrophilic amino acid containing peptides may not be able to pass through the cell membrane [14]. The advantages associated with peptides, such as less systemic toxicity and lower potential for the development of resistance, render them a promising alternative to small antibiotics [15]. However, certain limitations such as enzymatic degradation, short half-life and poor oral bioavailability can be easily circumvented using modified/unnatural amino acids [16–18] or backbone modification [19,20].

Various reports suggest that introduction of a halogen group imparts overall hydrophobicity to a molecule, apart from inducing stability and modulating the biological activity. Jia et al. demonstrated that introduction of a halogen on naturally occurring Jelleine-I enhanced the antimicrobial and anti-biofilm activity of the peptide, with iodinated Jelleine-I showing the strongest in vitro activity while its chloro and bromo counterparts showed the best in vivo efficacies [21]. Similarly, another study demonstrated that addition of a fluorine atom on the C-terminal amidated tritrpticin analogue, tritrp1, showed similar activities against *E. coli* when compared to the parent peptide [22]. Cruz et al. demonstrated that the replacement of chlorine with bromine produced a variant of lantibiotic NAI-107 with improved bactericidal activity against gram-positive pathogens [23]. On a similar note, Molchanova et al. demonstrated that incorporation of halogen atoms into otherwise inactive peptoids led to improved antimicrobial activities. However, the activities were strongly dependent on the choice of halogen atom, as chlorine or bromine led to higher activity than the parent peptoid while introduction of fluorine did not alter the activity [24]. In line with this, Gottler et al. reported that a hexafluoroleucine-containing variant of protegrin showed diminished activity against various bacterial strains [25]. Hence, the introduction of a halogen atom to peptides modulates the activities but the altered activities are largely dependent on the choice of halogen atom, type of peptide and the hydrophobic-hydrophilic balance obtained after the modifications.

Herein, we modulated the activity of a previously reported dipeptide **1** (Figure 1) [26] by incorporating an iodo group. In the previously reported series of Trp-His class of dipeptides, introduction of various substituted benzyl groups at the *N*-1 position led to the identification of an anticryptococcal peptide (**1**). The peptide **1** possesses a 3,5-di-*tert*-butylbenzyl group at the *N*-1 position of histidine and NHBzl group at the C-terminal providing hydrophobic character in the peptide. In the current study, we replaced the NHBzl with a methyl ester group and in an attempt to keep the hydrophobicity intact or balanced, an iodo group was introduced at the C-5 position of the histidine ring (**2**). In our recent work, we observed that the most active dipeptides possessed an NHBzl group at the C-terminal and free N-terminal. Further replacement of the C-terminal NHBzl with OMe and introduction of Boc at the N-terminal led to peptides with similar activities to that of the most active peptides. The slight difference in activities was dependent on the substitutions at the N-1 position of histidine [27]. Therefore, in the present work, a less bulky C-terminal, i.e., OMe was chosen, as a bulky halogen group was introduced at the C-5 position of histidine.

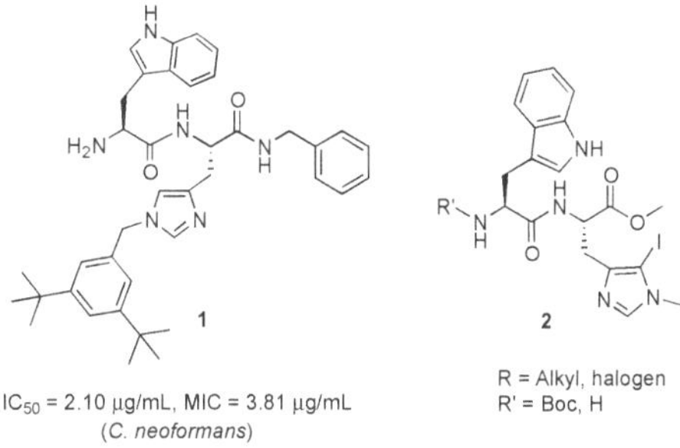

Figure 1. Structures of dipeptides.

A series of dipeptides **2** (Figure 1) were synthesized by utilizing the backbone of peptide **1** and introducing an iodo group at the C-5 position of the histidine along with speculating the effect of various electron donating and electron withdrawing groups on the N-1 benzyl group in the modulation of antimicrobial activities.

2. Results and Discussion
2.1. Synthesis

Synthesis of Boc-His (1-Bzl-5-iodo)-OMe: The N-terminal of His-OMe (**3**) was protected with a Boc group in the presence of di-*tert*-butyl dicarbonate (Boc$_2$O) to obtain Boc-His-OMe (**4**, Scheme 1) which was further subjected to iodination by direct electrophilic halogenation in the presence of N-iodosuccinimide at ambient temperatures under dark and inert conditions [28]. Under these conditions, both C-2,5-diiodo (**5**) and C-5-iodo (**6**) products were obtained. The crude products were purified using a silica gel column with hexane:ethyl acetate as a solvent system. Boc-His-5-iodo-OMe (**6**) was then benzylated at the N-1 position using various substituted benzyl bromides and the final derivatives (**7a–o**) were isolated in 72–92% yield (Figure 2).

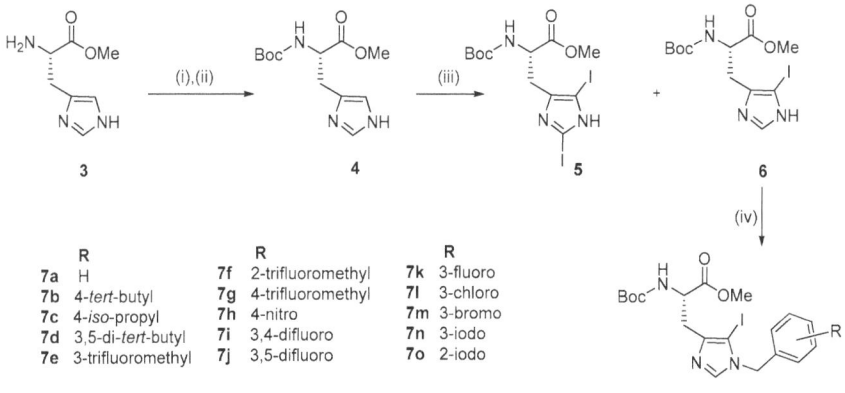

Reaction conditions: (i) Boc$_2$O (2.3 equiv.), TEA (2 equiv.), MeOH, rt, 2 h; (ii) K$_2$CO$_3$ (0.1 equiv.), MeOH, reflux, 3 h; (iii) NIS (1.2 equiv.), CH$_3$CN, dark, inert, rt, 24 h; (iv) K$_2$CO$_3$ (1.5 equiv.), BnBr (1.5 equiv.), DMF, rt, 4 h.

Scheme 1. Synthesis of N-benzylated 5-iodohistidine derivatives.

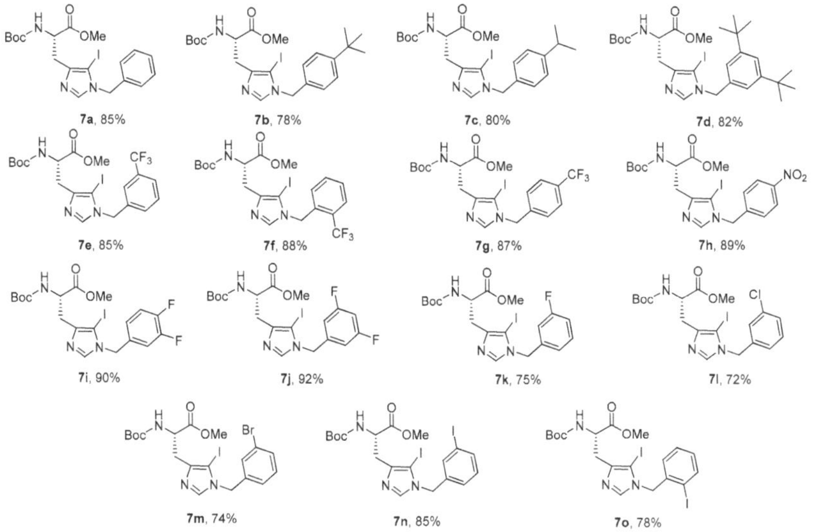

Figure 2. *N*-benzylated 5-iodohistidine derivatives.

Synthesis of peptides (Series 1–2): Synthesis of the Trp-His(1-Bzl-5-iodo)-OMe class of peptides was carried out from the *C*- to the *N*-terminus by sequential deprotection and coupling reactions (Scheme 2). Acidolysis of **7a–o** was accomplished with 6 M HCl to obtain **8a–o**, and then neutralized with DIEA.

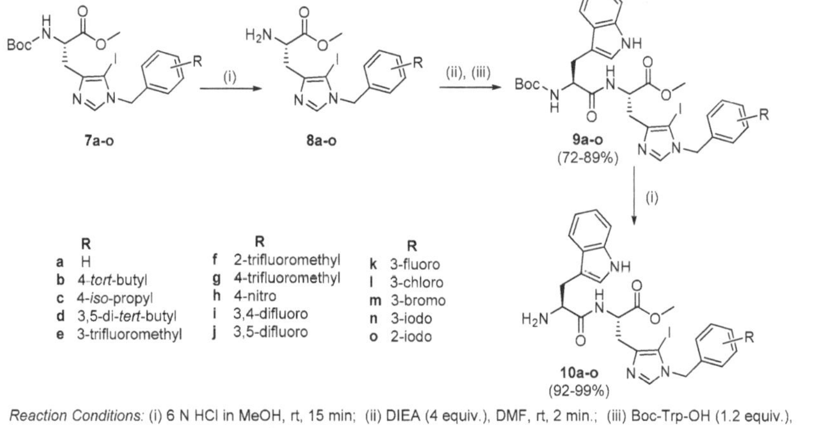

Reaction Conditions: (i) 6 N HCl in MeOH, rt, 15 min; (ii) DIEA (4 equiv.), DMF, rt, 2 min.; (iii) Boc-Trp-OH (1.2 equiv.), DIC (1.2 equiv.), HATU (1.2 equiv.), 60 °C, 30 min, MW.

Scheme 2. Synthesis of Trp-His (1-Bzl)-NHBzl class of dipeptides.

The coupling of **8a–o** with Boc-Trp-OH was executed in the presence of a coupling cocktail combination of HOAt and DIC in DMF under microwave irradiation. The crude peptides were purified on a fully automated flash column chromatography system with solvent system of CH_2Cl_2:MeOH. Deprotection at the *N*-terminal of purified dipeptides (**9a–o**) was performed with methanolic HCl to obtain dipeptides **10a–o**. The purity of all the synthesized peptides was analyzed by HPLC on a LC-18 column with a run time of 40 min with a flow of 1 mL/min using a gradient system of 95–5% (A:B) where buffer A and B were 0.1% CF_3COOH in H_2O and CH_3CN (see SI).

2.2. Antimicrobial Susceptibility Testing

Peptides **9a–o** and **10a–o** were tested against selected strains of fungi and bacteria and the results are summarized in Tables 1–3. In Series 1, with all Boc-protected peptides **9a–o** (Table 1), moderate to low activities were observed against *C. neoformans*. Most of the peptides with moderately bulky groups such as **9a** (R = benzyl), **9c** (R = 4-*iso*-propyl), **9e** (R = 3-trifluoromethyl) and with halogenated benzyl groups **9i–9n** showed weak fungicidal effects (IC$_{50}$ values ranging from 17.62 to 23.58 µg/mL) in comparison to the reference standard amphotericin B. The peptides **9a–o** were found to be inactive against all other fungal strains.

In Series 2, removal of a Boc group (Table 2) led to a significant increase in the anticryptococcal activity of the peptides. With an overall increase in the bulk from a benzyl group (**10a**, IC$_{50}$ = 17.68 µg/mL) to 3,5-di-*tert*-butylbenzyl (**10d**, IC$_{50}$ = 2.20 µg/mL, MIC = 4.01 µg/mL), a substantial increase in bioactivity was observed. Other peptides with electron donating groups such as **10b** (R = 4-*tert*-butyl) and **10c** (R = 4-*iso*-propyl) exhibited moderate activity with IC$_{50}$ values of 5.15 µg/mL (MIC = 9.36 µg/mL) and 8.81 µg/mL (MIC = 16.02 µg/mL), respectively. Hence, it is concluded that in peptides with electron donating side chains, the activity decreased with the decrease in bulk in the order: 3,5-di-*tert*-butylbenzyl > 4-*tert*-butyl > 4-*iso*-propyl > benzyl.

Table 1. In vitro antifungal screening of peptides (Series 1).

No.	R	C. neoformans		C. albicans		C. glabrata		C. parapsilosis		C. krusei	
		IC$_{50}$ [a]	MIC [b]	IC$_{50}$	MIC	IC$_{50}$	MIC	IC$_{50}$	MIC	IC$_{50}$	MIC
9a	H	17.78	32.34	>35.2	>64.0	>35.2	>64.0	>35.2	>64.0	>35.2	>64.0
9b	4-*tert*-butyl	>35.2	>64.0	>35.2	>64.0	>35.2	>64.0	>35.2	>64.0	>35.2	>64.0
9c	4-*iso*-propyl	20.39	37.08	>35.2	>64.0	>35.2	>64.0	>35.2	>64.0	>35.2	>64.0
9d	3,5-di-*tert*-butyl	>35.2	>64.0	>35.2	>64.0	>35.2	>64.0	>35.2	>64.0	>35.2	>64.0
9e	3-trifluoromethyl	20.71	37.65	>35.2	>64.0	>35.2	>64.0	>35.2	>64.0	>35.2	>64.0
9f	2-trifluoromethyl	30.56	55.57	>35.2	>64.0	>35.2	>64.0	>35.2	>64.0	>35.2	>64.0
9g	4-trifluoromethyl	>35.2	>64.0	>35.2	>64.0	>35.2	>64.0	>35.2	>64.0	>35.2	>64.0
9h	4-nitro	>35.2	>64.0	>35.2	>64.0	>35.2	>64.0	>35.2	>64.0	>35.2	>64.0
9i	3,4-difluoro	17.62	32.05	>35.2	>64.0	>35.2	>64.0	>35.2	>64.0	>35.2	>64.0
9j	3,5-difluoro	17.73	32.25	>35.2	>64.0	>35.2	>64.0	>35.2	>64.0	>35.2	>64.0
9k	3-fluoro	18.16	32.02	>35.2	>64.0	>35.2	>64.0	>35.2	>64.0	>35.2	>64.0
9l	3-chloro	18.59	33.80	>35.2	>64.0	>35.2	>64.0	>35.2	>64.0	>35.2	>64.0
9m	3-bromo	18.63	33.88	>35.2	>64.0	>35.2	>64.0	>35.2	>64.0	>35.2	>64.0
9n	3-iodo	23.58	42.87	>35.2	>64.0	>35.2	>64.0	>35.2	>64.0	>35.2	>64.0
9o	2-iodo	>35.2	>64.0	>35.2	>64.0	>35.2	>64.0	>35.2	>64.0	>35.2	>64.0
Amphotericin B		0.50	1.00	0.36	0.72	0.18	0.36	0.36	0.72	0.36	0.72

[a] IC$_{50}$ is the concentration in µg/mL that leads to ~50% inhibition of growth; [b] MIC (minimum inhibitory concentration) is the lowest test concentration (µg/mL) at which there is no detectable growth; Amphotericin B was use as standard antifungal drug.

Table 2. In vitro antifungal screening of peptides (Series 2).

10a-o

No.	R$_1$	C. neoformans		C. albicans		C. glabrata		C. parapsilosis		C. krusei	
		IC$_{50}$ [a]	MIC [b]	IC$_{50}$	MIC	IC$_{50}$	MIC	IC$_{50}$	MIC	IC$_{50}$	MIC
10a	H	17.68	32.15	>35.2	>64.0	>35.2	>64.0	>35.2	>64.0	>35.2	>64.0
10b	4-*tert*-butyl	5.15	9.358	>35.2	>64.0	>35.2	>64.0	>35.2	>64.0	>35.2	>64.0
10c	4-*iso*-propyl	8.81	16.02	>35.2	>64.0	>35.2	>64.0	>35.2	>64.0	>35.2	>64.0
10d	3,5-di-*tert*-butyl	2.20	4.01	>35.2	>64.0	>35.2	>64.0	>35.2	>64.0	>35.2	>64.0
10e	3-trifluoromethyl	4.87	8.86	>35.2	>64.0	>35.2	>64.0	>35.2	>64.0	>35.2	>64.0
10f	2-trifluoromethyl	17.70	32.18	>35.2	>64.0	>35.2	>64.0	>35.2	>64.0	>35.2	>64.0
10g	4-trifluoromethyl	13.53	24.60	>35.2	>64.0	>35.2	>64.0	>35.2	>64.0	>35.2	>64.0
10h	4-nitro	>35.2	>64.0	>35.2	>64.0	>35.2	>64.0	>35.2	>64.0	>35.2	>64.0
10i	3,4-difluoro	10.28	18.70	>35.2	>64.0	>35.2	>64.0	>35.2	>64.0	>35.2	>64.0
10j	3,5-difluoro	6.09	11.08	>35.2	>64.0	>35.2	>64.0	>35.2	>64.0	>35.2	>64.0
10k	3-fluoro	2.78	4.64	>35.2	>64.0	>35.2	>64.0	>35.2	>64.0	>35.2	>64.0
10l	3-chloro	17.66	32.11	>35.2	>64.0	>35.2	>64.0	>35.2	>64.0	>35.2	>64.0
10m	3-bromo	9.23	16.79	>35.2	>64.0	>35.2	>64.0	>35.2	>64.0	>35.2	>64.0
10n	3-iodo	17.62	32.05	>35.2	>64.0	>35.2	>64.0	>35.2	>64.0	>35.2	>64.0
10o	2-iodo	2.59	4.59	>35.2	>64.0	>35.2	>64.0	>35.2	>64.0	>35.2	>64.0
Amphotericin B		0.50	1.00	0.36	0.72	0.18	0.36	0.36	0.72	0.36	0.72

[a] IC$_{50}$ is the concentration in μg/mL that leads to ~50% inhibition of growth; [b] MIC (minimum inhibitory concentration) is the lowest test concentration (μg/mL) at which there is no detectable growth; Amphotericin B was use as standard antifungal drug.

Table 3. In vitro antibacterial screening of peptides (Series 1–2).

R$_2$= Boc (9a-o)
R$_2$= H (10a-o)

No.	R$_1$	R$_2$	E. faecalis		S. aureus		S. pyogens		E. coli		P. aeruginosa	
			IC$_{50}$ [a]	MIC [b]	IC$_{50}$	MIC	IC$_{50}$	MIC	IC$_{50}$	MIC	IC$_{50}$	MIC
10b	4-*tert*-butylbenzyl	H	>35.2	>64.0	35.2	64.0	>35.2	>64.0	35.2	64.0	>35.2	>64.0
10c	4-*n*-butylbenzyl	H	>35.2	>64.0	>35.2	>64.0	>35.2	>64.0	>35.2	>64.0	>35.2	>64.0
10d	3,5-di-*tert*-butylbenzyl	H	17.6	32.0	17.6	32.0	>35.2	>64.0	17.6	32.0	>35.2	>64.0
10e	3-trifluoromethyl	H	>35.2	>64.0	>35.2	>64.0	>35.2	>64.0	>35.2	>64.0	>35.2	>64.0
10k	3,5-difluoro	H	>35.2	>64.0	>35.2	>64.0	>35.2	>64.0	>35.2	>64.0	>35.2	>64.0
10l	3-fluoro	H	>35.2	>64.0	>35.2	>64.0	>35.2	>64.0	>35.2	>64.0	>35.2	>64.0
10n	3-bromo	H	>35.2	>64.0	>35.2	>64.0	>35.2	>64.0	>35.2	>64.0	>35.2	>64.0
10o	2-iodo	H	17.6	32.0	>35.2	>64.0	>35.2	>64.0	>35.2	>64.0	>35.2	>64.0
Rifampicin			1.00	2.00	2.00	4.00	1.00	2.00	1.00	2.00	16.00	32.00

[a] IC$_{50}$ is the concentration in μg/mL that leads to ~50% inhibition of growth; [b] MIC (minimum inhibitory concentration) is the lowest test concentration (μg/mL) at which there is no detectable growth; Rifampicin was use as standard antibacterial drug.

However, when the methyl group of the *tert*-butyl moiety was replaced with the less hydrophobic and highly electron withdrawing fluorine atom **10g** (IC$_{50}$ = 13.53 µg/mL, MIC = 24.6 µg/mL), the activity was reduced by 2.6-fold. The position of the trifluoromethyl group on the benzyl ring also affected the activity, such that 3-CF$_3$ (**10e**) was found to be moderately active with an IC$_{50}$ value of 4.87 µg/mL (MIC = 8.86 µg/mL) whereas the 2-CF$_3$ group containing peptide, **10f**, exhibited a much lower activity with an IC$_{50}$ value of 17.70 µg/mL (MIC = 32.18 µg/mL). Hence, the activity decreased in order 3-CF$_3$ > 4-CF$_3$ > 2-CF$_3$. The effect of the fluorine group was observed by direct introduction at different positions on the benzyl ring. The derivatives of 3,4-difluorobenzyl (**10i**) and 3,5-difluorobenzyl (**10j**) exhibited moderate activities with IC$_{50}$ values of 10.28 µg/mL (MIC = 18.7 µg/mL) and 6.09 µg/mL (MIC = 11.08 µg/mL), respectively. However, the 3-fluorobenzyl derivative (**10k**) displayed a significant increase in activity with an IC$_{50}$ value of 2.78 µg/mL (MIC = 4.64 µg/mL). This prompted us to evaluate various other 3-halobenzyl substituted derivatives. Peptides **10l, 10m** and **10n** containing 3-chloro, 3-bromo, 3-iodo groups, respectively, were moderately active with IC$_{50}$ values of 17.6, 9.23 and 17.6 µg/mL, respectively. However, when iodo was placed at the *ortho* position of the benzyl ring, a significant increase in activity was observed with an IC$_{50}$ value of 2.59 µg/mL (MIC = 4.59 µg/mL). Furthermore, the incorporation of an electron withdrawing nitro group (**10h**) at the fourth position of the benzyl ring drastically reduced the activity of the peptide (IC$_{50}$ < 20 µg/mL). In a nutshell, with an optimum balance of hydrophobicity, electronegativity and polarity, peptides tend to show enhanced activity. All the peptides were found to be inactive against *C. albicans, C. glabrata, C. parapsilosis* and *C. krusei* at the highest tested concentrations. Peptides with IC$_{50}$ values less than 20 µg/mL from both series were further tested against bacterial strains (Table 3) but none showed very significant activity.

To summarize, peptides **10d** (R = 3,5-di-*tert*-butylbenzyl) and **10o** (R = 2-iodobenzyl) showed the best activities of the two series with IC$_{50}$ values of 2.20 µg/mL (MIC = 4.01 µg/mL) and 2.59 µg/mL (MIC = 4.59 µg/mL), respectively. The presence of an iodo group at the C-5 position of the histidine in this series of dipeptides imparts the quintessential hydrophobicity, therefore aiding the fungicidal activity of the peptides. The presence of different halogen groups (Br, Cl and F) at C-5 and their impact on the biological activities will be further explored in future.

2.3. Cytotoxicity Assay

Cytotoxicity assays were carried out to determine the selectivity of the most active peptides **10d** and **10o** towards fungal cells and their toxicity towards mammalian cells. The peptides showed a non-cytotoxic nature against human cancer cells line (HeLa) and a non-cancerous mammalian cell line (HEK 293) at their MIC concentration and higher (Figure 3, Table 4).

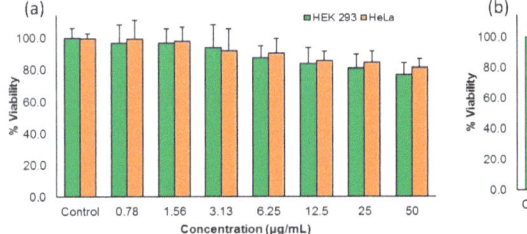
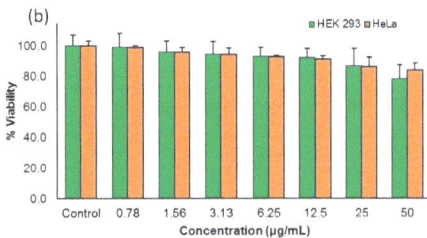

Figure 3. Mammalian cell cytotoxicity of peptide (**a**) **10d** and (**b**) **10o** as percentage viability of HEK-293 and HeLa cells at different concentrations.

Table 4. Cytotoxicity and hemolytic activities of the active peptides.

Peptides	MIC (µg/mL)	Cytotoxicity (TC$_{50}$) [a] (µg/mL)		% Hemolysis (µg/mL)	
		HEK 293	HeLa	HC$_{10}$ [b]	HC$_{50}$ [c]
10d	4.01	>100	>100	50.53	>100
10o	4.59	>100	>100	52.17	>100

[a] TC$_{50}$ = concentration of peptides causing 50% cytotoxicity, [b] HC$_{10}$ = concentration of peptides causing 10% hemolysis, [c] HC$_{50}$ = concentration of peptides causing 50% hemolysis.

2.4. Hemolytic Assay

Non-selective peptides do not differentiate between fungal cells and human erythrocytes and thereby interact with both, causing hemolysis. A hemolytic study was carried out to demonstrate the selectivity of the synthesized peptides towards fungal cells. Peptides **10d** and **10o** exhibited non-hemolytic behavior at their MIC values and above, as evident from the HC$_{10}$ and HC$_{50}$ values (Table 4); therefore, they show high selectivity towards *C. neoformans* cells.

2.5. Time Kill Kinetics

To determine the time-dependent fungicidal action of peptides **10d** and **10o**, their time–kill profile was studied. The assay was carried out with the active peptides **10d** and **10o**-treated cryptococcal cells while corresponding inactive counterparts **9d** and **9o**-treated cells along with untreated cells were taken as negative controls. Amphotericin B-treated cells were used as the positive control. The growth profile of fungal cells was determined for each sample over a period of 24 h.

The growth pattern of amphotericin B-treated cryptococcal cells showed a significant drop in colony forming units (CFUs) after 4 h. Peptide **10d** displayed significant fungicidal activity and inhibited the growth of cryptococcal cells after 12 h (Figure 4a). However, inactive peptide **9d**-treated cells did not show any growth inhibition and exhibited the growth curve similar to that of a standard curve shown by untreated cells. Furthermore, time–kill kinetics of the active peptide **10o** revealed a gradual decrease followed by complete inhibition of CFUs after 12 h (Figure 4b). However, negative peptide **9o**-treated and untreated cells showed similar growth curves. The results confirmed the fungicidal action of the tested peptides.

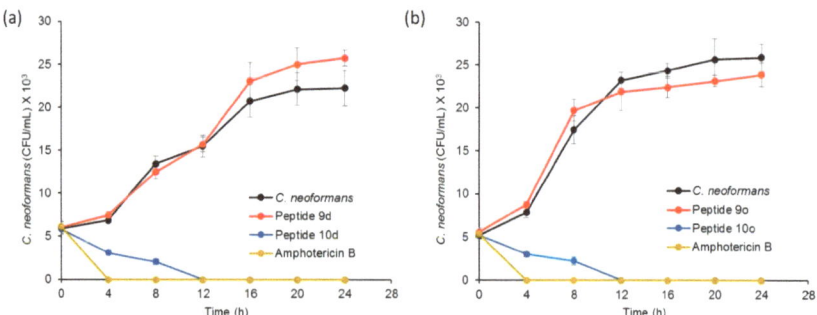

Figure 4. Time–kill kinetics profile for (**a**) peptide **10d**, with amphotericin B as positive control, while *C. neoformans* cells and peptide **9d** were negative controls; (**b**) peptide **10o**, with amphotericin B as positive control while *C. neoformans* cells and peptide **9o** were negative controls.

2.6. Drug Combination Study

The fungicidal nature of the active peptides was further evaluated when given in combination with clinical standards that are used for the treatment of invasive cryptococcal infections. Cryptococcal cells were treated with different concentrations of peptides **10d** and **10o** in combination with varying concentrations of amphotericin or fluconazole and the fractional inhibitory concentration (FIC) index was calculated (Table 5) [29].

$$\text{FIC index (FICI)} = \text{FIC of A} + \text{FIC of B} = \frac{\text{MIC}^A_{Comb}}{\text{MIC}^A_{alone}} + \frac{\text{MIC}^B_{Comb}}{\text{MIC}^B_{alone}} \quad (1)$$

Table 5. Evaluation of combinative effect of bioactive peptides with amphotericin B (Amp B) and fluconazole (Flu).

Treatment	MIC (µg/mL) Alone	MIC (µg/mL) In Combination	Fold Decrease in MIC	FICI	Effect
10d	4.01	0.250	16	0.18	Synergistic
Amp B	1.00	0.125	8		
10d	4.01	0.501	8	0.19	Synergistic
Flu	10.0	0.625	16		
10o	4.59	0.287	16	0.31	Synergistic
Amp B	1.00	0.250	4		
10o	4.59	2.999	1.5	1.00	Additive
Flu	10.0	5.0	2		

FICI ≤ 0.5: synergistic; FICI > 4: antagonistic; and FICI 0.6–4.0: additive or indifferent.

Peptide **10d**, when used in combination with amphotericin B, exhibited a significant synergistic action with an FICI value of 0.18. The MIC value of peptide **10d** showed a 16-fold decrease from 4.01 to 0.25 µg/mL, whereas that of amphotericin B showed an 8-fold decrease in the MIC value. Furthermore, **10d** also exhibited synergism with fluconazole, showing an FICI value of 0.19. An approx. 8-fold decrease in the MIC of **10d** (from 4.01 to 0.501 µg/mL) was observed and fluconazole showed an approx. 16-fold decrease in the MIC value (from 10 to 0.625 µg/mL). Peptide **10o**, at a non-cidal concentration, resulted in the 4-fold potentiation of amphotericin B in combination, while the MIC of peptide **10o** was lowered by around 16-fold (MIC from 4.59 to 0.285 µg/mL). The FICI value of this combination was found to be 0.31, indicating synergistic action. However, with fluconazole, peptide **10o** exhibited an additive effect with an FICI value of 1.0.

2.7. Mechanistic Investigations

The mechanism of action of the bioactive peptides was determined by analyzing the cell death pattern, by establishing the morphological changes after the treatment using electron microscopy and by identifying the broad intracellular targets using confocal imaging.

2.7.1. Cell Death Pattern Analysis Using Flow Cytometry

Apoptosis includes a series of events occurring inside the cell, causing changes in plasma membrane, genetic material and various internal proteins, therefore leading to programmed cell death. One of the early markers of apoptosis is the translocation of a membrane phospholipid, phosphatidylserine, from the inner to the outer leaflet of the plasma membrane without altering the integrity of the plasma membrane [30]. Annexin V-FITC interacts with the externalized phosphatidylserine, therefore showing the cell change towards apoptosis which can be analyzed using flow cytometry [31,32]. The four quadrants in flow cytometry indicate different stages of the cells. The percentage depicts the population of the cells in a specific stage. Q1 corresponds to the percentage of cells undergoing necrosis, Q2 depicts the early apoptotic stage of the cells whereas Q4 corresponds to the cells in late-stage apoptosis and Q3 depicts the cells in the native state [33].

The control samples for peptide **10o** showed cryptococcal cells alone, exhibiting 100% population in native state Q3 (Figure 5a), whereas PI incubated samples (Figure 5b), showed 99.3% of cell population in the native state and 0.7% were in Q1. After incubation with annexin V-FITC (Figure 5c), the population of cryptococcal cells scattered more towards Q4 (6.4%), while 93.6% were in native quadrant Q3. Further incubation of cells with both PI and annexin V-FITC (Figure 5d) did not have a significant effect on the redistribution of the cell population over all quadrants, as more than 95% cells were in native state Q3, Q1 had 0.6% cells, Q2 showed 0.1% and Q4 constituted 3.3% of total cell population. However, when peptide **10d**-treated fungal cells were incubated with both PI and annexin V-FITC (Figure 5e), a marked variation in the pattern of distribution of cells was observed over the four quadrants, as 52.2% of cell population was pushed towards the Q4 quadrant showing late-stage apoptosis, while 1.7% cells exhibited necrosis (Q1), 1.3% were in Q2 and 44.8% of cell population remained in native state Q3. On a similar note, when cells were treated with **10o** and incubated with PI and annexin V-FITC (Figure 5f), 2% necrosis was observed (Q1), 48.1% exhibited late stage apoptosis and only 1% were in Q2, whereas 48.9% were in the native state Q3.

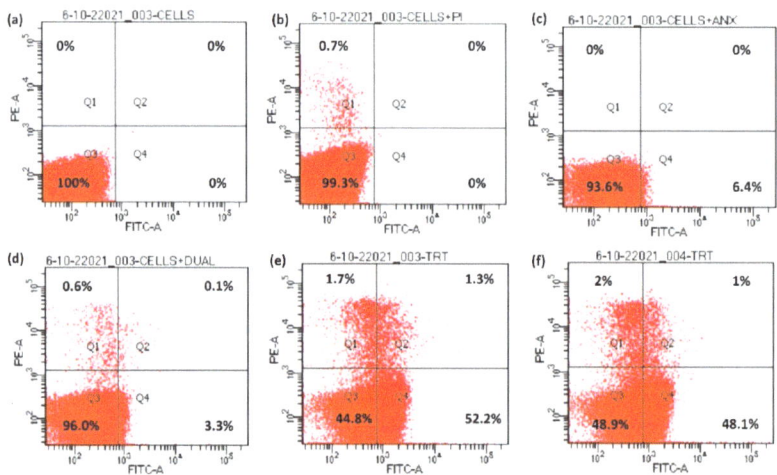

Figure 5. Externalization of phosphatidylserine in bioactive peptide-treated cells. (**a**) Unstained cells, (**b**) cells + PI, (**c**) cells + Annexin V-FITC, (**d**) cells with Annexin V-FITC + PI, (**e**) cells treated with Annexin V-FITC + PI + peptide **10d** and (**f**) cells treated with Annexin V-FITC + PI + peptide **10o**.

2.7.2. Surface Morphology Analysis Using Scanning Electron Microscopy (SEM)

A comparative analysis of the surface morphologies of treated and untreated cells was carried out using scanning electron microscopy (SEM). The untreated cells appeared as oval-shaped with smooth surfaces and intact cell membranes (Figure 6a–c) when observed in SEM. However, cells treated with peptide **10d** showed large pores in the middle of the cells (Figure 6d–f) giving a doughnut-shaped appearance. The cell surface comparatively became highly wrinkled and a blatant change in morphology of the cells was observed in comparison to the untreated cells. Likewise, cryptococcal cells treated with peptide **10o** showed a highly wrinkled cell surface with pores in the middle making their overall appearance doughnut-like (Figure 6g–i) when compared to the untreated cells. The cells were highly deformed and the intracellular contents appear to have come outside the cell, thereby causing cell death.

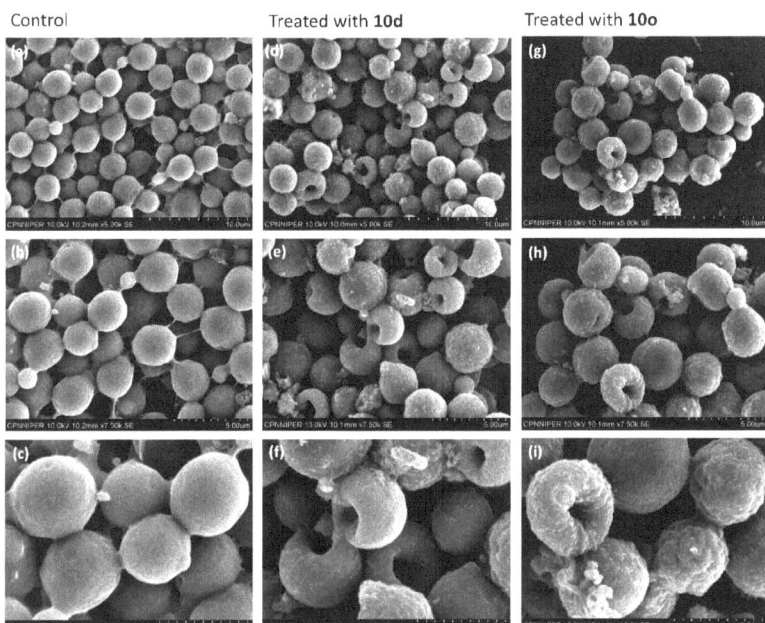

Figure 6. SEM-based surface morphological analysis of **10d** and **10o** treated and untreated *C. neoformans* cells. Images (**a–c**) represent the morphology of untreated cells; images (**d–f**) represent the morphology of cells treated with **10d**; images (**g–i**) represent the morphology of cells treated with **10o**. The scale bar for images (**a,d,g**) is 10 μm, for images (**b,e,h**) it is 5 μm and for images (**c,f,i**) it is 3 μm.

2.7.3. Internal Cell Morphology Analysis Using Transmission Electron Microscopy (TEM)

High-resolution transmission electron microscopy (HRTEM) provided an explicit view of the structural details of cells along with intricate changes that occur during the cell wall disruption. The cryptococcal cells in Figure 7a–c display a distinct inner plasma membrane covered with a layer of outer membrane followed by a faded capsule. The cell organelles can also be distinguished faintly from the images. However, the cells treated with peptide **10d** (Figure 7d–f) show complete lysis of the cell membrane. The outer membrane and capsule are not clearly distinguishable. The intracellular content of cells have oozed out and the cells appear as a stack of non-distinguishable structures lying one over the other. However, the level of cell membrane disruption was much more severe in the case of the 10o-treated cells (Figure 7g–i). The cells lost their shape completely and appear to have fused intracellular material. The cells were highly shrunken and the cell membrane was completely damaged as compared to the untreated cells.

Scanning transmission electron microscopy (STEM) analysis provides high contrast images of the cells and the results were in coherence with the HRTEM. The STEM images of untreated cells (Figure 8a,b) depict smooth walled, rounded cells with cell organelles intact, whereas the images of cells treated with peptide **10d** (Figure 8c,d) show highly shrunken cells with irregular cell membranes. The intracellular material has oozed out and a clear distinct cell was not observed. The deformed cells have merged to appear similar to a mass of highly irregular structure. Similarly, cryptococcal cells treated with **10o** (Figure 8e,f) were highly deformed and shrunken. The membrane separating the cells seemed to have disappeared and merged to form a cluster of deformed cells.

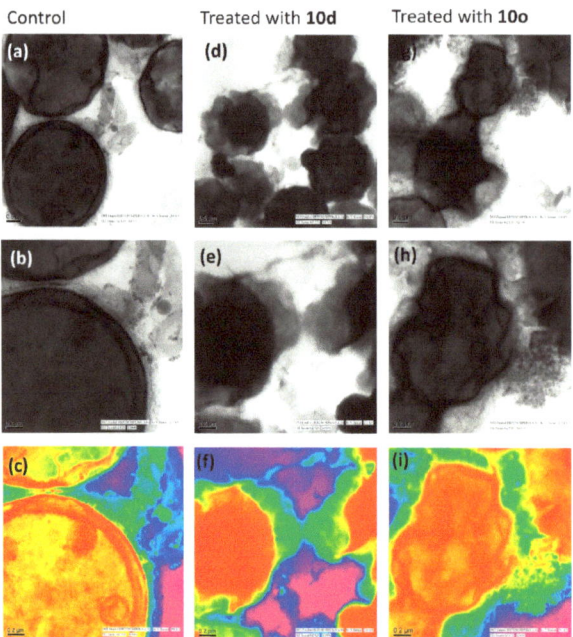

Figure 7. Morphological study of *C. neoformans* cells and cells treated with bioactive peptides by high-resolution transmission electron microscopy. Images (**a–c**) represent the morphology of untreated/healthy cells; images (**d–f**) represent the cells treated with **10d** and images (**g–i**) represent the cells treated with **10o**; images (**c,f,i**) are the rainbow form of images (**b,e,h**), respectively. The scale bar for images (**a,d,e**) is 0.5 μm and for images (**b,c,e,f,h,i**) it is 0.2 μm.

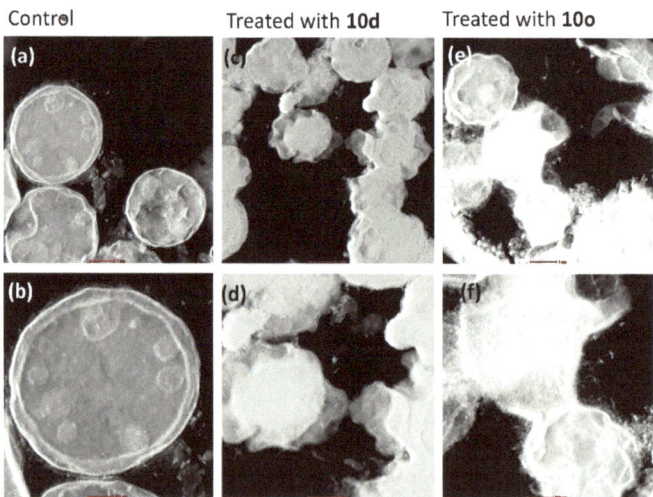

Figure 8. Morphological study of *C. neoformans* cells and cells treated with bioactive peptides by STEM. Images (**a,b**) represent the morphology of untreated/healthy cells; images (**c,d**) represent the cells treated with **10d**; and images (**e,f**) represent the cells treated with **10o**. The scale bar for images (**a,c,e**) is 1 μm and for images (**b,d,f**) it is 0.5 μm.

2.7.4. Confocal Laser Scanning Microscopy (CLSM)

(a) Membrane permeabilization and localization of FITC-labeled peptide

The bioactive peptides **10d** and **10o** along with an inactive peptide **10h** were labeled with FITC (fluorescein isothiocyanate, a green, fluorescent dye, with excitation at 480 nm). The permeabilization of peptides inside the cell was analyzed by incubating the FITC-labeled peptides with *C. neoformans* cells and observing the incubated slides under CLSM. The FITC-tagged inactive peptide, on incubation with cryptococcal cells, did not show any fluorescence when observed under CLSM (Figure 9a), depicting their inability to cross the cell membrane. However, the images of cells incubated with FITC-tagged peptides **10d** (Figure 9b) and **10o** (Figure 9c) showed prominent green fluorescence. Hence, it was concluded that peptides act via membrane permeabilization; therefore, the membrane integrity of the cells is lost leading to permeabilization of the FITC-peptide inside the cells followed by localization, providing a bright green fluorescence.

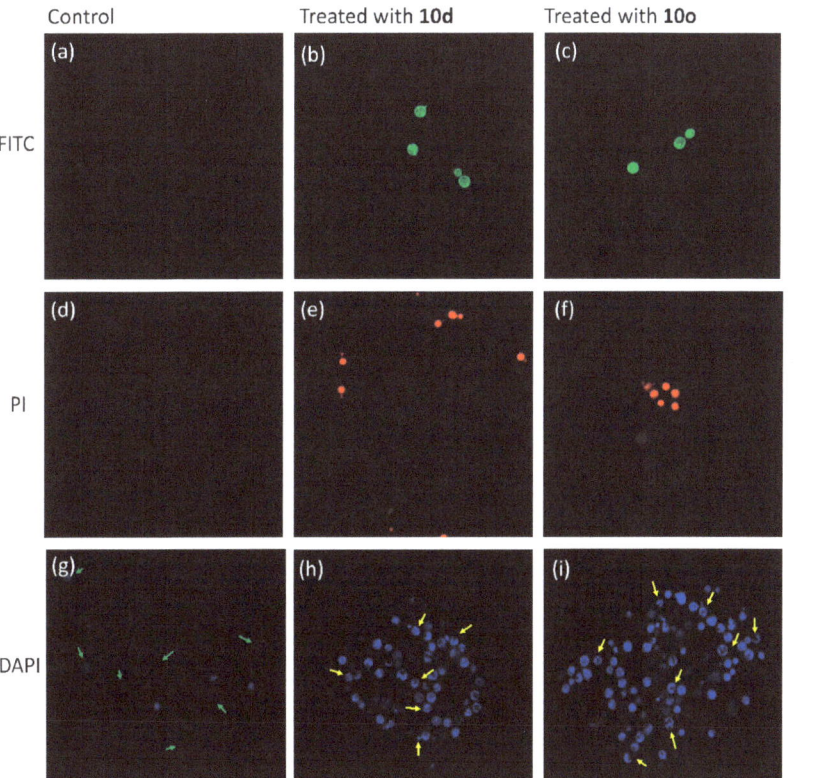

Figure 9. Confocal micrographs. Image (**a**) was obtained after incubating cells with inactive FITC-labeled peptide **10h**, while image (**b**) was obtained after treatment with active peptide **10d** tagged with FITC and image (**c**) was obtained after treatment with active peptide **10o** tagged with FITC. PI uptake assay: image (**d**) was obtained after incubating cells with PI, while image (**e**) was obtained after treatment with active peptide **10d** and image (**f**) was obtained after treatment with active peptide **10o**. DAPI uptake assay: image (**g**) was obtained after incubating cells with DAPI, while image (**h**) was obtained after incubating cells treated with **10d** with DAPI and image (**i**) was obtained after incubating cells treated with **10o** with DAPI.

(b) Membrane disruption and DNA interaction analysis by propidium iodide (PI) uptake

Propidium iodide (PI) dye cannot permeate the walls of healthy cells; hence, when cryptococcal cells were incubated with PI and observed under CLSM (excitation at 480 nm), they did not show any fluorescence (Figure 9d). However, when the cells were treated with peptide **10d** (Figure 9e) and **10o** (Figure 9f) and then incubated with PI, a prominent red fluorescence was observed. The results indicated that the peptides acted by lysis of the cell wall, which allowed the dye to penetrate the cell and intercalate with the DNA giving the whole cell a bright red fluorescence.

(c) Detection of nuclear fragmentation

The molecule 4′,6-diamidino-2-phenylindole (DAPI) easily permeates inside cells and interacts with the DNA giving a pinpoint blue fluorescence when observed under CLSM. It selectively binds to the minor groove of the DNA; therefore, any change in the fluorescence intensity pattern reveals the degree of damage to DNA. Untreated cells, when incubated with DAPI, showed faint blue pinpoint fluorescence (Figure 9g) indicating staining of the nucleus (marked by green arrows). However, cells treated with **10d** (Figure 9h) and **10o** (Figure 9i) exhibited fragmented bright blue fluorescence showing destroyed cells (marked by yellow arrows). Therefore, it can be concluded that after entering the cells, the peptides interact with the genetic material, triggering the event of cell death.

2.7.5. Possible Mechanism

Primarily, the negatively charged surface of fungi demands a positively charged moiety for easy interaction; hence, an overall positive charge was introduced in the peptides while designing them by incorporating charged amino acids. Upon interaction with the fungal cell membrane, the hydrophobicity of peptides plays a crucial role and helps the peptide to permeate inside the lipophilic membrane of the fungal cell. During permeation, the peptide induces morphological changes in the otherwise intact fungal cell membrane leading to the appearance of wrinkles on the cell surface, as evident from SEM. The peptide then interacts with various intracellular components inside the cell leading to depletion of cytoplasm (TEM), and triggering various apoptotic pathways as confirmed by flow cytometry. The depletion leads to an altered morphology of the cell, making it appear doughnut-shaped (SEM). Consequently, the intact membrane become indistinguishable from cytoplasm (TEM). The collective effect of different interactions result in distortion of the cell surface integrity, membrane permeabilization, pore formation, cell lysis and death.

3. Conclusions and Summary

In a series of *N*-substituted histidine-containing His-Trp class of dipeptides, we found that an additional substitution at the C-5 position with an iodo group influenced the biological activity against *C. neoformans*. In vitro antifungal susceptibility assays revealed that peptides Trp-His[1-(3,5-di-*tert*-butylbenzyl)-5-iodo]-OMe (**10d**) and Trp-His[1-(2-iodophenyl)-5-iodo)]-OMe (**10o**) exhibited the most significant antifungal activities against *C. neoformans* among the whole series and showed high selectivity and safety profiles. The mechanistic studies revealed that the peptides are membrane active in nature as evident from SEM and TEM analyses, which demonstrated the contrasting morphologies of healthy and bioactive peptide-treated cells. Perfectly intact oval-shaped cryptococcal cells attained a highly deformed structure with a large pore in the middle which gave it a doughnut-like appearance. Furthermore, CLSM analysis showed that the peptides easily moved across the cell membrane by increasing fluidity, thereby causing membrane lysis and disruption and interaction with various intracellular targets expediting the cell death. Furthermore, flow cytometry showed that the cell death was hastened by the induction of apoptotic pathways.

4. Material and Methods

Microbial strains: Microbial strains were procured from National Culture Collection of Pathogenic Fungi (NCCPF) at the Postgraduate Institute of Medical Education & Research (PGIMER), Chandigarh and Microbial Type Culture Collection and Gene bank (MTCC) at the Institute of Microbial Technology (IMTECH), Chandigarh, India. Peptides were screened against five different strains of fungi: *viz. Candida albicans* (NCCPF400034), *Candida glabrata* (MTCC 3019), *Candida parapsilosis* (NCCPF 440002), *Candida krusei* (NCCPF 440002) and *Cryptococcus neoformans* (NCCPF250316), and five strains of bacteria: *viz. Escherichia coli* (MTCC 2961), *Staphylococcus aureus* (MTCC 3160), *Enterococcus faecalis* (MTCC 439), *Streptococcus pyogenes* (MTCC 442) and *Pseudomonas aeruginosa* (MTCC 3542).

Growth media: Antifungal susceptibility testing was carried out using standard broth microdilution assays as per the Clinical and Laboratory Standards Institute (CLSI) guidelines for fungi [34,35]. RPMI 1640 (Sigma), yeast extract, peptone and dextrose (YPED, Himedia) were used as the incubation broths. The cells were diluted to a cell density of 10^3 colony forming unit (CFU/mL) and incubated at 30 °C for 48 h. Furthermore, Muller Hinton (Himedia) media was utilized for bacterial strains and antibacterial activity was evaluated per CLSI guidelines for bacteria [36]. Bacterial cells were diluted to a cell density of 10^5 CFU/mL and incubated at 37 °C for 24 h. Amphotericin B (Himedia, India) and rifampicin (Himedia, India) were used as standard drugs for the evaluation of activity against all the fungal and bacterial strains, respectively.

For the detailed synthetic procedures and characterization data please refer to supplementary information.

4.1. Broth Microdilution Assay

The stock solutions of peptides (2 mg/mL) were prepared in DMSO. Specific amounts of peptide from stock solution were added to a 96-well microtiter plate containing 100 µL of growth media and then serially diluted two-fold. A further 100 µL of growth media containing microbial cells were added to each well and incubated at 30–37 °C for 24–48 h. The optical density (OD) was measured at 600 nm using a BioStack Ready (BioTek Instruments, Winooski, VT, USA) microplate reader to analyze microbial growth inhibition, and IC_{50} and MIC values were calculated. To visualize the growth and inhibition pattern, a solution of 3-(4,5-dimethylthiazol-2-yl)-2,5-diphenyltetrazolium bromide (MTT) in water was added to the plate and incubated for 2–3 h. MTT reacts with the mitochondrial dehydrogenases, which are present only in a viable cell, to give blue colored formazan crystals. Therefore, a darker color indicates a high number of viable cells; however, non-viable cells appear pale or colorless.

4.2. Cytotoxicity Assay

The cytotoxicity studies of peptides **10d** and **10o** were carried out in standard 96-well cell culture plates against HEK-293 and HeLa cells. The cells (50,000 cells/well) were seeded to the wells of the plate in Dulbecco's Modified Eagle Medium (DMEM) supplemented with 10% fetal bovine serum at 37 °C overnight and incubated for 24 h to achieve confluency. Peptides at different concentrations of 50, 25, 12.5, 6.25, 3.12, 1.56 and 0.78 µg/mL were added to the cells in separate wells and incubated at 37 °C for 18 h. A further 20 µL MTT solution (5 mg/mL stock conc. in PBS) was added and the plate was incubated for another 3–4 h. To detect the viable cells that react with MTT to make formazan crystals, 120 µL of supernatant was removed and 100 µL DMSO was added to dissolve the crystals. Untreated cells and DMSO (10%) were used as negative and positive controls, respectively [37]. The percent viability of cells was calculated using equation:

$$\% \text{ Cell viability} = \frac{\text{Av. Absorbance of treated cells}}{\text{Av. Absorbance of control cells}} \times 100 \qquad (2)$$

4.3. Hemolytic Assay

Human blood in 10% citrate phosphate dextrose was obtained from Government Hospital, Chandigarh, India. Red blood cells (RBCs) were harvested by spinning at $1000\times g$ for 5 min followed by washing with PBS 3–5 times. The packed cell volume was obtained and utilized to make a 0.8% (v/v) suspension of RBCs in PBS. The suspension (100 µL) was transferred to each well of a 96-well microtiter plate and mixed with peptides **10d** and **10o** (100 µL) at concentrations of 50, 25, 12.5, 6.25, 3.12, 1.56 and 0.78 µg/mL. The plate was incubated at 37 °C for 60 min followed by centrifugation at $1000\times g$ for 5 min at 25 °C. The supernatant (100 µL) was transferred to a fresh microtiter plate and absorbance was recorded at 414 nm (Varioskan LUX multimode microplate reader, Thermo Scientific, Waltham, MS, USA) to analyze RBC lysis. Untreated RBCs in PBS and lysed RBCs in 0.1% Triton X-100 were used as negative and positive controls, respectively [29]. Percent hemolysis was calculated using following equation [38].

$$\% \text{ Hemolysis} = \frac{\text{Absorbance of treated sample} - \text{Absorbance of negative control}}{\text{Absorbance of positive control} - \text{Absorbance of negative control}} \times 100 \quad (3)$$

4.4. Time Kill Assay

C. neoformans cells ($\sim 1 \times 10^3$ CFU/mL) were inoculated in media and four samples for each test peptide were prepared, where the cryptococcal cells were either (i) incubated with test peptides (**10d** or **10o**), (ii) negative peptides (**9d** or **9o**), (iii) amphotericin B or (iv) left untreated in separate tubes with incubation broth. The tubes were then incubated for 24 h at 30 °C with $150\times g$ in a shaking incubator. Aliquots of 100 µL were removed from each sample at predetermined time intervals of 0, 4, 8, 12, 16, 20 and 24 h. Aliquots of 10 µL were serially diluted (10-fold) in saline and plated on nutrient agar plates. The plates were then incubated at 30 °C for 24 h and the colony forming units (CFUs) of C. neoformans cells were counted [29].

4.5. Drug Combination Study

Various dilutions of standard drugs, i.e., amphotericin B, fluconazole and bioactive peptides (**10d** and **10o**) were prepared. Incubation broth was added to 96-well microplates, followed by addition of different concentrations of the standard drugs across the rows, and different concentrations of bioactive peptides across the columns of the microtiter plates. Hence, a unique combination of concentrations of standard drug and test peptide were obtained in each well. Inocula were added to the microplate by correcting the OD600 of fungal suspension in incubation broth. The plate was then incubated for 48–72 h at 30 °C. The optical density of each well of the plate was recorded on an ELISA plate reader to calculate the FIC index.

4.6. Flow Cytometry

C. neoformans cells were treated with the bioactive peptides (**10d** or **10o**) at MIC value and incubated at 30 °C at $200\times g$ for 12 h. The treated cells along with a batch of untreated cells were centrifuged at $2000\times g$ for 10 min at 4 °C and suspended in cold phosphate-buffered saline (PBS), followed by 2–3 washings with PBS. The harvested treated and untreated cells were then incubated with zymolyase for 1 h at ambient temperature to obtain cell protoplasm. The staining of obtained protoplasm was done using an Annexin V-FITC detection kit (Sigma-Aldrich, Saint Louis, DE, USA). The protoplasm of untreated cells was divided into 4 tubes (2 mL) and into 3 tubes a different staining agent was added while one was kept unstained. Hence, four samples of untreated cells were prepared with (i) unstained cells alone, (ii) cells with propidium iodide (PI), (iii) cells with annexin V-FITC and (iv) cells with both PI and annexin V-FITC. Furthermore, two more samples were prepared where protoplasm of **10d**- and **10o**-treated cells were stained with both PI and annexin V-FITC. All 6 samples were then analyzed by using an FACS Calibur (Becton-

Dickinson, San Jose, CA, USA) at excitation of 488 nm (for FITC) and 560 nm (for PI) band filter. Approximately 10,000 cells were used for counting [29].

4.7. SEM

The bioactive peptides (**10d** or **10o**) were added at their MIC value to a suspension of *C. neoformans* cells (~10^3) in an incubation broth at 30 °C for 12 h. Then, the treated, as well as untreated, cells were centrifuged separately at 2000× *g* for 10 min at 4 °C and suspended in cold PBS and followed by 2–3 washings with PBS. The cells were fixed with 2% glutaraldehyde in 0.1% phosphate buffer for 1 h at ambient temperature and washed 2–3 times with PBS. An amount of 1% osmium tetroxide in 0.1 M PBS was added to the cells to further fix and stain them. The cells were incubated with OsO_4 for 1 h at 4 °C. The samples were then dehydrated by incubating them with increasing gradients of 10%, 30%, 50% and 70% of ethanol in water followed by 100% ethanol. The samples were placed on a round glass cover slip previously attached to the aluminum stub by adhesive carbon tape. The samples were dried using a vacuum freeze-drier HITACHI 2030 at ambient temperature, then sputter-coated with gold using a HITACHI E1010 and observed under the SEM (Hitachi S-3400N, Tokyo, Japan) [39].

4.8. TEM

The samples were prepared in a similar manner to as mentioned in the procedure for SEM sample preparation, up until the dehydration of cells with increasing gradients of ethanol. The dehydrated samples were then embedded in resin which was prepared from an epoxy embedding medium kit (Sigma, 45359-1EA-F). Increasing gradients (10%, 20%, 30%, 50%, 70% and 90%) of resin were added to the samples followed by incubation for 1–2 h at room temperature after addition of each gradient. Undiluted resin (100%) was added to the sample and incubated for 24 h at 70 °C. Semi-thin and ultrathin sections were cut with an ultramicrotome (Ultramicotome Lecia EM UC6). The sections of samples were placed on a 3.05 mm diameter and 200 mesh copper grid and stained with uranyl acetate or lead acetate, before observation under the HRTEM (FEI Technai G2 F20, Eindhoven, The Netherlands) and analysis at 120 KV.

4.9. CLSM

(a) FITC-labeled peptide uptake assay

Active and inactive peptides tagged with fluorescein isothiocyanate were incubated with *C. neoformans* cells (~1×10^3 CFU/mL) at their MIC for 12 h. After incubation, cells were harvested by centrifugation at 2000× *g* for 10 min at 4 °C and suspended in PBS and mounted on a slide for visualization under a confocal microscope with excitation and emission wavelengths of 488 nm and 515 nm, respectively.

(b) PI uptake assay

The samples for PI were prepared by incubating *C. neoformans* (ATCC350) cells (~1×10^3 CFU/mL) with test peptides (**10d** and **10o**) for 12 h at their MIC values. After incubation, treated and untreated cells were centrifuged at 2000× *g* for 10 min at 4 °C and suspended in cold PBS and followed by 2–3 washings with PBS. The cells were then incubated with PI (1.49 µM) for 1 h at room temperature with constant shaking (150× *g* rpm), and later harvested by centrifugation and suspended in PBS. Then, the cells were examined using confocal microscopy (Olympus Fluoview™ FV1000 SPD; Olympus, Tokyo, Japan) with a wavelength of >560 nm for PI. *C. neoformans* cells without treatment of active peptides served as a control.

(c) DAPI uptake assay

C. neoformans (ATCC350) cells (~1×10^3 CFU/mL) were incubated with test peptides for 12 h at their MIC values. After incubation, treated and untreated cells were centrifuged at 2000× *g* for 10 min at 4 °C and suspended in cold PBS and followed by 2–3 washings with

PBS. The cells were then incubated with DAPI (3.01 µM) for 10 min at room temperature with constant shaking, harvested by centrifugation and suspended in PBS. Then, the fungal cells were examined using confocal microscopy (Olympus Fluoview™ FV1000 SPD; Olympus, Tokyo, Japan) with excitation at 350 nm and emission at 470 nm [40].

Supplementary Materials: The following supporting information can be downloaded at: https://www.mdpi.com/article/10.3390/molecules28010087/s1. General procedure for the synthesis of histidine derivatives and peptides, characterization data, ^{1}H and ^{13}C-NMR spectra, HRMS data and analytical HPLC of peptides are included in the supplementary information [41,42].

Author Contributions: Investigation, K.S., S.A., I.K.M., S.S., S.M.R., V.K. and K.T.; Data curation, K.S. and R.J.; Writing—original draft, K.S.; Supervision, R.J.; Project administration, R.J. All authors have read and agreed to the published version of the manuscript.

Funding: Doctoral fellowship and research facilities were provided by National Institute of Pharmaceutical Education and Research, S.A.S. Nagar, India funded by Ministry of Chemicals and Fertilizers, Government of India.

Institutional Review Board Statement: Not applicable.

Informed Consent Statement: Informed consent was obtained for hemolytic study.

Data Availability Statement: The data will be made available by the corresponding author on reasonable request.

Acknowledgments: Komal Sharma thanks the National Institute of Pharmaceutical Education and Research, S.A.S. Nagar, India, for providing the doctoral fellowship and all research facilities.

Conflicts of Interest: The authors declare no competing financial interests.

References

1. Rajasingham, R.; Govender, N.P.; Jordan, A.; Loyse, A.; Shroufi, A.; Denning, D.W.; Meya, D.B.; Chiller, T.M.; Boulware, D.R. The global burden of HIV-associated cryptococcal infection in adults in 2020: A modelling analysis. *Lancet Infect. Dis.* **2022**, *22*, 1748–1755. [CrossRef] [PubMed]
2. Ngan, N.T.T.; Flower, B.; Day, J.N. Treatment of Cryptococcal Meningitis: How Have We Got Here and Where are We Going? *Drugs* **2022**, *82*, 1237–1249. [CrossRef] [PubMed]
3. Jarvis, J.N.; Lawrence, D.S.; Meya, D.B.; Kagimu, E.; Kasibante, J.; Mpoza, E.; Rutakingirwa, M.K.; Ssebambulidde, K.; Tugume, L.; Rhein, J. Single-Dose Liposomal Amphotericin B Treatment for Cryptococcal Meningitis. *N. Engl. J. Med.* **2022**, *386*, 1109–1120. [CrossRef] [PubMed]
4. Muhaj, F.F.; George, S.J.; Nguyen, C.D.; Tyring, S.K. Antimicrobials and resistance part II: Antifungals, antivirals, and antiparasitics. *J. Am. Acad. Dermatol.* **2022**, *86*, 1207–1226. [CrossRef] [PubMed]
5. Magana, M.; Pushpanathan, M.; Santos, A.L.; Leanse, L.; Fernandez, M.; Ioannidis, A.; Giulianotti, M.A.; Apidianakis, Y.; Bradfute, S.; Ferguson, A.L.; et al. The value of antimicrobial peptides in the age of resistance. *Lancet Infect. Dis.* **2020**, *20*, e216–e230. [CrossRef] [PubMed]
6. Mahindra, A.; Sharma, K.K.; Rathore, D.; Khan, S.I.; Jacob, M.R.; Jain, R. Synthesis and antimicrobial activities of His(2-aryl)-Arg and Trp-His(2-aryl) classes of dipeptidomimetics. *MedChemComm* **2014**, *5*, 671–676. [CrossRef] [PubMed]
7. Iyer, K.R.; Revie, N.M.; Fu, C.; Robbins, N.; Cowen, L.E. Treatment strategies for cryptococcal infection: Challenges, advances and future outlook. *Nat. Rev. Microbiol.* **2021**, *19*, 454–466. [CrossRef]
8. Struyfs, C.; Cammue, B.P.A.; Thevissen, K. Membrane-interacting antifungal peptides. *Front. Cell Dev. Biol.* **2021**, *9*, 649875. [CrossRef]
9. Sharma, K.K.; Maurya, I.K.; Khan, S.I.; Jacob, M.R.; Kumar, V.; Tikoo, K.; Jain, R. Discovery of a membrane-active, ring-modified histidine containing ultrashort amphiphilic peptide that exhibits potent inhibition of *Cryptococcus neoformans*. *J. Med. Chem.* **2017**, *60*, 6607–6621. [CrossRef]
10. Sharma, K.K.; Ravi, R.; Maurya, I.K.; Kapadia, A.; Khan, S.I.; Kumar, V.; Tikoo, K.; Jain, R. Modified histidine containing amphipathic ultrashort antifungal peptide, His-[2-*p*-(*n*-butyl) phenyl]-Trp-Arg-OMe exhibits potent anticryptococcal activity. *Eur. J. Med. Chem.* **2021**, *223*, 113635. [CrossRef]
11. Mahindra, A.; Bagra, N.; Wangoo, N.; Jain, R.; Khan, S.I.; Jacob, M.R.; Jain, R. Synthetically modified L-histidine-rich peptidomimetics exhibit potent activity against *Cryptococcus neoformans*. *Bioorg. Med. Chem. Lett.* **2014**, *24*, 3150–3154. [CrossRef]
12. Mahindra, A.; Bagra, N.; Wangoo, N.; Khan, S.I.; Jacob, M.R.; Jain, R. Discovery of short peptides exhibiting high potency against *Cryptococcus neoformans*. *ACS Med. Chem. Lett.* **2014**, *5*, 315–320. [CrossRef] [PubMed]

13. Sharma, K.K.; Sharma, K.; Kudwal, A.; Khan, S.I.; Jain, R. Peptide-Heterocycle Conjugates as Antifungals against Cryptococcosis. *Asian J. Org. Chem.* **2022**, *11*, e202200196. [CrossRef]
14. Greco, I.; Molchanova, N.; Holmedal, E.; Jenssen, H.; Hummel, B.D.; Watts, J.L.; Håkansson, J.; Hansen, P.R.; Svenson, J. Correlation between hemolytic activity, cytotoxicity and systemic in vivo toxicity of synthetic antimicrobial peptides. *Sci. Rep.* **2020**, *10*, 1–13. [CrossRef] [PubMed]
15. Sharma, K.; Sharma, K.K.; Sharma, A.; Jain, R. Peptide-based drug discovery: Current status and recent advances. *Drug Discov. Today* **2022**, 103464. [CrossRef] [PubMed]
16. Mahindra, A.; Bagra, N.; Jain, R. Palladium-catalyzed regioselective C-5 arylation of protected L-histidine: Microwave-assisted C–H activation adjacent to donor arm. *J. Org. Chem.* **2013**, *78*, 10954–10959. [CrossRef] [PubMed]
17. Sharma, K.K.; Mandloi, M.; Jain, R. Regioselective copper-catalyzed N(1)-(hetero)arylation of protected histidine. *Org. Biomol. Chem.* **2016**, *14*, 8937–8941. [CrossRef]
18. Sharma, K.K.; Mandloi, M.; Jain, R. Regioselective access to 1,2-diarylhistidines through the copper-catalyzed n1-arylation of 2-arylhistidines. *Eur. J. Org. Chem.* **2017**, *2017*, 984–988. [CrossRef]
19. Song, L.; Ojeda-Carralero, G.M.; Parmar, D.; González-Martínez, D.A.; Van Meervelt, L.; Van der Eycken, J.; Goeman, J.; Rivera, D.G.; Van der Eycken, E.V. Chemoselective Peptide Backbone Diversification and Bioorthogonal Ligation by Ruthenium-Catalyzed C—H Activation/Annulation. *Adv. Synth. Catal.* **2021**, *363*, 3297–3304. [CrossRef]
20. O'Brien, E.A.; Sharma, K.K.; Byerly-Duke, J.; Camacho, L.A., III; VanVeller, B. A General Strategy to Install Amidine Functional Groups Along the Peptide Backbone. *J. Am. Chem. Soc.* **2022**, *144*, 22397–22402. [CrossRef]
21. Jia, F.; Zhang, Y.; Wang, J.; Peng, J.; Zhao, P.; Zhang, L.; Yao, H.; Ni, J.; Wang, K. The effect of halogenation on the antimicrobial activity, antibiofilm activity, cytotoxicity and proteolytic stability of the antimicrobial peptide Jelleine-I. *Peptides* **2019**, *112*, 56–66. [CrossRef] [PubMed]
22. Arias, M.; Hoffarth, E.R.; Ishida, H.; Aramini, J.M.; Vogel, H.J. Recombinant expression, antimicrobial activity and mechanism of action of tritrpticin analogs containing fluoro-tryptophan residues. *Biochim. Biophys. Acta Biomembr.* **2016**, *1858*, 1012–1023. [CrossRef] [PubMed]
23. Cruz, J.o.C.S.; Iorio, M.; Monciardini, P.; Simone, M.; Brunati, C.; Gaspari, E.; Maffioli, S.I.; Wellington, E.; Sosio, M.; Donadio, S. Brominated variant of the lantibiotic NAI-107 with enhanced antibacterial potency. *J. Nat. Prod.* **2015**, *78*, 2642–2647. [CrossRef] [PubMed]
24. Molchanova, N.; Nielsen, J.E.; Sørensen, K.B.; Prabhala, B.K.; Hansen, P.R.; Lund, R.; Barron, A.E.; Jenssen, H. Halogenation as a tool to tune antimicrobial activity of peptoids. *Sci. Rep.* **2020**, *10*, 1–10. [CrossRef] [PubMed]
25. Gottler, L.M.; de la Salud Bea, R.; Shelburne, C.E.; Ramamoorthy, A.; Marsh, E.N.G. Using Fluorous Amino Acids to Probe the Effects of Changing Hydrophobicity on the Physical and Biological Properties of the β-Hairpin Antimicrobial Peptide Protegrin-1. *Biochemistry* **2008**, *47*, 9243–9250. [CrossRef]
26. Sharma, K.; Aaghaz, S.; Maurya, I.K.; Rudramurthy, S.M.; Singh, S.; Kumar, V.; Tikoo, K.; Jain, R. Antifungal evaluation and mechanistic investigations of membrane active short synthetic peptides-based amphiphiles. *Bioorg. Chem.* **2022**, *127*, 106002. [CrossRef]
27. Sharma, K.; Aaghaz, S.; Maurya, I.K.; Sharma, K.K.; Singh, S.; Rudramurthy, S.M.; Kumar, V.; Tikoo, K.; Jain, R. Synthetic amino acids-derived peptides target *Cryptococcus neoformans* by inducing cell membrane disruption. *Bioorg. Chem.* **2023**, *130*, 106252. [CrossRef]
28. Jain, R.; Avramovitch, B.; Cohen, L.A. Synthesis of ring-halogenated histidines and histamines. *Tetrahedron* **1998**, *54*, 3235–3242. [CrossRef]
29. Maurya, I.K.; Thota, C.K.; Sharma, J.; Tupe, S.G.; Chaudhary, P.; Singh, M.K.; Thakur, I.S.; Deshpande, M.; Prasad, R.; Chauhan, V.S. Mechanism of action of novel synthetic dodecapeptides against Candida albicans. *Biochim. Biophys. Acta* **2013**, *1830*, 5193–5203. [CrossRef]
30. Vermes, I.; Haanen, C.; Steffens-Nakken, H.; Reutelingsperger, C. Flow cytometric detection of phosphatidylserine expression on early apoptotic cells using fluorescein labelled Annexin V. *J. Immunol. Methods* **1995**, *184*, 39–51. [CrossRef]
31. Adan, A.; Alizada, G.; Kiraz, Y.; Baran, Y.; Nalbant, A. Flow cytometry: Basic principles and applications. *Crit. Rev. Biotechnol.* **2017**, *37*, 163–176. [CrossRef] [PubMed]
32. Liu, T.; Zhu, W.; Yang, X.; Chen, L.; Yang, R.; Hua, Z.; Li, G. Detection of apoptosis based on the interaction between annexin V and phosphatidylserine. *Anal. Chem.* **2009**, *81*, 2410–2413. [CrossRef]
33. Henry, C.M.; Hollville, E.; Martin, S.J. Measuring apoptosis by microscopy and flow cytometry. *Methods* **2013**, *61*, 90–97. [CrossRef] [PubMed]
34. CLSI. *Reference Method for Broth Dilution Antifungal Susceptibility Testing of Yeasts, CLSI Supplement M27*; Clinical and Laboratory Standards Institute: Wayne, PA, USA, 2017.
35. CLSI. *Reference Method for Broth Dilution Antifungal Susceptibility Testing of Filamentous Fungi, CLSI Supplement M38*; Clinical and Laboratory Standards Institute: Wayne, PA, USA, 2017.
36. CLSI. *Methods for Dilution Antimicrobial Susceptibility Tests for Bacteria That Grow Aerobically, CLSI Supplement M07*; Clinical and Laboratory Standards Institute: Wayne, PA, USA, 2018.
37. Sharma, A.; Singh, S.; Tewari, R.; Bhatt, V.P.; Sharma, J.; Maurya, I.K. Phytochemical analysis and mode of action against Candida glabrata of Paeonia emodi extracts. *J. Mycol. Med.* **2018**, *28*, 443–451. [CrossRef] [PubMed]

38. Green, R.M.; Bicker, K.L. Evaluation of peptoid mimics of short, lipophilic peptide antimicrobials. *Int. J. Antimicrob. Agents* **2020**, *56*, 106048. [CrossRef]
39. Mares, D. Electron microscopy of *Microsporum cookei* after 'in vitro' treatment with protoanemonin: A combined SEM and TEM study. *Mycopathologia* **1989**, *108*, 37–46. [CrossRef] [PubMed]
40. Park, C.; Lee, D.G. Melittin induces apoptotic features in *Candida albicans*. *Biochem. Biophys. Res. Commun.* **2010**, *394*, 170–172. [CrossRef]
41. Abdo, M.-R.; Joseph, P.; Boigegrain, R.-A.; Liautard, J.-P.; Montero, J.-L.; Köhler, S.; Winum, J.-Y. Brucella suis histidinol dehydrogenase: Synthesis and inhibition studies of a series of substituted benzylic ketones derived from histidine. *Bioorg. Med. Chem.* **2007**, *15*, 4427–4433. [CrossRef]
42. Meena, C.L.; Thakur, A.; Nandekar, P.P.; Sangamwar, A.T.; Sharma, S.S.; Jain, R. Synthesis of CNS active thyrotropin-releasing hormone (TRH)-like peptides: Biological evaluation and effect on cognitive impairment induced by cerebral ischemia in mice. *Bioorg. Med. Chem.* **2015**, *23*, 5641–5653. [CrossRef]

Disclaimer/Publisher's Note: The statements, opinions and data contained in all publications are solely those of the individual author(s) and contributor(s) and not of MDPI and/or the editor(s). MDPI and/or the editor(s) disclaim responsibility for any injury to people or property resulting from any ideas, methods, instructions or products referred to in the content.

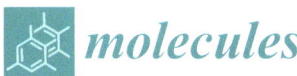

Article

Coumarin-Based Dual Inhibitors of Human Carbonic Anhydrases and Monoamine Oxidases Featuring Amino Acyl and (*Pseudo*)-Dipeptidyl Appendages: In Vitro and Computational Studies

Mariangela Agamennone [1], Marialuigia Fantacuzzi [1], Simone Carradori [1,*], Anél Petzer [2], Jacobus P. Petzer [2], Andrea Angeli [3], Claudiu T. Supuran [3] and Grazia Luisi [1]

[1] Department of Pharmacy, "G. d'Annunzio" University of Chieti-Pescara, 66100 Chieti, Italy
[2] Pharmaceutical Chemistry, School of Pharmacy and Centre of Excellence for Pharmaceutical Sciences, North-West University, Potchefstroom 2520, South Africa
[3] Neurofarba Department, Section of Pharmaceutical and Nutraceutical Sciences, University of Florence, Sesto Fiorentino, 50019 Florence, Italy
* Correspondence: simone.carradori@unich.it

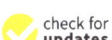

Citation: Agamennone, M.; Fantacuzzi, M.; Carradori, S.; Petzer, A.; Petzer, J.P.; Angeli, A.; Supuran, C.T.; Luisi, G. Coumarin-Based Dual Inhibitors of Human Carbonic Anhydrases and Monoamine Oxidases Featuring Amino Acyl and (*Pseudo*)-Dipeptidyl Appendages: In Vitro and Computational Studies. *Molecules* 2022, 27, 7884. https://doi.org/10.3390/molecules27227884

Academic Editors: Imtiaz Khan and Sumera Zaib

Received: 17 October 2022
Accepted: 11 November 2022
Published: 15 November 2022

Publisher's Note: MDPI stays neutral with regard to jurisdictional claims in published maps and institutional affiliations.

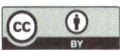

Copyright: © 2022 by the authors. Licensee MDPI, Basel, Switzerland. This article is an open access article distributed under the terms and conditions of the Creative Commons Attribution (CC BY) license (https://creativecommons.org/licenses/by/4.0/).

Abstract: The involvement of human carbonic anhydrase (hCA) IX/XII in the pathogenesis and progression of many types of cancer is well acknowledged, and more recently human monoamine oxidases (hMAOs) A and B have been found important contributors to tumor development and aggressiveness. With a view of an enzymatic dual-blockade approach, in this investigation, new coumarin-based amino acyl and (*pseudo*)-dipeptidyl derivatives were synthesized and firstly evaluated in vitro for inhibitory activity and selectivity against membrane-bound and cytosolic hCAs (hCA IX/XII over hCA I/II), as well as the hMAOs, to estimate their potential as anticancer agents. *De novo* design of peptide-coumarin conjugates was subsequently carried out and involved the combination of the widely explored coumarin nucleus with the unique biophysical and structural properties of native or modified peptides. All compounds displayed nanomolar inhibitory activities towards membrane-anchored hCAs, whilst they were unable to block the ubiquitous CA I and II isoforms. Structural features pertinent to potent and selective CA inhibitory activity are discussed, and modeling studies were found to support the biological data. Lower potency inhibition of the hMAOs was observed, with most compounds showing preferential inhibition of hMAO-A. The binding of the most potent ligands (**6** and **16**) to the hydrophobic active site of hMAO-A was investigated in an attempt to explain selectivity on the molecular level. Calculated Ligand Efficiency values indicate that compound **6** has the potential to serve as a lead compound for developing innovative anticancer agents based on the dual inhibition strategy. This information may help design new coumarin-based peptide molecules with diverse bioactivities.

Keywords: amino acyl coumarins; (*pseudo*)-dipeptidyl coumarins; carbonic anhydrases (CAs); monoamine oxidases (MAOs); molecular docking

1. Introduction

Due to its inherent biological relevance and chemical versatility, the coumarin skeleton has attracted significant interest in medicinal and organic chemistry, from as early as its isolation from tonka beans (*coumarou*) in 1820. The coumarin (benzopyran-2-one) scaffold, consisting of a benzene nucleus fused to the six-membered lactone ring or α-pyrone, is an extended electron-rich π-conjugated system with good charge transfer properties [1]. At the biomolecular level, it has been suggested that the binding strength of this aromatic heterocycle to its putative molecular targets is driven by hydrophobic interactions, particularly π-π interactions, as well as hydrogen bonding and dipole-dipole interactions involving the α-pyrone ring. Interestingly, due to the annular strain, which enhances the carbonyl reactivity, the opening of the lactone ring may be observed as a consequence of reactions with essential receptor/enzyme nucleophiles, or enzymes endowed with esterase activity. Furthermore, additional interactions with the specific targets are finely tuned by the different groups at variable positions of the coumarin skeleton. It should not be surprising then that natural and synthetic coumarins have encountered wide pharmaceutical applications such as antimicrobial, anticoagulant, analgesic, antidepressant, and anticancer agents, among others [2–4]. Over the past decades, numerous attempts have been made to modify the coumarin nucleus to develop novel biologically active molecules, and several chemical routes, starting from the simple single- or poly-substitution or the fusion with more complicated polycyclic systems to the hybridization approach with different pharmacophores, have been exploited [5].

Nonetheless, coumarins are not only interesting because of their bioactivity profiles, but also because of their metal chelating and optical properties. Particularly, substitution at the 7-position with electron-donating portions, such as hydroxy- or amino-groups, extends the π-π conjugated system of the nucleus, yielding highly fluorescent molecules, which have extensive applications in the investigation of enzyme activity [6,7].

A well-established method for the determination of protease specificity is based on the use of the 7-amino-4-methyl-coumarin (AMC) and similar fluorogenic moieties to label peptide substrates. It came to our attention that these biochemical probes, which are prototypical examples of peptidyl chains directly bound to the amino-coumarin scaffold through an anilido linkage, have not yet been exploited for a wider range of biological activities, such as inhibitory potential towards medicinally important enzymes that are sensitive to the coumarin class, such as carbonic anhydrases (CAs), monoamine oxidases (MAOs), cholinesterases and aromatase amongst others [6,8]. Considering the multitargeting approach in enzyme inhibition, and in order to explore in more detail this class of conjugates, with particular regard to the role of the peptidyl fragment in tuning drug-like properties such as selectivity and lipo/hydrophilicity balance, a small library of amino acyl and unprecedented (*pseudo*)-dipeptidyl coumarins were synthesized and firstly tested as inhibitors of selected CAs and MAOs.

This ongoing interest focused on the CA group, a large family of pH-regulatory metalloenzymes which catalyze the reversible hydration of carbon dioxide to yield bicarbonate and a proton, is encouraged by the crucial role of two membrane-anchored CAs, namely the IX and XII isoforms, in tumorigenesis, as a result of their ability to create an acidic extracellular *milieu* that promotes tumour survival and progression [9,10]. However, the design of specific CA inhibitors (CAIs) that target the tumor-related isoforms (IX and XII) is a challenging task because of the high structural homology among the 15 zinc-dependent human CAs (hCAs) known, whose three-dimensional structures have disclosed only subtle differences at the rim part of the active site cavity and the center region of the protein [11]. Consequently, the strategy to control the selectivity profile of CAIs towards hCA IX and XII over the widely distributed and physiologically relevant hCA I and hCA II isoforms has capitalized on molecules that have been reported to bind the protein in a position that is not essential for the Zn-chelating activity. In this context, coumarins have emerged as isoform-selective inhibitors for the CAs associated with tumorigenesis, by blocking the entrance of the CA active site in their opened, hydrolyzed form (similar to cinnamic acid derivatives). This is the consequence of specific interactions with regions where amino acids variability among the different classes is higher, and distant from the zinc ion.

Due to their central role in the oxidative deamination of neurotransmitters as well as other arylalkyl monoamines of xenobiotic origin, the MAOs represent attractive targets for the treatment of psychiatric and neurodegenerative disorders in humans. These are flavin adenine dinucleotide (FAD)-dependent enzymes attached to the outer membranes of mitochondria in neuronal, glial, and other cells. Human MAOs (hMAOs) consist of two fully characterized isoforms, hMAO-A and hMAO-B, which share approximately 70% sequence identity while differing in substrate specificity, tissue distribution, and inhibitor sensitivity. Selective hMAO-A inhibitors are in clinical use to treat depression and anxiety disorders. hMAO-B selective inhibitors are well-known coadjuvant agents for the treatment of Parkinson's disease (PD) and Alzheimer's disease (AD) and may possess neuroprotective properties by reducing oxidative injury due to the age-related increase of this isoform in the brain. In recent works, an exciting new role in cancer progression and metastasis has been highlighted for both MAOs [12], especially MAO-A [13]. The overexpression of the MAO-A isoform has been reported in several types of cancer, including prostate cancer (PCa), lung cancer, glioma, and Hodgkin lymphoma [14,15]. In particular, MAO-A is considered an important contributor in supporting PCa growth and development through epithelial-to-mesenchymal transition (EMT), elevation of ROS, and hypoxia.

A variety of coumarin-based MAO inhibitors have been reported to date, characterized by reversible and often selective inhibition. The chemical properties of the 2H-chromen-2-one nucleus explain the binding of coumarin derivatives to the hMAOs, and stabilization by H-bonds and π-π stacking interactions with the two crucial tyrosine residues (Tyr407 and Tyr444 for hMAO-A, and Tyr435 and Tyr398 for hMAO-B) are important factors. The introduction of substituents differing in size, length, and lipophilic or electronic characteristics at variable positions of the coumarin scaffold has been shown to modulate biological activity and isoform selectivity, enabling discrimination between the bipartite (hMAO-B) and monopartite (hMAO-A) substrate/inhibitor binding cavities of the two isoforms.

Pursuing our interest in bioactive coumarins, we have previously reported a chemical and biological investigation of new conjugates in which amino acids were linked to 6-amino-coumarin or AMC. These conjugates exhibited sub-micromolar inhibitory activity towards the membrane-bound hCA XII, with good selectivity ratios if compared to the CA I and CA II human isoforms [16].

In the present investigation, the selected coumarin scaffolds, AMC or 7-amino-4-metoxymethyl-coumarin (AMMC), were appropriately functionalized with enantiopure amino acids, to further define the impact of the stereochemistry of the peptide portion on conjugate recognition in the target active sites. The originally designed (*pseudo*)-dipeptidyl coumarin conjugates feature a urea unit placed between the components of the dipeptide portion, i.e., the internal residue, which forms an amide bond with the coumarin 7-amino group, and the terminal amino acid, protected in the ester form. It is worth noting that the central carbonyl of the urea divides the peptide substituent such that the external residue is linked as a retro-isomer, exposing its C-terminal functionality (Figure 1). In the field of peptide mimetics, the replacement of regularly arranged peptide bonds with a nonpeptide framework is a well-founded approach to introducing unique chemical and structural properties at the level of the individual backbone fragments [17–21]. This strategy is not only valuable for the rational design of peptide-based substrates and inhibitors for protein targets that will eventually be developed as therapeutics but also provides fundamental insights into the complexity of mutual dynamic interactions involving peptide ligands and their macromolecular acceptors, which leads to pharmacophore optimization and eventually translation of the peptide mimic into a small molecule drug. In this regard, the introduction of a carbonyldiamide (urea) NH-CO-NH linkage such as a peptide bond surrogate is a widely established method that exploits the structural and physico-chemical features of this moiety to improve target affinity and selectivity, as well as stability and bioavailability properties of the resulting *pseudo*-peptide compared to those of the native molecule [22–25]. Due to the delocalization of the nitrogen lone pair onto the urea carbonyl, which involves both NH functionalities, ureas present with reduced electrophilicity, enhanced chemical stability, and protease resistance relative to amides. The resonance effect gives rise to a more extended planarity of the NH-CO-NH junction and restricts the ω dihedral angle geometry of the two overlapping diamide groups, which results in rigidification of short linear peptide backbones. Furthermore, owing to an augmented H-bond donor capability vs. the amide counterpart, the urea moiety is routinely introduced into peptide backbones to form multiple stable hydrogen bonds with protein/receptor targets and water.

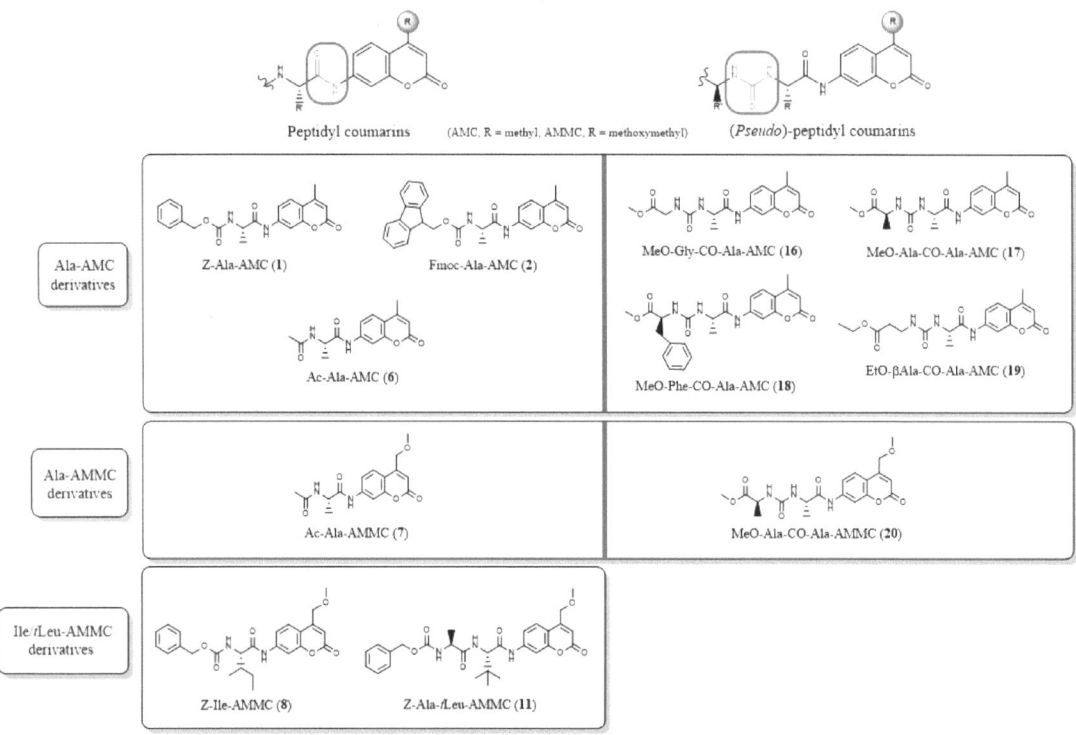

Figure 1. Amino acyl (compounds **1**, **2**, **6–8**) and (*pseudo*)-dipeptidyl (**11**, **16–20**) derivatives of 4-methyl (AMC)- and 4-methoxymethyl (AMMC)-substituted 7-amino-coumarins.

The underlying rationale for designing a peptidyl-extended coumarin scaffold resides in the potential of the chemically heterogeneous (*pseudo*)-peptide portion to create an additional stereo- specific pattern of interactions at the binding site, which is expected to produce improved selectivity between different enzyme isoforms, according to the tail approach [26].

2. Chemistry

Amino acyl (compounds **1**, **2**, **6–8**) and (*pseudo*)-dipeptidyl coumarins (compounds **11**, **16–20**), were synthesized in good overall yields employing solution phase procedures, as outlined in Schemes 1 and 2. Owing to the poor nucleophilic reactivity of the aromatic amino group, the acylation reactions of coumarins with the conveniently *N*-protected amino acids were preferably conducted by means of the mixed anhydride method. Thus, amino acyl coumarins **8**, **1**, **2**, **3**, and **9** were prepared by reacting the corresponding *N*-capped amino acid with isobutyl cloroformate (IBCF) and triethylamine (TEA) at −10 °C in tetrahydrofuran (THF) under inert atmosphere, followed by the addition of the appropriate coumarin nucleus. After removal of the ice bath, the reaction was completed in 20–24 h and resulted in a crop of the expected conjugate as a brown-red slurry. The work-up of the precipitate and the purification by chromatography and recrystallization gave the expected compounds in satisfactory yields.

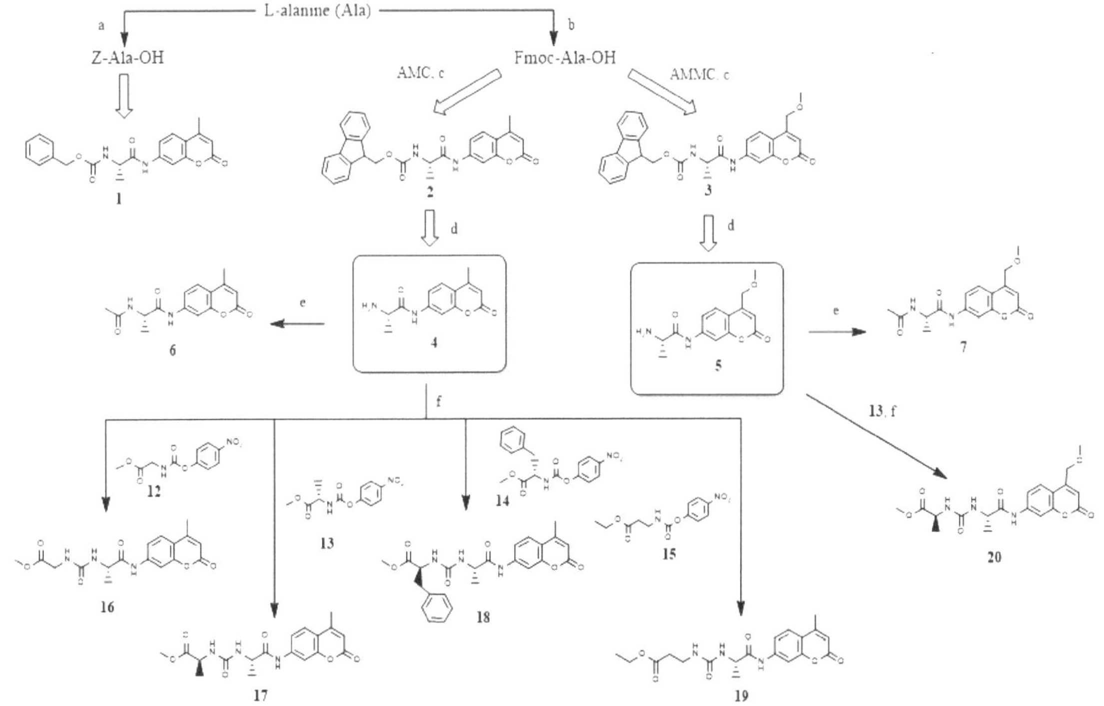

Scheme 1. Synthetic route to Ala-AMC/Ala-AMMC derivatives. Reagents and conditions: (**a**) Z-Cl, 1 N NaOH, 0 °C, 2 h, then r.t., 16 h; (**b**) Fmoc-OSu, TEA, H$_2$O/THF (2:1), r.t., 4 h; (**c**) IBCF, TEA, dry THF, −10 °C under N$_2$, 1 h, then r.t., 24 h; (**d**) DBU, dry DCM, r.t., 15 min; (**e**) Ac$_2$O, AcOH, r.t., 21 h; (**f**) DMAP, dry DMF, r.t., 72 h.

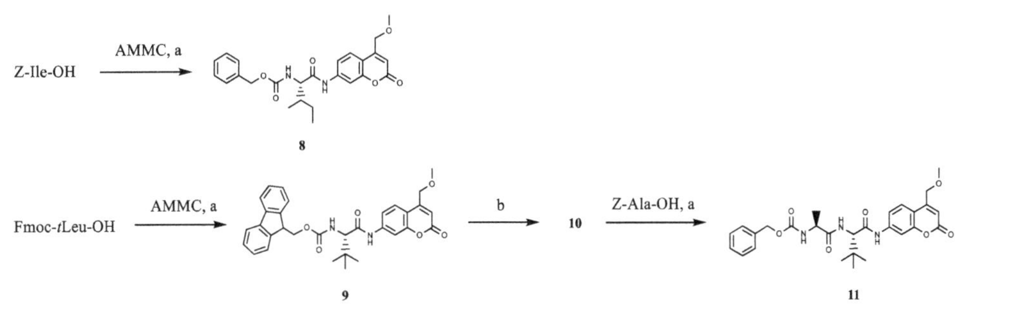

Scheme 2. Synthesis of amino acyl and dipeptidyl Ile/tLeu AMMC derivatives **8** and **11**. Reagents and conditions: (**a**) IBCF, TEA, dry THF, −10 °C under N$_2$, 1 h, then r.t., 20 h; (**b**) DBU, dry DCM, r.t., 15 min.

Amino acyl coumarins **2** and **3** were the precursors, via 1,8-diazabiciclo[5.4.0]undec-7-ene (DBU)-catalyzed removal of the protecting group under mild conditions [27], of the two key intermediates **4** and **5** required for the assemblage of the most substantial set of coumarin conjugates (amino acyl derivatives **6** and **7**, and (*pseudo*)-peptidyl coumarins **16–20**). Acetyl derivatives **6** and **7** were routinely prepared in excellent yields by room temperature reaction of alanyl coumarins **4** and **5**, respectively, with Ac$_2$O in acetic acid.

The preparation of dipeptidyl coumarin **11** was accomplished by starting from **9**, which was easily N-deprotected by DBU to afford compound **10**. Subsequent acylation was conducted following the mixed anhydride strategy with IBCF-activated Z-Ala-OH, resulting in satisfactory yields of **11**.

The route to the backbone-modified dipeptidyl coumarins **16–20**, featuring a urea bridge connecting the two amino acyl moieties, involved the preliminary activations of the external residues as the corresponding p-nitro-phenyl carbamates **12–15**. They were smoothly obtained in adequate yields by reacting at room temperature for 24 h with the appropriate H-Xaa-OMe/OEt hydrochloride with p-nitro-phenyl chloroformate in the presence of pyridine (Py). Subsequent acylation of the suitable alanyl coumarin core (**4/5**) with the proper active carbamate (**12/13/14/15**), carried on at room temperature in the presence of catalytic amounts of 4-(dimethylamino)pyridine (DMAP) in N,N-dimethylformamide (DMF), was completed in 72 h, giving rise to the expected (pseudo)-dipeptidyl coumarins **16–20** in very good yields.

Final compounds were purified to apparent homogeneity by column chromatography and fully characterized by ^{1}H- and ^{13}C-NMR spectroscopy. Spectral data are congruent with the expected structures of conjugates. In particular, a diagnostic signal in the range 157.2–158.4 δ could be seen in the ^{13}C-NMR spectra of the (pseudo)-dipeptidyl coumarins (compounds **16–20**), consistent with the presence of the urea carbonyl.

3. Biochemical Assays and SAR Analysis

3.1. CA Inhibition Results

Compounds **1, 2, 6–8, 11, 16–20** were initially tested in enzyme inhibition assays against hCA I, II, IX, and XII, and compared with the reference compound acetazolamide (AAZ). The bioactivity results and corresponding selectivity index (SI) between membrane-bound over cytosolic hCAs, as well as of hCA XII compared to hCA IX are reported in Table 1.

Table 1. Inhibitory activities, reported as K_i (nM) values [a], of amino acyl-(compounds **1, 2, 6–8**) and (pseudo)-dipeptidyl coumarins (**11, 16–20**) towards hCA I, hCA II, hCA IX, and hCA XII, and corresponding selectivities among the selected hCA isoforms.

Compound	K_i hCA I	K_i hCA II	K_i hCA IX	K_i hCA XII	SI hCA IX over hCA I or hCA II [b]	SI hCA XII over hCA I or hCA II [b]	SI hCA XII over hCA IX [c]
Z-Ala-AMC (**1**)	>10,000	>10,000	30.5	110.0 [d]	>327.9	>90.9	0.3
Fmoc-Ala-AMC (**2**)	>10,000	>10,000	91.0	37.2	>109.9	>268.8	2.4
Ac-Ala-AMC (**6**)	>10,000	>10,000	23.4	30.5	>427.3	>327.9	0.8
Ac-Ala-AMMC (**7**)	>10,000	>10,000	29.4	46.8	>340.1	>213.7	0.6
Z-Ile-AMMC (**8**)	>10,000	>10,000	78.7	41.5	>127.1	>241.0	1.9
Z-Ala-tLeu-AMMC (**11**)	>10,000	>10,000	171.5	336.3	>58.3	>29.7	0.5
MeO-Gly-CO-Ala-AMC (**16**)	>10,000	>10,000	183.3	38.2	>54.6	>261.8	4.8
MeO-Ala-CO-Ala-AMC (**17**)	>10,000	>10,000	163.3	9.6	>61.2	>1041.7	17.0
MeO-Phe-CO-Ala-AMC (**18**)	>10,000	>10,000	93.6	40.0	>106.8	>250.0	2.3
EtO-βAla-CO-Ala-AMC (**19**)	>10,000	>10,000	260.5	9.5	>38.4	>1052.6	27.4
MeO-Ala-CO-Ala-AMMC (**20**)	>10,000	>10,000	27.0	54.7	>370.4	>182.8	0.5
AAZ	250.0	12.1	25.8	5.7	9.7 / 0.5	43.8 / 2.1	4.5

[a] Data are the mean of three independent experiments, conducted by a stopped-flow technique (errors were in the range of ±5–10% of the reported values). [b] SI hCA IX or XII = K_i hCA I or II (nM)/K_i hCA IX or XII (nM). [c] SI hCA XII = K_i hCA IX (nM)/ K_i hCA XII (nM). [d] Ref. [16].

Significantly, the whole set of conjugates was found to possess good to excellent inhibitory activity towards the membrane-bound isoforms IX and XII, with K_i values in the submicromolar to low nanomolar range (K_i values of 23.4–260.5 nM for hCA IX, and 9.5–336.3 nM for the XII isoform). On the other hand, all the tested compounds were inactive towards the ubiquitous isoenzymes hCA I and II (K_i >10.000 nM), thus disclosing very high isoform selectivity with respect to AAZ.

The first series of derivatives (compounds **1**, **2**, **6**–**8**) are the simpler *N*-protected amino acyl-coumarins, with smaller molecular sizes compared to the other tested inhibitors. Apart from **8**, they all possess the alanine residue (compounds **1**, **2**, **6**, and **7**) combined with different *N*-protecting groups (conjugates **1**, **2**, **6**) or variable coumarin scaffolds (AMC for inhibitors **1**, **2**, **6**, and AMMC for **7**). They all exhibit a two-digit nanomolar inhibition against both target isoforms, except inhibitor **1**, which exhibits a K_i value of 110.0 nM vs. hCA XII. It is worth noting that in the alanyl-AMC/-AMMC main group of derivatives, independently from the coumarin type, the presence of a small acetyl group as *N*-capping substituent gave rise to an efficient and almost comparable inhibition of both hCA IX and hCA XII (as in compounds **6** and **7**, SI = 0.8 and 0.6, respectively). This behavior is not maintained in inhibitors bearing larger and more lipophilic *N*-protecting groups (see compounds **1** and **2**), suggesting that interactions at the protein clefts involving the ligand terminal appendage might be affected by the steric clash and/or electronic issues.

The AMMC-derivative **11** represents the only conjugate with an unmodified dipeptidyl skeleton obtained by incorporating a *t*Leu residue directly linked to the coumarin nucleus. Rather interestingly, **11** displays a significant decrease in inhibitory activity towards both membrane-bound isoforms, particularly towards hCA XII, compared to the above smaller compounds. The activity of **11** may be compared to the shorter, although structurally related, compound **8**, which also possesses a branched, lipophilic side chain. With regard to hCA XII, a large difference in inhibitory activity between compound **8** (still a good inhibitor, with a K_i value of 41.5 nM), and the approximately nine-fold weaker inhibitor **11** (K_i = 336.3 nM) was observed. In this case, peptide elongation seems to play a substantial role in reducing binding affinity. In contrast, the difference in the inhibitory constants of **8** and **11** towards hCA IX is smaller (K_i values of 78.7 nM and 171.5 nM, respectively); it may be suggested that the sterically demanding and highly lipophilic *t*Leu residue, a well-known conformational inducer, perturbs the binding to hCA IX and is here the main contributor to detrimental effects on inhibition.

The most interesting findings were among the (*pseudo*)-dipeptidyl coumarin series (compounds **16**–**20**), with the two low nanomolar hCA XII inhibitors **17** and **19** (K_i values of 9.6 nM and 9.5 nM, respectively) showing a noticeable gain in selectivity for the hCA XII isoform over the hCA IX (SI hCA XII values of 17.0 for compound **17**; 27.4 for inhibitor **19**). Both compounds possess the Ala-AMC scaffold, linked through the urea bridge to a small, aliphatic residue. It has been argued that the length and/or flexibility of the amino acid backbone, increasing from alanine (see compound **17**) to β-alanine (analogue **19**), may account, albeit partially, for the weaker binding affinity of **19** to hCA IX compared to **17** (K_i = 260.5 and 163.3 nM, respectively). The relative importance of substitution at the 4-position of the coumarin scaffold (methoxyl vs. the larger methoxymethyl group) for inhibitory activity of the ureic derivatives is exemplified by comparing **17** with the corresponding AMMC counterpart **20**. The latter compound displays a six-fold increase in hCA IX inhibitory activity (K_i = 27.0 nM against the K_i value of 163.3 nM for compound **17**). Due to the presence of the conformational constraint imposed by the NH-CO-NH junction, the 4-methoxymethyl group (conjugate **20**) may be forced into a favorable orientation that forms more productive interactions inside the hCA IX active site compared to the 4-methyl homolog, which represents a critical difference in binding to this isoform compared to inhibitor **17**. On the other hand, derivative **17** is an approximate six-fold more efficient inhibitor of hCA XII (K_i = 9.6 nM) compared to congener **20** (K_i = 54.7 nM), which demonstrates the opposite effects of the structural and electronic features of the 4-methoxymethyl AMC substituent on hCA XII binding.

It should be noted that this effect is not as pronounced with the smaller inhibitors **6** and **7**, where, conversely, the replacement of AMC for AMMC gives rise to only a very small reduction in both hCA IX and XII inhibitory activities. Here a plausible explanation may be found in the smaller molecular sizes of these ligands (compared to **17** and **20**), which allows the dynamic accommodation of the larger coumarin substituent inside the cleft of both isoforms.

In general, regarding hCA IX inhibitory activity, none of the (*pseudo*)-dipeptidyl derivatives **16–20** were found to be superior to the amino acyl coumarins **1, 2, 6–8**, with compounds **18** and **20** being almost equipotent to **2** and **7**, respectively, and derivatives **16, 17**, and **19** showing K_i values that are approximately seven to eleven-fold greater than the value of the best hCA IX inhibitor **6**. In contrast, the hCA XII inhibitory profiles of both series (compounds **1, 2, 6–8**, and **16–20**) partially overlap (with K_i values ranging from 30.5 to 54.7 nM, except for the three one-digit nanomolar inhibitors **1, 17** and **19**). It is worth noting that the pairs **2/18** and **7/20** possess similar inhibitory properties towards either hCA IX or hCA XII, respectively; this may be the result of similarities in structural and physico-chemical properties, such as the presence of the Fmoc/Phe aryl moiety (pair **2/18**), or the common AMMC nucleus (pair **7/20**).

Overall, the following conclusions may be drawn for this new panel of hCA inhibitors:

- Due to the complete lack of activity towards hCA I and II showing a K_i >10,000 nM, the test compounds fulfill the primary goal of selectivity towards membrane-anchored hCAs vs. the cytosolic enzymes;
- All molecules, apart from **1** and **11**, present the structural requisites that are compatible with a potent (one-/two-digit nanomolar K_i values) hCA XII inhibition;
- hCA IX inhibitory activity is maintained in the low nanomolar range for the smaller amino acyl-coumarin series (compounds **1, 2, 6–8**), whereas the extension of the (*pseudo*)-peptidyl chain results in up to an eleven-fold reduction of K_i values when compared to the most effective inhibitor **6** (excluding compounds **18** and **20**, which is similar in potency to **2** and **7**, respectively);
- In the amino acyl coumarin series, hCA inhibitory potency decreases from compounds with small N-protecting groups to analogs bearing more extended and lipophilic moieties;
- The general inhibitory profile discloses a significant selectivity towards hCA XII compared to the other isoform that is relevant to cancer; the most remarkable SI values are found in the (*pseudo*)-dipeptidyl coumarin series of derivatives (except **20**), which all share the urea structural motif;
- The replacement of AMC for AMMC in similar structures (pairs **6/7** and **17/20**) gives rise to unexpected effects, with a slight reduction of activity against both isoforms for the amino acyl-coumarin derivatives, whereas for the (*pseudo*)-dipeptidyl coumarin analogs the same replacement was found to cause a six-fold increase in hCA IX inhibition and a similar reduction in inhibitory activity towards hCA XII;
- The external amino acid also affects activity as observed with the (*pseudo*)-dipeptidyl AMC conjugates. The inhibition potency towards CA IX increases in the order βAla, Gly, Ala, and Phe, suggesting that, in the active site, a larger space is available for additional hydrophobic interactions involving the side chain; Ala and βAla, on the other hand, are the preferred residues for potent hCA XII inhibitory activity, which may be explained by suitable conformational rearrangements into the isoform binding site.

3.2. MAO Inhibition Results

Compounds **1, 2, 6–8, 11, 16–20** were further evaluated for their ability to inhibit human MAO-A and MAO-B. The inhibition activities are reported in Table 2 (as IC_{50} values) and compared to the reference inhibitors isatin and harmine.

Except for derivative **19**, which was found completely devoid of activity, the tested compounds were able to inhibit either one or both hMAO isoforms. The inhibition potencies were moderate with IC_{50} values in the low micromolar range (IC_{50} = 1.92–79.5 µM). The most potent inhibition was observed for the hMAO-A isoform with inhibitors **6, 1**, and **16** showing low micromolar IC_{50} values, whilst compounds **7, 8, 2, 11, 17**, and **18** presented inhibitions in the range 12.0–69.6 µM. The inhibition results suggest that steric size of the coumarin derivatives is an important determinant of MAO-A inhibition. The smallest derivative **6** is thus the most potent MAO-A inhibitor endowed with a 52-fold selectivity for this isoform, while replacement of the 4-methyl with a methoxymethyl (e.g., **7**) and increasing the (*pseudo*)-peptidyl side chain (e.g., **16**) reduce inhibition potency and isoform selectivity. For hMAO-B, only conjugates **7, 11, 17, 18**, and **20** were found to be inhibitors, although with lower potencies compared to hMAO-A (IC$_{50}$ = 45.6–79.5 µM). It is worth noting that compound **7** is the only active compound among amino acyl coumarins **1, 2, 6–8**, compared to the (*pseudo*)-dipeptidyl series.

Table 2. Inhibitory activities reported as IC$_{50}$ µM values [a] of amino acyl (compounds **1, 2, 6–8**) and (*pseudo*)-dipeptidyl coumarins **11, 16–20** against hMAO-A and hMAO-B.

Compound	MAO-A (IC$_{50}$ µM)	MAO-B (IC$_{50}$ µM)
Z-Ala-MAC (**1**)	9.31 ± 0.132	>100
Fmoc-Ala-MAC (**2**)	54.8 ± 0.028	>100
Ac-Ala-MAC (**6**)	1.92 ± 0.247	>100
Ac-Ala-MMAC (**7**)	12.0 ± 0.693	45.6 ± 1.85
Z-Ile-MMAC (**8**)	47.0 ± 13.5	>100
Z-Ala-*t*Leu-MMAC (**11**)	41.3 ± 17.8	79.5 ± 7.24
MeO-Gly-CO-Ala-MAC (**16**)	5.910 ± 0.155	>100
MeO-Ala-CO-Ala-MAC (**17**)	69.6 ± 9.28	58.6 ± 24.0
MeO-Phe-CO-Ala-MAC (**18**)	21.8 ± 0.092	78.0 ± 22.3
EtO-βAla-CO-Ala-MAC (**19**)	>100	>100
MeO-Ala-CO-Ala-MMAC (**20**)	>100	75.3 ± 0.976
Harmine	0.0041 ± 0.00007	-
Isatin	8.43 ± 0.245	3.90 ± 0.792

[a] Data are given as the mean ± SD of three independent experiments.

3.3. Computational Studies

Structure-based computational studies were carried out to obtain more insight into the inhibition activity of studied coumarins toward human CAs and MAOs.

For CAs inhibition, it has been demonstrated that coumarins can be hydrolyzed to E/Z 2-hydroxycinnamic acid by hCAs because of their esterase activity [28]. The hydrolysis of the coumarin lactone ring directly yields the hydroxycinnamic acid in the Z configuration, as observed in the X-ray complex of a naturally occurring coumarin derivative with hCA II (PDB ID: 3F8E) [29]. The isomerization to the E form (Scheme 3), which is more stable, has been observed for the simple coumarin in a complex with hCA II (PDB ID: 5BNL) [30]. However, this conversion may not be possible for large ligands in the CA binding site because of their steric hindrance [30]. As we have no experimental evidence on the stabilities (hydrolyzed E or Z/non-hydrolyzed) of the studied compounds in the binding pocket of hCAs, docking calculations were carried out on the amino-acyl and (*pseudo*)-dipeptidyl coumarins in the non-hydrolyzed and hydrolyzed forms, generating both E and Z configurations [9]. It may be postulated that, because of their dimensions, the Z form could be the most probable active isomer.

In the X-ray complexes of hCA II with coumarin derivatives mentioned above, the hydrolyzed ligands do not coordinate to the zinc ion despite the carboxylate function that could work as the zinc-binding group. Due to the fact that this experimental evidence, we carried out more docking calculations with and without the water molecule as the fourth ligand of the zinc ion. The presence of the water molecule prevents the ligand from binding to the catalytic cation and can serve as an anchoring point for hydrolyzed coumarins. Moreover, to account for the flexibility of the peptide chain and binding to a solvent-exposed region, a previously applied protocol that exploited the SP-peptide docking in Glide [31] was used that allows for expansion of the conformational sampling of the studied ligands [32,33]. The docked poses of ligands into the hCA IX and hCA XII catalytic sites confirm that peptidyl coumarin derivatives in the hydrolyzed form do not bind to the zinc ion, which is also the case when docking was performed without the coordination of the water molecules, as previously demonstrated by De Luca et al. [9]. The ligands occupy the rim portion of the binding site in the region that corresponds to that of hCA II in complex with the hydrolysis products of tetrahydrodehydrogeijerin [6-(1S-hydroxy-3-methylbutyl)-7-methoxy-2H-chromen-2-one] and the unsubstituted coumarin (PDB IDs: 3F8E and 5BNL, respectively) [29,30], which were selected as reference compounds (Supplementary Materials: Figure S1).

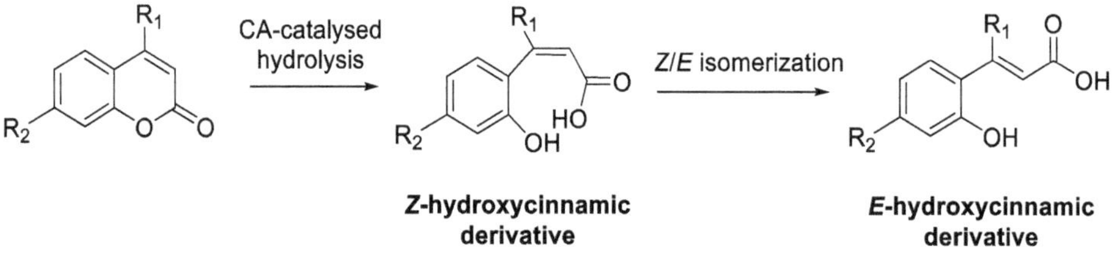

Scheme 3. hCA-mediated hydrolysis of coumarin derivatives and successive Z/E isomerization.

Furthermore, the results show that the docking scores for the hydrolyzed forms are, on average, higher than that obtained for the non-hydrolyzed coumarin derivatives; therefore, we can envision these forms as being responsible for the actual inhibition of hCA IX and hCA XII, particularly when considering their nanomolar potencies [29]. Consequently, the following discussion is mainly centered on ligands in the hydrolyzed form.

Focusing on hCA XII, the binding modes of the E and Z hydrolyzed forms of compound **19** are reported (Figure 2). A detailed analysis of the ligand docked poses in the hCA XII binding site shows different geometries for the two configurations: the *cis* form has a more extended binding geometry which hampers access to the zinc ion and establishes mainly polar contacts with the Lys3, Trp4, Pro200, Thr88, Gln89, and Ala129 residues. The ligand in the *trans* hydrolyzed form presents a bent geometry interacting with Leu60, Lys69, Asn71, Leu72, and Gln89. The docked geometries and contacts described here are conserved among almost all ligands, as demonstrated by the Interaction diagrams (Figure S2).

To further validate our prediction, the most conserved docked pose of compound **19**, as the hydrolyzed Z-form, in the hCA XII binding site was submitted to MD simulation to verify its stability and reliability. A 100 ns MD simulation was carried out where the protein maintains a stable conformation (maximum RMSD 2.00 Å, Figure 3), while the ligand slightly moves from the above-described docked pose and reaches a stable geometry throughout the simulation as well, apart from a short conformational rearrangement at 27.4 ns where the ligand urea function loses its interaction with Thr88 to form two intramolecular H-bonds with the β-Ala carbonyl group.

The alignment of representative geometries obtained from MD frames clustering, reported in Figure S7, further highlights the stable binding of compound **19** in the hCA XII binding region. One of the most representative geometries is depicted in Figure 4A. In the docking pose, the ligand establishes an ionic interaction between the carboxylic acid and Lys3 (Figure 2A). Embedding the complex in the box of explicit water molecules while running the simulation, H-bonding between the two urea NHs and Thr88 is favored.

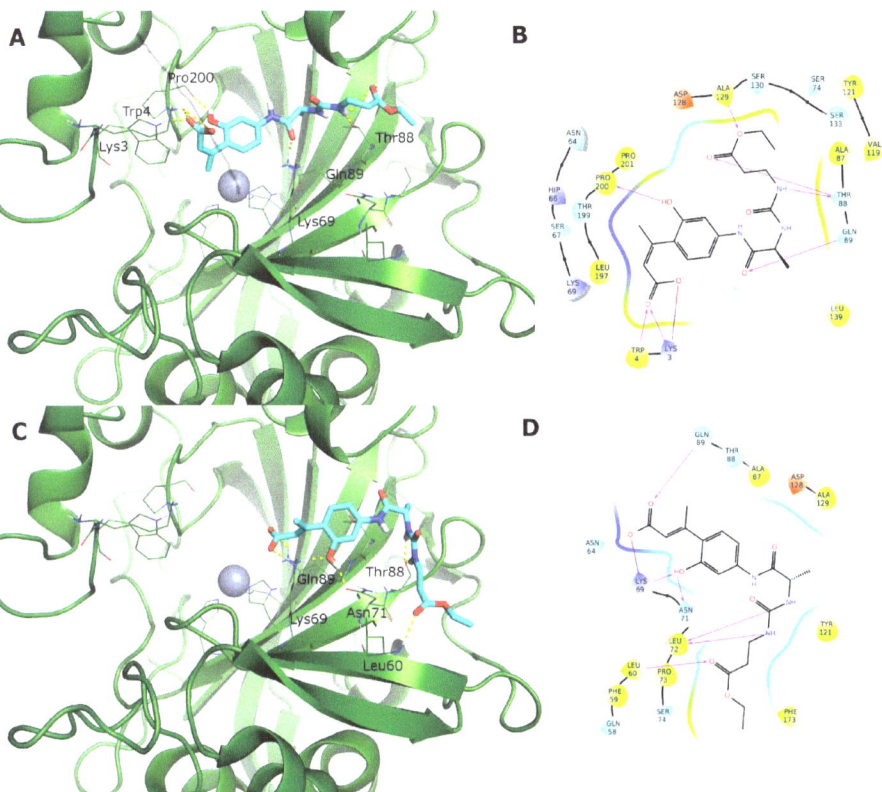

Figure 2. Docked poses of ligand **19** (stick, cyan C atoms) in the Z (panel (**A**)) and E (panel (**C**)) hydrolyzed forms complexed to hCA XII (dark green cartoon). The most relevant residues are represented as lines. Corresponding 2D ligand interaction diagrams are reported in panels (**B,D**), respectively.

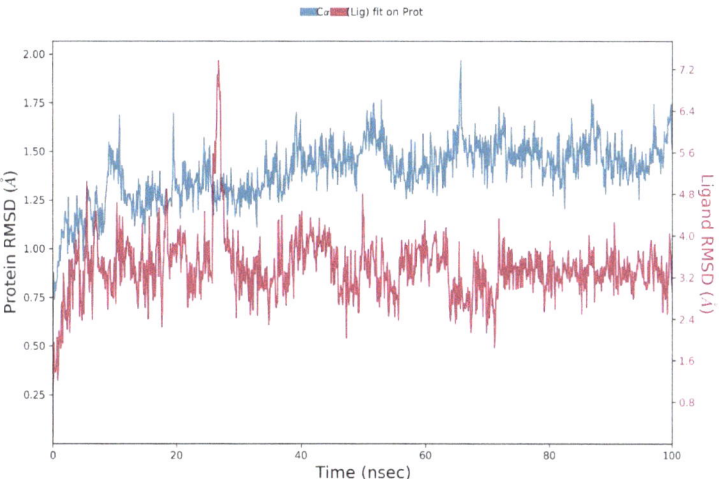

Figure 3. RMSD evolution during the MD simulation of the protein (light blue, calculated on the C-alpha, left Y-axis) and the ligand (compound **19**) (purple, calculated on all atoms, right Y-axis).

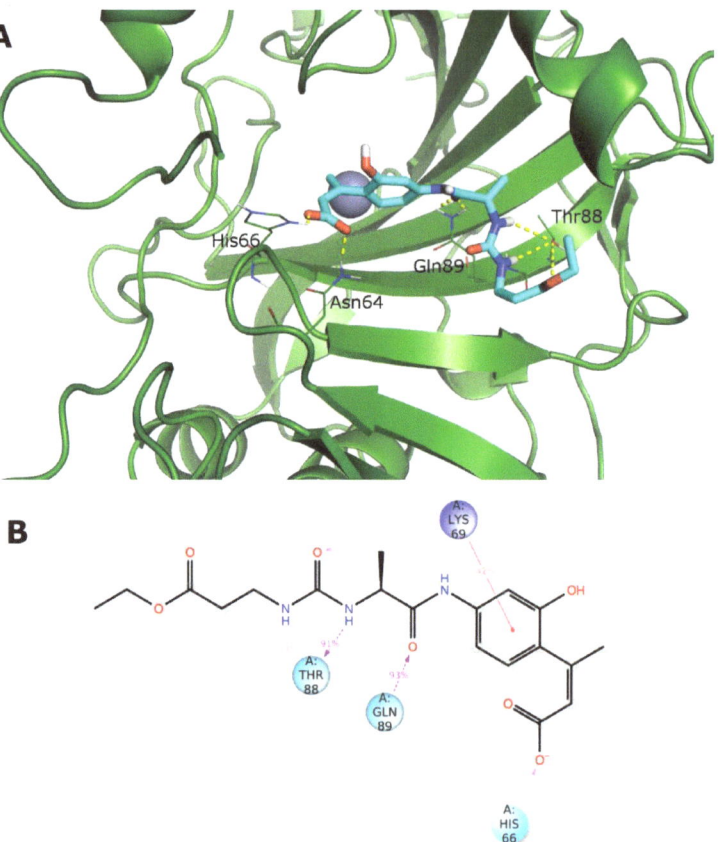

Figure 4. (**A**) Depiction of the binding geometry explored by ligand **19** in a representative frame of the MD simulation. (**B**) 2D representation of most conserved ligand-protein interactions with an indication of the persistence (%) along the simulation.

The carboxylic function can alternatively bind to His66, in a more extended conformation or to Lys69 in a bent geometry. Additionally, the latter residue forms a relatively stable cation-π contact with the aromatic ring of the hydroxycinnamic acid and an H-bond with urea carbonyl oxygen. The high stability of H-bonding contacts to Thr88 and Gln89 makes these latter the anchoring residues with a persistence of 90% during the simulation (Figure 4B). The stability of these H-bonds which involves the urea internal NH and the other polar contacts formed by the distal NH and the carbonyl oxygen, can contribute to explaining the better activity profile shown by (*pseudo*)-dipeptidyl derivatives with respect to amino acyl derivatives toward hCA XII.

The MD simulation confirms that, as already observed for the docked compounds, almost all ligand-protein contacts are polar (Figure S3), and the ligand is solvent-exposed. Assuming that all studied ligands share this behavior, this observation can provide an explanation for the improved activity profile shown by smaller and less hydrophobic ligands, while the presence of large and hydrophobic sidechains or protecting groups are less favored.

The above docking protocol was applied to study the binding of peptidyl coumarins to hCA IX as well. The docked poses of the ligands share some similarities to those retrieved in hCA XII: the hydrolyzed forms of the ligands do not bind the zinc ion and occupy the corresponding region of the binding site. Additionally, in this instance, the binding geometry is well conserved among hCA IX ligands (data not shown). The docked pose of the most active ligand **6** is reported in Figure 5. The terminal amidic NH forms a hydrogen bond with the carbonyl oxygen of Leu206 (corresponding to Thr88 of hCA XII), the carboxylic function binds the terminal NH_2 of Gln224 (that corresponds to Gln89 of hCA XII), while the phenolic OH is H-bound to the terminal C=O of Gln203 (corresponding to Lys69 of hCA XII).

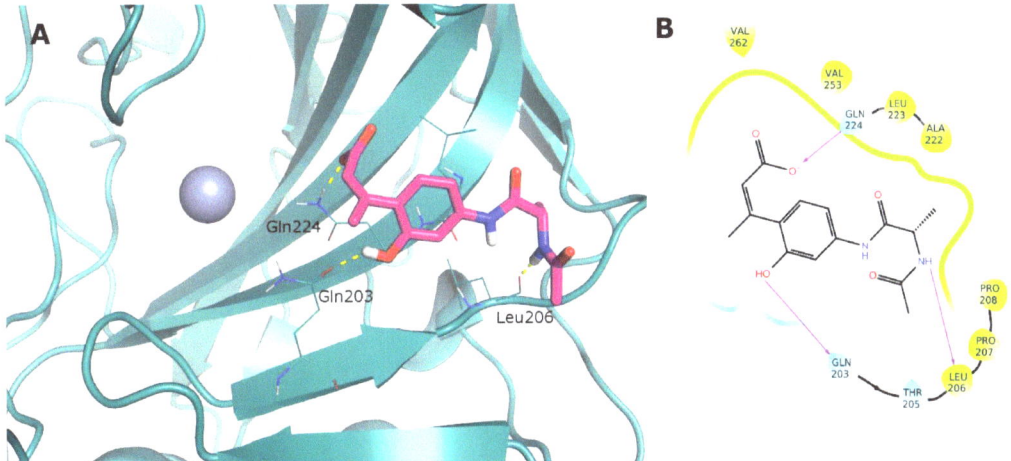

Figure 5. (**A**) Docked pose of ligand **6** (stick, magenta C atoms) in the hydrolyzed Z form in the hCA IX binding site (cartoon, dark cyan). (**B**) Corresponding 2D ligand interaction diagram.

It is known from the literature that the binding regions reported for coumarins are the most variable among hCAs, which can be exploited to obtain selective inhibitors [34–38]. To further confirm this observation and to obtain a more detailed explanation of the activity profiles of the studied compounds, the sequence similarity of the hCA I, II, IX, and XII isoforms was evaluated. The multiple sequence alignment based on the whole structure superposition, carried out in Maestro, provided an identity/similarity percentage of 40/54% for hCA IX, 36/52% for hCA II, and 37/53% for hCA I using the hCA XII as the reference.

When limiting the comparison to hCA XII residues that are mainly involved in the ligand binding (Lys3, Trp4, Lys57-Phe59, Asn64, His66, Lys69, Asn71, Leu72, Ala87, Thr88, and Gln89 in hCA XII), the identity/similarity further reduces to 33/33% and 31/31% for hCA II and hCA I, respectively, which is noteworthy since this region is formed by most diverse residues for the cytosolic hCAs. Similarity remains the same (38/54%) for hCA IX, which provides a possible explanation for the observed high selectivity (Selectivity Index hCA I or II/hCA XII > 30). Furthermore, we focused on the four most stable interactions retrieved from the MD simulation, which involved His66, Ly69, Thr88, and Gln89 in the hCA XII binding site. It has been verified that His66 and Gln89 are conserved among the studied isoforms, while hCA XII Lys69 is substituted by His67 in hCA I, Asn67 in hCA II and Gln203 in CA IX, and hCA XII Thr88 by Phe91 in hCA I, Ile91 in hCA II, and Leu223 in hCA IX. Therefore, these residues could be responsible for isoform selectivity. Residue variation between hCA XII and hCA IX, moreover, can explain the selectivity profile shown by ligands **16**, **17**, and **19** toward hCA IX; in fact, MD simulation indicates that the promising activity of these compounds as inhibitors of hCA XII is mainly due to the H-bonding between the ligand urea function and protein residue, Thr88. Therefore, the substitution of Thr88 with Leu206 eliminates the productive contact observed in the hCA XII binding site.

With regard to MAOs, molecular docking calculations were performed with human MAO-A and MAO-B in an attempt to explain the binding modes of the most potent and selective compounds toward hMAO-A (**6** and **16**), and to discover differences that could explain their selectivity profiles. It is well-known that the hMAO-B binding site is gated by residue Ile199 and can be longer and more hydrophobic compared to the hMAO-A binding site [39].

The docking poses in the hMAO-A pocket show coumarins **6** and **16** enclosed within the hydrophobic portion produced by the FAD and residues Tyr407, Tyr444, Phe352, and Tyr69. Furthermore, the terminal amide NH of **6** forms an H-bond with the carbonyl oxygen of Phe208, whereas three H-bonds stabilize compound **7**: the urea NH with the carbonyl oxygen of Ala111, the urea C=O with the thiol of Cys32, and the terminal carbonyl with the NH of Val210 (Figure 6).

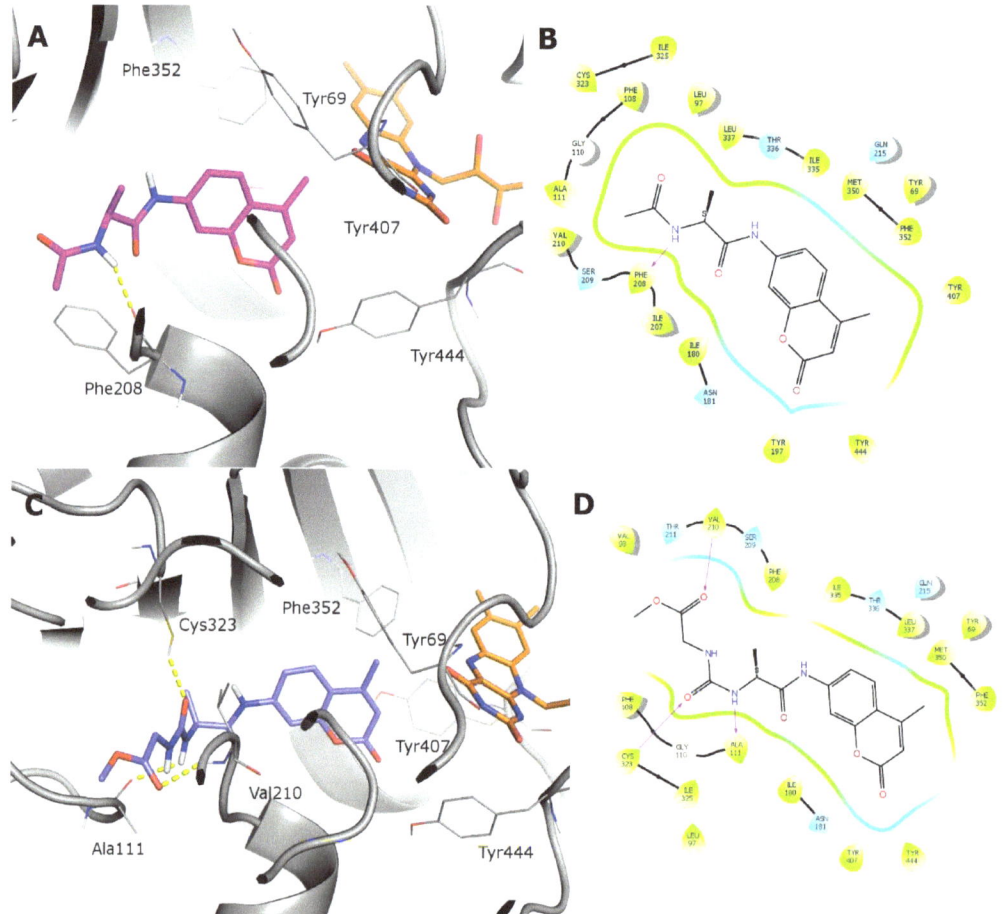

Figure 6. Panels (**A,C**) show the catalytic site of hMAO-A (grey cartoon) in complex with compounds **6** (magenta C atoms) and **16** (pale purple C atoms), respectively. Panels (**B,D**) show the corresponding 2D interaction diagrams.

Since the hydrophobic area of hMAO-B is more extended than in hMAO-A, in hMAO-B coumarins **6** and **16** are bound within the hydrophobic cage formed by FAD, Tyr326, Tyr398, and Tyr435. However, they do not find productive H-bonding interactions or π-π stacking with Tyr398 and Tyr435 as commonly described for coumarin derivatives [7,39,40]. In an attempt to find optimal binding orientations and interactions, the docking algorithm fits the ligands in a reversed orientation compared to their orientations in hMAO-A. Furthermore, for compound **16**, an H-bond is predicted to form between the amine of the urea and the carbonyl oxygen of Leu171 (Figure S7).

The activity profile of studied ligands is affected by the substitution pattern of the coumarin ring: by comparing these results with those already studied and more potent coumarin derivatives [40,41], it is evident that the substitution in 7-position of the 2*H*-chromen-2-one ring is not optimal for hMAO-B inhibition: the most active compounds usually are 3-substituted coumarins with small hydrophobic portions that occupy the longer hydrophobic pocket of hMAO-B, while the coumarin ring is stacked between Tyr398 and Tyr495. Fewer examples of potent 7-substituted ligands are known [42]. The 4,7-substitution pattern appears to be responsible for the relative lower potencies of the study compounds for both isoforms and, in particular, toward MAO-B. This is due to the steric hindrance that occurs when placing the ligand in the correct orientation in the enzyme active site. To further investigate this observation of the role of the substitution pattern, the fit of compounds **6** and **16** in the calculated hydrophobic interaction regions of the SiteMap for both enzyme binding sites are reported in Figure S9. In hMAO-A, both ligands occupy the binding site almost completely with the coumarin ring and its substituent in position four fitting into the hydrophobic site, while the peptide chain bends to reach H-bonding interactions outside the hydrophobic pocket. In hMAO-B, the reversed binding mode of the ligand produces an unfavorable occupation of the binding site by the peptide portion; the coumarin ring is partially embedded in the hydrophobic region with the 4-methyl substituent falling outside the calculated apolar site of the SiteMap.

To explore the possible dual activity of peptidyl coumarins toward both human Cas and MAOs, the Ligand Efficiency was calculated (Table S1). Compound **6** showed the best values for all enzymes. This confirms the validity of the core structure and provides an opportunity to start from this compound for future optimization studies.

To conclude these experiments, an in silico ADME predictive study was conducted (Table S2), which disclosed some issues concerning the drug-likeness profiles of the studied ligands. Their predicted physico-chemical properties are consistent with only moderate oral bioavailability, which may be due to limited cell permeability. On the contrary, the predicted blood-brain distribution is low, which would be detrimental only for hMAO inhibitors that act in the brain [43], and not in other body tissues.

4. Conclusions

The potential of linking the coumarin nucleus to a distinctive (*pseudo*)-peptide portion to target tumor-associated hCAs (IX/XII) and the hMAOs have been demonstrated in this study exploring an emerging field of interest of dual modulators [44]. The novel molecules have proven to potently inhibit hCAs IX/XII in vitro, without affecting the I and II cytosolic human isoforms. SAR analysis, in combination with computational studies, provided some interesting insights into structural determinants of the peptide fragment which contribute to the inhibitory profiles and isoform-selectivity of derivatives.

In the two diverging series of compounds, binding affinity for hCA is essentially driven by polar interactions, which mainly involve the peptide backbone functionalities, and secondly the hydroxycinnamic acid moiety, as corroborated by in silico results. Accordingly, in the group of amino acyl coumarins, the smallest and less hydrophobic protecting groups at the amino-terminal position of compounds appear to be beneficial for the inhibition of both isoforms, with alanine being the most optimal size for the residue directly bound to the 7-amino-coumarin core (compounds **6** and **7**). Most interestingly, the urea motif plays a key role in the (*pseudo*)-peptide inhibitors' selectivity towards the hCA XII isoform. Here molecular docking and MD simulations performed for the most active compound **19** provided a plausible explanation for the observed enzymatic selectivity, which is based on the stability of the peculiar H-bonding network which characterizes the ligand-hCA XII complex. In conclusion, given their prevalent and significant hCA IX and XII inhibitory activities, the study compounds appear to be promising leads for the search for tumor-selective agents. Besides compound **19**, other urea-based peptidyl derivatives can be investigated to gain further insights into how structural changes contribute to isoform-selectivity between the two isoforms.

Furthermore, the novel compounds behave as moderate inhibitors of hMAOs, with selectivity for the MAO-A isoform. While all compounds were found to be weak hMAO-B inhibitors, three compounds (**1**, **6**, and **16**) exhibited moderate hMAO-A inhibition with $IC_{50} < 10$ µM. The smaller steric size of both the coumarin and (*pseudo*)-peptidyl moieties was favorable for MAO-A inhibition.

In summary, this work resulted in the identification of dual inhibitors of cancer-related hCAs and hMAOs. In particular, compound **6** can be considered a valid starting point for the optimization of activity toward both targets and improving the physicochemical and pharmacokinetic profile of this scaffold.

5. Experimental Section
5.1. Chemical Synthesis

Solvents and other reagents were purchased from Merck (Milan, Italy) and used as supplied without further purification. Coumarins and amino acids were provided by Iris Biotech GmbH (Marktredwitz, Germany) and Merck (Milan, Italy). Boc-Ala-OH and HCl · H-Leu-OMe were purchased from Merck-Millipore (Milan, Italy). Esters H-β-Ala-OMe, H-β-Ala-OEt, and H-Leu-OMe, commercially available as hydrochlorides, were provided by Bachem (Bubendorf, Switzerland). Mixtures of solvents are specified with the stated ratios as volume/volume. All reactions involving air- or moisture-sensitive compounds were performed under a nitrogen atmosphere using dried glassware and syringe techniques to transfer solutions. Melting points were determined on a Büchi B-450 apparatus and are uncorrected. Chromatographic purifications were performed by Merck 60 (70–230 mesh ASTM) silica gel column. Analytical thin layer chromatography (TLC) was carried out on Merck 60 F_{254} silica gel PET plates. Next, ^{1}H-(300 MHz) and ^{13}C-(75.43 MHz) NMR spectra were recorded on a 300 MHz Varian VXR spectrometer using a suitable deuterated solvent. Chemical shifts are expressed as parts per million (δ) downfield from the internal standard tetramethylsilane (Me$_4$Si), and multiplicities are indicated as s (singlet), d (doublet), dd (doublet of doublets), ddd (doublet of doublets of doublets), t (triplet), q (quartet), m (multiplet), and br (broad signal); coupling constants (J) are reported in Hertz (Hz).

5.1.1. General Procedure for the Synthesis of Z/Fmoc-Xaa-AMC/AMMC Derivatives (**1–3**, **8**, and **9**)

A stirred solution of Z/*Fmoc*-Xaa-OH (0.97 mmol) in dry THF (3 mL) was kept under nitrogen at -10 °C, and IBCF (0.13 g, 0.97 mmol) and TEA (0.098 g, 0.97 mmol) were added portion-wise over a period of 5 min, followed after 10 min by a solution of AMC/AMMC (0.97 mmol) in dry THF (6 mL). After stirring for 1 h at -10 °C and 20–24 h at room temperature, the reaction mixture was evaporated to dryness under a *vacuum*, the residue taken up in CHCl$_3$, and the organic layer washed with 5% KHSO$_4$ and H$_2$O. The raw materials obtained after solvent drying and evaporation were chromatographed on silica gel, using a gradient of CHCl$_3$/MeOH as eluent. Solid products were furtherly purified by crystallization with the opportune solvent(s).

Z-Ala-AMC (**1**)

White solid (32% yield); R_f (CHCl$_3$/MeOH 98:2) = 0.4; m.p. 175–177 °C (MeOH). Chromatography eluent: CHCl$_3$/MeOH (98:2). ^{1}H-NMR (DMSO-d$_6$): δ 10.45 (s, 1H, AMC NH), 7.76 (s, 1H, ArH), 7.71 (d, 1H, J = 8.3 Hz, ArH), 7.49 (d, 1H, J = 8.3 Hz, ArH), 7.38–7.30 (m, 5H, ArH), 7.18 (br, 1H, Ala NH), 6.25 (s, 1H, C=CH), 5.01 (s, 2H, OCH$_2$), 4.19 (app t, 1H, Ala α-CH), 2.38 (s, 3H, AMC CH$_3$), 1.29 (d, 3H, J = 6.6 Hz, Ala CH$_3$ ^{3}C-NMR (DMSO-d$_6$): δ 172.9 (CONH), 160.6 (AMC COO), 156.3 (OCONH), 154.1, 153.6,

142.7, 137.3, 128.8, 128.3, 128.2, 126.4, 115.7, 115.5, 112.7, and 106.1 (aromatics), 65.9 (OCH$_2$), 51.4 (Ala C$^\alpha$), 18.4, and 18.2 (Ala C$^\beta$ and CH$_3$).

Fmoc-Ala-AMC (**2**)

White solid (68% yield). R_f (CHCl$_3$/MeOH 98:2) = 0.3; m.p. 153–155 °C (MeOH/AcOEt). Gradient chromatography eluent: CHCl$_3$/MeOH (99:1 → 95:5). ^{1}H-NMR (DMSO-d$_6$): δ 10.45 (s, 1H, AMC NH), 7.87 (d, 2H, J = 7.0 Hz, ArH), 7.79–7.69 (m, 5H, ArH), 7.54 (d, 1H, J = 7.0 Hz, ArH), 7.42–7.29 (m, 4H, ArH and Ala NH), 6.25 (s, 1H, C=CH), 4.28–4.26 (m, 3H, OCH$_2$CH), 4.21 (q, 1H, J = 7.0 Hz, Ala α-CH), 2.38 (s, 3H, AMC CH$_3$), 1.31 (d, 3H, J = 7.0 Hz, Ala CH$_3$). ^{13}C-NMR (DMSO-d$_6$): δ 173.0 (CONH), 160.9 (AMC COO), 156.3 (OCONH), 154.0, 144.2, 142.6, 141.1, 136.0, 130.0, 128.2, 127.6, 125.6, 124.4, 121.6, 120.5, and 115.6 (aromatics), 69.4 (OCH$_2$), 47.00 (Ala C$^\alpha$), 18.4, and 18.1 (Ala C$^\beta$ and CH$_3$).

Fmoc-Ala-AMMC (**3**)

Pale yellow sticky solid (67% yield). R_f (CHCl$_3$/MeOH 90:10) = 0.7. Gradient chromatography eluent: CHCl$_3$/MeOH (97:3 → 90:10). ^{1}H-NMR (DMSO-d$_6$): δ 10.52 (s, 1H, AMMC NH), 7.86 (d, 2H, J = 7.3 Hz, ArH), 7.79 (s, 1H, ArH), 7.77–7.64 (m, 4H, ArH), 7.62 (d, 1H, J = 8.8 Hz, ArH), 7.48–7.31 (m, 4H, ArH and Ala NH), 6.28 (s, 1H, C=CH), 4.64 (s, 2H, AMMC OCH$_2$), 4.29–4.27 (m, 3H, OCH$_2$CH), 4.21 (q, 1H, J = 7.0 Hz, Ala α-CH), 3.39 (s, 3H, AMMC OCH$_3$), 1.32 (d, 3H, J = 7.0 Hz, Ala CH$_3$).

Z-Ile-AMMC (**8**)

Pale yellow solid (32% yield). R_f (CHCl$_3$/MeOH 98:2) = 0.6; m.p. 78–80 °C (AcOEt). Chromatography eluent: CHCl$_3$/MeOH (99:1). ^{1}H-NMR (CDCl$_3$): δ 9.26 (s, 1H, AMMC NH), 7.71 (s, 1H, ArH), 7.32–7.26 (m, 6H, ArH), 7.12 (d, 1H, J = 8.7 Hz, ArH), 6.35 (s, 1H, C=CH), 5.79 (d, 1H, J = 8.7 Hz, Ile NH), 5.12 (ABq, 2H, J = 12.3 Hz, OCH$_2$), 4.50 (ABq, 2H, J = 15.0 Hz, AMMC OCH$_2$), 4.26 (app t, 1H, Ile α-CH), 3.49 (s, 3H, OCH$_3$), 1.95 (m,1H, Ile β-CH), 1.62 (m, 1H, Ile γ-CH$_A$), 1.21 (m, 1H, Ile γ-CH$_B$), 0.99 (d, 3H, J = 6.6 Hz, Ile γ'-CH$_3$), 0.90 (t, 3H, J = 7.2 Hz, Ile δ-CH$_3$). ^{13}C-NMR (CDCl$_3$): δ 171.0 (CONH), 161.1 (AMC COO), 157.1 (OCONH), 154.0, 151.6, 141.0, 135.9, 124.2, 115.6, 113.4, 111.2, and 107.3 (aromatics), 70.0 (AMMC OCH$_2$), 67.4 (OCH$_2$), 60.6 (AMMC OCH$_3$), 59.1 (Ile C$^\alpha$), 37.0 (Ile C$^\beta$), 24.9 (Ile C$^\gamma$), 15.5 (Ile C$^{\gamma'}$), 10.9 (Ile C$^\delta$).

Fmoc-tLeu-AMMC (**9**)

Yellow oil (53% yield). R_f (CHCl$_3$/MeOH 98:2) = 0.4. Chromatography eluent: CHCl$_3$/MeOH (98:2). ^{1}H-NMR (CDCl$_3$): δ 8.94 (s, 1H, AMMC NH), 7.74 (d, 2H, J = 6.9 Hz, ArH), 7.56 (d, 2H, J = 7.2 Hz, ArH), 7.38 (t, 2H, J = 7.2 Hz, ArH), 7.31–7.24 (m, 5H, ArH), 6.39 (s, 1H, C=CH), 5.86 (d, 1H, J = 9.0 Hz, tLeu NH), 4.58–4.35 (m, 4H, AMMC OCH$_2$, OCH$_2$CH, and tLeu α-CH), 4.20 (ABq, 2H, J = 9.9 Hz, OCH$_2$CH), 3.47 (s, 3H, AMMC OCH$_3$), 1.08 (s, 9H, tLeu CH$_3$). ^{13}C-NMR (CDCl$_3$): δ 170.1 (CONH), 161.1 (AMC COO), 157.0 (OCONH), 154.2, 151.4, 143.6, 142.4, 141.3, 140.8, 127.8, 127.1, 125.0, 124.9, 124.3, 120.0, 115.7, 111.4, and 107.6 (aromatics), 70.1 (AMMC OCH$_2$), 67.5 (OCH$_2$), 63.7 (AMMC OCH$_3$), 59.0 (tLeu C$^\alpha$), 34.6 (tLeuC$^\beta$), 26.5 (tLeu C$^\gamma$).

5.1.2. General Protocol for the N-Deprotection of Fmoc-Xaa-AMC/AMMC Derivatives (**2**, **3**, **9**): Preparation of **4**, **5**, and **10**

To a stirred solution of Fmoc-Xaa-AMC/AMMC (4.66 mmol) in DCM (30 mL), DBU (0.71 g, 4.66 mmol) in DCM (4 mL) was added dropwise at room temperature. After 15 min the solution was evaporated to dryness and the residue was chromatographed on silica gel using an appropriate solvent mixture as eluent, to give the pure N-deprotected derivative. Spectral characterization is reported only for compound **4**.

H-Ala-AMC (**4**)

Pale yellow solid (83% yield). R_f (CHCl$_3$/MeOH 90:10) = 0.2; m.p. 214–216 °C (MeOH). Gradient chromatography eluent: CHCl$_3$/MeOH (95:5 → 85:15). ^{1}H-NMR (DMSO-d$_6$) (amine protons are not observable): δ 10.59 (br, 1H, AMC NH), 8.01 (s, 1H, ArH), 7.70 (d, 1H, J = 9.0 Hz, ArH), 7.47 (d, 1H, J = 9.0 Hz, ArH), 6.25 (s, 1H, C=CH), 4.51 (q, 1H, J = 6.9 Hz, Ala α-CH), 2.38 (s, 3H, AMC CH$_3$), 1.30 (d, 3H, J = 6.9 Hz, Ala CH$_3$). ^{13}C-NMR

(DMSO-d$_6$): δ 172.4 (CONH), 160.9 (AMC COO), 153.9, 142.4, 126.4, 118.8, 116.0, 112.6, and 106.2 (aromatics), 51.2 (Ala C$^\alpha$), 20.9 (Ala C$^\beta$), 18.4 (CH$_3$).

H-Ala-AMMC (5)

Pale yellow solid (96% yield). R$_f$ (CHCl$_3$/MeOH 90:10) = 0.3; m.p. 158–160 °C (MeOH). Gradient chromatography eluent: CHCl$_3$/MeOH (95:5 → 90:10).

H-tLeu-AMMC (10) Yellow oil (81% yield). Gradient chromatography eluent: CHCl$_3$/MeOH (95:5 → 85:15). R$_f$ (CHCl$_3$/MeOH 85:15) = 0.15.

5.1.3. General Procedure for the Synthesis of Ac-Ala-AMC/AMMC (6 and 7)

The N-deprotected derivative (0.81 mmol) was solved in glacial AcOH (5 mL) and the stirred solution was treated with Ac$_2$O (0.10 g, 0.97 mmol). After 21 h under stirring at room temperature, the solution was evaporated *in vacuo*, and the resulting material was repeatedly taken up in dry Et$_2$O before being chromatographed on a silica gel column using a CHCl$_3$/MeOH (90:10) mixture as the eluent.

Ac-Ala-AMC (6)

Pale yellow powder (87% yield). R$_f$ (CHCl$_3$/MeOH 90:10) = 0.45; m.p. 237–238 °C (MeOH). ^{1}H-NMR (CD$_3$OD) (rapidly exchanging amide protons are not observable): δ 7.79 (s, 1H, ArH), 7.68 (d, 1H, J = 8.8 Hz, ArH), 7.45 (d, 1H, J = 8.8 Hz, ArH), 6.21 (s, 1H, C=CH), 4.46 (q, 1H, J = 7.3 Hz, Ala α-CH), 2.43 (s, 3H, AMC CH$_3$), 2.01 (s, 3H, COCH$_3$), 1.43 (d, 3H, J = 7.3 Hz, Ala CH$_3$). ^{13}C-NMR (CD$_3$OD): δ ^{13}C-NMR (DMSO-d$_6$): δ 171.7 (CONH), 170.1 (CONH), 160.1 (AMC COO), 153.3, 152.7, 141.6, 125.0, 114.8, 111.7, 110.0, and 105.5 (aromatics), 49.0 (Ala C$^\alpha$), 21.0 (CH$_3$CO), 16.8 and 16.6 (Ala C$^\beta$ and CH$_3$).

Ac-Ala-AMMC (7)

Yellow powder (76% yield). R$_f$ (CHCl$_3$/MeOH 90:10) = 0.5; m.p. 208–210 °C (MeOH). ^{1}H-NMR (CDCl$_3$): δ 9.96 (s, 1H, AMMC NH), 7.79 (s, 1H, ArH), 7.38 (d, 1H, J = 8.7 Hz, ArH), 7.27 (d, 1H, J = 8.7 Hz, ArH), 7.26 (d, 1H, J = 7.5 Hz, Ala NH), 6.41 (s, 1H, C=CH), 4.78 (app t, 1H, Ala α-CH), 4.56 (s, 2H, AMMC OCH$_2$), 3.44 (s, 3H, AMMC OCH$_3$), 2.01 (s, 3H, CH$_3$CO), 1.49 (d, 3H, J = 7.5 Hz, Ala CH$_3$). ^{13}C-NMR (CDCl$_3$): δ 171.9 (CONH), 171.3 (CONH), 161.2 (AMC COO), 154.1, 151.6, 141.5, 124.2, 120.1, 115.8, 111.1, and 107.4 (aromatics), 70.0 (AMMC OCH$_2$), 59.0 (AMMC OCH$_3$), 50.2 (Ala C$^\alpha$), 23.1 (CH$_3$CO), 18.1 (Ala C$^\beta$).

5.1.4. Synthesis of Z-Ala-tLeu-AMMC (11)

To a stirred solution of Z-Ala-OH (0.105 g, 0.47 mmol) in dry THF (2 mL), kept under nitrogen at −10 °C, IBCF (0.064 g, 0.47 mmol) and TEA (0.048 g, 0.47 mmol) were added portion-wise over a period of 5 min, followed after 10 min by a solution of 10 (0.149 g, 0.47 mmol) in dry THF (3 mL). After stirring for 1 h at −10 °C and 24 h at r.t., the reaction mixture was evaporated to dryness *in vacuo*, and the residue was taken up in CHCl$_3$. The organic layer was washed with 5% KHSO$_4$ and H$_2$O, dried, and evaporated under reduced pressure to furnish a raw material, which was eluted from a silica gel column using CHCl$_3$/MeOH (98:2) as the eluent, to give compound 11 as a pure white solid (0.11 g, 45%). R$_f$ (CHCl$_3$/MeOH 98:2) = 0.2; m.p. 205–209 °C (MeOH/AcOEt). ^{1}H-NMR (CDCl$_3$): δ 9.20 (s, 1H, AMMC NH), 7.71 (s, 1H, ArH), 7.42–7.25 (m, 8H, ArH and tLeu NH), 6.39 (s, 1H, C=CH), 5.79 (br, 1H, Ala NH), 5.15 (s, 2H, OCH$_2$), 4.55–4.47 (m, 4H, AMMC OCH$_2$, tLeu and Ala α-CH), 3.48 (s, 3H, AMMC OCH$_3$), 1.40 (d, 3H, J = 7.2 Hz, Ala CH$_3$), 1.04 (s, 9H, tLeu CH$_3$). ^{13}C-NMR (CDCl$_3$): δ 173.0 (CONH), 169.5 (CONH), 161.0 (AMC COO), 156.3 (OCONH), 154.2, 151.3, 141.0, 136.0, 128.5, 128.2, 128.0, 124.2, 116.0, 113.7, 111.4, and 107.7 (aromatics), 70.1 (AMMC OCH$_2$), 67.2 (OCH$_2$), 61.8 (AMMC OCH$_3$), 59.0 (tLeu C$^\alpha$), 50.8 (Ala C$^\alpha$), 34.7 (tLeu C$^\beta$), 26.6 (tLeu C$^\gamma$), 18.2 (Ala C$^\beta$).

5.1.5. General Protocol for the Preparation of Active Carbamates (12–15)

A stirred solution of H-Xaa-OMe/OEt.HCl (1.33 mmol) in dry DCM (2 mL) was treated with Py (0.11 g, 1.39 mmol) at room temperature, and a solution of p-NO$_2$-phenyl cloroformate (0.28 g, 1.39 mmol) in dry DCM (1 mL) was added. The reaction mixture was kept under stirring for 24 h, then evaporated under reduced pressure, and the residue was taken up in CHCl$_3$. The solution was repeatedly and successively washed with 5% KHSO$_4$, Na$_2$CO$_3$ (saturated), and H$_2$O. The residue obtained after drying and evaporation of the solvent was eluted from a silica gel column using CHCl$_3$/hexane (97:3) as eluent, to give the expected carbamate.

p-NO$_2$-Ph-OCO-Gly-OMe (12)

White foam (yield 34%). R_f (CHCl$_3$/hexane 97:3) = 0.1. ^{1}H-NMR (CDCl$_3$): δ 8.25 (d, 2H, J = 6.6 Hz, ArH), 7.33 (d, J = 6.6 Hz, 2H, ArH), 5.71 (br t, 1H, Gly NH), 4.1 (d, 2H, J = 5.7 Hz, Gly α-CH$_2$), 3.81 (s, 3H, COOCH$_3$).

p-NO$_2$-Ph-OCO-Ala-OMe (13)

White foam (yield 70%). R_f (CHCl$_3$/hexane 97:3) = 0.6. ^{1}H-NMR (CDCl$_3$): δ 8.23 (d, 2H, J = 8.7 Hz, ArH), 7.32 (d, 2H, J = 8.7 Hz, ArH), 5.79 (br d, 1H, Ala NH), 4.47 (app t, 1H, Ala α-CH), 3.79 (s, 3H, COOCH$_3$), 1.50 (d, 3H, J = 7.2 Hz, Ala CH$_3$).

p-NO$_2$-Ph-OCO-Phe-OMe (14)

White foam (yield 26%). R_f (CHCl$_3$/hexane 97:3) = 0.15). ^{1}H-NMR (CDCl$_3$): δ 8.22 (d, 2H, J = 7.2 Hz, ArH), 7.33 (d, 2H, J = 7.2 Hz, ArH), 7.29–7.25 (m, 3H, ArH), 7.18 (d, 2H, J = 7.5 Hz, ArH), 5.64 (d, 1H, J = 8.1 Hz, Phe NH), 4.7 (ddd, 1H, J = 6.0 Hz, J = 8.1 Hz, J = 13.8 Hz, Phe α-CH), 3.79 (s, 3H, COOCH$_3$), 3.2 (ddd, 2H, J = 6.0 Hz, J = 13.8 Hz, J = 29.1 Hz, Phe β-CH$_2$).

p-NO$_2$-Ph-OCO-βAla-OEt (15)

Pale yellow wax (yield 29%). R_f (CHCl$_3$/hexane 97:3) = 0.3. ^{1}H-NMR (CDCl$_3$): δ 8.22 (d, 2H, J = 8.9 Hz, ArH), 7.29 (d, 2H, J = 8.9 Hz, ArH), 5.80 (br t, 1H, βAla NH), 4.18 (q, 2H, J = 7.0 Hz, OCH$_2$CH$_3$), 3.55 (dd, 2H, J = 6.2 Hz, J = 11.9 Hz, βAla β-CH$_2$), 2.61 (dd, 2H, J = 6.2 Hz, J = 11.9 Hz, βAla α-CH$_2$), 1.28 (t, 3H, J = 7.0 Hz, OCH$_2$CH$_3$).

5.1.6. General Procedure for the Synthesis of (*Pseudo*)-Dipeptidyl Coumarins (16–20)

To a stirred solution of H-Ala-AMC/AMMC (6/7) (1.27 mmol) in dry DMF (10 mL) and catalytic amounts of DMAP (0.039 g, 0.32 mmol) a solution of carbamate (12–15) (1.27 mmol) in dry DMF (5 mL) was added portion-wise at room temperature. After stirring for 72 h at room temperature, the reaction mixture was evaporated under a vacuum and the residue was taken up in EtOAc. The organic layer was washed with 5% KHSO$_4$, Na$_2$CO$_3$ (saturated), and H$_2$O, dried, and evaporated under reduced pressure to furnish the expected compound as raw material. Purification by silica gel column chromatography of the resulting crude product, using CHCl$_3$/MeOH (95:5) as the eluent, afforded the expected pure urea derivatives.

MeO-Gly-CO-Ala-AMC (16)

White solid (yield 44%). R_f (CHCl$_3$/MeOH 95:5) = 0.15; m.p. 193–195 °C (MeOH). ^{1}H-NMR (DMSO-d_6): δ 10.46 (s, 1H, AMC NH), 7.76 (d, 1H, J = 2.0 Hz, ArH), 7.69 (d, 1H, J = 8.7 Hz, ArH), 7.45 (dd, 1H, J = 8.7 Hz, J = 2.0 Hz, ArH), 6.65 (d, 1H, J = 7.7 Hz, Ala NH) 6.41 (t, 1H, J = 6.2 Hz, Gly NH), 6.24 (s, 1H, C=CH), 4.32 (app t, 1H, Ala α-CH), 3.78 (d, 2H, J = 6.2 Hz, Gly α-CH$_2$), 3.59 (s, 3H, COOCH$_3$), 2.37 (s, 3H, MAC CH$_3$), 1.26 (d, 3H, J = 6.7 Hz, Ala CH$_3$). ^{13}C-NMR (DMSO-d_6): δ 173.5 (CONH), 172.0 (COO), 160.6 (AMC COO), 157.8 (NHCONH), 154.0, 153.7, 142.7, 126.4, 115.7, 115.5, 112.7, and 106.1 (aromatics), 52.0 (OCH$_3$), 50.1 (Ala C^α), 41.7 (Gly C^α), 19.4, and 18.4 (Ala C^β and CH$_3$).

MeO-Ala-CO-Ala-AMC (17)

White solid (yield 80%). R_f (CHCl$_3$/MeOH 95:5) = 0.4; m.p. 193–195 °C (MeOH). ^{1}H-NMR (DMSO-d_6): δ 10.45 (s, 1H, AMC NH), 7.76 (s, 1H, ArH), 7.71 (d, 1H, J = 8.7 Hz, ArH), 7.48 (d, 1H, J = 8.7 Hz, ArH), 6.48 (d, 1H, J = 7.8 Hz, Ala NH), 6.41 (d, 1H, J = 7.5 Hz, Ala NH), 6.25 (s, 1H, C=CH), 4.28 (m, 1H, Ala α-CH), 4.13 (m, 1H, Ala α-CH), 3.60 (s, 3H, COOCH$_3$), 2.38 (s, 3H, AMC CH$_3$), 1.24 (d, 3H, J = 7.2 Hz, Ala CH$_3$), 1.23 (d, 3H, J = 7.2 Hz, Ala CH$_3$). ^{13}C-NMR (DMSO-d_6): δ 173.5 (CONH), 173.4 (COO), 160.4 (AMC COO), 157.2 (NHCONH), 154.1, 153.5, 142.7, 126.4, 126.3, 115.6, 115.4, 112.7, and 106.0 (aromatics), 52.1 (OCH$_3$), 50.0 (Ala C^α), 48.5 (Ala C^α), 19.4, and 18.4 (Ala C^β and CH$_3$).

MeO-Phe-CO-Ala-AMC (**18**)

Pale orange solid (yield 91%). R_f (CHCl$_3$/MeOH 95:5) = 0.35; m.p. 177–183 °C (MeOH). ^{1}H-NMR (DMSO-d_6): δ 10.45 (s, 1H, AMC NH), 7.75 (d, 1H, J = 1.2 Hz, ArH), 7.70 (d, 1H, J = 8.7 Hz, ArH), 7.45 (dd, 1H, J = 8.7 Hz, J = 1.2 Hz, ArH), 7.29–7.14 (m, 5H, ArH), 6.58 (d, 1H, J = 7.8 Hz, Ala or Phe NH), 6.41 (d, 1H, J = 7.8 Hz, Phe or Ala NH), 6.25 (s, 1H, C=CH), 4.41–4.24 (m, 2H, Ala and Phe α-CH), 3.57 (s, 3H, COOCH$_3$), 2.98–2.82 (m, 2H, Phe β-CH$_2$), 2.37 (s, 3H, AMC CH$_3$), 1.24 (d, 3H, J = 6.9 Hz, Ala CH$_3$). ^{13}C-NMR (DMSO-d_6): δ 173.4 (CONH), 173.2 (COO), 160.6 (AMC COO), 157.3 (NHCONH), 154.0, 153.7, 142.7, 142.5, 137.2, 130.2, 129.6, 128.8, 127.1, 126.4, 115.7, 115.5, 112.7, and 106.1 (aromatics), 54.5 (Phe C^α), 50.2 and 50.1 (OCH$_3$ and Ala C^α), 37.8 (Phe C^β), 19.3, and 18.4 (Ala C^β and CH$_3$).

EtO-βAla-CO-Ala-AMC (**19**)

White solid (yield 66%). R_f (CHCl$_3$/MeOH 95:5) = 0.45. m.p. 182–183 °C (MeOH/AcOEt). ^{1}H-NMR (CDCl$_3$): δ 10.08 (s, 1H, AMC NH), 7.74 (s, 1H, ArH), 7.44 (d, 1H, J = 8.6 Hz, ArH), 7.3 (d, 1H, J = 8.6 Hz, ArH), 6.26 (br d, 1H, Ala NH), 6.10 (s, 1H, C=CH), 5.93 (br t, 1H, βAla NH), 4.61 (m, 1H, Ala α-CH), 4.10 (q, 2H, J = 7.1 Hz, OCH_2CH$_3$), 3.52–3.38 (m, 2H, βAla β-CH$_2$), 2.49 (app t, 2H, βAla α-CH$_2$), 2.38 (s, 3H, AMC CH$_3$), 1.45 (d, 3H, J = 7.2 Hz, Ala CH$_3$), 1.22 (t, 3H, J = 7.1 Hz, OCH$_2$CH_3). ^{13}C-NMR (CDCl$_3$): δ 173.8 (CONH), 172.5 (COO), 161.1 (AMC COO), 158.4 (NHCONH), 153.9, 152.6, 141.7, 125.0, 115.9, 115.7, 113.0, and 107.3 (aromatics), 60.7 (OCH$_2$), 50.8 (Ala C^α), 35.9 (βAla C^α), 34.8 (βAla C^β), 18.5, and 18.3 (Ala C^β and CH$_3$), 14.1 (CH$_3$).

MeO-Ala-CO-Ala-AMMC (**20**)

White solid (yield 54%). R_f (CHCl$_3$/MeOH 95:5) = 0.3; m.p. 148–150 °C (MeOH). ^{1}H-NMR (DMSO-d_6): δ 10.43 (s, 1H, AMMC NH), 7.76 (s, 1H, ArH), 7.61 (d, 1H, J = 9.0 Hz, ArH), 7.42 (d, 1H, J = 9.0 Hz, ArH), 6.45 (d, 1H, J = 7.5 Hz, Ala NH), 6.37 (d, 1H, J = 7.5 Hz, Ala NH), 6.26 (s, 1H, C=CH), 4.62 (s, 2H, AMMC OCH$_2$), 4.26 (m, 1H, Ala α-CH), 4.10 (m, 1H, Ala α-CH), 3.57 (s, 3H, COOCH$_3$), 3.37 (s, 3H, AMMC OCH$_3$), 1.27 (d, 3H, J = 7.2 Hz, Ala CH$_3$), 1.22 (d, 3H, J = 7.2 Hz, Ala CH$_3$). ^{13}C-NMR (DMSO-d_6): δ 174.5 (CONH), 173.5 (COO), 161.0 (AMC COO), 157.2 (NHCONH), 152.7, 142.7, 126.6, 125.7, 115.7, 113.0, 110.4, and 106.2 (aromatics), 69.7 (AMMC OCH$_2$), 58.8 (AMMC OCH$_3$), 52.2 (OCH$_3$), 50.0 (Ala C^α), 48.5 (Ala C^α), 19.4, and 18.4 (Ala C^β).

5.2. Biological Methods

5.2.1. hCA Inhibition Assay

An Applied Photophysics stopped-flow instrument was used for measuring hCA-catalyzed CO$_2$ hydration activity [45]. Phenol red (at a concentration of 0.2 mM) was used as an indicator, the reactions were monitored at a wavelength of 557 nm, and 20 mM Hepes (pH 7.4) containing 20 mM Na$_2$SO$_4$ (for maintaining constant ionic strength) was used as a buffer. The initial rates of the CA-catalyzed CO$_2$ hydration reaction were measured for a period of 10–100 s. The CO$_2$ concentrations ranged from 1.7 to 17 mM for the determination of the kinetic parameters and inhibition constants. The non-catalyzed CO$_2$ hydration was not subtracted from these curves and accounted for the remaining observed activity, which, even at a high concentration of inhibitors, was in the range of 16–25%. However, the background activity from the uncatalyzed reaction was always subtracted when IC$_{50}$ values were obtained by using the data analysis software for the stopped-flow instrument. Enzyme concentrations ranged between 5 nM and 12 nM. For each inhibitor, at least six graphs of the initial 5–10% of the reaction were used to determine the initial velocity. The uncatalyzed rates were measured in the same manner and were subtracted from the total observed rates. Stock solutions of the inhibitor (0.1 mM) were prepared in distilled-deionized water, and dilutions up to 0.01 nM were performed thereafter with the assay buffer. Inhibitor and enzyme solutions were preincubated together for 15 min at room temperature prior to the assay, to allow for the formation of the E–I complex. The inhibition constants (K_i) were obtained by the nonlinear least-squares methods using PRISM 3 and the Cheng-Prusoff equation as reported earlier and are presented as the mean from at least three different determinations. All hCA isoforms were recombinant proteins obtained in-house, as reported earlier [46].

5.2.2. hMAO Inhibition Studies

Activity measurements (IC_{50}) for hMAO-A and hMAO-B were carried out as reported in the literature [47,48]. Recombinant human MAO-A and MAO-B were obtained commercially (Sigma-Aldrich, Cape Town, South Africa) and were used as enzyme sources. Kynuramine is a non-specific substrate and serves as a substrate for both hMAO isoforms. The hMAOs metabolize kynuramine to produce 4-hydroxyquinoline, which was measured at the endpoint of the enzyme reactions by fluorescence spectrophotometry.

5.3. Computational Studies

5.3.1. Ligand Preparation

All molecular modeling experiments were performed on Schrödinger Life-Sciences Suite 2021-4 [49]. Ligand structures were built in Maestro using the 2D sketcher. For the hCA docking studies, the hydrolyzed forms of both in *E* and *Z* configurations were also produced. The ligand 3D geometry was obtained using LigPrep to find all possible tautomers and protonation states at pH 7.0 ± 0.4. The obtained structures were energy-minimized with MacroModel, using the OPLS4 force field, and applying 5000 steps of PRCG algorithm with a convergence criterion of 0.001 KJ/molÅ.

5.3.2. hCA Structure Preparation and Docking

The 3D structures of the studied hCAs were retrieved from the Protein Data Bank; protein structures with PDB ID 6F3B for hCA I, 5BNL for hCA II, 6G9U for hCA IX and 5LL5 for hCA XII (resolution 1.40, 2.00, 1.75, and 1.42, respectively) were selected for the structure-based studies. The proteins were prepared using the Protein Preparation routine in Maestro [50] which prepares the protein structure by adding hydrogen atoms, removing water molecules, adjusting the protonation states of ionizable groups, optimizing the H-bond network, and performing a constrained minimization of the final structure. All proteins were aligned to each other using the Protein Structure Alignment module in Maestro. A water molecule that coordinates with the zinc ion was copied from the 5BNL structure to the other hCAs as the fourth zinc ligand to complete its coordination sphere.

Docking calculations were carried out using Glide [51,52]. The Glide Grid suitable for the SP-peptide docking protocol was generated and the center of the grid was set on the X-ray ligand of 5BNL [(2*E*)-3-(2-hydroxy-phenyl)acrylic acid] for all receptors. The grid box dimension of up to 25 Å was set for three ligands. The Glide SP-peptide docking calculation was carried out saving 100 poses for each ligand. Following a previously applied procedure, ligand poses were clustered, and the highest-scored binding geometry of the most populated cluster was further analyzed for each ligand [29,30]. The Multiple Sequence Alignment tool was exploited to measure the sequence identity and similarity among studied hCAs.

5.3.3. Molecular Dynamics of the CA XII:Ligand **19** Complex

The docked complex of compound **19** in the hCA XII protein was submitted to Molecular Dynamics simulation using Desmond [53]. The complex was embedded in an orthorombic box of TIP4P water molecules. The system was neutralized by adding 8 Na^+ ions.

The solvated complex was submitted to six relaxation steps of 20 ns that preceded the production phase by default. The 100 ns simulation was then carried out recording frames every 100 ps using a normal pressure-temperature (NPT) ensemble with a Nosé-Hoover thermostat at 300 K and Martyna-Tobias-Klein barostat at 1.01325 bar pressure. The Smooth Particle Mesh Ewald method was also applied to analyze the electrostatic interactions with a cut-off distance set to 9.0 Å. The trajectory was analyzed using the Simulation interaction diagram facility in Maestro.

5.3.4. hMAO-A and hMAO-B Protein Structure Preparation and Docking

The X-ray structures of hMAO-A and hMAO-B with PDB ID 2Z5X and 2V5Z were retrieved from the Protein Data Bank (resolution 2.20 Å and 1.60 Å, respectively).

The crystal structures were corrected and minimized using the Protein Preparation wizard in Maestro as already described. Water molecules not directly linked to FAD were removed. Molecular docking analyses were performed using Glide [46]. The Glide grid box was generated by using the center of mass of crystallographic ligands. The following rotatable OH and SH bonds were set: Cys323, Tyr407, Tyr444 for hMAO-A, and Cys172, Tyr398, Tyr435, for MAO-B. The SP docking protocol was applied with the OPLS4 force field. The reliability of the docking protocol was assessed by docking the crystallographic ligands. The Root Mean Square Deviation (RMSD), based on the maximum common structure, of the best-docked poses from the position of the crystallographic ligands were 0.1363 Å, and 0.2279 Å for hMAO-A (2Z5X) and hMAO-B (2V5Z), respectively. SiteMap calculations [54,55] were carried out on the hMAO-A and hMAO-B binding sites to analyze the binding site, and to calculate a fine grid.

Supplementary Materials: The following supporting information can be downloaded at: https://www.mdpi.com/article/10.3390/molecules27227884/s1, Figure S1: Alignment of 3F8E and 5BNL CA II X-ray complexes, and docked posed of compound **19** in CA XII and compound **6** in CA IX; Figure S2: Ligand interaction diagrams; Figure S3: Ligand RMSF; Figure S4: Protein RMSF; Figure S5: Timeline representation of ligand-protein contacts; Figure S6: Depiction of frequency and type of ligand-protein interaction along with the MD simulation; Figure S7: Alignment of CA XII:**19** representative binding geometries obtained from clustering the MD frames; Figure S8: Docked poses of ligands **6** and **16** in MAO-B binding site; Figure S9: SiteMap hydrophobic sites in MAO-A and MAO-B binding site; Table S1: Ligand efficiency values calculated from the inhibition data of studied coumarin derivatives against CAs and MAOs; Table S2: Physico-chemical and pharmacokinetic properties of studied ligands calculated by QuikProp.

Author Contributions: Conceptualization, G.L., C.T.S. and S.C.; syntheses, G.L. and S.C.; software, M.A. and M.F.; formal analysis, A.A., A.P. and J.P.P.; resources, G.L. and S.C.; writing—original draft preparation, G.L. and M.A.; writing—review and editing, J.P.P. and C.T.S.; supervision, C.T.S. All authors have read and agreed to the published version of the manuscript.

Funding: This work was supported by research funds from the "G. d'Annunzio" University of Chieti-Pescara (MIUR, FAR 2020 grants to S.C. and G.L.).

Institutional Review Board Statement: Not applicable.

Informed Consent Statement: Not applicable.

Data Availability Statement: Data are contained within the article.

Conflicts of Interest: The authors declare that they have no conflict of interest.

Sample Availability: Samples of all compounds are available from the authors.

References

1. Matos, M.J.; Santana, L.; Uriarte, E.; Abreu, O.A.; Molina, E.; Yordi, E.G. Coumarins—An Important Class of Phytochemicals. In *Phytochemicals—Isolation, Characterisation and Role in Human Health*; Rao, V., Rao, L., Eds.; InTech: Rijeka, Croatia, 2015; Chapter 5, pp. 113–140.
2. Hoult, J.R.S.; Payá, M. Pharmacological and biochemical actions of simple coumarins: Natural products with therapeutic potential. *Gen. Pharmacol.* **1996**, *27*, 713–722. [CrossRef]
3. Sadeghpour, M.; Olyaei, A.; Adl, A. 4-Aminocoumarin derivatives: Synthesis and applications. *New J. Chem.* **2021**, *45*, 5744–5763. [CrossRef]
4. Emami, S.; Dadashpour, S. Current developments of coumarin-based anti-cancer agents in medicinal chemistry. *Eur. J. Med. Chem.* **2015**, *102*, 611–630. [CrossRef] [PubMed]
5. Carneiro, A.; Matos, M.J.; Uriarte, E.; Santana, L. Trending Topics on Coumarin and Its Derivatives in 2020. *Molecules* **2021**, *26*, 501. [PubMed]

6. Chimenti, F.; Secci, D.; Bolasco, A.; Chimenti, P.; Bizzarri, B.; Granese, A.; Carradori, S.; Yáñez, M.; Orallo, F.; Ortuso, F.; et al. Synthesis, molecular modeling, and selective inhibitory activity against human monoamine oxidases of 3-carboxamido-7-substituted coumarins. *J. Med. Chem.* **2009**, *52*, 1935–1942. [CrossRef] [PubMed]
7. Secci, D.; Carradori, S.; Bolasco, A.; Chimenti, P.; Yáñez, M.; Ortuso, F.; Alcaro, S. Synthesis and selective human monoamine oxidase inhibition of 3-carbonyl, 3-acyl, and 3-carboxyhydrazido coumarin derivatives. *Eur. J. Med. Chem.* **2011**, *46*, 4846–4852.
8. Carotti, A.; Altomare, C.; Catto, M.; Gnerre, C.; Summo, L.; De Marco, A.; Rose, S.; Jenner, P.; Testa, B. Lipophilicity plays a major role in modulating the inhibition of monoamine oxidase B by 7-substituted coumarins. *Chem. Biodivers.* **2006**, *3*, 134–149. [CrossRef]
9. De Luca, L.; Mancuso, F.; Ferro, S.; Buemi, M.R.; Angeli, A.; Del Prete, S.; Capasso, C.; Supuran, C.T.; Gitto, R. Inhibitory effects and structural insights for a novel series of coumarin-based compounds that selectively target human CA IX and CA XII carbonic anhydrases. *Eur. J. Med. Chem.* **2018**, *143*, 276–282. [CrossRef]
10. McDonald, P.C.; Chafe, S.C.; Supuran, C.T.; Dedhar, S. Cancer Therapeutic Targeting of Hypoxia Induced Carbonic Anhydrase IX: From Bench to Bedside. *Cancers* **2022**, *14*, 3297. [CrossRef]
11. Supuran, C.T. Carbonic anhydrase inhibitors: An update on experimental agents for the treatment and imaging of hypoxic tumors. *Expert Opin. Investig. Drugs* **2021**, *30*, 1197–1208. [CrossRef]
12. Marconi, G.D.; Gallorini, M.; Carradori, S.; Guglielmi, P.; Cataldi, A.; Zara, S. The Up-Regulation of Oxidative Stress as a Potential Mechanism of Novel MAO-B Inhibitors for Glioblastoma Treatment. *Molecules* **2019**, *24*, 2005. [CrossRef] [PubMed]
13. Shui, X.; Ren, X.; Xu, R.; Xie, Q.; Hu, Y.; Qin, J.; Meng, H.; Zhang, C.; Zhao, J.; Shi, C. Monoamine oxidase A drives neuroendocrine differentiation in prostate cancer. *Biochem. Biophys. Res. Commun.* **2022**, *606*, 135–141. [PubMed]
14. Wu, J.B.; Shao, C.; Li, X.; Li, Q.; Hu, P.; Shi, C.; Li, Y.; Chen, Y.T.; Yin, F.; Liao, C.P.; et al. Monoamine oxidase A mediates prostate tumorigenesis and cancer metastasis. *J. Clin. Investig.* **2014**, *124*, 2891–2908. [CrossRef] [PubMed]
15. Bardaweel, S.; Aljanabi, R.; Sabbah, D.; Sweidan, K. Design, Synthesis, and Biological Evaluation of Novel MAO-A Inhibitors Targeting Lung Cancer. *Molecules* **2022**, *27*, 2887.
16. Küçükbay, F.Z.; Küçükbay, H.; Tanc, M.; Supuran, C.T. Synthesis and carbonic anhydrase inhibitory properties of amino acid—Coumarin/quinolinone conjugates incorporating glycine, alanine and phenylalanine moieties. *J. Enzym. Inhib. Med. Chem.* **2016**, *31*, 1198–1202. [CrossRef]
17. Spatola, A.F. *Chemistry and Biochemistry of Amino Acids, Peptides and Proteins*; Weinstein, B., Ed.; Marcel Dekker, Inc.: New York, NY, USA, 1983; Volume 7, pp. 267–357.
18. Hruby, V.J. Conformational and topographical considerations in the design of biologically active peptides. *Biopolymers* **1993**, *33*, 1073–1082. [CrossRef]
19. Marraud, M.; Aubry, A. Crystal structures of peptides and modified peptides. *Biopolymers* **1996**, *40*, 45–83. [CrossRef]
20. Calcagni, A.; Rossi, D.; Paglialunga Paradisi, M.; Lucente, G.; Luisi, G.; Gavuzzo, E.; Mazza, F.; Pochetti, G.; Paci, M. Peptides containing the sulfonamide junction: Synthesis, structure, and conformation of Z-Tau-Pro-Phe-NHiPr. *Biopolymers* **1997**, *41*, 555–567. [CrossRef]
21. Luisi, G.; Mollica, A.; Carradori, S.; Lenoci, A.; De Luca, A.; Caccuri, A.M. Nitrobenzoxadiazole-based GSTP1-1 inhibitors containing the full peptidyl moiety of (pseudo)glutathione. *J. Enzym. Inhib. Med. Chem.* **2016**, *31*, 924–930.
22. Calcagni, A.; Duprè, S.; Lucente, G.; Luisi, G.; Pinnen, F.; Rossi, D. Synthesis and activity of the glutathione analogue-(L-azaglutamyl)-L-cisteinyl-glycine. *Int. J. Peptide Prot. Res.* **1995**, *46*, 434–439.
23. Semetey, V.; Hemmerlin, C.; Didierjean, C.; Schaffner, A.P.; Giner, A.G.; Aubry, A.; Briand, J.P.; Marraud, M.; Guichard, G. Unexpected stability of the urea cis-trans isomer in urea-containing model pseudopeptides. *Org. Lett.* **2001**, *3*, 3843–3846. [CrossRef] [PubMed]
24. Myers, A.C.; Kowalski, J.A.; Lipton, M.A. Facile incorporation of urea pseudopeptides into protease substrate analogue inhibitors. *Bioorg. Med. Chem. Lett.* **2004**, *14*, 5219–5222. [CrossRef] [PubMed]
25. Fayad, A.A.; Pubill-Ulldemolins, C.; Sharma, S.V.; Day, D.; Goss, R.J.M. A One-Pot Synthesis of Symmetrical and Unsymmetrical Dipeptide Ureas. *Eur. J. Org. Chem.* **2015**, *2015*, 5603–5609. [CrossRef]
26. Kumar, A.; Siwach, K.; Supuran, C.T.; Sharma, P.K. A decade of tail-approach based design of selective as well as potent tumor associated carbonic anhydrase inhibitors. *Bioorg. Chem.* **2022**, *126*, 105920. [CrossRef] [PubMed]
27. Calcagni, A.; Duprè, S.; Lucente, G.; Luisi, G.; Pinnen, F.; Rossi, D.; Spirito, A. Synthesis and activity of the glutathione analogue gamma-(L-gamma-oxaglutamyl)-L-cisteinyl-glycine. *Arch. Pharm. Pharm. Med. Chem.* **1996**, *329*, 498–502. [CrossRef] [PubMed]
28. Supuran, C.T. Carbonic anhydrases: Novel therapeutic applications for inhibitors and activators. *Nat. Rev. Drug Discov.* **2008**, *7*, 168–181. [CrossRef]
29. Maresca, A.; Temperini, C.; Vu, H.; Pham, N.B.; Poulsen, S.-A.; Scozzafava, A.; Quinn, R.J.; Supuran, C.T. Non-zinc mediated inhibition of carbonic anhydrases: Coumarins are a new class of suicide inhibitors. *J. Am. Chem. Soc.* **2009**, *131*, 3057–3062. [CrossRef]
30. Maresca, A.; Temperini, C.; Pochet, L.; Masereel, B.; Scozzafava, A.; Supuran, C.T. Deciphering the mechanism of carbonic anhydrase inhibition with coumarins and thiocoumarins. *J. Med. Chem.* **2010**, *53*, 335–344. [CrossRef]
31. Tubert-Brohman, I.; Sherman, W.; Repasky, M.; Beuming, T. Improved docking of polypeptides with Glide. *J. Chem. Inf. Model.* **2013**, *53*, 1689–1699. [CrossRef]

32. Scala, M.C.; Agamennone, M.; Pietrantoni, A.; Di Sarno, V.; Bertamino, A.; Superti, F.; Campiglia, P.; Sala, M. Discovery of a Novel Tetrapeptide Against Influenza A Virus: Rational Design, Synthesis, Bioactivity Evaluation and Computational Studies. *Pharmaceuticals* **2021**, *14*, 959.
33. Agamennone, M.; Superti, F. Broad-Spectrum Activity of Small Molecules Acting against Influenza A Virus: Biological and Computational Studies. *Pharmaceuticals* **2022**, *15*, 301. [CrossRef] [PubMed]
34. Carta, F.; Maresca, A.; Scozzafava, A.; Supuran, C.T. Novel coumarins and 2-thioxo-coumarins as inhibitors of the tumor-associated carbonic anhydrases IX and XII. *Bioorg. Med. Chem.* **2012**, *20*, 2266–2273. [PubMed]
35. Krishnamurthy, V.M.; Kaufman, G.K.; Urbach, A.R.; Gitlin, I.; Gudiksen, K.L.; Weibel, D.B.; Whitesides, G.M. Carbonic Anhydrase as a Model for Biophysical and Physical-Organic Studies of Proteins and Protein-Ligand Binding. *Chem. Rev.* **2008**, *108*, 946–1051. [PubMed]
36. Snyder, P.W.; Mecinovic, J.; Moustakas, D.T.; Thomas, S.W., 3rd; Harder, M.; Mack, E.T.; Lockett, M.R.; Héroux, A.; Sherman, W.; Whitesides, G.M. Mechanism of the hydrophobic effect in the biomolecular recognition of arylsulfonamides by carbonic anhydrase. *Proc. Natl. Acad. Sci. USA* **2011**, *108*, 17889–17894. [CrossRef]
37. Alterio, V.; Hilvo, M.; Di Fiore, A.; Supuran, C.T.; Pan, P.; Parkkila, S.; Scaloni, A.; Pastorek, J.; Pastorekova, S.; Pedone, C.; et al. Crystal structure of the catalytic domain of the tumor-associated human carbonic anhydrase IX. *Proc. Natl. Acad. Sci. USA* **2009**, *106*, 16233–16238. [CrossRef]
38. Thacker, P.S.; Mohammed, A.; Supuran, C.T.; Tiwari, P.L.; Goud, N.S.; Srikanth, D.; Angeli, A. Synthesis and biological evaluation of coumarin carboxamides as selective and potent inhibitors of carbonic anhydrases IX and XII. *Anticancer Agents Med. Chem.* **2022**, *22*, 2647–2654. [CrossRef]
39. Guglielmi, P.; Mathew, B.; Secci, D.; Carradori, S. Chalcones: Unearthing their therapeutic possibility as monoamine oxidase B inhibitors. *Eur. J. Med. Chem.* **2020**, *205*, 112650. [CrossRef]
40. Mathew, B.; Carradori, S.; Guglielmi, P.; Uddin, M.S.; Kim, H. New aspects of monoamine oxidase B inhibitors: The key role of halogens to open the golden door. *Curr. Med. Chem.* **2021**, *28*, 266–283.
41. Bester, E.; Petzer, A.; Petzer, J.P. Coumarin derivatives as inhibitors of d-amino acid oxidase and monoamine oxidase. *Bioorg. Chem.* **2022**, *123*, 105791. [CrossRef]
42. Koyiparambath, V.P.; Prayaga Rajappan, K.; Rangarajan, T.M.; Al-Sehemi, A.G.; Pannipara, M.; Bhaskar, V.; Nair, A.S.; Sudevan, S.T.; Kumar, S.; Mathew, B. Deciphering the detailed structure-activity relationship of coumarins as Monoamine oxidase enzyme inhibitors—An updated review. *Chem. Biol. Drug. Des.* **2021**, *98*, 655–673.
43. Pardridge, W.M. The blood-brain barrier: Bottleneck in brain drug development. *NeuroRx* **2005**, *2*, 3–14. [CrossRef] [PubMed]
44. Provensi, G.; Costa, A.; Rani, B.; Becagli, M.V.; Vaiano, F.; Passani, M.B.; Tanini, D.; Capperucci, A.; Carradori, S.; Petzer, J.P.; et al. New β-arylchalcogeno amines with procognitive properties targeting Carbonic Anhydrases and Monoamine Oxidases. *Eur. J. Med. Chem.* **2022**, *244*, 114828. [CrossRef] [PubMed]
45. Khalifah, R.G. The carbon dioxide hydration activity of carbonic anhydrase. *J. Biol. Chem.* **1971**, *246*, 2561–2573. [PubMed]
46. D'Ascenzio, M.; Secci, D.; Carradori, S.; Zara, S.; Guglielmi, P.; Cirilli, R.; Pierini, M.; Poli, G.; Tuccinardi, T.; Angeli, A.; et al. 1,3-Dipolar Cycloaddition, HPLC Enantioseparation, and Docking Studies of Saccharin/Isoxazole and Saccharin/Isoxazoline Derivatives as Selective Carbonic Anhydrase IX and XII Inhibitors. *J. Med. Chem.* **2020**, *63*, 2470–2488.
47. Weissbach, H.; Smith, T.E.; Daly, J.W.; Witkop, B.; Udenfriend, S. A rapid spectrophotometric assay of mono-amine oxidase based on the rate of disappearance of kynuramine. *J. Biol. Chem.* **1960**, *235*, 1160–1163. [CrossRef]
48. Mostert, S.; Petzer, A.; Petzer, J.P. Indanones as high-potency reversible inhibitors of monoamine oxidase. *ChemMedChem* **2015**, *10*, 862–873. [CrossRef]
49. Schrödinger. *Schrödinger Release 2021-4: Maestro, Glide, Prime, Desmond, Protein Preparation Wizard, Epik; SiteMap* Schrödinger, LLC: New York, NY, USA, 2021.
50. Sastry, G.M.; Adzhigirey, M.; Day, T.; Annabhimoju, R.; Sherman, W. Protein and ligand preparation: Parameters, protocols, and influence on virtual screening enrichments. *J. Comput. Aided Mol. Des.* **2013**, *27*, 221–234. [CrossRef]
51. Halgren, T.A.; Murphy, R.B.; Friesner, R.A.; Beard, H.S.; Frye, L.L.; Pollard, W.T.; Banks, J.L. Glide: A New Approach for Rapid, Accurate Docking and Scoring. 2. Enrichment Factors in Database Screening. *J. Med. Chem.* **2004**, *47*, 1750–1759. [CrossRef]
52. Friesner, R.A.; Banks, J.L.; Murphy, R.B.; Halgren, T.A.; Klicic, J.J.; Mainz, D.T.; Repasky, M.P.; Knoll, E.H.; Shaw, D.E.; Shelley, M.; et al. Glide: A new approach for rapid, accurate docking and scoring. 1. Method and assessment of docking accuracy. *J. Med. Chem.* **2004**, *47*, 1739–1749. [CrossRef]
53. Bowers, K.J.; Chow, E.; Xu, H.; Dror, R.O.; Eastwood, M.P.; Gregersen, B.A.; Klepeis, J.L.; Kolossvary, I.; Moraes, M.A.; Sacerdoti, F.D.; et al. Scalable Algorithms for Molecular Dynamics Simulations on Commodity Clusters. In Proceedings of the ACM/IEEE Conference on Supercomputing (SC06), Tampa, FL, USA, 11–17 November 2006; p. 43.
54. Halgren, T. Identifying and characterizing binding sites and assessing druggability. *J. Chem. Inf. Model.* **2009**, *49*, 377–389.
55. Halgren, T. New method for fast and accurate binding-site identification and analysis. *Chem. Biol. Drug Des.* **2007**, *69*, 146–148. [CrossRef] [PubMed]

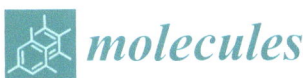

Article

Design, Synthesis, In Silico and In Vitro Studies of New Immunomodulatory Anticancer Nicotinamide Derivatives Targeting VEGFR-2

Reda G. Yousef [1], Wagdy M. Eldehna [2], Alaa Elwan [1], Abdelaziz S. Abdelaziz [1], Ahmed B. M. Mehany [3], Ibraheem M. M. Gobaara [3], Bshra A. Alsfouk [4], Eslam B. Elkaeed [5], Ahmed M. Metwaly [6,7,*] and Ibrahim H. Eissa [1,*]

[1] Pharmaceutical Medicinal Chemistry and Drug Design Department, Faculty of Pharmacy (Boys), Al-Azhar University, Cairo 11884, Egypt; redayousof@azhar.edu.eg (R.G.Y.); alaaelwan34@azhar.edu.eg (A.E.); zi.17.sh@gmail.com (A.S.A.)
[2] Department of Pharmaceutical Chemistry, Faculty of Pharmacy, Kafrelsheikh University, Kafrelsheikh 33516, Egypt; wagdy2000@gmail.com
[3] Zoology Department, Faculty of Science (Boys), Al-Azhar University, Cairo 11884, Egypt; abelal_81@azhar.edu.eg (A.B.M.M.); ibraheemgobaara@azhar.edu.eg (I.M.M.G.)
[4] Department of Pharmaceutical Sciences, College of Pharmacy, Princess Nourah bint Abdulrahman University, P.O. Box 84428, Riyadh 11671, Saudi Arabia; baalsfouk@pnu.edu.sa
[5] Department of Pharmaceutical Organic Chemistry, Faculty of Pharmacy (Boys), Al-Azhar University, Cairo 11884, Egypt; eslamkaeed@azhar.edu.eg
[6] Pharmacognosy and Medicinal Plants Department, Faculty of Pharmacy (Boys), Al-Azhar University, Cairo 11884, Egypt
[7] Biopharmaceutical Products Research Department, Genetic Engineering and Biotechnology Research Institute, City of Scientific Research and Technological Applications (SRTA-City), Alexandria 21934, Egypt
* Correspondence: ametwaly@azhar.edu.eg (A.M.M.); ibrahimeissa@azhar.edu.eg (I.H.E.)

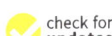

Citation: Yousef, R.G.; Eldehna, W.M.; Elwan, A.; Abdelaziz, A.S.; Mehany, A.B.M.; Gobaara, I.M.M.; Alsfouk, B.A.; Elkaeed, E.B.; Metwaly, A.M.; Eissa, I.H. Design, Synthesis, In Silico and In Vitro Studies of New Immunomodulatory Anticancer Nicotinamide Derivatives Targeting VEGFR-2. *Molecules* 2022, 27, 4079. https://doi.org/10.3390/molecules27134079

Academic Editors: Imtiaz Khan and Sumera Zaib

Received: 4 May 2022
Accepted: 20 June 2022
Published: 24 June 2022

Publisher's Note: MDPI stays neutral with regard to jurisdictional claims in published maps and institutional affiliations.

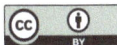

Copyright: © 2022 by the authors. Licensee MDPI, Basel, Switzerland. This article is an open access article distributed under the terms and conditions of the Creative Commons Attribution (CC BY) license (https://creativecommons.org/licenses/by/4.0/).

Abstract: VEGFR-2, the subtype receptor tyrosine kinase (RTK) responsible for angiogenesis, is expressed in various cancer cells. Thus, VEGFER-2 inhibition is an efficient approach for the discovery of new anticancer agents. Accordingly, a new set of nicotinamide derivatives were designed and synthesized to be VEGFR-2 inhibitors. The chemical structures were confirmed using IR, ^{1}H-NMR, and ^{13}C-NMR spectroscopy. The obtained compounds were examined for their anti-proliferative activities against the human cancer cell lines (HCT-116 and HepG2). VEGFR-2 inhibitory activities were determined for the titled compounds. Compound **8** exhibited the strongest anti-proliferative activities with IC$_{50}$ values of 5.4 and 7.1 µM against HCT-116 and HepG2, respectively. Interestingly, compound **8** was the most potent VEGFR-2 inhibitor with an IC$_{50}$ value of 77.02 nM (compare to sorafenib: IC$_{50}$ = 53.65 nM). Treatment of HCT-116 cells with compound **8** produced arrest of the cell cycle at the G0–G1 phase and a total apoptosis increase from 3.05 to 19.82%—6.5-fold in comparison to the negative control. In addition, compound **8** caused significant increases in the expression levels of caspase-8 (9.4-fold) and Bax (9.2-fold), and a significant decrease in the Bcl-2 expression level (3-fold). The effects of compound **8** on the levels of the immunomodulatory proteins (TNF-α and IL-6) were examined. There was a marked decrease in the level of TNF-α (92.37%) compared to the control (82.47%) and a non-significant reduction in the level of IL-6. In silico docking, molecular dynamics simulations, and MM-PBSA studies revealed the high affinity, the correct binding, and the optimum dynamics of compound 8 inside the active site of VEGFR-2. Finally, in silico ADMET and toxicity studies indicated acceptable values of drug-likeness. In conclusion, compound **8** has emerged as a promising anti-proliferative agent targeting VEGFR-2 with significant apoptotic and immunomodulatory effects.

Keywords: anticancer; immunomodulatory; apoptosis; in silico studies; nicotinamide; VEGFR-2

1. Introduction

Cancer is a pernicious disease characterized by uncontrolled and overexcited cell differentiation and division, along with the possibility of such cells invading other parts of the body, leading to death [1]. While progress has been made in treatment and prevention, the global burden of cancer mortality is increasing tremendously. Epidemiological studies revealed the responsibility of cancer for one-fifth of all deaths [1]. In 2020, more than 19 million new cancer cases were estimated, and almost 10.0 million deaths because of cancer occurred. The most diagnosed cancer was female breast cancer with an yearly estimated incidence of 2.3 million. Additionally, the incidences of lung, colorectal, prostate, and stomach cancers were 11.4%, 10.0%, 7.3%, and 5.6%, respectively [2]. In response, research contentious work to discover new anticancer agents that have maximum effectiveness and minimal toxicity is still a vitaltrend in anticancer drug development and research [3].

Cancer cells are characterized by biochemical abnormalities [4]. Oxygen and nutrients are fundamental to cancer cells' survival and proliferation; hence, cancer cells have to be located be near to blood vessels to have a high accessibility to the blood circulation [5]. Angiogenesis, the sprouting of new blood vessels from pre-existing vasculatures, is an essential factor in the process of cancer development and growth [6]. Current evidence confirmed that the primary tumor and the resulted metastasis depend on angiogenesis [7,8]. The angiogenesis process is under the control of various protein kinases, including the growth factors [7]. Amidst that growth factors, the vascular endothelial growth factor (VEGF) is of the most effective angiogenic determinants that can regulate angiogenesis and be engaged in the progression of a tumor [9,10].

VEGFs exert their angiogenic effects via binding with the different types of kinase domains of vascular endothelial growth factor receptors (VEGFRs 1, 2, and 3) [11]. VEGFR-2, the subtype receptor tyrosine kinase (RTK) responsible for angiogenesis [7], is expressed in various cancer cells and is responsible for the mediation of almost all the cellular responses to VEGF [12]. Thus, the VEGF/VEGFER-2 pathway is an competent target having vital selectivity for cancer cells [13]. The inhibition of the VEGFR-2/VEGF signaling pathway or the down-regulation of its response is a practical method for the discovery of new drugs for the treatment of several cancer types [12,14].

One of the hallmarks of cancer cells is their ability to avoid apoptosis, permitting unchecked and uncontrolled proliferation. Accordingly, the activation of apoptosis in cancer cells is a favorable strategy with which to defeat cancer [15]. The Bcl-2 family comprises members that are pro-apoptotic, such as Bax protein, which promotes cell apoptosis; and other members are antiapoptotic, such as Bcl-2 protein, which inhibits cell apoptosis [16]. The regulation of anti-apoptotic and pro-apoptotic proteins (Bax/Bcl-2 ratio) determines cell fate [16,17].

Several reports have detailed various small-molecule inhibitors of VEGFR-2 that target the ATP binding sites of the RTKs, resulting in diminished VEGF signal transduction [18–24]. These VEGFR-2 inhibitors can be broadly categorized into three types according to their modes of binding to the ATP binding pocket [14,18]. Type I inhibitors bind competitively to the adenine binding region of the ATP binding site in the active conformation (DFG-in) [18,25]. Type II inhibitors act on the ATP binding pocket and additionally function in the new allosteric hydrophobic pocket to stabilize the inactive conformation (DFG-out) [18]. Type II inhibitors provide better activity than type I by avoiding competitive inhibition [16]. Type III inhibitors adopt the inactive DFG-out conformation and bind covalently to the ATP binding site beyond the gatekeeper residue [25].

Over the last few years, a diverse range of VEGFR-2 inhibitors were designed, including sunitinib **I**, pazopanib **II**, sorafenib **III**, regorafenib **IV**, and trametinib **V** (Figure 1). However, drug resistance leads to decreased effectiveness and undesirable side effects. Therefore, it is essential to discover novel VEGFR-2 inhibitors for the treatment of cancer that have low toxicity and can overcome drug resistance [26].

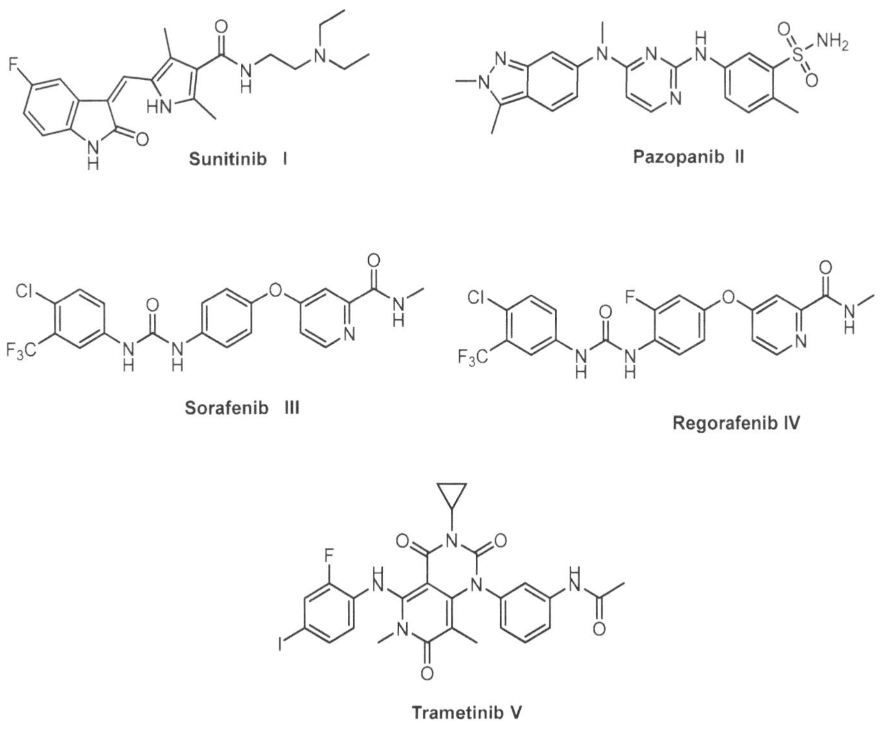

Figure 1. Some reported VEGFR inhibitors.

Rationale and Design

The study of the SAR of various VEGFR-2 inhibitors revealed that the core structures of most of them shared four fundamental features [16,26]: (i) A hetero aromatic ring (head) to occupy the catalytic ATP binding domain and participate in H-bonding interactions with the Cys919 amino acid residue the hinge region [18]. (ii) A "linker" segment occupying the gatekeeper residues that connects between the DFG domain and the ATP-binding domain. (iii) A hydrogen-bonding moiety (pharmacophore), such as urea or amide, interacts with the amino acids (Glu885 and Asp1046) via H-bonds in the DFG motif of the protein [4,15]. (iv) A terminal hydrophobic (tail) moiety directed toward the allosteric hydrophobic pocket, and binding with it through various hydrophobic interactions [15,16].

In continuation of our previous work on synthesizing new, potent, and safe anticancer agents [12,27–32], new nicotinamide derivatives were synthesized that keep the essential pharmacophoric features of VEGFR-2 inhibitors, aiming for the development of efficient anticancer agents that target VEGFR-2 inhuman cancer cell lines.

The designs of the new derivatives depend on the bioisosteric modifications at the four pharmacophoric features of the reported VEGFR-2 inhibitors. Firstly, it was reported that the nitrogen atom of the pyridine ring of sorafenib is a critical point for H-bonding interactions with Cys919 at the ATP binding domain. In addition, nicotinamidescaffold is required to occupy the hinge region (compound **VI**) [14]. Accordingly, nicotinamidemoiety was utilized as a head in the synthesized compounds to maintain the essential H-bonding interaction at the hinge region. In addition, it was reported that amide moiety may exert an anticancer effect [33]. With respect to the linker segment, it is usually 3–5 bond lengths [34]. The designed compounds involve a phenyl ring as a linker moiety to keep a tight fit in the gatekeeper area through hydrophobic interactions. Regarding the H-bonding pharmacophore moiety, we used a hydrazone moiety as an H-bonding center. This was based on the significant effect of the hydrazone moiety in the binding with VEGFR-2. Previously, our team developed compound **VII**, which has a promising VEGFR-2 inhibitory effect and comprises a hydrazone moiety as a pharmacophore group [35]. Finally, the terminal phenyl ring was kept to play its vital role and occupy the allosteric lipophilic pocket. The phenyl ring was substituted by diverse groups. Additionally, the hydrophobic moieties were modified to be amide moieties, in hopes of making extra binding interactions (Figure 2).

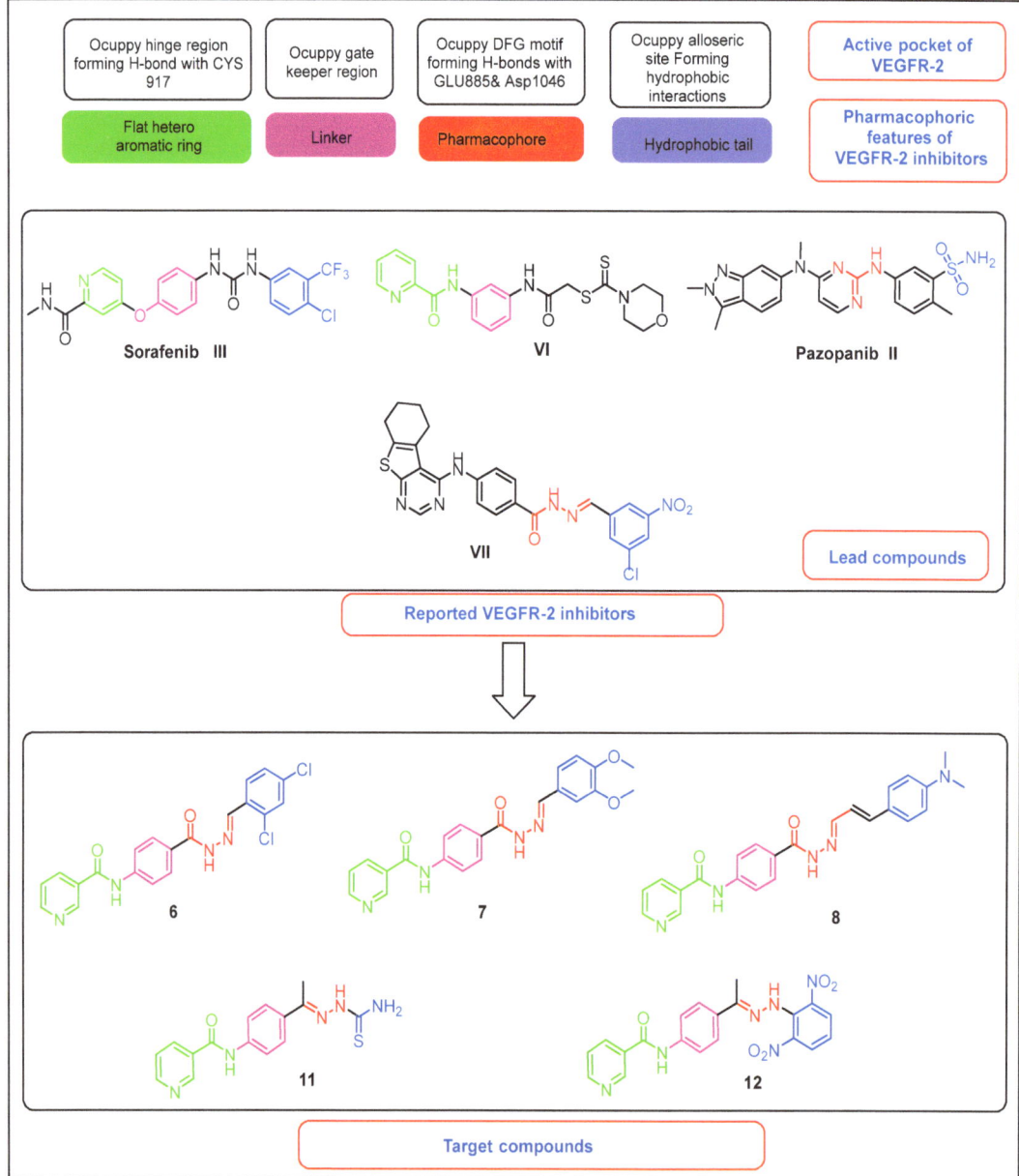

Figure 2. The design rationale of the targeted compounds.

2. Results and Discussion

2.1. Chemistry

Schemes 1 and 2 demonstrate the synthetic pathways of the target compounds. Firstly, heating of nicotinic acid **1** with a thionyl chloride in 1,2 dichloroethane and DMF (catalytic amount) furnished nicotinoyl chloride **2** [16,28]. Reflux of nicotinoyl chloride **2** with 4-aminomethylbenzoate **3** in the presence of triethylamine in acetonitrile afforded the corresponding methyl ester derivative N-(4-acetylphenyl)nicotinamide **4** [16], which was treated with hydrazine hydrate to produce N-(4-(hydrazinecarbonyl)-phenyl)nicotinamide **5** [28]. The produced hydrazide derivative **5** was then reacted with appropriate aldehydes, namely, 2,4-dichlorobenzaldehyde, 3,4-dimethoxybenzaldehyde, and 3-(4-(dimethylamino)-phenyl) acrylaldehyde to afford the target compounds **6–8**, respectively (Scheme 1).

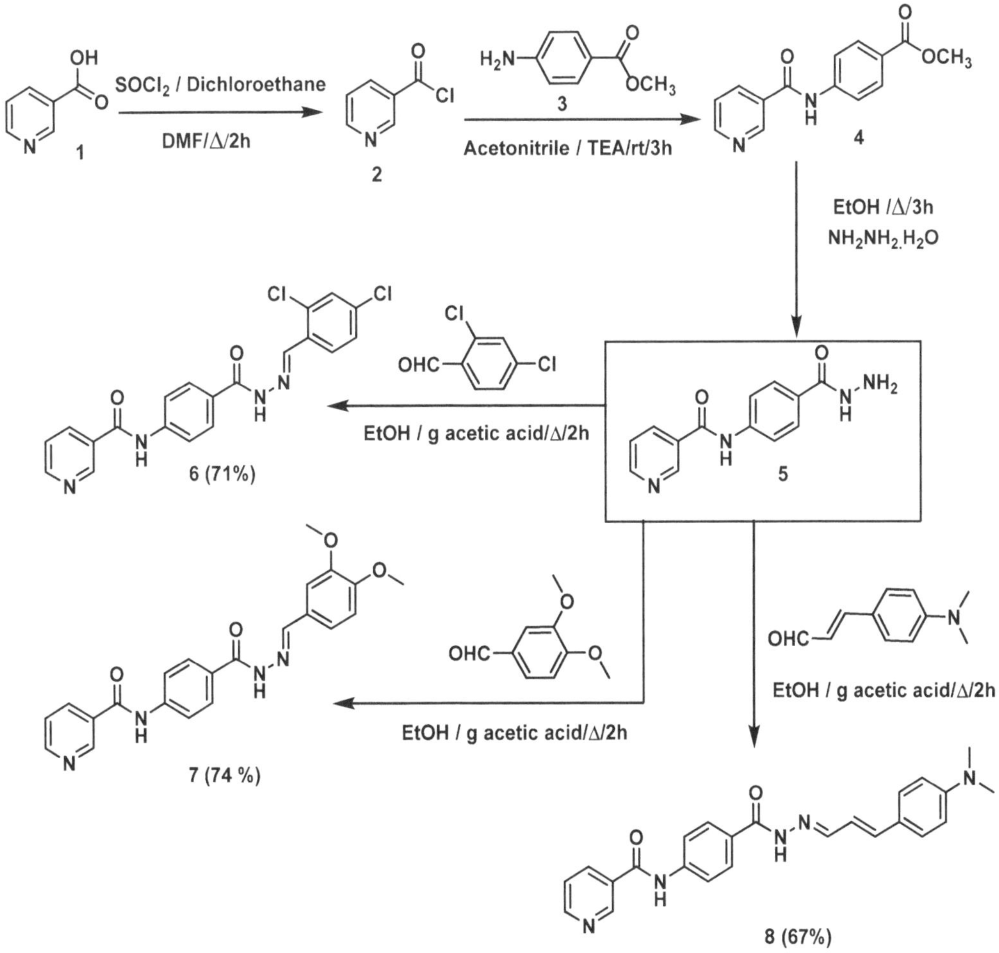

Scheme 1. Synthetic route of target compounds **6–8**.

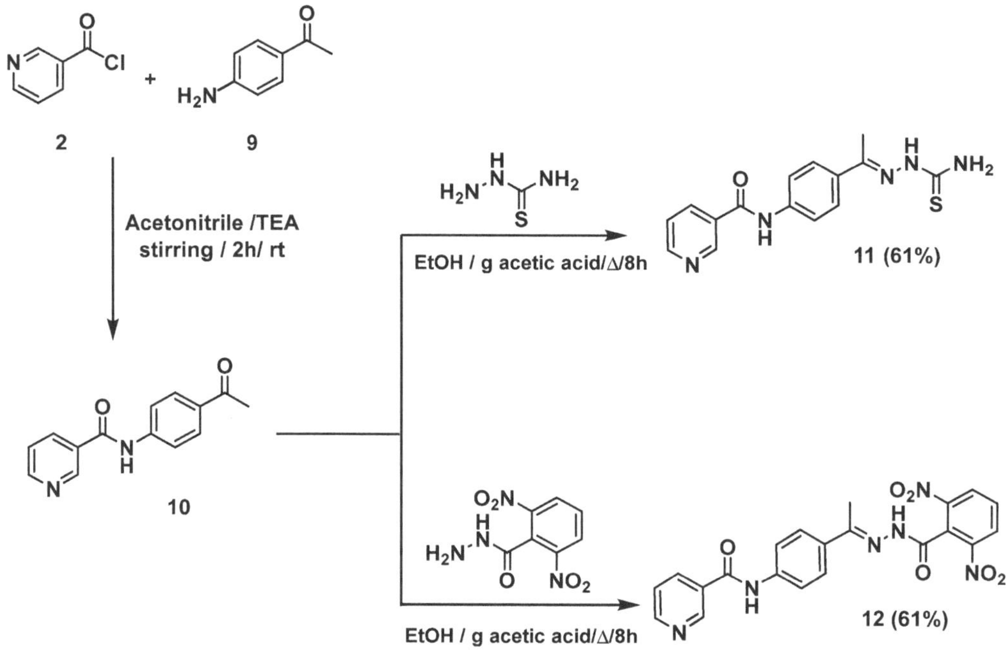

Scheme 2. Synthetic route of final target compounds, **11** and **12**.

Furthermore, nicotinoyl chloride **2** was further allowed to react with the commercially available *p*-aminoacetophenone **9** to yield the equivalent *N*-(4-acetylphenyl)nicotinamide **10** [27,28]. The latter was refluxed in ethanol and a catalytic amount of glacial acetic acid with appropriate amines, namely, thiosemicarbazide and 2,6-dinitrobenzohydrazide to give the target compounds **11** and **12**, respectively (Scheme 2).

The structures of the synthesized compounds **6**, **7**, **8**, **11**, and **12** were authenticated by ^{1}H-NMR, which showed the presence of two downfield singlet signals attributed to the NH protons. Taking compound **8** as a representative example, it showed two singlet signals at δ 11.57 and 10.71 ppm. The aromatic and olefinic protons appeared in the aromatic region from 9.14 to 6.73 ppm. The six protons of the two methyl groups appeared at the aliphatic area at 2.97 ppm as singlet signals.

2.2. Biological Testing

2.2.1. In Vitro Anti-Proliferative Activities

Two human cancer cell lines (HCT-116; colorectal rectal cancer, and HepG2; hepatocellular carcinoma) were utilized to examine the anti-proliferative effects of the synthesized compounds. The VEGFR-2 protein is usually overexpressed in the HCT-116 and HepG-2 cell lines [36,37]. Accordingly, these two types of cancer cell lines were utilized in the presented work. MTT assay was employed with sorafenib as a standard anti-proliferative drug [35]. The results of cytotoxic activities (Table 1) revealed that compound **8** is the most active member showing strong cytotoxicity against HCT-116 and HepG2 with IC_{50} values of 5.4 and 7.1 µM, respectively. These results are comparable to sorafenib's results (IC_{50} = 9.30 ± 0.201 and 7.40 ± 0.253 µM, respectively). Other members showed moderate activities with IC_{50} values ranging from 16.5 to 25.07 µM.

Table 1. In vitro cytotoxic of compounds **6, 7, 8, 11**, and **12** against HCT-116 and HepG2 cell lines and in vitro inhibitory activities against VEGFR-2.

Compounds	Cytotoxicity IC$_{50}$ (µM) [a]		VEGFR-2 IC$_{50}$ (nM) [a]
	HCT-116	HepG2	
6	17.8 ± 0.059	16.5 ± 0.057	172.3 ± 10.20
7	19.2 ± 0.062	18.8 ± 0.061	112.6 ± 7.23
8	5.4 ± 0.02	7.1 ± 0.03	77.02 ± 4.25
11	25.07 ± 0.07	20.3 ± 0.064	83.41 ± 5.53
12	18.2 ± 0.06	17.5 ± 0.058	115.2 ± 7.33
Sorafenib	9.30 ± 0.201	7.40 ± 0.235	53.65 ± 3.87

[a] IC$_{50}$ value is the mean ± S.D. (standard deviation) of three separate experiments.

2.2.2. In Vitro Vegfr-2 Enzyme Assay Inhibition

The obtained compounds were also investigated for their inhibitory potential against VEGFR-2 to examine the design and predict their inhibitory effect [16]. The VEGFR-2 inhibitory assay results (Table 1) indicated that compound **8** was the strongest inhibitor with an IC$_{50}$ value of 77.02 nM (compare to sorafenib: IC$_{50}$ = 53.65 nM). In addition, the other compounds showed moderate inhibitory effects with IC$_{50}$ values ranging from 83.41 to 172.3 nM.

Depending on the outputs of cytotoxicity and VEGFR-2 kinase inhibition, compound **8**, was selected for further biological investigations.

Safety Pattern of the Tested Compounds

An in-vitro viability test was used to investigate the safety patterns of the tested compounds at different concentrations. The Vero cell lines were used as a non-cancerous model to investigate the safety of the targeted compounds. The results of the MTT assays indicate that the tested compounds have IC$_{50}$ values ranging from 85.24 to 127.91 µM. Such values are very high in comparison to the corresponding values on the cancer cell lines, which reflect the high in vitro safety profiles of the tested members towards the examined non-cancerous cell lines (Table 2).

Table 2. In vitro anti-proliferative activities of compounds **6, 7, 8, 11**, and **12** against Vero cell lines.

Compounds	Cytotoxicity Against Vero Cell Lines (IC$_{50}$ µM)
6	84.72
7	127.91
8	85.24
11	105.28
12	95.37

Selectivity Index (SI)

The selectivity index (SI) of a particular compound is the ratio of its toxic and effective concentrations (SI = IC$_{50}$ against non-cancer cells/IC$_{50}$ against cancer cells) [38]. Relatively, low SI (<1) means that the tested compound is toxic and cannot be used as a safe drug [39]. All the tested hybrids showed decreased potency against Vero cell lines. This finding encouraged us to investigate the selectivity profiles of the synthetized compounds. The selectivity index values of the synthesized compounds against cancer cells are indicated in Table 3. In general, all compounds showed SI of more than 4.2, indicating high selectivity of the tested compounds against cancer cell lines.

Table 3. Selectivity indices (SI) of the synthesized compounds against different cancer cell lines.

Compounds	(HCT-116) [a]	(HepG2) [b]
6	4.76	5.13
7	6.66	6.80
8	15.79	12.01
11	4.20	5.19
12	5.24	5.45

[a] SI = Cytotoxicity against Vero cells/cytotoxicity against HCT-116 cell lines. [b] SI = cytotoxicity against Vero cells/cytotoxicity against HepG2 cell lines.

2.2.3. Cell Cycle Analysis

Anticancer compounds exert their cytotoxicity by aborting the cellular growth at certain points. These points, phases, are distinguishable in the cell cycle, whose suppression causes the cessation of cell proliferation [15]. The ability of a compound to arrest the cell cycle is directly linked to apoptosis induction [40].

Flow cytometry analysis was utilized to investigate the efficacy of compound **8** on the cell cycle progression and apoptosis induction in the HCT-116 colon cancer cell line [41]. In the test, the HCT-116 cells were treated with compound **8** at a concentration of 5.4 µM, then incubated for 24 h. The cell cycle distribution was analyzed to identify the definite phase at which compound **8** can arrest the cell cycle. The results showed that compound **8** significantly declined the cell populations at G2/M and Pre-G1 phases, which were 12.91% (2.11-fold) and 3.05% (6.49-fold), compared to 27.29 and 19.82% for the control, respectively. Moreover, marked augmentation was observed in G0–G1 phase (55.62%; 1.42-fold) compared to the control (38.96%). This finding suggests that **8** arrested the cell cycle proliferation of the HCT-116 cell line at the G0–G1 phase (Table 4 and Figure 3).

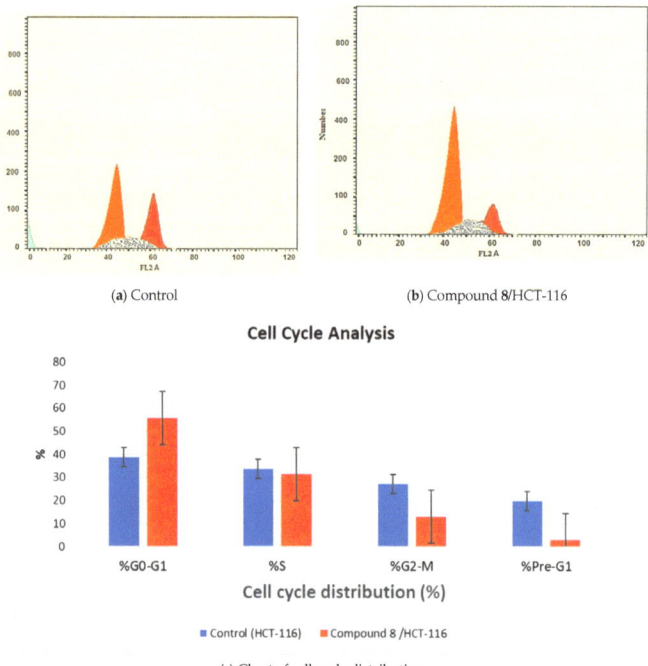

Figure 3. Flow cytometric analysis of cell cycle phases of HCT-116 cells after exposure to compound **8** (5.4 µM) after treatment for 24 h.

Table 4. Effects of compound **8** (5.4 µM) on cell cycle phases of HCT-116 cells after treatment for 24 h.

Sample	Cell Cycle Distribution (%)			
	%G0-G1	% S	%G2-M	%Pre-G1
Control (HCT-116)	38.96	33.75	27.29	19.82
Compound 8/HCT-116	55.62	31.47	12.91	3.05

2.2.4. Induction of Apoptosis

As compound **8** produced arrest of HCT-116 cells at the G0–G1 phase, it is highly important to investigate its ability to induce apoptosis in the experienced cells. Its apoptosis induction ability was estimated using the Annexin V and PI double staining assay [42]. The results revealed significant elevations in cell percentages in both early (from 0.7 to 3.74%) and late apoptosis (from 1.73 to 14.23%) phases. These results indicate an increase in the total apoptosis from 3.05 to 19.82%—6.5-fold in comparison to the control. These findings clearly confirm that the cell death was attributable to functional apoptosis (Table 5 and Figure 4).

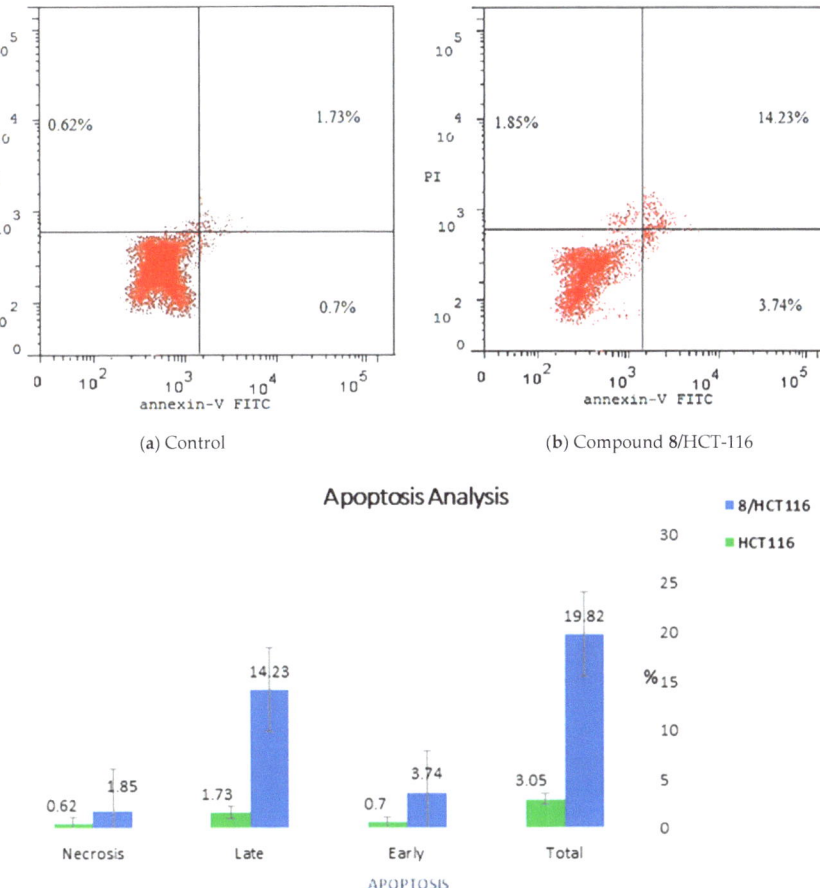

(a) Control

(b) Compound 8/HCT-116

(c) Chart of apoptosis distribution

Figure 4. Flow cytometric analysis of apoptosis in HCT-116 cells after exposure to compound **8** (5.4 µM) after treatment for 24 h.

Table 5. Stages of cell death in HCT-116 cells after exposure to compound 8 (5.4 µM) for 24 h.

Sample	Apoptosis			Necrosis
	Total	Early	Late	
Control (HCT-116)	3.05	0.7	1.73	0.62
Compound 8/HCT-116	19.82	3.74	14.23	1.85

2.2.5. Effects of Compound 8 on the Apoptotic Markers (Bax, Bcl-2, and caspase-8)

The effects of compound 8 on the levels of protein expression of the apoptotic markers (Bax, Bcl-2, and caspase-8) were estimated. HCT-116 cells were exposed to compound 8 at a concentration of 5.4 µM for 24 h; then the concentrations of the examined proteins were estimated using quantitative Real-Time Reverse-Transcriptase PCR (qRT-PCR). The results display high increases in caspase-8 levels (9.4-fold) and Bax (9.2-fold) compared to the control cells. Additionally, the Bcl-2 level was decreased by 3-fold comparing the control cells (Table 6). Such results indicate the significant apoptotic effect of the tested compound.

Table 6. Effects of compound 8 (5.4 µM) on the expression levels of caspase 8, Bax, and Bcl-2; and TNF-α and IL-6 inhibition in the treated HCT-116 cells for 24 h.

Sample	Caspase-8 (Pg/mL)	Bax (Pg/mL)	Bcl-2 (Pg/mL)	TNF-α (% Inhibition)	IL-6 (% Inhibition)
8	472.3	387.26	1.844	92.37	94.06
Control	50.317	42.19	5.603	82.47	93.15

2.2.6. Effects of Compound 8 on the Levels of the Immunomodulatory Proteins (TNF-α and IL-6)

Further investigations were conducted to assess the effects of compound 8 on the levels of immunomodulatory proteins (TNF-α and IL-6). HCT-116 cells were exposed to compound 8 at a concentration of 5.4 µM for 24 h, and then the concentrations of the examined proteins were determined using qRT-PCR. The results revealed a significant decrease in the level of TNF-α (92.37%) compared to the control (82.47%). On the other hand, compound 8 exerted a non-significant reduction in the level of IL-6. This suggests that compound 8 might induce apoptosis in HCT-116 cancer cells through immunomodulatory-dependent pathways (Table 4).

2.3. In Silico Studies

2.3.1. Molecular Docking

A molecular docking experiment gives deep insight into the binding affinity between a specific compound and the target receptor [43]. The biological efficacy of a compound is linked to its better binding energy value and the degree of similarity in the binding mode compared the reference ligand [43]. To investigate the binding hallmarks of the targeted compounds against VEGFR-2, molecular docking studies were fulfilled by MOE. 2019.01 (Montreal, QC, Canada). The X-ray structure of VEGFR-2 co-crystallized with sorafenib was obtained from the Protein Data Bank (PDB ID: 4ASD) [14]. The docking process was firstly verified by re-docking of sorafenib inside the active pocket of VEGFR-2 (Figure 5). The low value (≤ 2.0 Å) of root mean square deviation (RMSD) of the docked conformer of sorafenib in the experimental crystal validates the utilized scoring function [27,44]. In the current study, the RMSD between the co-crystallized conformer and the re-docked one is 0.79 Å. This indicates the correctness of the employed docking protocol. The docking scores of the tested ligands are summarized in Table 7, and their binding features inside the active site of the target protein are depicted. The binding poses with the highest energy scores were selected for analysis. The outputted files from MOE software were visualized with Discovery Studio 4.0 software (San Diego, CA, USA).

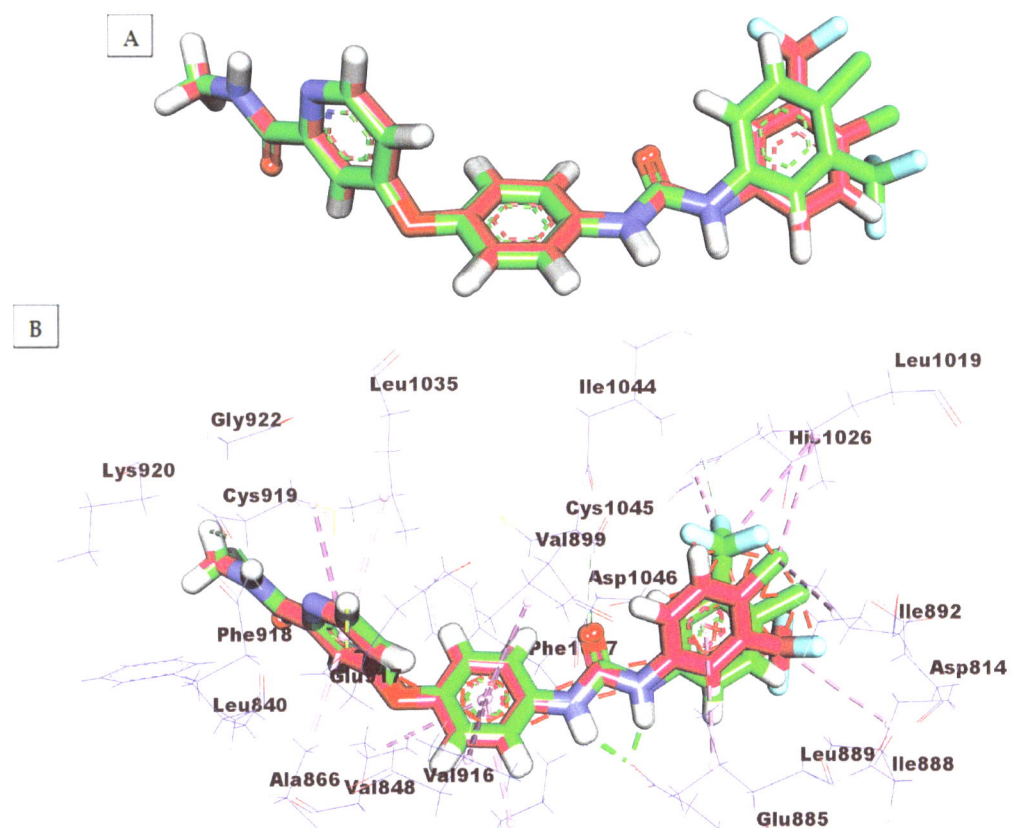

Figure 5. (**A**) the superimposition of the re-docked conformer (green) of sorafenib over the co-crystallized (original) one (pink) with an RMSD value of 0.79 Å. (**B**) the superimposition of the re-docked conformer (green) of sorafenib over the co-crystallized (original) one (pink) showing the essential binding against the active site.

Table 7. The calculated S scores (binding free energies) of the examined compounds and sorafenib against VEGFR-2 (ΔG in Kcal/mole).

Compounds	S [a] [Kcal/mole]	RMSD [b]	RMSD_refine [c]	E_conf [d]	E_place [e]	E_refine [f]
6	−16.45	2.03	2.03	1.23	−130.99	−16.45
7	−20.57	0.06	0.06	0.89	−119.49	−20.57
8	−22.71	0.65	0.65	1.45	−152.95	−22.71
11	−16.02	0.60	0.60	1.34	−85.84	−16.02
12	−15.25	2.20	2.20	1.08	−78.21	−15.25
Sorafenib	−36.23	1.91	1.91	1.60	−130.18	−36.23

[a] S: The placement score of the tested compound inside the binding pocket of the target enzyme utilizing the ASE scoring function. [b] RMSD: RMSD in Å, of the examined pose, from the pose of the original ligand. [c] RMSD_refine: RMSD between the heavy atoms of the predicted pose after and before refinement. [d] E_conf: The conformer's energy. [e] E_place: Score from the placement stage. [f] E_refine: The sum of solvation energies and the van der Waals electrostatics, under the model of generalized Born solvation (GB/VI).

Tyrosine kinase inhibitors have been divided into two types of binding patterns, (type I and II). Type I inhibitors bind to the kinase's active form's adenosine triphosphate (ATP) binding site, resulting in reduced selectivity, whereas type II inhibitors bind to the ATP site and the allosteric, hydrophobic site, resulting in great selectivity. This interaction takes place when the kinases are inactive. The kinase enzymes' active and inactive phases are controlled by the conserved triad Asp–Phe–Gly (DGF). DGF-in conformation was observed in the active state, whereas DFG-out conformation was observed in the inactive state. The front and back pockets make up the VEGFR-2 active site's basic architecture. A crucial residue related to the ATP binding front pocket is Cys919. Glu885 and Asp1046 are found in the back hydrophobic pocket. The Glu885 is located on the C helix, and Asp1046 is a crucial component of the triad [16].

A molecular docking study of sorafenib was carried out to study its binding interactions and orientation. This binding pattern showed a docking score of −36.23 kcal/mol with ten hydrogen bonds (H-bonds) and nine hydrophobic interactions. The carbonyl group of the N- methylpicolinamide head was involved in an H-bond with the vital amino acid Cys919 in the hinge region. Likewise, the pyridine ring was involved in three hydrophobic interactions against the hydrophobic pocket built by the amino acid, Leu1035, Phe918 (pi–pi stacking), and Ala866. Additionally, the spacer phenyl ring is bound to another hydrophobic pocket comprised of Lys 868, Val916, and Val899. Further, the urea moiety was involved in three H-bonds at the DFG motif, where the two NH made two H-bonds with Glu885 and the carbonyl group of the urea interacted with Asp1046. Finally, the terminal phenyl ring was involved in hydrophobic interactions (pi–pi stacking) with Leu1019, Ile1044, and His1026 (Figure 6).

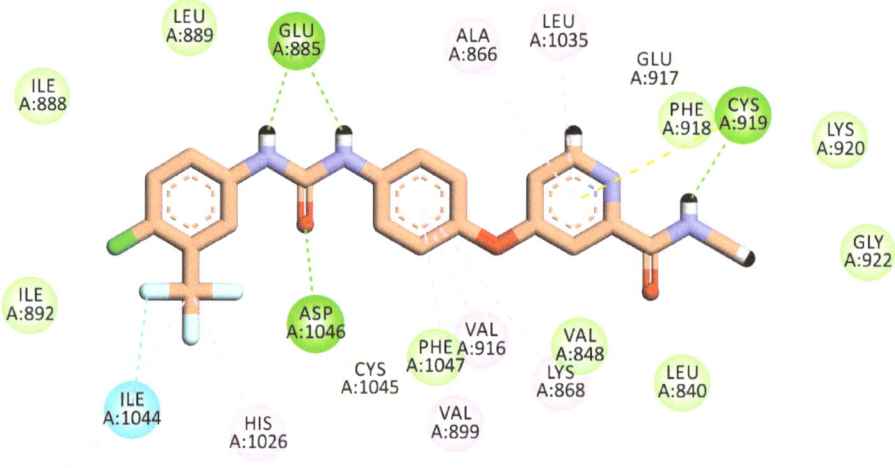

Figure 6. 2D binding mode of sorafenib in the VEGFR-2 active site. H-bonds (dashed green) were formed with Cys919, Glu885, and Asp1046. Hydrophobic interactions (dashed organ) were formed with Leu1035, Phe918, Ala866, Lys 868, Val916, Val899, Leu1019, Ile1044, and His1026.

All the newly synthesized compounds exhibited an interesting binding mode. Two representative compounds (**7** and **8**) were selected for analyzing their binding interactions and orientations against the active pocket of VEGFR-2.

Compound **7** demonstrated a promising binding pattern like that of sorafenib. This compound bonded tightly to the receptor with a binding energy value of −20.57 kcal/mol. In its binding, the pyridinyl group engaged with the hinge region forming a H-bond interaction with the vital amino acid Cys919. In addition, three hydrophobic interactions were displayed between this head and the hydrophobic pocket of (Leu840, Leu1035, and Ala866). The phenyl ring was stabilized in the gatekeeper district through four hydrophobic interactions with Val916, Val899, Lys868, and Cys1045. However, the pharmacophore hydrazone moiety achieved its required job by binding to the vital amino acids Glu885 and Asp1046 in the DGF motif. Moreover, the terminal dimethoxyphenyl hydrophobic tail completely fits in the allosteric site (Figure 7).

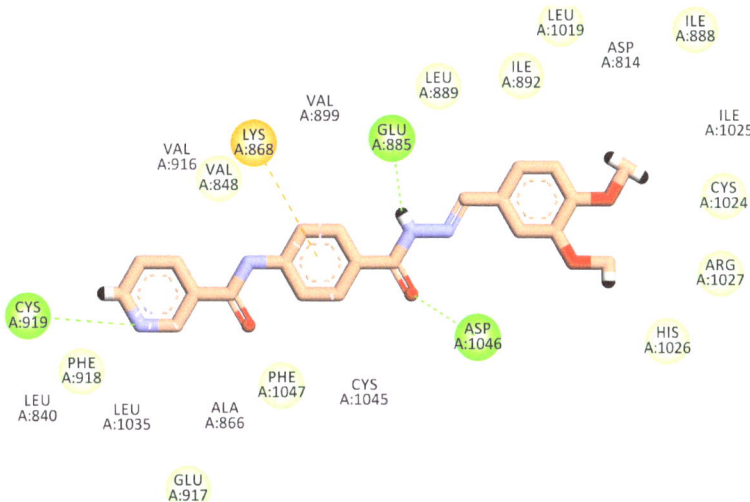

Figure 7. 2D binding mode of compound **7** into the VEGFR-2 active site. H-bonds (dashed green) were formed with Cys919, Glu885, and Asp1046. Hydrophobic interactions (dashed organ) were formed with Leu840, Leu1035, Ala866, Val916, Val899, Lys868, and Cys1045.

The best-scored pose (−22.71 kcal/mol) of compound **8** mimicked sorafenib's key interactions. It kept the H-bonding interaction with the essential amino acid Cys919 in the hinge region via the nitrogen of the pyridine ring. The pyridine head was much more stabilized by many hydrophobic interactions generated with Leu840, Leu1035, Cys919, and Ala866. Moreover, the phenyl linker was enclosed in the gatekeeper area through four hydrophobic interactions with Val899, Val916, Lys868, and Cys1045. Furthermore, the hydrazone moiety interacted as an H-bond donor and acceptor, producing essential H-bonding interactions with Glu885 and Asp1046 at the DGF motif. Finally, the *N,N*-dimethyl aniline tail occupied the hydrophobic allosteric site (Figure 8).

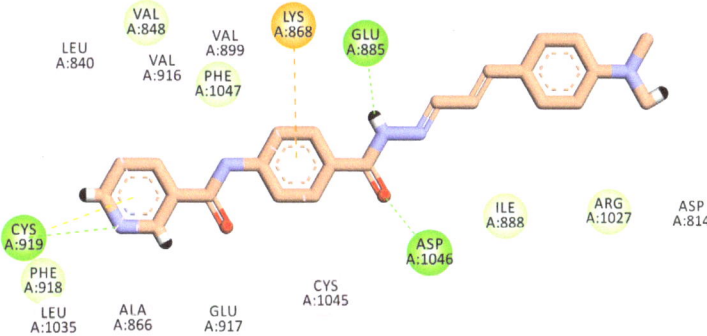

Figure 8. 2D binding mode of compound **8** in the VEGFR-2 active site. H-bonds (dashed green) were formed with Cys919, Glu885, and Asp1046. Hydrophobic interactions (dashed organ) were formed with Leu840, Leu1035, Cys919, Ala866, Val899, Val916, Lys868, and Cys1045.

2.3.2. In Silico ADMET Analysis

The pharmacokinetic characteristics of the prepared compounds were analyzed by applying Discovery Studio 4.0 [45–47]. Sorafenib was utilized as a reference. The results of the ADME studies are listed in Table 8 and Figure 9. Except for compound **6**, all the investigated compounds demonstrated low or very low blood–brain barrier penetration. Compounds **7**, **8**, and **11** demonstrated good aqueous solubility; compounds **6** and **12** showed weak aqueous solubility. All synthesized compounds enjoyed high levels of absorption, whereas compound **13** showed a moderate one. All the tested members were anticipated to be CYP2D6 non-inhibitors. Finally, compounds **6**, **7**, **8**, and **12** can bind the plasma protein at a rate greater than 90%, and compound **11** was predicted to bind at a rate less than 90%.

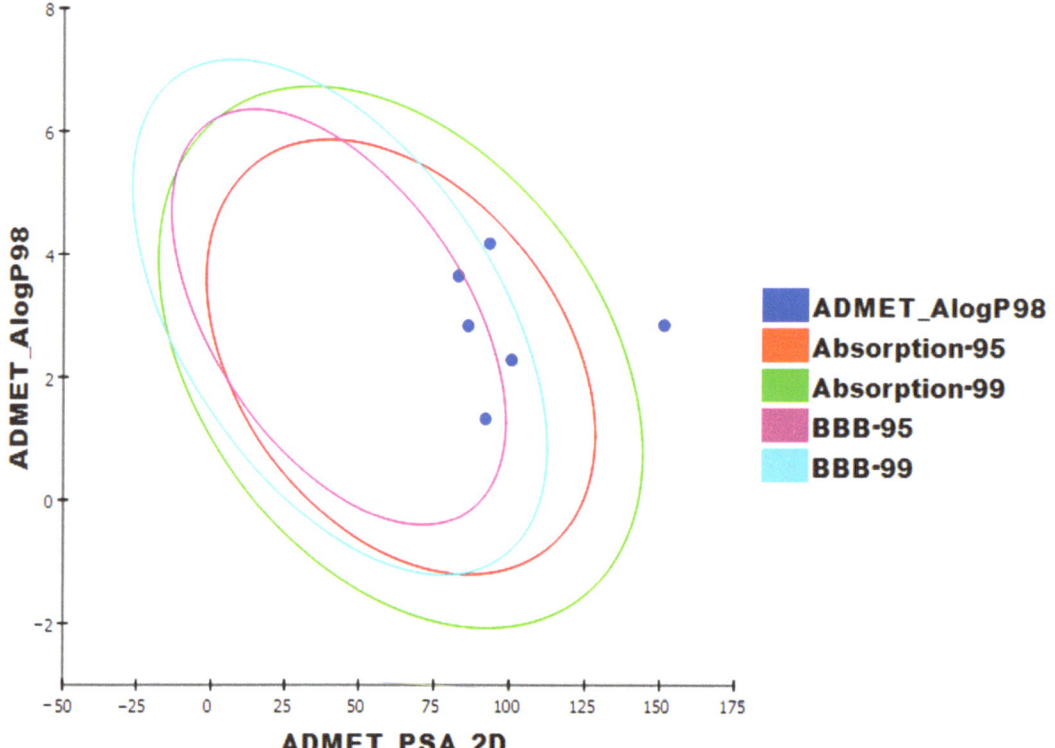

Figure 9. The predicted ADMET parameters. ADMET_PSA_2D is the polar molecular surface area. ADMET_AlogP98 is the lipid-water partition coefficient. PSA_2D is 2D polar surface area. Each examined compound is plotted against the calculated atom-type partition coefficient (ALogP98). The area enclosed by the ellipse constitutes good absorption without violation of other ADMET features. Based on Egan et al.'s [48] absorption, the 95% and 99% confidence limits' ellipses corresponding to the BBB and intestinal absorption models are demonstrated.

Table 8. In silico ADMET features of the considered compounds and sorafenib.

Comp.	BBB Level [a]	Solubility Level [b]	Absorption Level [c]	CYP2D6 Prediction [d]	PPB Prediction [e]
6	M	L	G	NIN	M
7	L	G	G	NIN	M
8	L	G	G	NIN	M
11	L	G	G	NIN	L
12	VL	L	VP	NIN	M
Sorafenib	VL	VL	G	NIN	M

[a] BBB level, l, 0 = VH, 1 = H, 2 = M, 3 = L, 4 = VL. [b] Solubility level, 1 = VL, 2 = L, 3 = G, 4 = O. [c] Absorption level, 0 = G, 1 = M, 2 = P, 3 = VP. [d] CYP2D6, cytochrome P2D6, IN = inhibitor, X = NIN. [e] PBB, plasma protein binding, (L) = less than 90%, (M) = more than 90%.

2.3.3. Lipinski's Rule of Five and Veber's Rule

The oral absorption of a certain compound is normally better if that compound satisfies at least three of the four Lipinski rules, listed below. (i) H-bond donors $\leq$ 5; (ii) H-bond acceptors $\leq$ 10; (iii) molecular weight < 500; (iv) logP < 5. The results revealed that all the synthesized compounds given in Table 9, and sorafenib, showed no violation of Lipinski's rules.

Table 9. Lipinski's rule of five and Veber's rule for the synthesized compounds and sorafenib.

Compound			Lipinski's Rule of 5			Veber's Rule	
	Log P	Mole. Wt.	HBD	HBA	Lipinski's Rule Violation	No. of Rotatable Bonds	TPSA
6	3.646	413.257	2	4	0	5	83.45
7	2.284	404.419	2	6	0	7	101.91
8	2.839	413.472	2	5	0	7	86.69
11	1.414	313.377	3	4	0	5	124.49
12	2.852	420.378	2	9	0	7	158.01
Sorafenib	4.175	464.825	3	4	0	6	92.35

Moreover, Veber's rule was applied to the synthesized compounds. Veber's rule depends on the molecular flexibility, as indicated by rotatable bonds number, and polar surface area to predict the oral bioavailability [49]. Compounds that have 10 or less rotatable bonds and a total polar surface area of 140 Å or less are predicted to have good oral bioavailability [49,50]. The results revealed that all the synthesized compounds obey Veber's rule, except compound **12**, which has a total polar surface area of 158.01 Å.

2.3.4. Toxicity Studies

Furthery, the toxicity profile of the considered compounds was estimated using Discovery studio software. The results are demonstrated in Table 10. The results reveal that all compounds are non-mutagenic, except compounds **8** and **12**. Compounds **6**, **8**, **11**, and **12** showed carcinogenic potency TD_{50} values of 11.304, 29.149, 71.809, and 22.976 g/kg, respectively. These values are higher than that of sorafenib (14.244 g/kg). On the contrary, compound **7** showed lowers values of carcinogenic potency, TD_{50} (10.934 g/kg). Compounds **6**, **11**, and **12** showed maximum tolerated dose values of 0.125, 0.145, and 0.111 g/kg, respectively, which are higher than that of sorafenib (0.089 g/kg); compounds **7** (0.058 g/kg) and **8** (0.064 g/kg) were less tolerated than sorafenib. In addition, except for compound **11** (0.477 g/kg), the considered compounds showed oral LD_{50} values ranging from 1.282 to 2.143 g/kg, which are higher than that of sorafenib (0.823 g/kg). Additionally, the chronic lowest observed adverse effect level (LOAEL) was determined for all compounds. The results indicate LOAEL values ranging from 0.055 to 0.231 g/kg, higher than that of sorafenib (0.0048 g/kg). Finally, all the considered compounds were found to be non-irritant against the skin but to have mild irritant effects on the eye.

Table 10. In silico toxicity potential of the synthesized compounds.

Comp.	Ames Prediction	Carcinogenic Potency TD_{50} (Rat) [a]	Rat Maximum Tolerated Dose (Feed) [b]	Rat Oral LD_{50} [b]	Rat Chronic LOAEL [b]	Skin Irritancy	Ocular Irritancy
6	Non-Mutagen	11.304	0.125	1.486	0.120	None	Mild
7	Non-Mutagen	10.934	0.058	4.507	0.103	None	Mild
8	Mutagen	29.149	0.064	1.282	0.055	None	Mild
11	Non-Mutagen	71.809	0.146	0.477	0.131	None	Mild
12	Mutagen	22.976	0.111	2.143	0.231	None	Mild
Sorafenib	Non-Mutagen	14.244	0.089	0.823	0.005	None	Mild

[a] Unit: g/kg. [b] Unit: mg/kg/day.

2.3.5. MD Simulations

Molecular dynamics (MD) simulations are close to becoming routine in silico tools for drug design and discovery [51]. These studies have two major advantages. First is their explicit ability to examine any change that occurs in the ligand and the protein target, whether that change is structural or entropic. Second, MD studies compute the changes occurring at determined time steps over a very short period with atomic-level revolution [52]. Consequently, MD studies can correctly determine the kinetic and thermodynamic changes that occur through the process of ligand-protein binding [53]. These advantages present MD studies as a powerful tool to reveal the structure–function changes of the studied ligand–protein complex. They explore essential factors, such as ligand–target stability, in addition to ligand binding kinetics and energy [54].

The dynamic and conformational changes of backbone atoms of the VEGFR-2–compound **8** complex were evaluated by RMSD to explore the stability upon apo and **8** bonding states. Figure 10A reveals low RMSD values for VEGFR-2, compound **8**, and the VEGFR-2–compound **8** complex over 100 ns, except for a minor fluctuation after 60 ns. VEGFR-2 flexibility was inspected in terms of RMSF to investigate the fluctuated regions of the examined VEGFR-2 protein over the simulation. Figure 10B shows that compound **8** binding of VEGFR-2 does not make VEGFR-2 highly flexible. The radius of gyration (Rg) of the examined VEGFR-2 enzyme was explored. As shown in Figure 10C, a slight degree of fluctuation of the VEGFR-2 enzyme throughout 100 ns indicates the compactness of the VEGFR-2 -compound **8** complex. Additionally, solvent accessible surface area (SASA) was investigated over 100 ns to investigate the VEGFR-2–compound **8** complex's interaction with the surrounding solvents. Amazingly, the VEGFR-2 enzyme featured a reduced SASA value at 100 ns compared to 0 ns (Figure 10D), indicating the stability of the VEGFR-2–compound **8** complex. Finally, H-bonding in the VEGFR-2–compound **8** complex was revealed to be up to three H-bonds (Figure 10E).

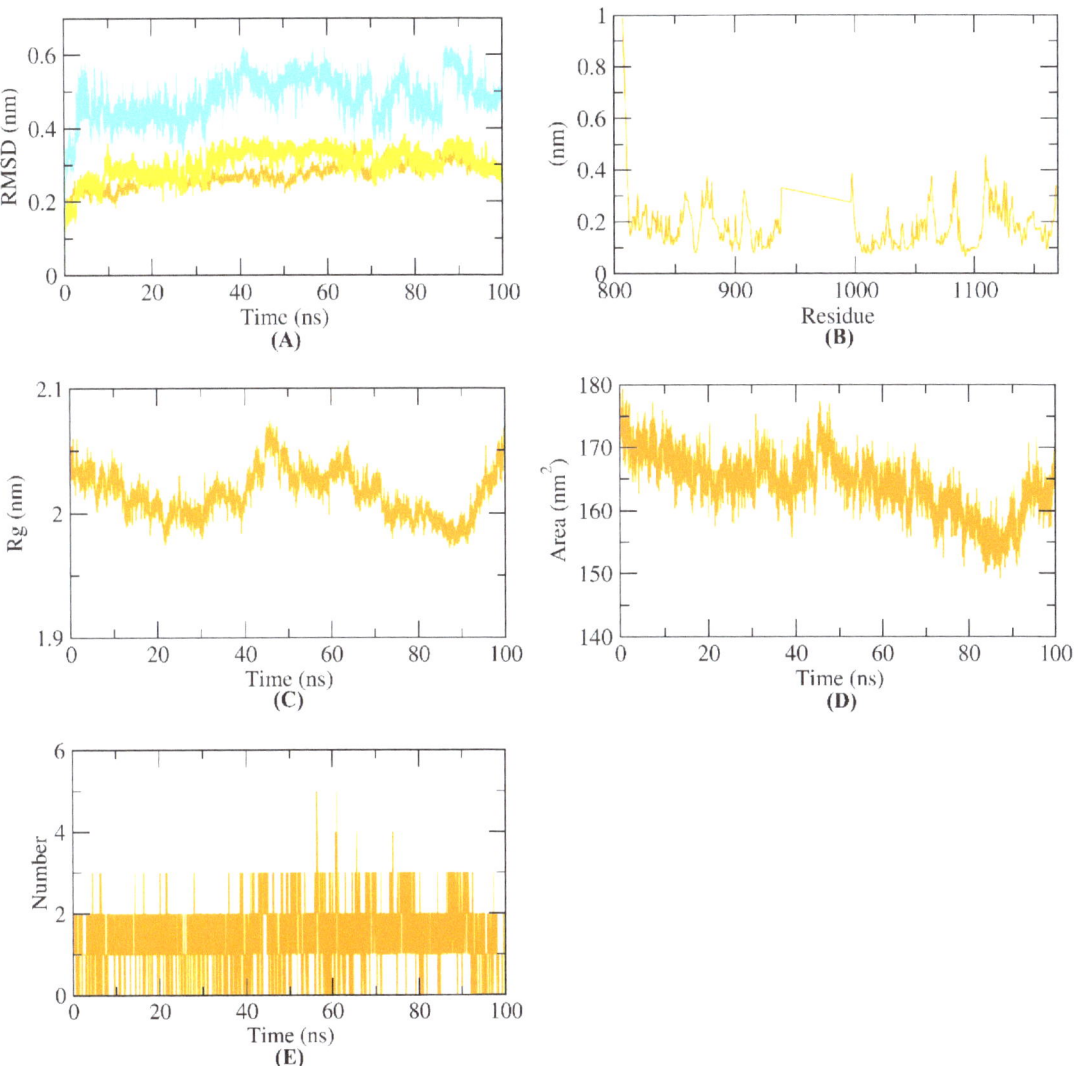

Figure 10. MD simulations. (**A**) RMSD values, (**B**) RMSF, (**C**) R_g, (**D**) SASA, and (**E**) H-bonding of VEGFR-2–compound **8** complex.

2.3.6. MM-PBSA Studies

The molecular mechanical energies with the Poisson–Boltzmann Born and surface area continuum solvation (MM-PBSA) method is an accurate approach to computing the exact free energy of the binding of an examined compound inside a specific protein [55]. The exact binding energy of the VEGFR-2–compound **8** complex in the final 20 ns of the MD was found with an interval of 100 ps from the resulted MD trajectories. Compound **8** demonstrated binding free energy of 220 KJ/mol with the VEGFR-2 enzyme (Figure 11A). Furthermore, the contribution of every amino acid of VEGFR-2 in the obtained binding free energy after the interaction with compound **8** was analyzed. The achieved findings gave an insight into the fundamental residues that had a pivotal role in the binding of the VEGFR-2–compound **8** complex. It was found that ASP-852, ASP-857, GLU-917, GLU-934, and GLU-1038 residues of the VEGFR-2 contributed to the binding energy by more than −20 KJ/mol (Figure 11B).

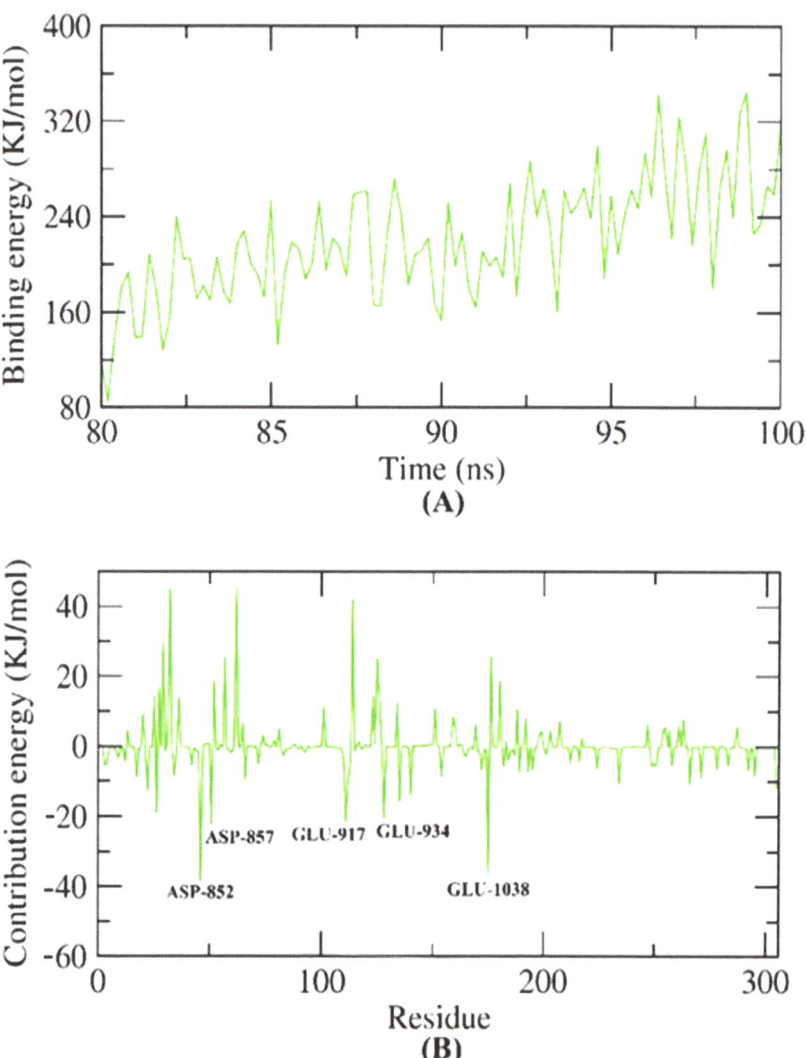

Figure 11. MM-PBSA results. (**A**) The exact binding energy of the VEGFR-2–compound **8** complex. (**B**) Amino acid residues that contributed in the binding process against VEGFR-2.

2.3.7. Flexible Alignment

3D flexible alignment of compound **8** with sorafenib was studied. The result of flexible alignment revealed the general good overlap of compound **8** with sorafenib with the same spatial orientation. In detail, nicotinamide, phenyl, hydrazone, and 3-(4-(dimethylamino)phenyl)allylidene moieties of compound **8** showed the same orientation of the *N*-methylpicolinamide, phenoxy, urea, and 4-chloro-3-(trifluoromethyl)phenyl) moieties as sorafenib, respectively (Figure 12).

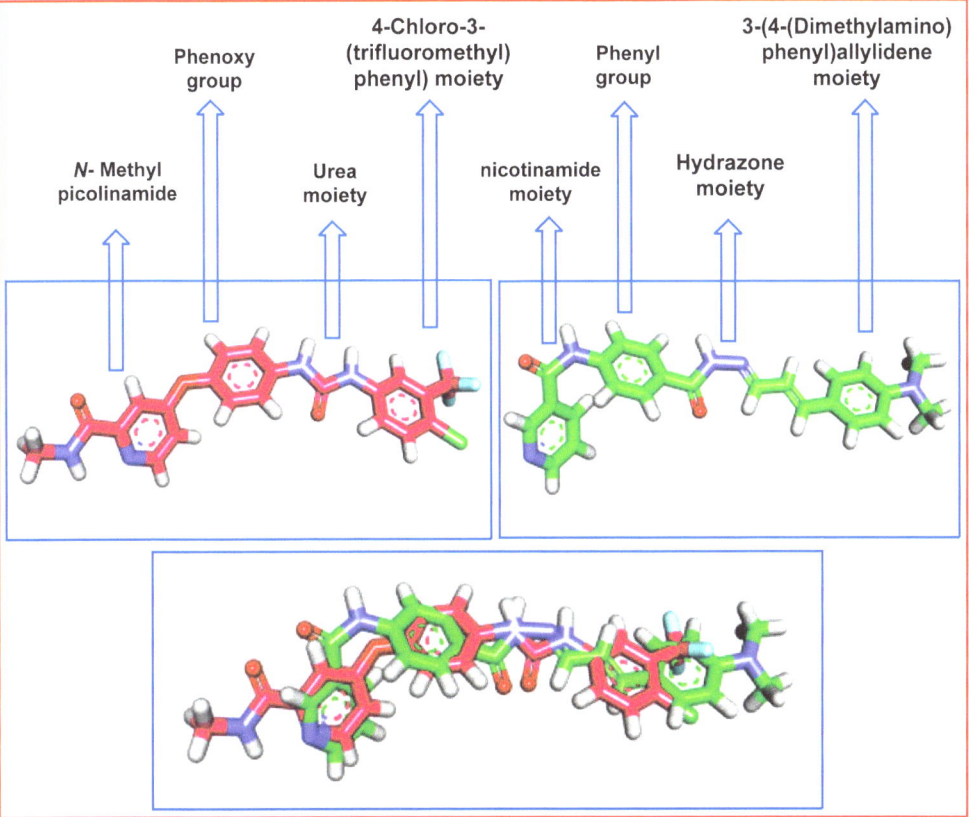

Figure 12. Flexible alignment of compound **8** (green) with sorafenib (pink), showing the same orientation.

3. Conclusions

Five new nicotinamide derivatives were designed and synthesized as anti-proliferative VEGFR-2 inhibitors. The synthesized compounds showed promising antiproliferative activities against (HCT-116 and HepG2) cell lines, and good VEGFR-2 inhibitory activities. The most active member, **8**, exhibited IC$_{50}$ values of 5.4 and 7.1 µM against HCT-116 and HepG2, respectively, and an IC$_{50}$ value of 77.02 nM against VEGFR-2. Deep biological studies were conducted for compound **8**. It showed a promising apoptotic ability (6.5-fold in comparison to the control) to arrest the cell cycle at the G0–G1 phase. In addition, compound **8** produced significant increases in the expression levels of Bax (9.2-fold) and caspase-8 (9.4-fold) compared to the control cells. Furthermore, it caused a significant reduction in the anti-apoptotic factor (Bcl-2) by 3-fold compared to the control cells. Furthermore, it caused a significant reduction in the level of TNF-α (92.37%) compared to the control (82.47%), and a non-significant reduction in the level of IL-6. Docking studies explained the binding modes of the considered compounds. They showed binding modes like that of sorafenib. In silico ADMET and toxicity studies indicated the low toxicity of the considered compounds, and a good range of pharmacokinetic properties. The molecular dynamics simulations revealed the high stability of the most active member, **8**, in the active site of VEGFR−2. Compound **8** is considered a good lead for further chemical modifications and deep biological testing.

4. Experimental

4.1. Chemistry

4.1.1. General

All reagents, chemicals, and apparatus are shown in the Supplementary data. The solvents and chemicals were purchased from El-Gomhouria Co. For Trading Drugs, Chemicals and Medical Supplies, Cairo, Egypt. Compounds **2, 3, 4, 5,** and **10** were previously reported [56,57].

4.1.2. Synthesis of Compounds 6, 7, and 8

A mixture of hydrazide derivative **5** (0.256 g, 0.001 mol) and 0.001 mol of the suitable aromatic aldehyde (0.001 mol), namely, 2,4-dichlorobenzaldehyde, 3,4-dimethoxybenzaldehyde, or 4-(dimethylamino)cinnamaldehyde, were refluxed in 30 mL of ethanol (absolute) containing glacial acetic acid (0.15 mL) for 2 h. After reaction accomplishment, the reaction mixture was cooled, filtered, dried, and recrystallized from ethanol to afford compounds **6, 7,** and **8**, respectively.

(*E*)-*N*-(4-(2-(2,4-Dichlorobenzylidene)hydrazine-1-carbonyl)phenyl)-nicotinamide (**6**)

White crystal (yield, 71%); m.p. = 278–280 °C; $C_{20}H_{14}Cl_2N_4O_2$ (413.2580 g/mol); IR (KBr) ν cm^{-1}: 3301, 3228 (NH), 3034 (CH aromatic), 1644 (C=O), 1593 (C=N); ^{1}H-NMR (400 MHz, DMSO-d_6) δ 12.08 (s, 1H), 10.73 (s, 1H), 9.14 (d, *J* = 2.3 Hz, 1H), 8.92–8.68 (m, 2H), 8.33 (dt, *J* = 7.9, 2.0 Hz, 1H), 8.05–8.03 (d, *J* = 8 Hz, 1H), 8.00–7.98 (d, *J* = 8 Hz 2H), 7.96–7.94(d, *J* = 8 Hz, 2H), 7.70 (d, *J* = 2.2 Hz, 1H), 7.59 (dd, *J* = 8.0, 4.8 Hz, 1H), 7.52 (dd, *J* = 8.6, 2.2 Hz, 1H); ^{13}C-NMR (101 MHz, DMSO-d_6) δ 164.92, 163.13, 152.78, 149.18, 142.84, 142.66, 136.06, 135.50, 134.29(2C), 131.22, 130.77(2C), 129.81, 129.07(2C), 128.54, 128.46, 124.03, 120.10.

(*E*)-*N*-(4-(2-(3,4-Dimethoxybenzylidene)hydrazine-1-carbonyl)phenyl)-nicotinamide (**7**)

Off-white crystal (yield, 74%); m.p. = 250–252 °C; $C_{22}H_{20}N_4O_4$ (404.4260 g/mol); IR (KBr) ν cm^{-1}: 3311, 3248 (NH), 3037 (CH aromatic), 2945 (CH aliphatic), 1644 (C=O), 1598 (C=N); ^{1}H-NMR (400 MHz, DMSO-d6) δ 11.75 (s, 1H), 10.75 (s, 1H), 9.16 (d, *J* = 2.2 Hz, 1H), 8.80 (dd, *J* = 4.8, 1.6 Hz, 1H), 8.52–8.27 (m, 2H), 7.99–7.97 (d, *J* = 8 Hz, 2H), 7.96–7.94 (d, *J* = 8 Hz, 2H), 7.60 (dd, *J* = 7.9, 4.8 Hz, 1H), 7.37 (s, 1H), 7.22 (d, *J* = 8.2 Hz, 1H), 7.04 (d, *J* = 8.3 Hz, 1H), 3.82 (s, 6H); ^{13}C-NMR (101 MHz, DMSO-d6) δ 164.89, 162.91, 152.80, 151.20, 149.55, 149.24, 148.26, 142.39, 136.06, 130.82(2C), 129.04, 128.93, 127.57, 124.02, 122.38, 120.08, 111.95, 108.65, 56.04, 55.92.

N-(4-(2-((1*E*,2*E*)-3-(4-(Dimethylamino)phenyl)allylidene)hydrazine-1-carbonyl) phenyl)nicotinamide (**8**)

White crystal (yield, 67%); m.p. = 260–262 °C; $C_{24}H_{23}N_5O_2$ (413.4810 g/mol); IR (KBr) ν cm^{-1}: 3308, 3239 (NH), 3033 (CH aromatic), 2895 (CH aliphatic), 1643 (C=O), 1608 (C=N); ^{1}H-NMR (400 MHz, DMSO-d_6) δ 11.57 (s, 1H), 10.71 (s, 1H), 9.14 (s, 1H), 8.80 (d, *J* = 4.7 Hz, 1H), 8.33 (d, *J* = 8.0 Hz, 1H), 8.19 (d, *J* = 9.1 Hz, 1H), 7.94 (s, 4H), 7.61 (t, *J* = 6.5 Hz, 1H), 7.47 (d, *J* = 8.3 Hz, 2H), 6.92 (d, *J* = 16.0 Hz, 1H), 6.83 (d, *J* = 9.3 Hz, 1H), 6.73 (d, *J* = 8.4 Hz, 2H), 2.97 (s, 6H); ^{13}C-NMR (101 MHz, DMSO-d6) δ 164.89, 162.58, 152.82, 151.16, 150.89, 149.23, 144.29, 142.29, 140.19, 138.74, 136.08, 133.38, 130.85, 129.09(2C), 128.89(2C), 124.13, 124.05, 121.05, 120.01, 112.49, 38.79.

4.1.3. Synthesis of Compounds 11 and 12

To a solution of compound **10** (0.24 g, 0.001 mol) in absolute ethanol (20 mL) and 0.15 mL of glacial acetic acid, the appropriate amine derivative, namely, thiosemicarbazide or 2,5-dinitrobenzohydrazide (10 mmol), was added. The reaction mixture was refluxed for 8 h. The obtained solids were filtered, washed dried, and recrystallized from ethanol to give the target compounds **11** and **12**.

N-(4-(1-(2-Carbamothioylhydrazono)ethyl)phenyl)nicotinamide (**11**)

Brownish white crystal (yield, 61%); m.p. = 239–241 °C; $C_{15}H_{15}N_5OS$ (313.3790 g/mol); IR (KBr) ν cm^{-1}: 3346, 3261 (NH), 3171 (CH aromatic), 1659 (C=O), 1594 (C=N); ^{1}H-NMR (400 MHz, DMSO-d6) δ 10.56 (s, 1H), 10.18 (s, 1H), 9.13 (d, *J* = 2.8 Hz, 1H), 8.78 (dd, *J* = 4.8, 1.7 Hz, 1H), 8.33–8.30 (m, 1H), 8.00–7.93 (m, 3H), 7.84–7.79 (m, 2H), 7.71–7.62 (m, 1H), 7.59 (dd, *J* = 8.0, 4.7 Hz, 1H), 2.30 (s, 3H); ^{13}C-NMR (101 MHz, DMSO-d6) δ 179.19, 170.39, 164.62, 152.67, 149.18, 147.86, 140.30, 136.01, 133.47, 131.76, 130.96, 127.64, 124.01, 120.10, 14.23. This compound has Z and E forms at 1:0.5

(*E*)-*N*-(4-(1-(2-(2,6-Dinitrophenyl)hydrazono)ethyl)phenyl)nicotinamide (**12**)

Reddish crystal (yield, 61%); m.p. = 265–267 °C; $C_{21}H_{16}N_6O_6$ (420.3850 g/mol); IR (KBr) ν cm^{-1}: 3299 (NH), 3095 (CH aromatic), 2927 (CH aliphatic) 1679 (C=O), 1611 (C=N); ^{1}H-NMR (400 MHz, DMSO-*d$_6$*) δ 11.15 (s, 1H), 10.67 (s, 1H), 9.14 (s, 1H), 8.92 (s, 1H), 8.80 (s, 1H), 8.43 (d, *J* = 9.5 Hz, 1H), 8.33 (s, 1H), 8.15 (d, *J* = 9.6 Hz, 1H), 8.01 (d, *J* = 7.7 Hz, 2H), 7.92 (d, *J* = 8.8 Hz, 2H), 7.61 (s, 1H), 2.48 (s, 3H); ^{13}C-NMR (101 MHz, DMSO-d6) δ 164.77, 153.39, 152.76, 149.22, 144.93, 142.92, 137.69, 136.04, 132.80, 130.63, 130.23, 127.73(2C), 127.70, 124.03, 123.56, 120.80(2C), 120.41, 117.09, 13.99.

4.2. Biological Testing

4.2.1. In Vitro Anti-Proliferative Activity

MTT procedure [58,59] was applied as represented in the Supplementary Materials.

4.2.2. In Vitro VEGFR-2 Enzyme Inhibition Assay

VEGFR-2 inhibitory activity was explored using the Human VEGFR-2 ELISA kit [60], as represented in Supplementary Materials.

4.2.3. Flow Cytometry Analysis for Cell Cycle

This was explored utilizing propidium iodide (PI) staining and flow cytometry analysis for compound **8**, as represented in Supplementary Materials [61].

4.2.4. Flow Cytometry Analysis for Apoptosis

Flow cytometry cell apoptosis analysis was applied for compound **8**, as represented in Supplementary Materials [62–64].

4.2.5. Quantitative Real-Time Reverse-Transcriptase PCR (qRT-PCR) Technique

The effects of compound **8** on the expression of cleaved caspase-3, Bax, Bcl-2, TNF-α, and IL-6 were determined using qRT-PCR as represented in Supplementary Materials [65–67].

4.3. In Silico Studies

4.3.1. Docking Studies

The synthesized compounds were docked against the crystal structure of VEGFR-2 [PDB: 4ASD, resolution: 2.03 Å] using MOE2019.01 software as represented in Supplementary Materials [24].

4.3.2. ADMET Studies

ADMET descriptors were determined using Discovery studio 4.0 [23] as represented in (Supplementary Materials).

4.3.3. Toxicity Studies

The toxicity parameters were calculated using Discovery studio 4.0 [22], as represented in Supplementary Materials.

Molecular Dynamics Simulation & MM/PBSA

MD simulations and MM/PBSA (molecular mechanics/Poisson Boltzmann surface Area) were performed using GROMACS [68] as represented in the Supplementary Materials.

Supplementary Materials: The following supporting information can be downloaded at: https://www.mdpi.com/article/10.3390/molecules27134079/s1. Refs. [69–77] are cited in the Supplementary Materials.

Author Contributions: Conceptualization, I.H.E. and A.M.M.; methodology, R.G.Y., A.S.A. and A.E; software, I.H.E. and A.E.; validation, A.B.M.M., B.A.A. and W.M.E.; formal analysis, A.B.M.M. and I.M.M.G.; investigation, E.B.E.; resources, A.E.; data curation, I.E and A.E.; writing—original draft preparation, R.G.Y.; writing—review and editing, A.M.M. and W.M.E.; visualization, I.H.E.; supervision, I.H.E.; project administration, A.M.M.; funding acquisition, B.A.A. All authors have read and agreed to the published version of the manuscript.

Funding: This research was funded by Princess Nourah bint Abdulrahman University Researchers Supporting Project PNURSP2022R142, Princess Nourah bint Abdulrahman University, Riyadh, Saudi Arabia.

Institutional Review Board Statement: Not applicable.

Informed Consent Statement: Not applicable.

Data Availability Statement: Not applicable.

Conflicts of Interest: The authors declare no conflict of interest.

Sample Availability: Samples of the compounds are available from the authors.

References

1. Siegel, R.L.; Miller, K.D.; Jemal, A. Cancer statistics, 2020. *CA A Cancer J. Clin.* **2020**, *70*, 7–30. [CrossRef] [PubMed]
2. Sung, H.; Ferlay, J.; Siegel, R.L.; Laversanne, M.; Soerjomataram, I.; Jemal, A.; Bray, F. Global cancer statistics 2020: GLOBOCAN estimates of incidence and mortality worldwide for 36 cancers in 185 countries. *CA A Cancer J. Clin.* **2021**, *71*, 209–249. [CrossRef] [PubMed]
3. Fabbro, D.; Parkinson, D.; Matter, A. Protein tyrosine kinase inhibitors: New treatment modalities? *Curr. Opin. Pharmacol.* **2002**, *2*, 374–381. [CrossRef]
4. Abdallah, A.E.; Mabrouk, R.R.; Al Ward, M.M.S.; Eissa, S.I.; Elkaeed, E.B.; Mehany, A.B.; Abo-Saif, M.A.; El-Feky, O.A.; Alesawy, M.S.; El-Zahabi, M.A. Synthesis, biological evaluation, and molecular docking of new series of antitumor and apoptosis inducers designed as VEGFR-2 inhibitors. *J. Enzym. Inhib. Med. Chem.* **2022**, *37*, 573–591. [CrossRef] [PubMed]
5. Lugano, R.; Ramachandran, M.; Dimberg, A. Tumor angiogenesis: Causes, consequences, challenges and opportunities. *Cell. Mol. Life Sci.* **2020**, *77*, 1745–1770. [CrossRef]
6. Phillips, C.M.; Lima, E.A.; Woodall, R.T.; Brock, A.; Yankeelov, T.E. A hybrid model of tumor growth and angiogenesis: In silico experiments. *PLoS ONE* **2020**, *15*, e0231137. [CrossRef]
7. Patel, H.M.; Bari, P.; Karpoormath, R.; Noolvi, M.; Thapliyal, N.; Surana, S.; Jain, P. Design and synthesis of VEGFR-2 tyrosine kinase inhibitors as potential anticancer agents by virtual based screening. *RSC Adv.* **2015**, *5*, 56724–56771. [CrossRef]
8. Folkman, J. Role of angiogenesis in tumor growth and metastasis. *Semin. Oncol.* **2002**, *29*, 15–18. [CrossRef]
9. Shibuya, M. Vascular endothelial growth factor and its receptor system: Physiological functions in angiogenesis and pathological roles in various diseases. *J. Biochem.* **2013**, *153*, 13–19. [CrossRef]
10. Frezzetti, D.; Gallo, M.; Roma, C.; D'Alessio, A.; Maiello, M.R.; Bevilacqua, S.; Normanno, N.; De Luca, A. Vascular endothelial growth factor a regulates the secretion of different angiogenic factors in lung cancer cells. *J. Cell. Physiol.* **2016**, *231*, 1514–1521. [CrossRef]
11. Stuttfeld, E.; Ballmer-Hofer, K. Structure and function of VEGF receptors. *IUBMB Life* **2009**, *61*, 915–922. [CrossRef] [PubMed]
12. Shi, L.; Zhou, J.; Wu, J.; Shen, Y.; Li, X. Anti-angiogenic therapy: Strategies to develop potent VEGFR-2 tyrosine kinase inhibitors and future prospect. *Curr. Med. Chem.* **2016**, *23*, 1000–1040. [CrossRef] [PubMed]
13. Shahin, M.I.; Abou El Ella, D.A.; Ismail, N.S.; Abouzid, K.A. Design, synthesis and biological evaluation of type-II VEGFR-2 inhibitors based on quinoxaline scaffold. *Bioorganic Chem.* **2014**, *56*, 16–26. [CrossRef] [PubMed]
14. Zeidan, M.A.; Mostafa, A.S.; Gomaa, R.M.; Abou-Zeid, L.A.; El-Mesery, M.; Magda, A.-A.; Selim, K.B. Design, synthesis and docking study of novel picolinamide derivatives as anticancer agents and VEGFR-2 inhibitors. *Eur. J. Med. Chem.* **2019**, *168*, 315–329. [CrossRef]
15. Kassab, A.E.; Gedawy, E.M.; Hamed, M.I.; Doghish, A.S.; Hassan, R.A. Design, synthesis, anticancer evaluation, and molecular modelling studies of novel tolmetin derivatives as potential VEGFR-2 inhibitors and apoptosis inducers. *J. Enzym. Inhib. Med. Chem.* **2021**, *36*, 922–939. [CrossRef]

16. Pal, M.K.; Jaiswar, S.P.; Srivastav, A.K.; Goyal, S.; Dwivedi, A.; Verma, A.; Singh, J.; Pathak, A.K.; Sankhwar, P.L.; Ray, R.S. Synergistic effect of piperine and paclitaxel on cell fate via cyt-c, Bax/Bcl-2-caspase-3 pathway in ovarian adenocarcinomas SKOV-3 cells. *Eur. J. Pharmacol.* **2016**, *791*, 751–762. [CrossRef]
17. Ling, Y.; Lu, N.; Gao, Y.; Chen, Y.; Wang, S.; Yang, Y.; Guo, Q. Endostar induces apoptotic effects in HUVECs through activation of caspase-3 and decrease of Bcl-2. *Anticancer Res.* **2009**, *29*, 411–417.
18. Alsaif, N.A.; Elwan, A.; Alanazi, M.M.; Obaidullah, A.J.; Alanazi, W.A.; Alasmari, A.F.; Albassam, H.; Mahdy, H.A.; Taghour, M.S. Design, synthesis and molecular docking of new [1, 2, 4] triazolo [4, 3-a] quinoxaline derivatives as anticancer agents targeting VEGFR-2 kinase. *Mol. Divers.* **2021**, *347*, 1–18. [CrossRef]
19. Eissa, I.H.; El-Helby, A.-G.A.; Mahdy, H.A.; Khalifa, M.M.; Elnagar, H.A.; Mehany, A.B.; Metwaly, A.M.; Elhendawy, M.A.; Radwan, M.M.; ElSohly, M.A. Discovery of new quinazolin-4 (3H)-ones as VEGFR-2 inhibitors: Design, synthesis, and antiproliferative evaluation. *Bioorganic Chem.* **2020**, *105*, 104380. [CrossRef]
20. El-Adl, K.; Ibrahim, M.K.; Khedr, F.; Abulkhair, H.S.; Eissa, I.H. N-Substituted-4-phenylphthalazin-1-amine-derived VEGFR-2 inhibitors: Design, synthesis, molecular docking, and anticancer evaluation studies. *Arch. Der Pharm.* **2021**, *354*, 2000219. [CrossRef]
21. El-Adl, K.; Sakr, H.M.; Yousef, R.G.; Mehany, A.B.; Metwaly, A.M.; Elhendawy, M.A.; Radwan, M.M.; ElSohly, M.A.; Abulkhair, H.S.; Eissa, I.H. Discovery of new quinoxaline-2 (1H)-one-based anticancer agents targeting VEGFR-2 as inhibitors: Design, synthesis, and anti-proliferative evaluation. *Bioorganic Chem.* **2021**, *114*, 105105. [CrossRef] [PubMed]
22. Wang, R.; Liu, H.; You, Y.-Y.; Wang, X.-Y.; Lv, B.-B.; Cao, L.-Q.; Xue, J.-Y.; Xu, Y.-G.; Shi, L. Discovery of novel VEGFR-2 inhibitors embedding 6, 7-dimethoxyquinazoline and diarylamide fragments. *Bioorganic Med. Chem. Lett.* **2021**, *36*, 127788. [CrossRef] [PubMed]
23. Parmar, D.R.; Soni, J.Y.; Guduru, R.; Rayani, R.H.; Kusurkar, R.V.; Vala, A.G.; Talukdar, S.N.; Eissa, I.H.; Metwaly, A.M.; Khalil, A.; et al. Discovery of new anticancer thiourea-azetidine hybrids: Design, synthesis, in vitro antiproliferative, SAR, in silico molecular docking against VEGFR-2, ADMET, toxicity, and DFT studies. *Bioorganic Chem.* **2021**, *115*, 105206. [CrossRef] [PubMed]
24. Alanazi, M.M.; Eissa, I.H.; Alsaif, N.A.; Obaidullah, A.J.; Alanazi, W.A.; Alasmari, A.F.; Albassam, H.; Elkady, H.; Elwan, A. Design, synthesis, docking, ADMET studies, and anticancer evaluation of new 3-methylquinoxaline derivatives as VEGFR-2 inhibitors and apoptosis inducers. *J. Enzym. Inhib. Med. Chem.* **2021**, *36*, 1760–1782. [CrossRef]
25. Mohamed, T.K.; Batran, R.Z.; Elseginy, S.A.; Ali, M.M.; Mahmoud, A.E. Synthesis, anticancer effect and molecular modeling of new thiazolylpyrazolyl coumarin derivatives targeting VEGFR-2 kinase and inducing cell cycle arrest and apoptosis. *Bioorganic Chem.* **2019**, *85*, 253–273. [CrossRef]
26. Reddy, V.G.; Reddy, T.S.; Jadala, C.; Reddy, M.S.; Sultana, F.; Akunuri, R.; Bhargava, S.K.; Wlodkowic, D.; Srihari, P.; Kamal, A. Pyrazolo-benzothiazole hybrids: Synthesis, anticancer properties and evaluation of antiangiogenic activity using in vitro VEGFR-2 kinase and in vivo transgenic zebrafish model. *Eur. J. Med. Chem.* **2019**, *182*, 111609. [CrossRef]
27. El-Adl, K.; El-Helby, A.-G.A.; Sakr, H.; Elwan, A. Design, synthesis, molecular docking and anti-proliferative evaluations of [1, 2, 4] triazolo [4, 3-a] quinoxaline derivatives as DNA intercalators and Topoisomerase II inhibitors. *Bioorganic Chem.* **2020**, *105*, 104399. [CrossRef]
28. El-Adl, K.; El-Helby, A.-G.A.; Sakr, H.; Elwan, A. [1, 2, 4] Triazolo [4, 3-a] quinoxaline and [1, 2, 4] triazolo [4, 3-a] quinoxaline-1-thiol-derived DNA intercalators: Design, synthesis, molecular docking, in silico ADMET profiles and anti-proliferative evaluations. *New J. Chem.* **2021**, *45*, 881–897. [CrossRef]
29. Alsaif, N.A.; Dahab, M.A.; Alanazi, M.M.; Obaidullah, A.J.; Al-Mehizia, A.A.; Alanazi, M.M.; Aldawas, S.; Mahdy, H.A.; Elkady, H. New quinoxaline derivatives as VEGFR-2 inhibitors with anticancer and apoptotic activity: Design, molecular modeling, and synthesis. *Bioorganic Chem.* **2021**, *110*, 104807. [CrossRef]
30. Alanazi, M.M.; Mahdy, H.A.; Alsaif, N.A.; Obiadullah, A.J.; Alkahtani, H.M.; Al-Mehizia, A.A.; Alsubaie, S.M.; Dahab, M.A.; Eissa, I.H. New bis ([1, 2, 4] triazolo)[4, 3-a: 3′, 4′-c] quinoxaline derivatives as VEGFR-2 inhibitors and apoptosis inducers: Design, synthesis, in silico studies, and anticancer evaluation. *Bioorganic Chem.* **2021**, *112*, 104949. [CrossRef]
31. Mahdy, H.A.; Ibrahim, M.K.; Metwaly, A.M.; Belal, A.; Mehany, A.B.; El-Gamal, K.M.; El-Sharkawy, A.; Elhendawy, M.A.; Radwan, M.M.; Elsohly, M.A. Design, synthesis, molecular modeling, in vivo studies and anticancer evaluation of quinazolin-4 (3H)-one derivatives as potential VEGFR-2 inhibitors and apoptosis inducers. *Bioorganic Chem.* **2020**, *94*, 103422. [CrossRef] [PubMed]
32. Eissa, I.H.; Ibrahim, M.K.; Metwaly, A.M.; Belal, A.; Mehany, A.B.; Abdelhady, A.A.; Elhendawy, M.A.; Radwan, M.M.; ElSohly, M.A.; Mahdy, H.A. Design, molecular docking, in vitro, and in vivo studies of new quinazolin-4 (3H)-ones as VEGFR-2 inhibitors with potential activity against hepatocellular carcinoma. *Bioorganic Chem.* **2021**, *107*, 104532. [CrossRef] [PubMed]
33. Eid, A.M.; Hawash, M.; Amer, J.; Jarrar, A.; Qadri, S.; Alnimer, I.; Sharaf, A.; Zalmoot, R.; Hammoudie, O.; Hameedi, S. Synthesis and biological evaluation of novel isoxazole-amide analogues as anticancer and antioxidant agents. *BioMed Res. Int.* **2021**, *2021*, 6633297. [CrossRef] [PubMed]
34. Hassan, A.; Badr, M.; Hassan, H.A.; Abdelhamid, D.; Abuo-Rahma, G.E.D.A. Novel 4-(piperazin-1-yl) quinolin-2 (1H)-one bearing thiazoles with antiproliferative activity through VEGFR-2-TK inhibition. *Bioorganic Med. Chem.* **2021**, *40*, 116168. [CrossRef]
35. El-Metwally, S.A.; Abou-El-Regal, M.M.; Eissa, I.H.; Mehany, A.B.; Mahdy, H.A.; Elkady, H.; Elwan, A.; Elkaeed, E.B. Discovery of thieno [2, 3-d] pyrimidine-based derivatives as potent VEGFR-2 kinase inhibitors and anti-cancer agents. *Bioorganic Chem.* **2021**, *112*, 104947. [CrossRef]

36. Zhong, M.; Li, N.; Qiu, X.; Ye, Y.; Chen, H.; Hua, J.; Yin, P.; Zhuang, G. TIPE regulates VEGFR2 expression and promotes angiogenesis in colorectal cancer. *Int. J. Biol. Sci.* **2020**, *16*, 272. [CrossRef]
37. Han, L.; Lin, X.; Yan, Q.; Gu, C.; Li, M.; Pan, L.; Meng, Y.; Zhao, X.; Liu, S.; Li, A. PBLD inhibits angiogenesis via impeding VEGF/VEGFR2-mediated microenvironmental cross-talk between HCC cells and endothelial cells. *Oncogene* **2022**, *41*, 1851–1865. [CrossRef]
38. Pritchett, J.C.; Naesens, L.; Montoya, J. Treating HHV-6 infections: The laboratory efficacy and clinical use of ati-HHV-6 agents. In *Human Herpesviruses HHV-6A, HHV-6B & HHV-7*; Elsevier: Amsterdam, The Netherlands, 2014.
39. Indrayanto, G.; Putra, G.S.; Suhud, F. Validation of in-vitro bioassay methods: Application in herbal drug research. *Profiles Drug Subst. Excip. Relat. Methodol.* **2021**, *46*, 273–307.
40. Pucci, B.; Kasten, M.; Giordano, A. Cell cycle and apoptosis. *Neoplasia* **2000**, *2*, 291–299. [CrossRef]
41. Riccardi, C.; Nicoletti, I. Analysis of apoptosis by propidium iodide staining and flow cytometry. *Nat. Protoc.* **2006**, *1*, 1458–1461. [CrossRef]
42. Vermes, I.; Haanen, C.; Steffens-Nakken, H.; Reutellingsperger, C. A novel assay for apoptosis flow cytometric detection of phosphatidylserine expression on early apoptotic cells using fluorescein labelled annexin V. *J. Immunol. Methods* **1995**, *184*, 39–51. [CrossRef]
43. Sobhy, M.K.; Mowafy, S.; Lasheen, D.S.; Farag, N.A.; Abouzid, K.A. 3D-QSAR pharmacophore modelling, virtual screening and docking studies for lead discovery of a novel scaffold for VEGFR 2 inhibitors: Design, synthesis and biological evaluation. *Bioorganic Chem.* **2019**, *89*, 102988. [CrossRef] [PubMed]
44. Mena-Ulecia, K.; Tiznado, W.; Caballero, J. Study of the differential activity of thrombin inhibitors using docking, QSAR, molecular dynamics, and MM-GBSA. *PLoS ONE* **2015**, *10*, e0142774. [CrossRef] [PubMed]
45. Elkady, H.; Elwan, A.; El-Mahdy, H.A.; Doghish, A.S.; Ismail, A.; Taghour, M.S.; Elkaeed, E.B.; Eissa, I.H.; Dahab, M.A.; Mahdy, H.A.; et al. New benzoxazole derivatives as potential VEGFR-2 inhibitors and apoptosis inducers: Design, synthesis, anti-proliferative evaluation, flowcytometric analysis, and in silico studies. *J. Enzym. Inhib. Med. Chem.* **2022**, *37*, 397–410. [CrossRef]
46. Alanazi, M.M.; Elwan, A.; Alsaif, N.A.; Obaidullah, A.J.; Alkahtani, H.M.; Al-Mehizia, A.A.; Alsubaie, S.M.; Taghour, M.S.; Eissa, I.H. Discovery of new 3-methylquinoxalines as potential anti-cancer agents and apoptosis inducers targeting VEGFR-2: Design, synthesis, and in silico studies. *J. Enzym. Inhib. Med. Chem.* **2021**, *36*, 1732–1750. [CrossRef]
47. Yousef, R.G.; Sakr, H.M.; Eissa, I.H.; Mehany, A.B.; Metwaly, A.M.; Elhendawy, M.A.; Radwan, M.M.; ElSohly, M.A.; Abulkhair, H.S.; El-Adl, K. New quinoxaline-2 (1 H)-ones as potential VEGFR-2 inhibitors: Design, synthesis, molecular docking, ADMET profile and anti-proliferative evaluations. *New J. Chem.* **2021**, *45*, 16949–16964. [CrossRef]
48. Egan, W.J.; Merz, K.M.; Baldwin, J.J. Prediction of drug absorption using multivariate statistics. *J. Med. Chem.* **2000**, *43*, 3867–3877. [CrossRef]
49. Veber, D.F.; Johnson, S.R.; Cheng, H.-Y.; Smith, B.R.; Ward, K.W.; Kopple, K.D. Molecular properties that influence the oral bioavailability of drug candidates. *J. Med. Chem.* **2002**, *45*, 2615–2623. [CrossRef]
50. Lipinski, C.A.; Lombardo, F.; Dominy, B.W.; Feeney, P.J. Experimental and computational approaches to estimate solubility and permeability in drug discovery and development settings. *Adv. Drug Deliv. Rev.* **1997**, *23*, 3–25. [CrossRef]
51. Sousa, S.F.; Fernandes, P.A.; Ramos, M.J. Protein–ligand docking: Current status and future challenges. *Proteins Struct. Funct. Bioinform.* **2006**, *65*, 15–26. [CrossRef]
52. Hollingsworth, S.A.; Dror, R.O. Molecular dynamics simulation for all. *Neuron* **2018**, *99*, 1129–1143. [CrossRef] [PubMed]
53. Hansson, T.; Oostenbrink, C.; van Gunsteren, W. Molecular dynamics simulations. *Curr. Opin. Struct. Biol.* **2002**, *12*, 190–196. [CrossRef]
54. Durrant, J.D.; McCammon, J.A. Molecular dynamics simulations and drug discovery. *BMC Biol.* **2011**, *9*, 71. [CrossRef] [PubMed]
55. Genheden, S.; Ryde, U. The MM/PBSA and MM/GBSA methods to estimate ligand-binding affinities. *Expert Opin. Drug Discov.* **2015**, *10*, 449–461. [CrossRef] [PubMed]
56. Ran, F.; Li, W.; Qin, Y.; Yu, T.; Liu, Z.; Zhou, M.; Liu, C.; Qiao, T.; Li, X.; Yousef, R.G.; et al. Inhibition of vascular smooth muscle and cancer cell proliferation by new VEGFR inhibitors and their immunomodulator effect: Design, synthesis, and biological evaluation. *Oxidative Med. Cell. Longev.* **2021**, *2021*, 8321400. [CrossRef] [PubMed]
57. Chaitra, G.; Rohini, R. Synthesis and biological activities of [1, 3]-oxazine derivatives. *Der Pharma Chem.* **2018**, *10*, 96–101.
58. Eldehna, W.M.; Al-Rashood, S.T.; Al-Warhi, T.; Eskandrani, R.O.; Alharbi, A.; El Kerdawy, A.M. Novel oxindole/benzofuran hybrids as potential dual CDK2/GSK-3β inhibitors targeting breast cancer: Design, synthesis, biological evaluation, and in silico studies. *J. Enzym. Inhib. Med. Chem.* **2021**, *36*, 270–285. [CrossRef]
59. Al-Sanea, M.M.; Al-Ansary, G.H.; Elsayed, Z.M.; Maklad, R.M.; Elkaeed, E.B.; Abdelgawad, M.A.; Bukhari, S.N.A.; Abdel-Aziz, M.M.; Suliman, H.; Eldehna, W.M.; et al. Development of 3-methyl/3-(morpholinomethyl) benzofuran derivatives as novel antitumor agents towards non-small cell lung cancer cells. *J. Enzym. Inhib. Med. Chem.* **2021**, *36*, 987–999. [CrossRef]
60. Abou-Seri, S.M.; Eldehna, W.M.; Ali, M.M.; Abou El Ella, D.A. 1-Piperazinylphthalazines as potential VEGFR-2 inhibitors and anticancer agents: Synthesis and in vitro biological evaluation. *Eur. J. Med. Chem.* **2016**, *107*, 165–179. [CrossRef]
61. Kim, K.H.; Sederstrom, J.M. Assaying cell cycle status using flow cytometry. *Curr. Protoc. Mol. Biol.* **2015**, *111*, 28.6.1–28.6.11. [CrossRef]

62. Lo, K.K.-W.; Lee, T.K.-M.; Lau, J.S.-Y.; Poon, W.-L.; Cheng, S.-H. Luminescent biological probes derived from ruthenium (II) estradiol polypyridine complexes. *Inorg. Chem.* **2008**, *47*, 200–208. [CrossRef] [PubMed]
63. Sabt, A.; Abdelhafez, O.M.; El-Haggar, R.S.; Madkour, H.M.; Eldehna, W.M.; El-Khrisy, E.E.-D.A.; Abdel-Rahman, M.A.; Rashed, L.A. Novel coumarin-6-sulfonamides as apoptotic anti-proliferative agents: Synthesis, in vitro biological evaluation, and QSAR studies. *J. Enzym. Inhib. Med. Chem.* **2018**, *33*, 1095–1107. [CrossRef] [PubMed]
64. Hawash, M.; Qneibi, M.; Jaradat, N.; Abualhasan, M.; Amer, J.; Amer, E.-H.; Ibraheem, T.; Hindieh, S.; Tarazi, S.; Sobuh, S.; et al. The impact of filtered water-pipe smoke on healthy versus cancer cells and their neurodegenerative role on AMPA receptor. *Drug Chem. Toxicol.* **2021**, 1–9, online ahead of print. [CrossRef]
65. Balah, A.; Ezzat, O.; Akool, E.-S. Vitamin E inhibits cyclosporin A-induced CTGF and TIMP-1 expression by repressing ROS-mediated activation of TGF-β/Smad signaling pathway in rat liver. *Int. Immunopharmacol.* **2018**, *65*, 493–502. [CrossRef]
66. Aborehab, N.M.; Elnagar, M.R.; Waly, N.E. Gallic acid potentiates the apoptotic effect of paclitaxel and carboplatin via over-expression of Bax and P53 on the MCF-7 human breast cancer cell line. *J. Biochem. Mol. Toxicol.* **2020**, *35*, e22638. [CrossRef] [PubMed]
67. Elnagar, M.R.; Walls, A.B.; Helal, G.K.; Hamada, F.M.; Thomsen, M.S.; Jensen, A.A. Functional characterization of α7 nicotinic acetylcholine and NMDA receptor signaling in SH-SY5Y neuroblastoma cells in an ERK phosphorylation assay. *Eur. J. Pharmacol.* **2018**, *826*, 106–113. [CrossRef]
68. Yousef, R.G.; Ibrahim, A.; Khalifa, M.M.; Eldehna, W.M.; Gobaara, I.M.; Mehany, A.B.; Elkaeed, E.B.; Alsfouk, A.A.; Metwaly, A.M. Discovery of new nicotinamides as apoptotic VEGFR-2 inhibitors: Virtual screening, synthesis, anti-proliferative, immunomodulatory, ADMET, toxicity, and molecular dynamic simulation studies. *J. Enzym. Inhib. Med. Chem.* **2022**, *37*, 1389–1403. [CrossRef]
69. Jo, S.; Kim, T.; Iyer, V.G.; Im, W. CHARMM-GUI: A web-based graphical user interface for CHARMM. *J. Comput. Chem.* **2008**, *29*, 1859–1865. [CrossRef]
70. Brooks, B.; Brooks, C.; Mackerell, A.; Nilsson, L.; Petrella, R.; Roux, B.; Won, Y.; Archontis, G.; Bartels, C.; Boresch, S.; et al. CHARMM: The biomolecular simulation program. *J. Comput. Chem.* **2009**, *30*, 1545–1614. [CrossRef]
71. Lee, J.; Cheng, X.; Swails, J.M.; Yeom, M.S.; Eastman, P.K.; Lemkul, J.; Wei, S.; Buckner, J.; Jeong, J.C.; Qi, Y.; et al. CHARMM-GUI Input Generator for NAMD, GROMACS, AMBER, OpenMM, and CHARMM/OpenMM Simulations Using the CHARMM36 Additive Force Field. *J. Chem. Theory Comput.* **2015**, *12*, 405–413. [CrossRef]
72. Best, R.; Zhu, X.; Shim, J.; Lopes, P.; Mittal, J.; Feig, M. and MacKerell, A. Optimization of the Additive CHARMM All-Atom Protein Force Field Targeting Improved Sampling of the Backbone φ, ψ and Side-Chain χ_1 and χ_2 Dihedral Angles. *J. Chem. Theory Comput.* **2012**, *8*, 3257–3273. [CrossRef] [PubMed]
73. Phillips, J.; Braun, R.; Wang, W.; Gumbart, J.; Tajkhorshid, E.; Villa, E.; Chipot, C.; Skeel, R.; Kalé, L.; Schulten, K. Scalable molecular dynamics with NAMD. *J. Comput. Chem.* **2005**, *26*, 1781–1802. [CrossRef] [PubMed]
74. Jorgensen, W.L.; Chandrasekhar, J.; Madura, J.D.; Impey, R.W.; Klein, M.L. Comparison of simple potential functions for simulating liquid water. *J. Chem. Phys.* **1983**, *79*, 926–935. [CrossRef]
75. Yu, W.; He, X.; Vanommeslaeghe, K.; MacKerell, A.D. Extension of the CHARMM general force field to sulfonyl-containing compounds and its utility in biomolecular simulations. *J. Comput. Chem.* **2012**, *33*, 2451–2468. [CrossRef]
76. Nosé, S.; Klein, M. Constant pressure molecular dynamics for molecular systems. *Mol. Phys.* **1983**, *50*, 1055–1076. [CrossRef]
77. Nosé, S. A molecular dynamics method for simulations in the canonical ensemble. *Mol. Phys.* **1984**, *52*, 255–268. [CrossRef]

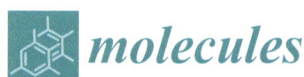 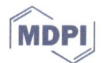

Article

Ligand and Structure-Based In Silico Determination of the Most Promising SARS-CoV-2 nsp16-nsp10 2′-o-Methyltransferase Complex Inhibitors among 3009 FDA Approved Drugs

Ibrahim H. Eissa [1,*], Mohamed S. Alesawy [1], Abdulrahman M. Saleh [1], Eslam B. Elkaeed [2], Bshra A. Alsfouk [3], Abdul-Aziz M. M. El-Attar [4] and Ahmed M. Metwaly [5,6,*]

[1] Pharmaceutical Medicinal Chemistry and Drug Design Department, Faculty of Pharmacy (Boys), Al-Azhar University, Cairo 11884, Egypt; mohammedalesawy@azhar.edu.eg (M.S.A.); abdo.saleh240@azhar.edu.eg (A.M.S.)
[2] Department of Pharmaceutical Sciences, College of Pharmacy, Almaarefa University, Riyadh 13713, Saudi Arabia; ikaeed@mcst.edu.sa
[3] Department of Pharmaceutical Sciences, College of Pharmacy, Princess Nourah Bint Abdulrahman University, P.O. Box 84428, Riyadh 11671, Saudi Arabia; baalsfouk@pnu.edu.sa
[4] Pharmaceutical Analytical Chemistry Department, Faculty of Pharmacy, Al-Azhar University, Cairo 11884, Egypt; zizoalattar@yahoo.com
[5] Pharmacognosy and Medicinal Plants Department, Faculty of Pharmacy (Boys), Al-Azhar University, Cairo 11884, Egypt
[6] Biopharmaceutical Products Research Department, Genetic Engineering and Biotechnology Research Institute, City of Scientific Research and Technological Applications (SRTA-City), Alexandria 21934, Egypt
* Correspondence: ibrahimeissa@azhar.edu.eg (I.H.E.); ametwaly@azhar.edu.eg (A.M.M.)

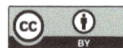

Citation: Eissa, I.H.; Alesawy, M.S.; Saleh, A.M.; Elkaeed, E.B.; Alsfouk, B.A.; El-Attar, A.-A.M.M.; Metwaly, A.M. Ligand and Structure-Based In Silico Determination of the Most Promising SARS-CoV-2 nsp16-nsp10 2′-o-Methyltransferase Complex Inhibitors among 3009 FDA Approved Drugs. *Molecules* **2022**, *27*, 2287. https://doi.org/10.3390/molecules27072287

Academic Editors: Anna Maria Almerico, Imtiaz Khan and Sumera Zaib

Received: 23 February 2022
Accepted: 28 March 2022
Published: 31 March 2022

Publisher's Note: MDPI stays neutral with regard to jurisdictional claims in published maps and institutional affiliations.

Copyright: © 2022 by the authors. Licensee MDPI, Basel, Switzerland. This article is an open access article distributed under the terms and conditions of the Creative Commons Attribution (CC BY) license (https://creativecommons.org/licenses/by/4.0/).

Abstract: As a continuation of our earlier work against SARS-CoV-2, seven FDA-approved drugs were designated as the best SARS-CoV-2 nsp16-nsp10 2′-o-methyltransferase (2′OMTase) inhibitors through 3009 compounds. The in silico inhibitory potential of the examined compounds against SARS-CoV-2 nsp16-nsp10 2′-o-methyltransferase (PDB ID: 6W4H) was conducted through a multi-step screening approach. At the beginning, molecular fingerprints experiment with **SAM** (S-Adenosylmethionine), the co-crystallized ligand of the targeted enzyme, unveiled the resemblance of 147 drugs. Then, a structural similarity experiment recommended 26 compounds. Therefore, the 26 compounds were docked against 2′OMTase to reveal the potential inhibitory effect of seven promising compounds (Protirelin, (**1187**), Calcium folinate (**1913**), Raltegravir (**1995**), Regadenoson (**2176**), Ertapenem (**2396**), Methylergometrine (**2532**), and Thiamine pyrophosphate hydrochloride (**2612**)). Out of the docked ligands, Ertapenem (**2396**) showed an ideal binding mode like that of the co-crystallized ligand (**SAM**). It occupied all sub-pockets of the active site and bound the crucial amino acids. Accordingly, some MD simulation experiments (RMSD, RMSF, R_g, SASA, and H-bonding) have been conducted for the 2′OMTase—Ertapenem complex over 100 ns. The performed MD experiments verified the correct binding mode of Ertapenem against 2′OMTase exhibiting low energy and optimal dynamics. Finally, MM-PBSA studies indicated that Ertapenem bonded advantageously to the targeted protein with a free energy value of −43 KJ/mol. Furthermore, the binding free energy analysis revealed the essential amino acids of 2′OMTase that served positively to the binding. The achieved results bring hope to find a treatment for COVID-19 via in vitro and in vivo studies for the pointed compounds.

Keywords: SARS-CoV-2 nsp16-nsp10 2′-o-methyltransferase; FDA approved drugs; molecular fingerprints; structural similarity; molecular docking; MD simulations; MMPBSA

1. Introduction

The WHO, addressed on 16 February 2022, confirmed that the worldwide infections of COVID-19 were 414,525,183. Grievously, this number includes 5,832,333 deaths [1]. Although 10,227,670,521 vaccinations have been administered [1], the virus can still infect and spread widely [2]. Responding to these numbers, massive work is demanded from scientists all over the world to find a cure.

The regular process of new drug discovery is highly expensive and takes much time. The average required time for the complete development of a new drug is about 12 years, with a cost of 2.6 billion USD [3]. In contrast, drug repurposing or repositioning is a much faster technique in which the exploration of new pharmacological use for an old or existing drug occurs [4]. The strategy of drug repurposing was applied successfully in the discovery of anti-cancer [5], COVID-19 [6], anti-inflammatory [7], antibacterial [8], anti-parasitic [9], and anti-viral [10] drugs.

The tremendous applications of computational chemistry in drug discovery are due to different factors. First, the exploration of accurate 3D structures of different protein targets in the human body [11]. Second, the vast advancements in the fields of computer hardware and software [12]. Finally, the development of structure–activity relationship (SAR) principles [13]. Consequently, computational chemistry methods were applied to estimate various pharmacodynamic and pharmacokinetic parameters that relate the chemical structure of compounds to its activity and also to characterize the interaction of compounds with biological targets such as structure similarity [14], molecular fingerprints [15], QSAR [16], pharmacophores [17], homology models [18], molecular modeling [19], drug molecular design [20], rational drug design [21,22], molecular docking [23], MD simulations [24], absorption [25], distribution [26], metabolism [27], excretion [28], and toxicity properties [29], as well as physicochemical characterization [30] and DFT [31].

In this regard, our team employed the strategies of computer-based chemistry to discover the potential inhibitive effects of the secondary metabolites of *Asteriscus hierochunticus* [32], *Monanchora* sp. [33], *Artemisia sublessingiana* [34], and *Artemisia* sp. [35], as well as 69 isoflavonoids [36] against SARS-CoV-2. Additionally, we designed a multi-step in silico selection method to prime the most active inhibitor drugs against a SASRS-CoV-2 protein amongst a vast number of compounds. As an exemplification, amongst 310 natural metabolite and 69 semisynthetic compounds, the highest potential inhibitors against SARS-CoV-2 nsp10 [37] and the SARS-CoV-2 PLpro [38], respectively, were decided

In this research, a panel of 3009 FDA-approved compounds was retrieved from the internet [39] to be screened depending on various computational methods to distinguish the most potent SARS-CoV-2 nsp16-nsp10 2′-o-methyltransferase complex inhibitor.

The starting point in our study was (S-Adenosylmethionine, **SAM**), the co-crystallized ligand of the essential COVID-19 protein, 2′OMTase (PDB ID: (6W4H), that showed high binding affinity against it. Firstly, the selected compounds were subjected to two ligand-based computational techniques (molecular fingerprints and similarity) successively to select the most similar candidates to **SAM**. Then, several structure-based computational methods (molecular docking and MD simulations) were conducted to confirm the binding modes, energies, and dynamic behaviors of the singled-out candidates.

2. Results and Discussion

2.1. Filter Using Fingerprint

Molecular fingerprint is a ligand-based computational (*in silico*) computational technique. This approach can predict the biological activity of a molecule based on its chemical structure [40]. The scientific base of ligand-based calculations is influenced by the principles of target–structure–activity relationships (SAR). It can set a relationship between the measured bio response/s exerted by a molecule and its chemical structure. Accordingly, compounds with similar chemical structures are expected to exert similar activities [41].

A co-crystallized ligand is one that exerts an excellent binding affinity with the corresponding protein forming a crystallizable ligand–protein complex [42]. In accordance, the chemical structure of that ligand could be employed as a model to design and develop an inhibitor that can bind strongly to the target protein. The molecular fingerprints study was performed using Discovery Studio against **SAM**. The experiment examined the next variables: H-bond acceptor and donor [43], charge [44], hybridization [45], positive and negative ionizable [46], halogen, aromatic, or none of the above besides the ALogP of atoms and fragments.

In structural terms, the chemical structures of the examined molecules are encoded and transformed binary bit strings (sequences of 0's and 1's). Every bit corresponds to a "pre-defined/determined" structural descriptor or feature of substructure or fragment. If the examined molecule has that feature, the bit position that corresponds to this descriptor is set to 1 (ON). If it is absent, it is set to 0 (OFF) [47].

SA describes the number bits that were computed in the FDA-approved drugs and the **SAM**. SB identifies the number bits that were found in the FDA-approved drugs, but not **SAM**. SC refers to the number bits that were discovered in **SAM**, but not in the FDA-approved drugs.

The study (Table 1) favored 147 compounds. These compounds showed the highest fingerprint similarity with **SAM**.

Table 1. Fingerprint similarity between the tested compounds and **SAM**.

Comp.	Similarity	SA	SB	SC	Comp.	Similarity	SA	SB	SC
SAM	1	237	0	0	1670	0.57	257	214	−20
4	0.497396	191	147	46	1694	0.5	191	145	46
42	0.597	138	−6	99	1737	0.506944	146	51	91
50	0.651	157	4	80	1740	0.491582	146	60	91
51	0.581	137	−1	100	1756	0.506912	220	197	17
56	0.665	171	20	66	1761	0.523404	246	233	−9
58	0.491525	174	117	63	1766	0.54321	176	87	61
74	0.495652	171	108	66	1778	0.511299	181	117	56
91	0.496241	132	29	105	1792	0.50211	238	237	−1
113	0.485714	170	113	67	1793	0.494792	285	339	−48
130	0.490463	180	130	57	1802	0.56	237	186	0
152	0.624	143	−8	94	1805	0.501433	175	112	62
158	0.5	189	141	48	1818	0.508475	210	176	27
186	0.644	150	−4	87	1860	0.494024	124	14	113
189	0.5	122	7	115	1886	0.493478	227	223	10
190	0.492958	175	118	62	1911	0.490683	158	85	79
214	0.515723	164	81	73	1913	0.494033	207	182	30
241	0.717	160	−14	77	1917	0.929	235	16	2
251	0.490956	190	150	47	1919	0.488701	173	117	64
272	0.508403	121	1	116	1927	0.489796	216	204	21
281	0.510806	260	272	−23	1928	0.488636	215	203	22
304	0.488938	221	215	16	1932	0.50303	166	93	71
310	0.717	160	−14	77	1949	0.505464	185	129	52
322	0.486154	158	88	79	1960	0.48995	195	161	42
380	0.514563	159	72	78	1993	0.522599	185	117	52
390	0.52862	157	60	80	1995	0.488998	200	172	37
404	0.535211	190	118	47	2002	0.49	147	63	90
428	0.498623	181	126	56	2009	0.511364	135	27	102
446	0.50641	158	75	79	2017	0.663	193	54	44

Table 1. Cont.

Comp.	Similarity	SA	SB	SC	Comp.	Similarity	SA	SB	SC
458	0.488136	144	58	93	2023	0.627	168	31	69
461	0.507837	162	82	75	2024	0.527378	183	110	54
470	0.491803	180	129	57	2031	0.57	147	21	90
515	0.501493	168	98	69	2036	0.487179	171	114	66
516	0.561	165	57	72	2042	0.664	172	22	65
539	0.519149	122	−2	115	2174	0.488318	209	191	28
562	0.489496	233	239	4	2176	0.661	199	64	38
573	0.491049	192	154	45	2232	0.642	265	176	−28
598	0.510504	243	239	−6	2233	0.701	202	51	35
659	0.540816	159	57	78	2256	0.543662	193	118	44
663	0.492537	198	165	39	2268	0.538776	132	8	105
672	0.48913	135	39	102	2303	0.503597	210	180	27
679	0.501661	151	64	86	2306	0.494737	188	143	49
683	0.488798	240	254	−3	2333	0.494595	183	133	54
711	0.566	137	5	100	2376	0.643	160	12	77
723	0.561	142	16	95	2396	0.491525	232	235	5
736	0.5	169	101	68	2410	0.513587	189	131	48
753	0.504425	228	215	9	2437	0.489189	181	133	56
771	0.486076	192	158	45	2467	0.503086	163	87	74
772	0.489703	214	200	23	2483	0.539185	172	82	65
781	0.487603	177	126	60	2488	0.542274	186	106	51
816	0.497297	184	133	53	2496	0.522099	189	125	48
821	0.493369	186	140	51	2501	0.496711	151	67	86
824	0.492958	175	118	62	2530	0.495468	164	94	73
874	0.553531	243	202	−6	2532	0.491667	236	243	1
919	0.504032	125	11	112	2538	0.501887	133	28	104
1129	0.5	186	135	51	2581	0.486141	228	232	9
1179	0.488701	173	117	64	2585	0.524	131	13	106
1185	0.571	348	372	−111	2612	0.504792	158	76	79
1187	0.510989	186	127	51	2618	0.489028	156	82	81
1249	0.497222	179	123	58	2717	0.555556	190	105	47
1274	0.502	251	263	−14	2732	0.571	140	8	97
1315	0.514368	179	111	58	2751	0.490667	184	138	53
1391	0.494005	206	180	31	2786	0.562	140	12	97
1401	0.490446	154	77	83	2831	0.603	155	20	82
1411	0.491803	180	129	57	2853	0.52214	283	305	−46
1444	0.495238	156	78	81	2861	0.522822	252	245	−15
1458	0.5	166	95	71	2876	0.635	223	114	14
1478	0.558074	197	116	40	2877	0.519651	238	221	−1

Table 1. *Cont.*

Comp.	Similarity	SA	SB	SC	Comp.	Similarity	SA	SB	SC
1587	0.485849	206	187	31	2879	0.7	168	3	69
1595	0.547414	127	−5	110	2884	0.486425	215	205	22
1604	0.489189	181	133	56	2894	0.494279	216	200	21
1642	0.603	225	136	12	2907	0.488889	220	213	17
1651	0.586	309	290	−72	2918	0.490028	172	114	65
1662	0.507576	134	27	103	2959	0.489362	230	233	7

SA: The number bits in both **SAM** and the test set. **SB**: The number bits in the test set, but not **SAM**. **SC**: The number bits in **SAM** but not the test set.

2.2. Molecular Similarity

The connection between chemical structures and biological activities of different compounds has always been an interesting area for research [48]. Consequently, the implementation of different molecular similarity strategies in drug design and development have been competently increased effectively [49]. Many descriptors have been considered in molecular similarity studies.

The examined descriptors are of a molecular type, such as molecular weight (M.W.) [50], hydrogen bond donors (HBA) [51], hydrogen bond acceptors (HBD) [52], partition coefficient (ALog p), which is the ratio of the concentration of a substance in the lipid phase to the concentration in the aqueous phase when the two concentrations are at equilibrium [53], number of rotatable bonds [54], number of rings, and aromatic rings [55], as well as the molecular fractional polar surface area (MFPSA) [56]. The examined compound is represented as a binary array (number of binary bits) to be computed.

The mentioned descriptors were calculated for the FDA-approved drugs then compared with the co-crystallized ligand of 2′OMTase (**SAM**) using Discovery studio software.

Figure 1 represented the co-crystalized ligand (**SAM**) (red ball), compounds with good similarities (green balls), and compounds with diminished similarities (blue balls). The degree of molecular likeness or similarity between two compounds depends on a similarity coefficient that is utilized to compute a quantitative score. That calculated score is equivalent to the degree of similarity and is based on the computed values of several structural descriptors. Similarity between two compounds is inversely proportional to the calculated distance between them in the descriptor space [57]. In this work, the distances between the several descriptors were computed to determine descriptor similarity among test compounds and **SAM** [58]. The computed distances describe the shortest distance between two points. Typed graph distances (Figure 1) show the overall similarity of behavior of the FDA-approved drugs compared to **SAM**. The study preferred 26 compounds among the most suitable 30 metabolites (Figures 1 and 2, and Table 2).

2.3. Docking Studies

Docking studies of the tested compounds were conducted using the MOE (Molecular Operating Environment) software [58] to understand the proposed binding mode and the orientations of such compounds with the prospective target 2′OMTase (PDB ID: 6W4H)).

The active site of 2′OMTase consists of some crucial amino acids which can form hydrogen bonds with the active ligands. These amino acids include: Asn6841, Gly6879, Gly6869, Asp6928, Asp6897, Met6929, and Cys6913. In addition, there are some hydrophobic amino acids which can be incorporated in hydrophobic attractions with the active ligand and the hydrophobic amnio acids such as Leu6898 and Met6929 (Figure 3).

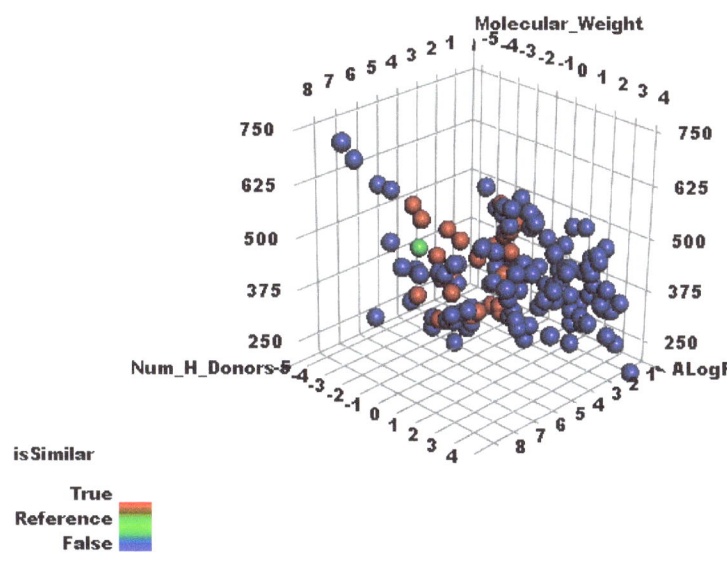

Figure 1. The molecular similarity of the examined compounds and **SAM**.

Table 2. Molecular descriptors of the examined 26 compounds and **SAM**.

Comp.	ALog p	MW	HBA	HBD	Rotatable Bonds	Rings	Aromatic Rings	MFPSA	Minimum Distance
SAM	−4.25	399.45	9	4	7	3	2	0.483	0
50	−1.38	297.27	9	4	3	3	2	0.508	0.768
56	−1.38	365.21	11	5	4	3	2	0.602	0.738
152	−0.77	287.21	8	3	5	2	2	0.502	0.836
186	−1.31	285.23	8	4	2	3	2	0.52	0.884
190	−1.04	435.43	11	4	7	2	1	0.576	0.874
214	−0.17	395.41	9	4	5	3	1	0.577	0.91
241	−1.88	267.24	8	4	2	3	2	0.539	0.877
310	−1.88	267.24	8	4	2	3	2	0.539	0.877
1129	−2.81	476.49	11	1	7	4	2	0.624	0.896
1187	−2.39	362.38	5	4	6	3	1	0.414	0.801
1444	−0.64	383.4	9	3	5	3	1	0.56	0.874
1478	−3.74	434.45	9	3	7	3	2	0.316	0.478
1913	−3.05	511.5	12	5	9	3	2	0.545	0.67
1995	−0.99	482.51	7	2	6	3	2	0.442	0.796
2017	−2.16	365.24	12	6	4	3	2	0.655	0.856
2036	−1.59	440.48	11	2	7	4	2	0.594	0.781
2042	−2.09	285.26	9	5	2	3	2	0.589	0.874
2176	−1.93	390.35	10	5	4	4	3	0.491	0.838
2376	−1.32	269.26	8	4	2	3	2	0.54	0.917
2396	−4.6	497.5	9	4	7	4	1	0.484	0.705
2467	−2.12	405.39	9	2	5	3	1	0.628	0.87

Table 2. *Cont.*

Comp.	ALog p	MW	HBA	HBD	Rotatable Bonds	Rings	Aromatic Rings	MFPSA	Minimum Distance
2532	−0.73	469.53	7	4	6	4	2	0.266	0.909
2612	−1.98	460.77	10	4	8	2	2	0.572	0.594
2732	−0.82	299.22	8	3	5	3	2	0.504	0.752
2831	−0.98	305.23	9	4	5	2	2	0.55	0.76
2879	−1.26	294.31	8	3	3	3	2	0.395	0.846

ALog p: lipid–water partition coefficient, MWt: molecular weight, HBA: hydrogen bond acceptor, HBD: hydrogen bond donor, Rotatable bonds: any single non-ring bond, attached to a non-terminal, non-hydrogen atom, Rings: non-aromatic rings, MFPSA: molecular fractional polar surface area, Minimum Distance: the shortest distance between a tested compound and the reference one.

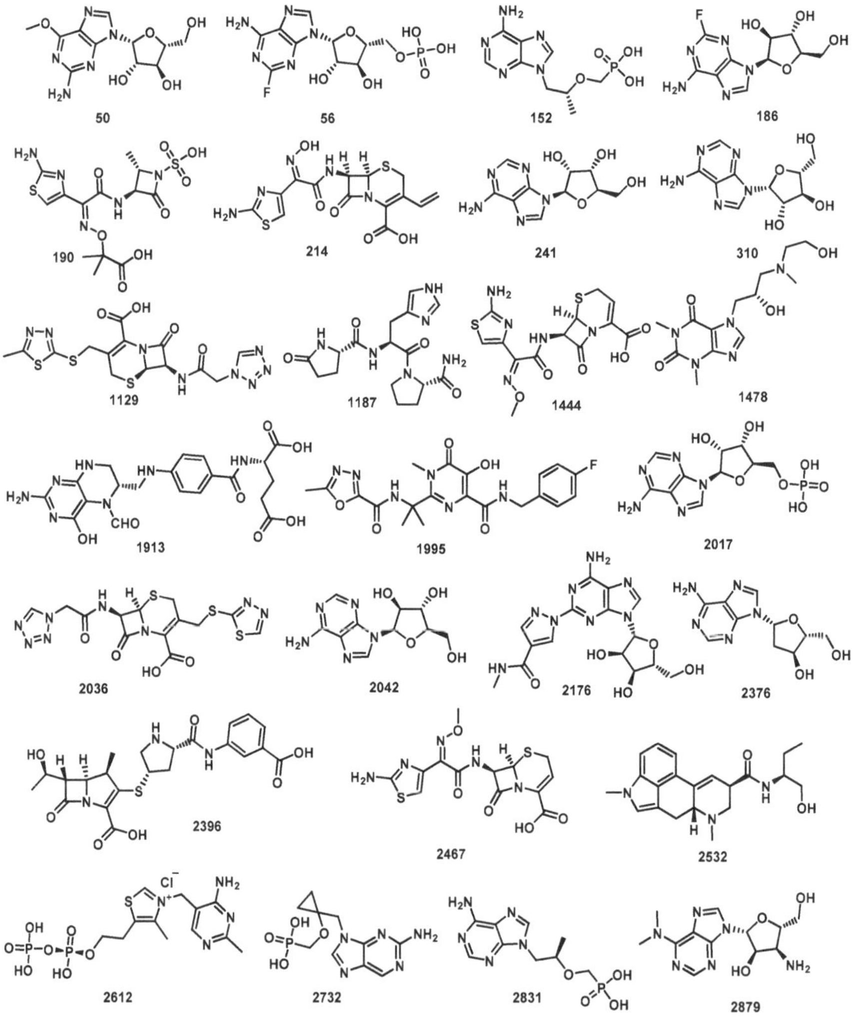

Figure 2. Twenty-six compounds with good molecular similarity with the co-crystallized ligand (**SAM**) of 2′OMTase (PDB ID: (6W4H).

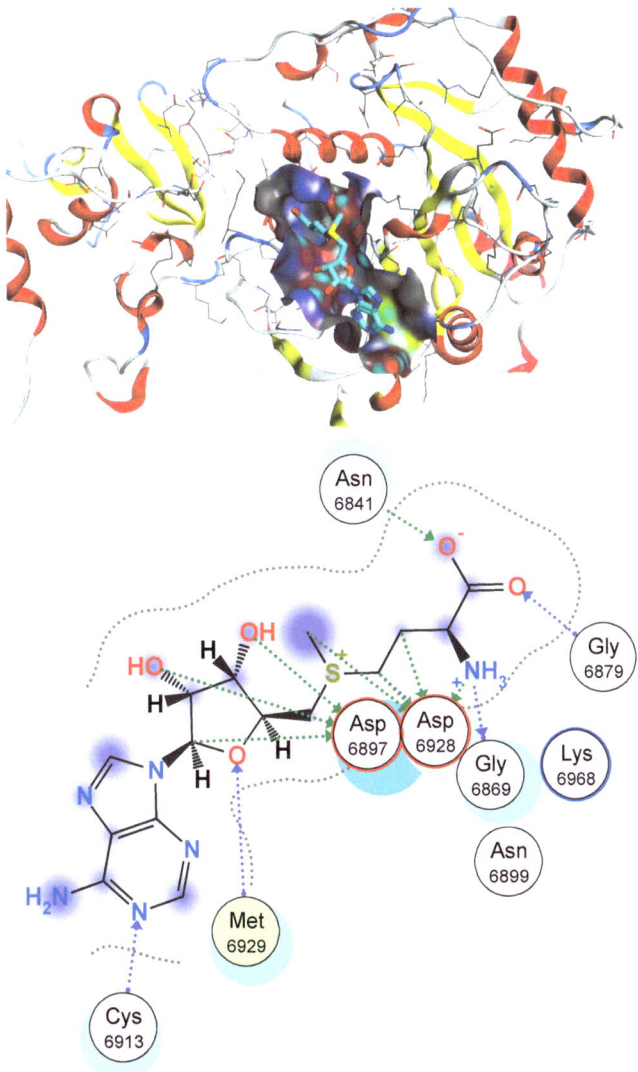

Figure 3. Active site (3D and 2D) of 2′OMTase (PDB ID: (6W4H)).

The co-crystalized ligand s-adenosylmethionine (**SAM**) was used as a reference compound. First, the validation process was carried out to confirm the validity of the docking algorithm in obtaining accurate docking results. This was achieved by redocking the co-crystallized ligand (**SAM**) with 2′OMTase. The obtained low values of root mean square deviation (RMSD = 1.15 Å) between the native and redocked pose, in addition to the symmetrical superimposition in orientation between both the native (turquoise) and redocked (magenta) co-crystallized poses in Figure 4, guaranteed the valid performance of the docking protocol [36,38], in addition to the docking algorithm's capability to obtain the reported binding mode of the co-crystallized ligand S-adenosylmethionine (**SAM**) [59].

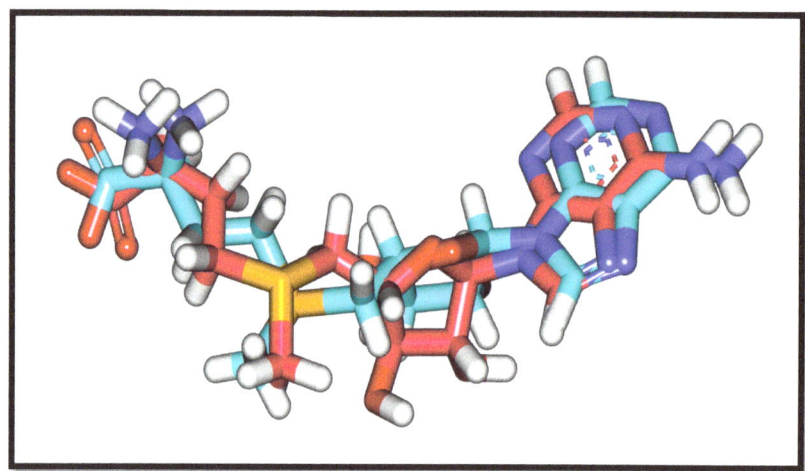

Figure 4. Alignment of the co-crystallized ligand (turquoise) and the docking pose (rose) of the same ligand (**SAM**) in the active site of 2′OMTase.

In comparing the tested compounds, the binding free energy (ΔG) between the docked molecules and the active site, and also the proper binding mode, were properly considered. The estimated (ΔG) (binding free energies) of the investigated drugs and the reference molecule (**SAM**) against the 2′OMTase are presented in Table 3.

Table 3. Binding free energies (calculated ΔG in kcal/mol) of the examined compounds and ligand SAM against 2′OMTase.

Comp.	Name	ΔG [kcal/mol]
SAM	S-Adenosylmethionine	−21.52
50	Arranon (Nelarabine)	−13.84
56	Fludara (Fludarabine)	−15.53
152	Tenofovir (PMPA)	−13.58
186	Fludarabine	−14.19
190	Azactam (aztreonam)	−14.88
214	Cefdinir (cefdinir)	−15.41
241	Adenosine	−14.09
310	VIRA-A (vidarabine)	−14.10
1129	Cefazolin	−16.66
1187	Protirelin	−18.68
1444	Ceftizoxime	−10.99
1478	Xanthinol Nicotinate	−16.19
1913	Calcium folinate	−19.09
1995	Raltegravir	−21.07
2017	Adenosine 5′-monophosphate	−15.34
2036	Ceftezole	−15.21
2042	Vidarabine	−13.41
2176	Regadenoson	−18.54

Table 3. *Cont.*

Comp.	Name	ΔG [kcal/mol]
2376	2′-Deoxyadenosine	−13.16
2396	Ertapenem	−20.73
2467	Ceftizoxime	−13.63
2532	Methylergometrine	−20.46
2612	Thiamine pyrophosphate hydrochloride	−18.03
2732	Besifovir	−13.47
2831	Tenofovir	−14.36
2879	Puromycin aminonucleoside	−15.33

The predicted binding mode of the redocked ligand (**SAM**) yielded an affinity value of −21.52 kcal/mol. It interacted with its 6-amino-purin moiety and formed one hydrogen bond with Asp6912, in addition to hydrophobic interactions with Leu6898 and Met6929. Moreover, the di hydroxy tetrahydrofuran moiety formed two hydrogen bonds with Tyr6930, and the sulfur atom was involved in electrostatic interaction with Asp6928. Additionally, the terminal NH_2 group was found to form one hydrogen bond with Gly6869, and two electrostatic interactions with Asp6928. Finally, the terminal carboxylic group formed one hydrogen bond with Gly6879 (Figure 5).

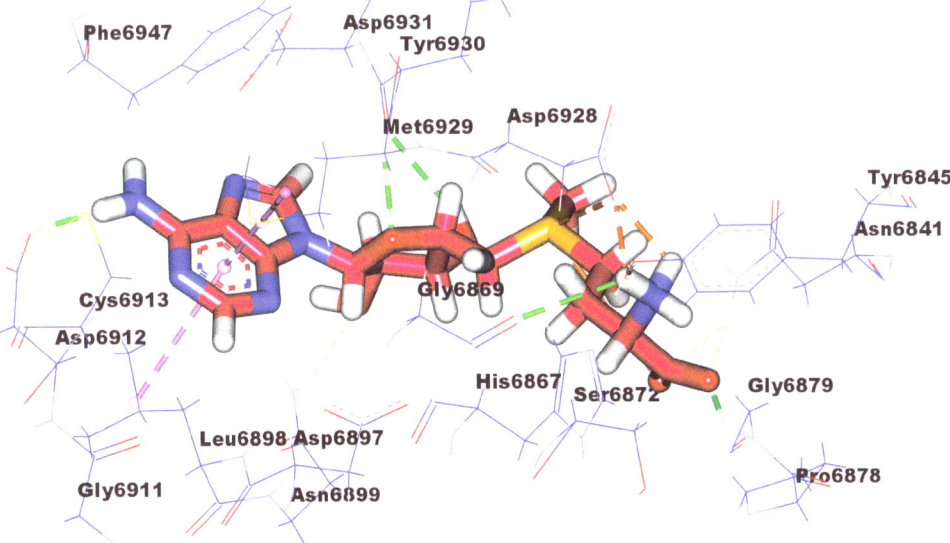

Figure 5. *Cont.*

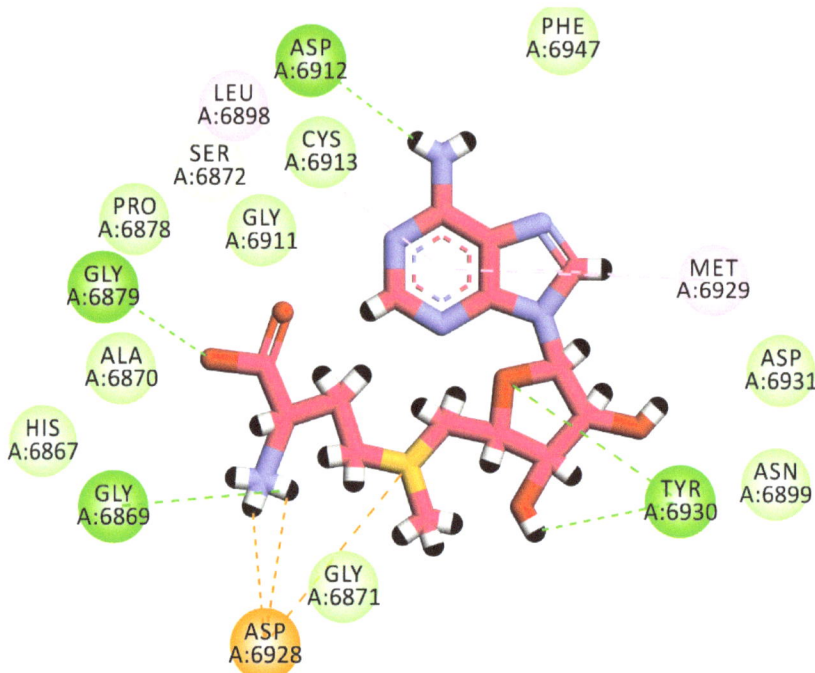

Figure 5. 3D and 2D binding mode of the redocked ligand (**SAM**) in the active site of the target protein.

From the tested compounds, seven members showed good binding mode with high binding energy. These compounds are **1187** (Protirelin), **1913** (Calcium folinate), **1995** (Raltegravir), **2176** (Regadenoson), **2396** (Ertapenem), **2532** (Methylergometrine), and **2612** (Methylergometrine).

Compound **1187** has a docking score of −18.68 kcal/mol and formed four hydrogen bonds with the crucial amino acids in the active site of the 2′OMTase enzyme. The pyrrolidin-2-one moiety formed two hydrogen bonds with Asp6928 and Lys6968 via its NH and C=O groups, respectively. Furthermore, the NH group of the central amide moiety formed one hydrogen bond with Tyr6930. Moreover, the (S)-pyrrolidine-2-carboxamide moiety formed one hydrogen with Tyr6930 and two hydrophobic bonds with Met6929 and Leu6898 (Figure 6).

Compound **1913** has a docking score of −19.09 kcal/mol, forming six hydrogen bonds within the active site. The 2-amino-4-hydroxy-7,8-dihydropteridine-5(6H)-carbaldehyde moiety formed three hydrogen bonds with Cys6913, Gly6911, and Asp6912 via its NH_2, OH groups, and the hetero nitrogen atom at 3-position. In addition, the glutamic acid moiety formed three hydrogen bonds with Asn6841, Gly6879, and Gly6871. Moreover, a carboxylate group of glutamic acid moiety formed one electrostatic interaction with Asp6873 (Figure 7).

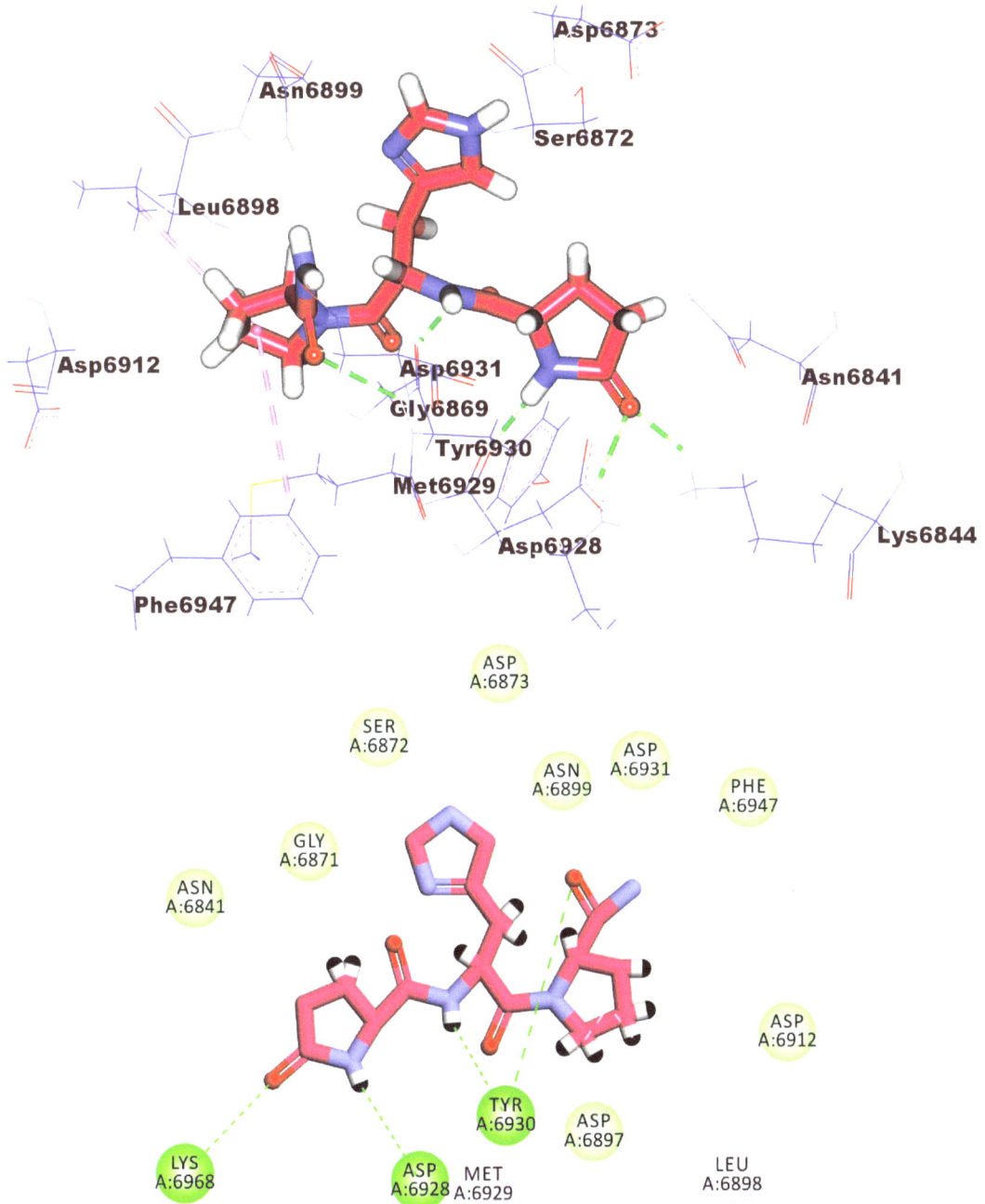

Figure 6. 3D and 2D binding mode of compound **1187** in the active site of the target protein.

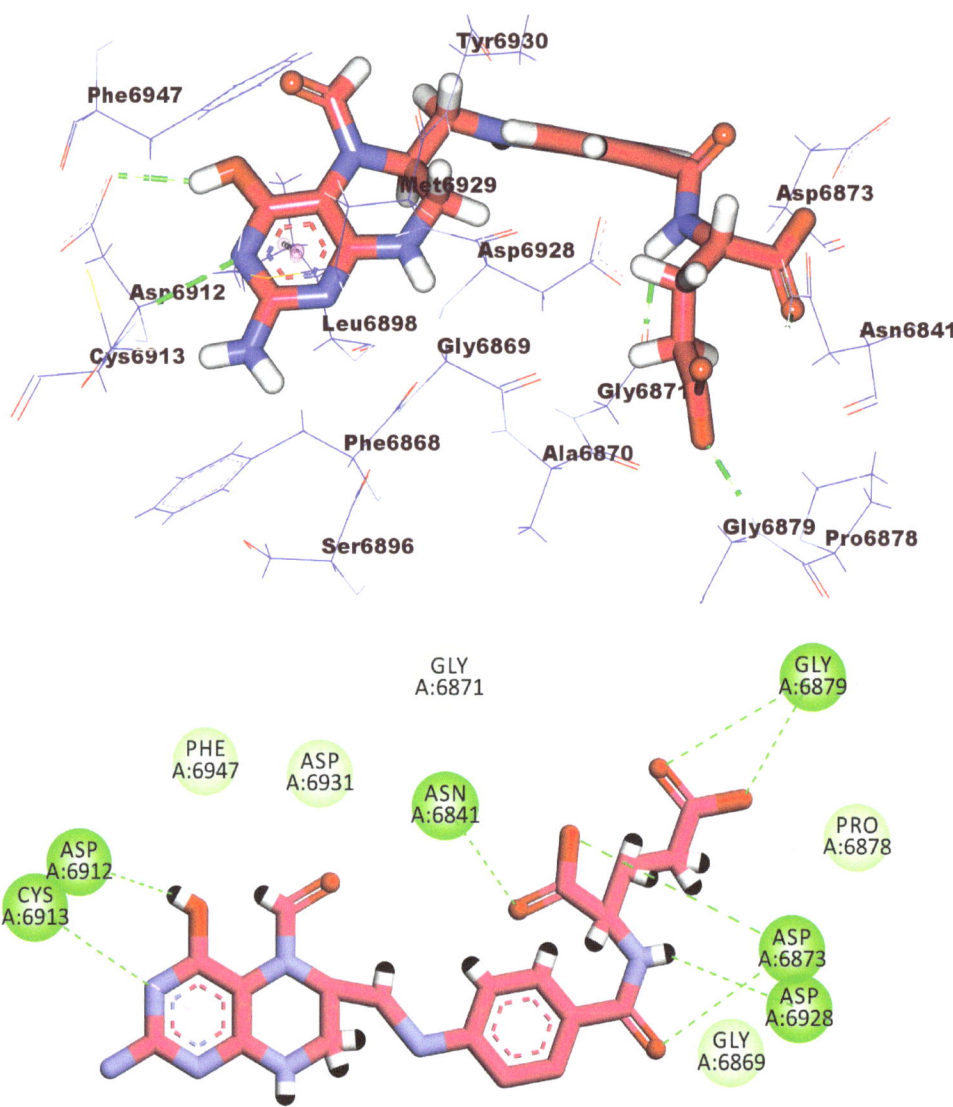

Figure 7. 3D and 2D binding mode of compound **1913** in the active site of the target protein.

With a docking score of −21.07 kcal/mol, compound **1995** fit well into the active site of the 2′OMTase enzyme and formed four hydrogen bonds. The fluorobenzene formed one hydrogen bond with Cys6913 and one hydrophobic interaction with Leu6898. The carbonyl group of the amide moiety formed one hydrogen bond with Tyr6930. The carbonyl group of 5-hydroxy-3-methylpyrimidin-4(3H)-one moiety formed one hydrogen bond with Asn6899. In addition, the 5-hydroxy-3-methylpyrimidin-4(3H)-one moiety formed hydrophobic bond with Gly6871. The NH group of 2-methyl-1,3,4-oxadiazole moiety formed one hydrogen bond with Lys6844 (Figure 8).

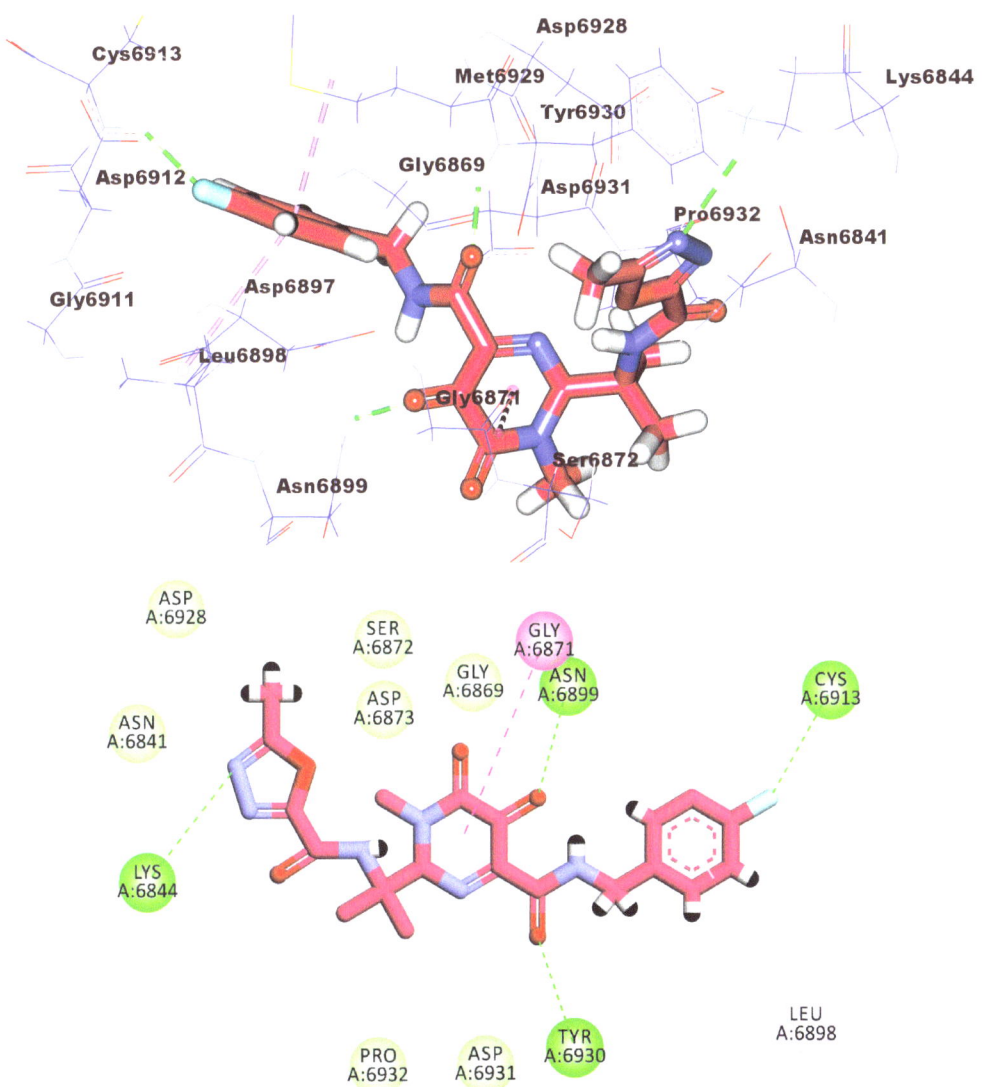

Figure 8. 3D and 2D binding mode of compound **1995** in the active site of the target protein.

Compound **2176** showed a binding energy of −18.54 kcal/mol. This compound formed four hydrogen bonds in the active site of the target protein. The ribose sugar moiety formed three hydrogen bonds with Gly6879, Ala6870, and Gly6871. Furthermore, the NH group of the 9H-purin-6-amine moiety formed a hydrogen bond with Ty6930. Moreover, the N-methyl-1H-pyrazole-4-carboxamide moiety was incorporated in hydrophobic interaction with Met6929 and one electrostatic interaction with Asp6897 (Figure 9).

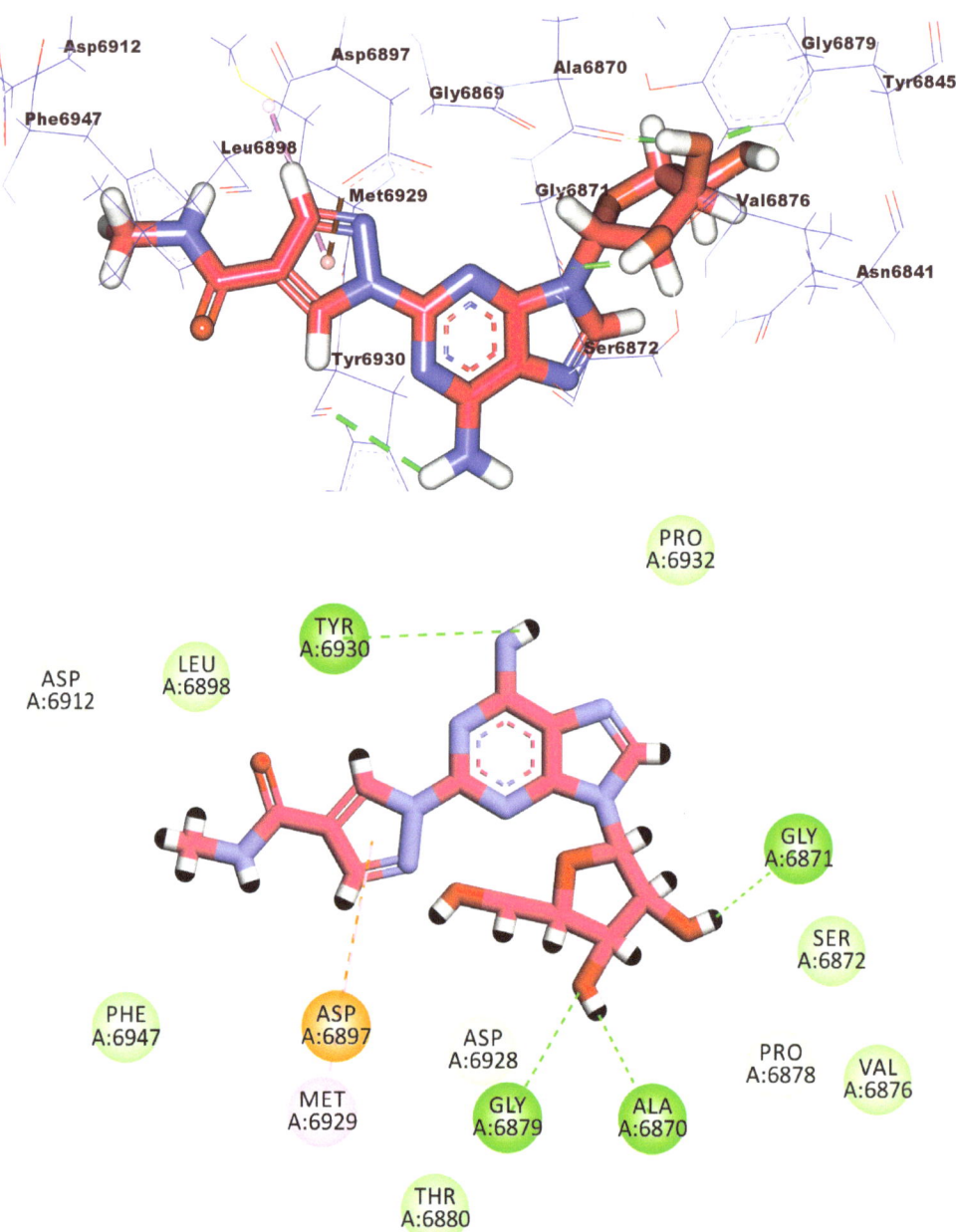

Figure 9. 3D and 2D binding mode of compound **2176** in the active site of the target protein.

Compound **2396** (Ertapenem) has a docking score of −20.73 kcal/mol and created five hydrogen bonds with the crucial amino acids in the active site of the 2′OMTase enzyme. The benzoic acid moiety formed one hydrogen bond with Cys6913 via its carboxylic group, and two hydrophobic interactions with Met6929 and Leu6898. Furthermore, the NH group formed another hydrogen bond with Asp6897. Moreover, the carboxylate group at 2-position of 1-azabicyclo[3.2.0]hept-2-ene moiety formed one hydrogen and one electrostatic bond with Asp6873. The terminal hydroxyl group formed two hydrogen bonds with Asp6928 and Gly6869 (Figure 10). Although Ertapenem showed a binding energy less than Raltegravir, it showed an ideal binding mode like that of the co-crystallized ligand (**SAM**). It occupied all sub pockets of the active site and bound the crucial amino acids. Accordingly, it was used for further in silico testing via MD simulations.

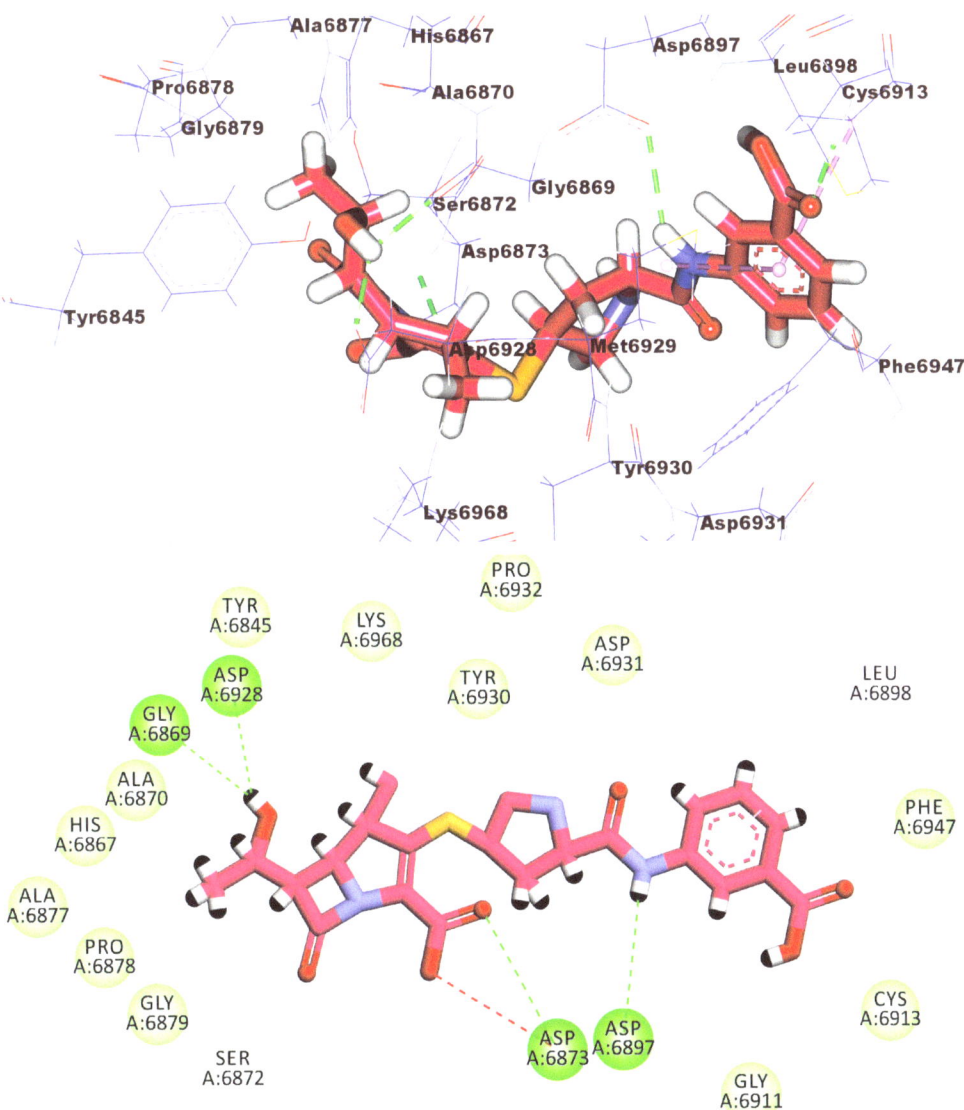

Figure 10. 3D and 2D binding mode of compound **2396** in the active site of the target protein.

The binding mode of compound **2532** (affinity value of −20.46 kcal/mol), which is extremely close to ligand **SAM**, revealed that the amide group formed two hydrogen bonds with fundamental amino acids Asp6928 and Gly6871. In addition, the OH group formed another hydrogen bond with the amino acid Asn6841. Furthermore, the terminal ethyl moiety was incorporated in hydrophobic interaction with His6867 and Tyr6845. The phenyl ring formed an electrostatic attraction with Asp6897 (Figure 11).

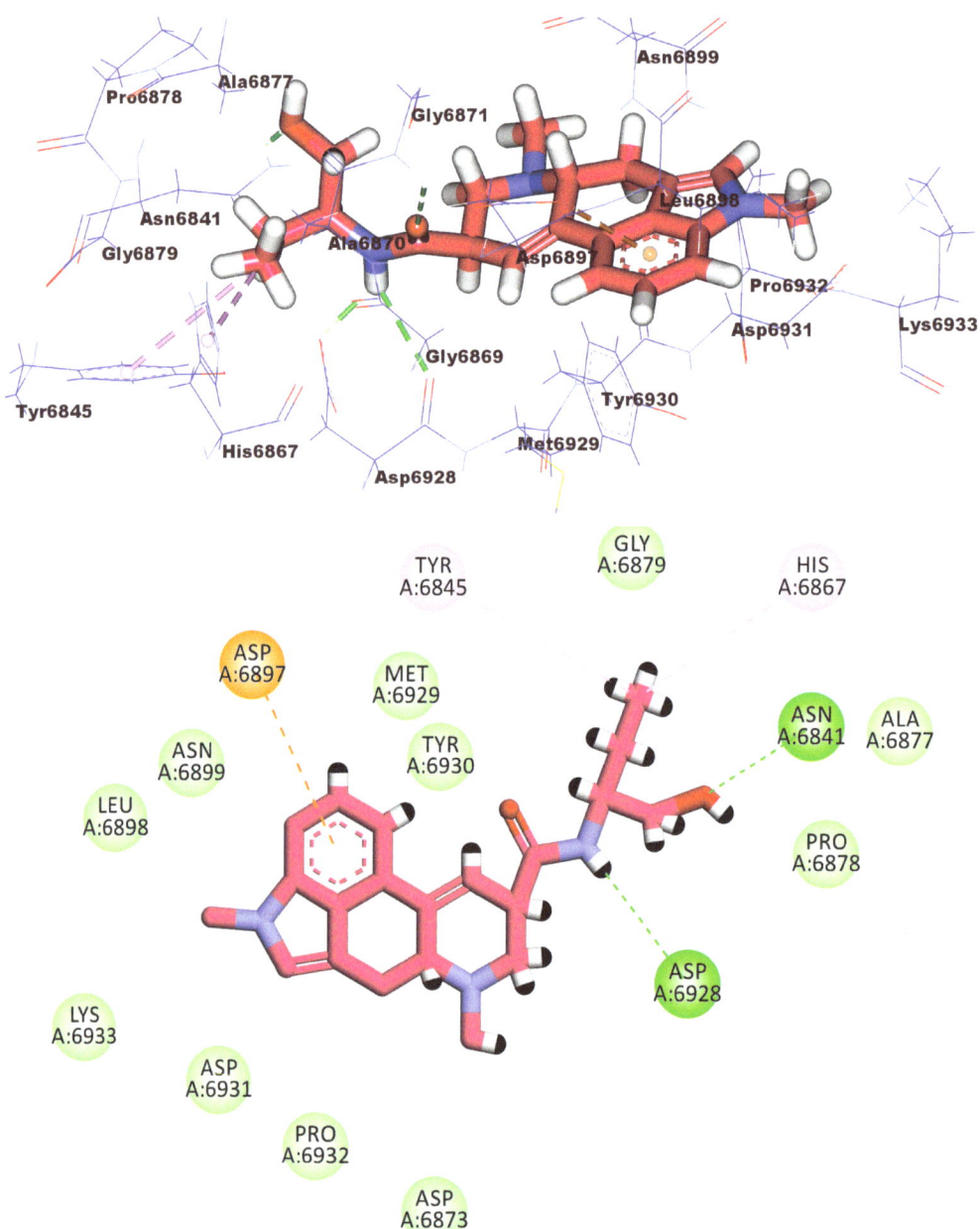

Figure 11. 3D and 2D binding mode of compound **2532** in the active site of the target protein.

As demonstrated in Figure 12, compound **2612** had a high potential binding affinity ($\Delta G = -18.03$ kcal/mol) with 2′OMTase enzyme active site. The strong binding affinity is assumed to be due to the formation of four hydrogen bonds in addition to many hydrophobic and electrostatic attractions. The terminal diphosphate moiety formed four hydrogen bonds with Gly6871, and Asn6841. It also formed three electrostatic attractions with Asp6928. In addition, the 4-methylthiazol-3-ium moiety formed a hydrophobic interaction with Gly6871 and an electrostatic attraction with Asp6897. Furthermore, the 2-methylpyrimidin-4-amine moiety was incorporated in a hydrophobic attraction with Phe6947.

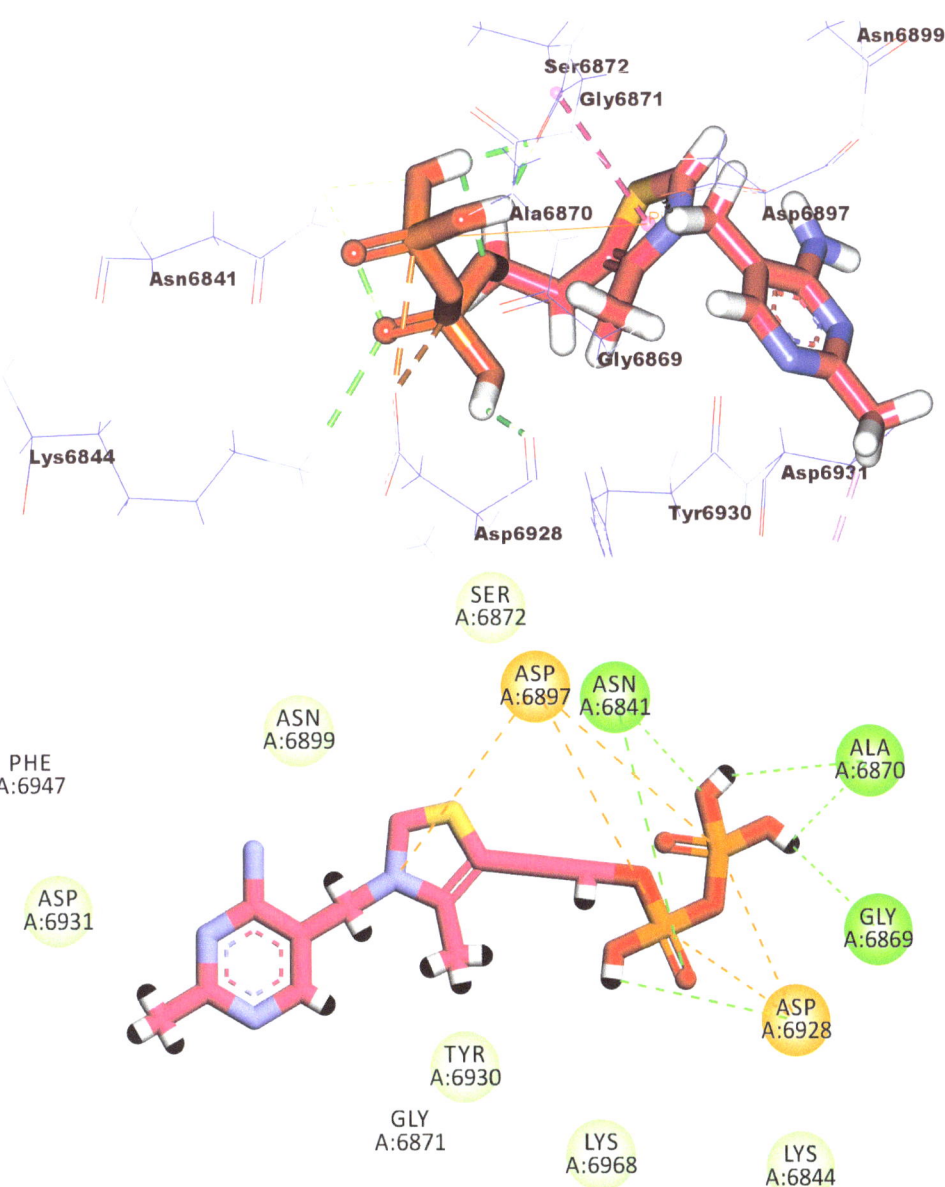

Figure 12. 3D and 2D binding mode of compound **2612** in the active site of the target protein.

2.4. Molecular Dynamic Simulation

Molecular dynamics (MD) simulations studies can be applied to examine almost every kind of biomacromolecule (protein, nucleic acid, or carbohydrate) of biological significance [60]. The MD experiments can afford abundant information regarding the dynamic structural of the studied system [61]. Additionally, it contributes large amounts of energetic data. Such data are essential to understand the structure–function relationship of the examined ligand, its target protein, as well as the protein–ligand interactions. Correspondingly, MD studies could be a vital guide in the drug design and discovery processes [62].

The dynamic, as well as conformational shifts of backbone atoms of 2'OMTase, Ertapenem in addition to 2'OMTase—Ertapenem complex, were estimated through the calculation of the root mean square deviation (RMSD) to distinguish the stability of the examined molecules before and after binding. RMSD investigation demonstrates both of conformational and dynamics changes [63] that occur after binding. Excitingly, the 2'OMTase—Ertapenem complex demonstrated low RMSD values with slight fluctuations from 40–70 ns~ and was stabilized later until the end of the study (Figure 13A) Fortunately, this slight fluctuation did not affect the integrity of the 2'OMTase—Ertapenem complex as the next experiments (R_g and SASA) did not record major changes in this time. However, the H-binding showed that the number of H-bonds decreased in this period (40–70 ns), from 3–4 bonds to 2 bonds. The study demonstrated that the number of H-bonds became 3–4 again after 70 ns. The flexibility of the evaluated complex was measured in the terms of RMSF to identify the fluctuated region of 2'OMTase during the 100 ns of the simulation. Favorably, the binding of Ertapenem does not make 2'OMTase very flexible (Figure 13B). The compactness of the 2'OMTase—Ertapenem complex was investigated by the computation of radius of gyration (R_g) of the evaluated enzyme. Complementarily, the Rg exhibited was noticed to be of lower value during the 100 ns of the experiment compared to the starting time (Figure 13C). In a similar manner, SASA (solvent accessible surface area) denotes the interaction between 2'OMTase—Ertapenem complex, and the surrounding solvents was measured. SASA value is an excellent indicator to the conformational changes that occurred during the simulation experiment because of binding interactions. Of note, the surface area of 2'OMTase (Figure 13D) displayed a considerable reduction in SASA values through the simulation time compared to the starting point. Finally, hydrogen bonding, as an essential factor in the binding of 2'OMTase—Ertapenem complex, was estimated. The greatest number of H-bonds that formed between 2'OMTase—Ertapenem complex was up to three H-bonds (Figure 13E).

2.5. Molecular Mechanics Poisson-Boltzmann Surface Area (MM-PBSA) Studies

The binding free energy of 2'OMTase—Ertapenem complex was investigated in the last 20 ns of the MD run with an interval of 100 ps from the produced MD trajectories. The MM/PBSA method was utilized with the MmPbSaStat.py script to compute the average free binding energy as well as its standard deviation/error. Interestingly, as shown in Figure 14A, Ertapenem demonstrated a low binding free energy with a value of −43 KJ/mol (equivalent to −10.28 kcal/mol) with 2'OMTase. The share of the different amino acid residues of 2'OMTase in respect of the binding energy compared to the binding with Ertapenem. Total binding free energy decomposing of the 2'OMTase—Ertapenem complex into per residue share energy was achieved. The following amino acid residues of 2'OMTase, GLY-6871, LEU-6898, ASP-6928, MET-6829, and GLU-7001, contributed the binding energy with values that are more than −3 KJ/mol (Figure 14B).

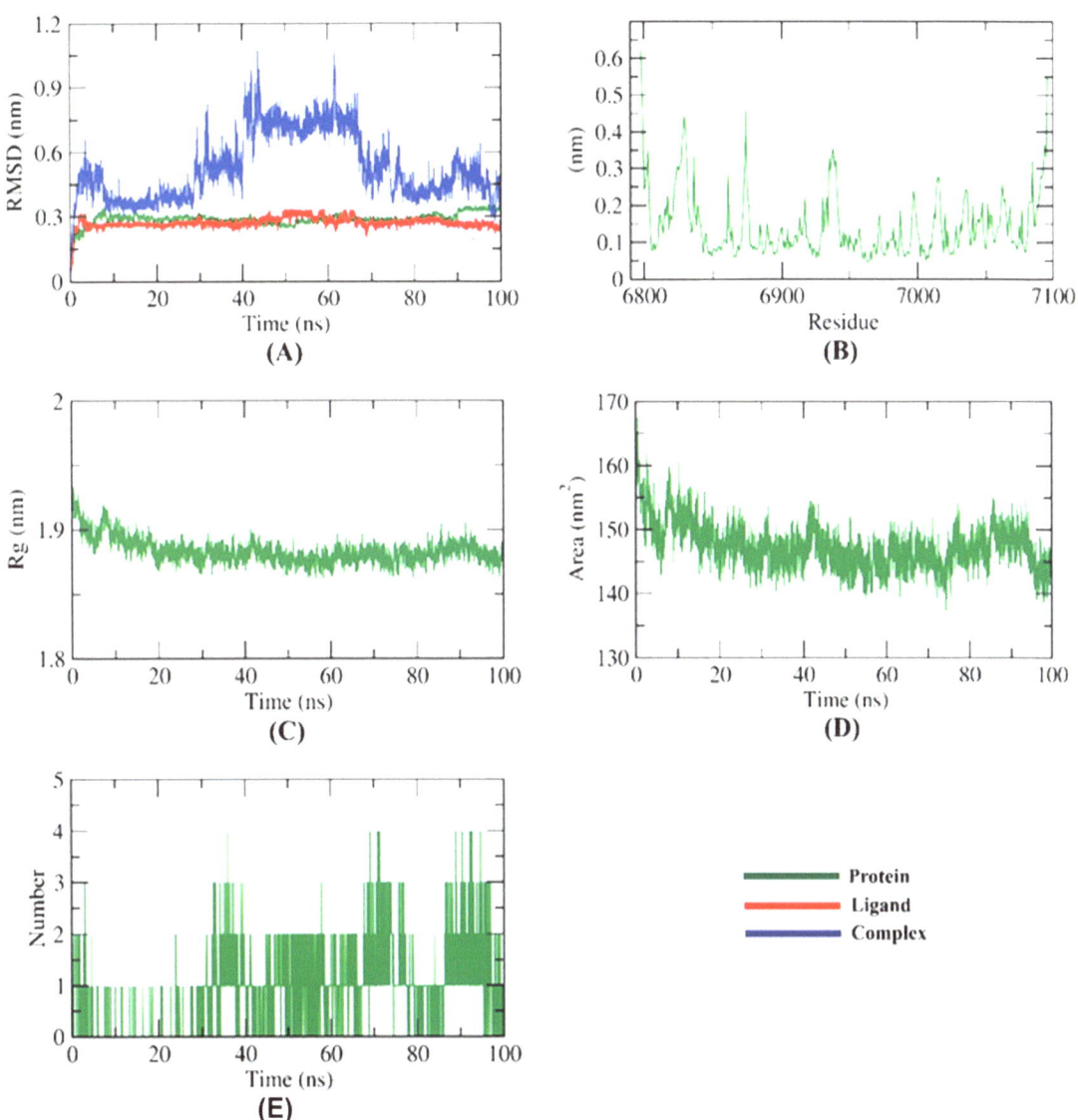

Figure 13. Results of M D simulations of 2′OMTase—Ertapenem complex; (**A**) RMSD, (**B**) RMSF, (**C**) R_g, (**D**) SASA, and (**E**) H-bonding.

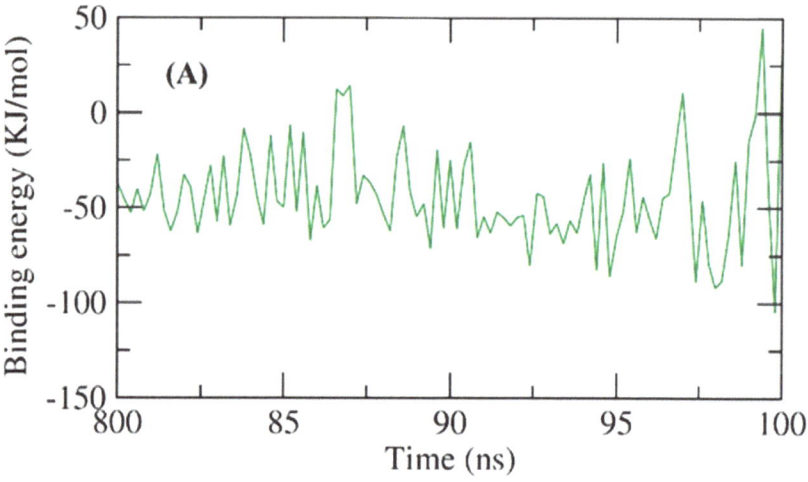
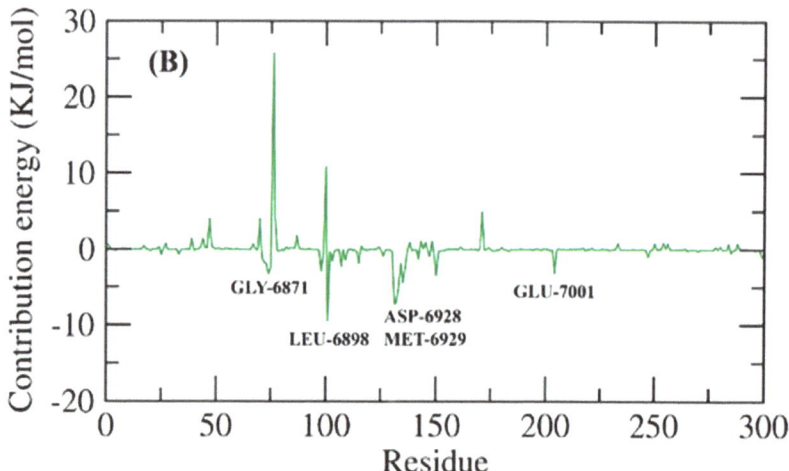

Figure 14. MM-PBSA study of 2′OMTase—Ertapenem; (**A**): total binding free energy, (**B**): analyzed binding free energy per amino acid residue.

3. Method

3.1. Molecular Similarity Detection

Discovery studio 4.0 software was used (see method part in Supplementary Materials).

3.2. Fingerprint Studies

Discovery studio 4.0 software was used (see method part in Supplementary Materials).

3.3. Docking Studies

Docking studies were performed against target enzymes using Discovery studio software [64] (see method part in Supplementary Materials).

3.4. Molecular Dynamics Simulation

The system was prepared using the web-based CHARMM-GUI [65–67] interface utilizing CHARMM36 force field [68] and NAMD 2.13 [69] package. The TIP3P explicit solvation model was used (see Supplementary Materials).

3.5. MM-PBSA Studies

The g_mmpbsa package of GROMACS was utilized to calculate the MM/PBSA (See Supplementary Materials).

4. Conclusions

Seven FDA-approved compounds (Protirelin, (**1187**), Calcium folinate (**1913**), Raltegravir (**1995**), Regadenoson (**2176**), Ertapenem (**2396**), Methylergometrine (**2532**), and Thiamine pyrophosphate hydrochloride (**2612**), out of 3009 were elected as the strongest 2′OMTase inhibitors. The selection of compounds was based on a multistep in silico study. The utilized studies included molecular fingerprints and structure similarity studies against **SAM**, the co-crystallized ligand of the targeted enzyme in addition to molecular docking studies. Ertapenem (**2396**) was subjected to MD simulation studies (RMSD, RMSF, R_g, SASA, and H-bonding) for 100 ns, confirming the excellent binding. These encouraging results could be a step to discover an effective cure against COVID-19 through further in vitro and in vivo studies for the pointed candidates.

Supplementary Materials: The following supporting information can be downloaded at: https://www.mdpi.com/article/10.3390/molecules27072287/s1, The method of Fingerprints; Molecular Similarity; Docking; Molecular dynamics; and MMPBSA studies.

Author Contributions: Conceptualization, I.H.E. and A.M.M.; Funding acquisition, B.A.A.; Project administration, I.H.E. and A.M.M.; Software, I.H.E., M.S.A., A.M.S. and E.B.E.; Writing—review and editing, E.B.E., B.A.A., A.-A.M.M.E.-A. and A.M.M. All authors have read and agreed to the published version of the manuscript.

Funding: This research was funded by Princess Nourah Bint Abdulrahman University Researchers Supporting Project number (PNURSP2022R142), Princess Nourah Bint Abdulrahman University, Riyadh, Saudi Arabia.

Institutional Review Board Statement: Not applicable.

Informed Consent Statement: Not applicable.

Data Availability Statement: All data is contained in the published article.

Conflicts of Interest: The authors declare no conflict of interest.

Sample Availability: Samples of the compoundsre not available from the authors.

References

1. WHO. WHO Coronavirus (COVID-19) Dashboard. Available online: https://covid19.who.int/ (accessed on 19 January 2022).
2. Wang, Q.; Yang, L.; Jin, H.; Lin, L. Vaccination against COVID-19: A systematic review and meta-analysis of acceptability and its predictors. *Prev. Med.* **2021**, *150*, 106694. [CrossRef] [PubMed]
3. Chan, H.S.; Shan, H.; Dahoun, T.; Vogel, H.; Yuan, S. Advancing drug discovery via artificial intelligence. *Trends Pharmacol. Sci.* **2019**, *40*, 592–604. [CrossRef] [PubMed]
4. Pushpakom, S.; Iorio, F.; Eyers, P.A.; Escott, K.J.; Hopper, S.; Wells, A.; Doig, A.; Guilliams, T.; Latimer, J.; McNamee, C. Drug repurposing: Progress, challenges and recommendations. *Nat. Rev. Drug Discov.* **2019**, *18*, 41–58. [CrossRef]
5. Sleire, L.; Førde, H.E.; Netland, I.A.; Leiss, L.; Skeie, B.S.; Enger, P.Ø. Drug repurposing in cancer. *Pharmacol. Res.* **2017**, *124*, 74–91. [CrossRef] [PubMed]
6. Singh, T.U.; Parida, S.; Lingaraju, M.C.; Kesavan, M.; Kumar, D.; Singh, R.K. Drug repurposing approach to fight COVID-19. *Pharmacol. Rep.* **2020**, *72*, 1479–1508. [CrossRef] [PubMed]
7. Hong, J.; Bang, M. Anti-inflammatory strategies for schizophrenia: A review of evidence for therapeutic applications and drug repurposing. *Clin. Psychopharmacol. Neurosci.* **2020**, *18*, 10. [CrossRef] [PubMed]
8. Konreddy, A.K.; Rani, G.U.; Lee, K.; Choi, Y. Recent drug-repurposing-driven advances in the discovery of novel antibiotics. *Curr. Med. Chem.* **2019**, *26*, 5363–5388. [CrossRef]

9. Shirley, D.-A.; Sharma, I.; Warren, C.A.; Moonah, S. Drug repurposing of the alcohol abuse medication disulfiram as an anti-parasitic agent. *Front. Cell. Infect. Microbiol.* **2021**, *11*, 165. [CrossRef]
10. Trivedi, J.; Mohan, M.; Byrareddy, S.N. Drug repurposing approaches to combating viral infections. *J. Clin. Med.* **2020**, *9*, 3777. [CrossRef]
11. Westbrook, J.D.; Burley, S.K. How structural biologists and the Protein Data Bank contributed to recent FDA new drug approvals. *Structure* **2019**, *27*, 211–217. [CrossRef]
12. Grimme, S.; Schreiner, P.R. Computational chemistry: The fate of current methods and future challenges. *Angew. Chem. Int. Ed.* **2018**, *57*, 4170–4176. [CrossRef] [PubMed]
13. Amin, S.; Banerjee, S.; Singh, S.; Qureshi, I.A.; Gayen, S.; Jha, T. First structure–activity relationship analysis of SARS-CoV-2 virus main protease (Mpro) inhibitors: An endeavor on COVID-19 drug discovery. *Mol. Divers.* **2021**, *25*, 1827–1838. [CrossRef] [PubMed]
14. Ranjan, S.; Devarapalli, R.; Kundu, S.; Saha, S.; Deolka, S.; Vangala, V.R.; Reddy, C.M. Isomorphism: Molecular similarity to crystal structure similarity'in multicomponent forms of analgesic drugs tolfenamic and mefenamic acid. *IUCrJ* **2020**, *7*, 173–183. [CrossRef] [PubMed]
15. Baidya, A.T.; Ghosh, K.; Amin, S.A.; Adhikari, N.; Nirmal, J.; Jha, T.; Gayen, S. In silico modelling, identification of crucial molecular fingerprints, and prediction of new possible substrates of human organic cationic transporters 1 and 2. *New J. Chem.* **2020**, *44*, 4129–4143. [CrossRef]
16. Shi, Y. Support vector regression-based QSAR models for prediction of antioxidant activity of phenolic compounds. *Sci. Rep.* **2021**, *11*, 8806. [CrossRef] [PubMed]
17. Idris, M.O.; Yekeen, A.A.; Alakanse, O.S.; Durojaye, O.A. Computer-aided screening for potential TMPRSS2 inhibitors: A combination of pharmacophore modeling, molecular docking and molecular dynamics simulation approaches. *J. Biomol. Struct. Dyn.* **2021**, *39*, 5638–5656. [CrossRef]
18. Lu, Y.; Li, M. A new computer model for evaluating the selective binding affinity of phenylalkylamines to T-Type Ca^{2+} channels. *Pharmaceuticals* **2021**, *14*, 141. [CrossRef]
19. Eissa, I.H.; Ibrahim, M.K.; Metwaly, A.M.; Belal, A.; Mehany, A.B.; Abdelhady, A.A.; Elhendawy, M.A.; Radwan, M.M.; ElSohly, M.A.; Mahdy, H.A. Design, molecular docking, in vitro, and in vivo studies of new quinazolin-4 (3H)-ones as VEGFR-2 inhibitors with potential activity against hepatocellular carcinoma. *Bioorgan. Chem.* **2021**, *107*, 104532. [CrossRef]
20. Zhanzhaxina, A.; Suleimen, Y.; Metwaly, A.M.; Eissa, I.H.; Elkaeed, E.B.; Suleimen, R.; Ishmuratova, M.; Akatan, K.; Luyten, W. In vitro and in silico cytotoxic and antibacterial activities of a diterpene from cousinia alata schrenk. *J. Chem.* **2021**, *2021*, 5542455. [CrossRef]
21. Jalmakhanbetova, R.; Elkaeed, E.B.; Eissa, I.H.; Metwaly, A.M.; Suleimen, Y.M. Synthesis and molecular docking of some grossgemin amino derivatives as tubulin inhibitors targeting colchicine binding site. *J. Chem.* **2021**, *2021*, 5586515. [CrossRef]
22. El-Adl, K.; El-Helby, A.-G.A.; Ayyad, R.R.; Mahdy, H.A.; Khalifa, M.M.; Elnagar, H.A.; Mehany, A.B.; Metwaly, A.M.; Elhendawy, M.A.; Radwan, M.M. Design, synthesis, and anti-proliferative evaluation of new quinazolin-4 (3H)-ones as potential VEGFR-2 inhibitors. *Biorgan. Med. Chem.* **2021**, *29*, 115872. [CrossRef] [PubMed]
23. Imieje, V.O.; Zaki, A.A.; Metwaly, A.M.; Eissa, I.H.; Elkaeed, E.B.; Ali, Z.; Khan, I.A.; Falodun, A. Antileishmanial derivatives of humulene from Asteriscus hierochunticus with in silico tubulin inhibition potential. *Rec. Nat. Prod.* **2021**, *16*, 150–171.
24. Rafi, M.O.; Al-Khafaji, K.; Tok, T.T.; Rahman, M.S. Computer-based identification of potential compounds from Salviae miltiorrhizae against Neirisaral adhesion A regulatory protein. *J. Biomol. Struct. Dyn.* **2020**, 1–13. [CrossRef] [PubMed]
25. Parmar, D.R.; Soni, J.Y.; Guduru, R.; Rayani, R.H.; Kusurkar, R.V.; Vala, A.G.; Talukdar, S.N.; Eissa, I.H.; Metwaly, A.M.; Khalil, A. Discovery of new anticancer thiourea-azetidine hybrids: Design, synthesis, in vitro antiproliferative, SAR, in silico molecular docking against VEGFR-2, ADMET, toxicity, and DFT studies. *Biorgan. Chem.* **2021**, *115*, 105206. [CrossRef]
26. El-Adl, K.; Sakr, H.M.; Yousef, R.G.; Mehany, A.B.; Metwaly, A.M.; Elhendawy, M.A.; Radwan, M.M.; ElSohly, M.A.; Abulkhair, H.S.; Eissa, I.H. Discovery of new quinoxaline-2 (1H)-one-based anticancer agents targeting VEGFR-2 as inhibitors: Design, synthesis, and anti-proliferative evaluation. *Biorgan. Chem.* **2021**, *114*, 105105. [CrossRef]
27. Suleimen, Y.M.; Metwaly, A.M.; Mostafa, A.E.; Elkaeed, E.B.; Liu, H.-W.; Basnet, B.B.; Suleimen, R.N.; Ishmuratova, M.Y.; Turdybekov, K.M.; Van Heckc, K. Isolation, Crystal Structure, and In Silico Aromatase Inhibition Activity of Ergosta-5, 22-dien-3β-ol from the Fungus Gyromitra esculenta. *J. Chem.* **2021**, *2021*, 5529786. [CrossRef]
28. Yousef, R.G.; Sakr, H.M.; Eissa, I.H.; Mehany, A.B.; Metwaly, A.M.; Elhendawy, M.A.; Radwan, M.M.; ElSohly, M.A.; Abulkhair, H.S.; El-Adl, K. New quinoxaline-2 (1 H)-ones as potential VEGFR-2 inhibitors: Design, synthesis, molecular docking, ADMET profile and anti-proliferative evaluations. *New J. Chem.* **2021**, *45*, 16949–16964. [CrossRef]
29. Amer, H.H.; Alotaibi, S.H.; Trawneh, A.H.; Metwaly, A.M.; Eissa, I.H. Anticancer activity, spectroscopic and molecular docking of some new synthesized sugar hydrazones, Arylidene and α-Aminophosphonate derivatives. *Arab. J. Chem.* **2021**, *14*, 103348. [CrossRef]
30. Husain, A.; Farooqui, A.; Khanam, A.; Sharma, S.; Mahfooz, S.; Shamim, M.; Akhter, F.; Alatar, A.A.; Faisal, M.; Ahmad, S. Physicochemical characterization of C-phycocyanin from Plectonema sp. and elucidation of its bioactive potential through in silico approach. *Cell. Mol. Biol.* **2021**, *67*, 68–82. [CrossRef]

31. Mohammed, S.O.; El Ashry, E.S.H.; Khalid, A.; Amer, M.R.; Metwaly, A.M.; Eissa, I.H.; Elkaeed, E.B.; Elshobaky, A.; Hafez, E.E. Expression, Purification, and Comparative Inhibition of Helicobacter pylori Urease by Regio-Selectively Alkylated Benzimidazole 2-Thione Derivatives. *Molecules* **2022**, *27*, 865. [CrossRef]
32. Imieje, V.O.; Zaki, A.A.; Metwaly, A.M.; Mostafa, A.E.; Elkaeed, E.B.; Falodun, A. Comprehensive In Silico Screening of the Antiviral Potentialities of a New Humulene Glucoside from Asteriscus hierochunticus against SARS-CoV-2. *J. Chem.* **2021**, *2021*, 5541876. [CrossRef]
33. El-Demerdash, A.; Metwaly, A.M.; Hassan, A.; El-Aziz, A.; Mohamed, T.; Elkaeed, E.B.; Eissa, I.H.; Arafa, R.K.; Stockand, J.D. Comprehensive virtual screening of the antiviral potentialities of marine polycyclic guanidine alkaloids against SARS-CoV-2 (COVID-19). *Biomolecules* **2021**, *11*, 460. [CrossRef] [PubMed]
34. Jalmakhanbetova, R.I.; Suleimen, Y.M.; Oyama, M.; Elkaeed, E.B.; Eissa, I.; Suleimen, R.N.; Metwaly, A.M.; Ishmuratova, M.Y. Isolation and In Silico Anti-COVID-19 Main Protease (Mpro) Activities of Flavonoids and a Sesquiterpene Lactone from Artemisia sublessingiana. *J. Chem.* **2021**, *2021*, 5547013. [CrossRef]
35. Suleimen, Y.M.; Jose, R.A.; Suleimen, R.N.; Arenz, C.; Ishmuratova, M.; Toppet, S.; Dehaen, W.; Alsfouk, A.A.; Elkaeed, E.B.; Eissa, I.H.; et al. Isolation and In Silico Anti-SARS-CoV-2 Papain-Like Protease Potentialities of Two Rare 2-Phenoxychromone Derivatives from Artemisia spp. *Molecules* **2022**, *27*, 1216. [CrossRef]
36. Alesawy, M.S.; Abdallah, A.E.; Taghour, M.S.; Elkaeed, E.B.; H Eissa, I.; Metwaly, A.M. In Silico Studies of Some Isoflavonoids as Potential Candidates against COVID-19 Targeting Human ACE2 (hACE2) and Viral Main Protease (Mpro). *Molecules* **2021**, *26*, 2806. [CrossRef]
37. Eissa, I.H.; Khalifa, M.M.; Elkaeed, E.B.; Hafez, E.E.; Alsfouk, A.A.; Metwaly, A.M. In Silico Exploration of Potential Natural Inhibitors against SARS-Cov-2 nsp10. *Molecules* **2021**, *26*, 6151. [CrossRef]
38. Alesawy, M.S.; Elkaeed, E.B.; Alsfouk, A.A.; Metwaly, A.M.; Eissa, I. In Silico Screening of Semi-Synthesized Compounds as Potential Inhibitors for SARS-CoV-2 Papain-like Protease: Pharmacophoric Features, Molecular Docking, ADMET, Toxicity and DFT Studies. *Molecules* **2021**, *26*, 6593. [CrossRef]
39. FDA-Approved Drug Library. Available online: https://www.selleckchem.com/screening/fda-approved-drug-library.html (accessed on 19 November 2021).
40. Briem, H.; Kuntz, I.D. Molecular similarity based on DOCK-generated fingerprints. *J. Med. Chem.* **1996**, *39*, 3401–3408. [CrossRef]
41. Vidal, D.; Garcia-Serna, R.; Mestres, J. Ligand-based approaches to in silico pharmacology. In *Chemoinformatics and Computational Chemical Biology*; Springer: Berlin/Heidelberg, Germany, 2011; pp. 489–502.
42. Hassell, A.M.; An, G.; Bledsoe, R.K.; Bynum, J.M.; Carter, H.L.; Deng, S.-J.; Gampe, R.T.; Grisard, T.E.; Madauss, K.P.; Nolte, R.T. Crystallization of protein–ligand complexes. *Acta Crystallogr. Sect. D Biol. Crystallogr.* **2007**, *63*, 72–79. [CrossRef]
43. Chu, H.; He, Q.-X.; Wang, J.; Hu, Y.; Wang, Y.-Q.; Lin, Z.-H. In silico design of novel benzohydroxamate-based compounds as inhibitors of histone deacetylase 6 based on 3D-QSAR, molecular docking, and molecular dynamics simulations. *New J. Chem.* **2020**, *44*, 21201–21210. [CrossRef]
44. Ieritano, C.; Campbell, J.L.; Hopkins, W.S. Predicting differential ion mobility behaviour in silico using machine learning. *Analyst* **2021**, *146*, 4737–4743. [CrossRef] [PubMed]
45. Taha, M.; Ismail, N.H.; Ali, M.; Rashid, U.; Imran, S.; Uddin, N.; Khan, K.M. Molecular hybridization conceded exceptionally potent quinolinyl-oxadiazole hybrids through phenyl linked thiosemicarbazide antileishmanial scaffolds: In silico validation and SAR studies. *Bioorgan. Chem.* **2017**, *71*, 192–200. [CrossRef] [PubMed]
46. Opo, F.A.D.M.; Rahman, M.M.; Ahammad, F.; Ahmed, I.; Bhuiyan, M.A.; Asiri, A.M. Structure based pharmacophore modeling, virtual screening, molecular docking and ADMET approaches for identification of natural anti-cancer agents targeting XIAP protein. *Sci. Rep.* **2021**, *11*, 4049. [CrossRef] [PubMed]
47. Durant, J.L.; Leland, B.A.; Henry, D.R.; Nourse, J.G. Reoptimization of MDL keys for use in drug discovery. *J. Chem. Inf. Comput. Sci.* **2002**, *42*, 1273–1280. [CrossRef]
48. Maggiora, G.; Vogt, M.; Stumpfe, D.; Bajorath, J. Molecular similarity in medicinal chemistry: Miniperspective. *J. Med. Chem.* **2014**, *57*, 3186–3204. [CrossRef]
49. Bender, A.; Glen, R.C. Molecular similarity: A key technique in molecular informatics. *Org. Biomol. Chem.* **2004**, *2*, 3204–3218. [CrossRef]
50. Sullivan, K.M.; Enoch, S.J.; Ezendam, J.; Sewald, K.; Roggen, E.L.; Cochrane, S. An adverse outcome pathway for sensitization of the respiratory tract by low-molecular-weight chemicals: Building evidence to support the utility of in vitro and in silico methods in a regulatory context. *Appl. Vitr. Toxicol.* **2017**, *3*, 213–226. [CrossRef]
51. Altamash, T.; Amhamed, A.; Aparicio, S.; Atilhan, M. Effect of hydrogen bond donors and acceptors on CO_2 absorption by deep eutectic solvents. *Processes* **2020**, *8*, 1533. [CrossRef]
52. Wan, Y.; Tian, Y.; Wang, W.; Gu, S.; Ju, X.; Liu, G. In silico studies of diarylpyridine derivatives as novel HIV-1 NNRTIs using docking-based 3D-QSAR, molecular dynamics, and pharmacophore modeling approaches. *RSC Adv.* **2018**, *8*, 40529–40543. [CrossRef]
53. Turchi, M.; Cai, Q.; Lian, G. An evaluation of in-silico methods for predicting solute partition in multiphase complex fluids—A case study of octanol/water partition coefficient. *Chem. Eng. Sci.* **2019**, *197*, 150–158. [CrossRef]

54. Escamilla-Gutiérrez, A.; Ribas-Aparicio, R.M.; Córdova-Espinoza, M.G.; Castelán-Vega, J.A. In silico strategies for modeling RNA aptamers and predicting binding sites of their molecular targets. *Nucleosides Nucleotides Nucleic Acids* **2021**, *40*, 798–807. [CrossRef] [PubMed]
55. Kaushik, A.C.; Kumar, A.; Bharadwaj, S.; Chaudhary, R.; Sahi, S. Ligand-Based Approach for In-silico Drug Designing. In *Bioinformatics Techniques for Drug Discovery*; Springer: Berlin/Heidelberg, Germany, 2018; pp. 11–19.
56. Zhang, H.; Ren, J.-X.; Ma, J.-X.; Ding, L. Development of an in silico prediction model for chemical-induced urinary tract toxicity by using naïve Bayes classifier. *Mol. Divers.* **2019**, *23*, 381–392. [CrossRef] [PubMed]
57. Sheridan, R.P.; Kearsley, S.K. Why do we need so many chemical similarity search methods? *Drug Discov. Today* **2002**, *7*, 903–911. [CrossRef]
58. MOE. MOE User Guide. Available online: https://www.easa.europa.eu/sites/default/files/dfu/B01.UG_.CAO_.00024-008%20User%20Guide%20for%20Maintenance%20Organisation%20Exposition.PDF (accessed on 1 October 2021).
59. Rosas-Lemus, M.; Minasov, G.; Shuvalova, L.; Inniss, N.L.; Kiryukhina, O.; Brunzelle, J.; Satchell, K.J. High-resolution structures of the SARS-CoV-2 2′-O-methyltransferase reveal strategies for structure-based inhibitor design. *Sci. Signal.* **2020**, *13*, eabe1202. [CrossRef]
60. Sousa, S.F.; Fernandes, P.A.; Ramos, M.J. Protein–ligand docking: Current status and future challenges. *Proteins Struct. Funct. Bioinform.* **2006**, *65*, 15–26. [CrossRef] [PubMed]
61. Hollingsworth, S.A.; Dror, R.O. Molecular dynamics simulation for all. *Neuron* **2018**, *99*, 1129–1143. [CrossRef]
62. Liu, X.; Shi, D.; Zhou, S.; Liu, H.; Liu, H.; Yao, X. Molecular dynamics simulations and novel drug discovery. *Expert Opin. Drug Discov.* **2018**, *13*, 23–37. [CrossRef]
63. Kuzmanic, A.; Zagrovic, B. Determination of ensemble-average pairwise root mean-square deviation from experimental B-factors. *Biophys. J.* **2010**, *98*, 861–871. [CrossRef]
64. Protein Data Bank. 2021. Available online: https://www.rcsb.org/structure/4OW0 (accessed on 5 January 2022).
65. Jo, S.; Kim, T.; Iyer, V.G.; Im, W. CHARMM-GUI: A web-based graphical user interface for CHARMM. *J. Comput. Chem.* **2008**, *29*, 1859–1865. [CrossRef]
66. Brooks, B.R.; Brooks, C.L., III.; Mackerell, A.D., Jr.; Nilsson, L.; Petrella, R.J.; Roux, B.; Won, Y.; Archontis, G.; Bartels, C.; Boresch, S.; et al. CHARMM: The biomolecular simulation program. *J. Comput. Chem.* **2009**, *30*, 1545–1614. [CrossRef]
67. Lee, J.; Cheng, X.; Swails, J.M.; Yeom, M.S.; Eastman, P.K.; Lemkul, J.A.; Wei, S.; Buckner, J.; Jeong, J.C.; Qi, Y.; et al. CHARMM-GUI Input Generator for NAMD, GROMACS, AMBER, OpenMM, and CHARMM/OpenMM Simulations Using the CHARMM36 Additive Force Field. *J. Chem. Theory Comput.* **2016**, *12*, 405–413. [CrossRef] [PubMed]
68. Best, R.B.; Zhu, X.; Shim, J.; Lopes, P.E.; Mittal, J.; Feig, M.; Mackerell, A.D., Jr. Optimization of the additive CHARMM all-atom protein force field targeting improved sampling of the backbone phi, psi and side-chain chi(1) and chi(2) dihedral angles. *J. Chem. Theory Comput.* **2012**, *8*, 3257–3273. [CrossRef] [PubMed]
69. Phillips, J.C.; Braun, R.; Wang, W.; Gumbart, J.; Tajkhorshid, E.; Villa, E.; Chipot, C.; Skeel, R.D.; Kale, L.; Schulten, K. Scalable molecular dynamics with NAMD. *J. Comput. Chem.* **2005**, *26*, 1781–1802. [CrossRef] [PubMed]

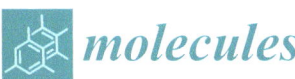

Article

Rhodamine 101 Conjugates of Triterpenoic Amides Are of Comparable Cytotoxicity as Their Rhodamine B Analogs

Niels V. Heise, Daniel Major, Sophie Hoenke, Marie Kozubek, Immo Serbian and René Csuk *

Department of Organic Chemistry, Martin-Luther University Halle-Wittenberg, Kurt-Mothes Str. 2, D-06120 Halle (Saale), Germany; niels.heise@chemie.uni-halle.de (N.V.H.); daniel.major@student.uni-halle.de (D.M.); sophie.hoenke@chemie.uni-halle.de (S.H.); marie.kozubek@chemie.uni-halle.de (M.K.); immoserbian@gmail.com (I.S.)
* Correspondence: rene.csuk@chemie.uni-halle.de; Tel.: +49-345-5525660

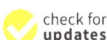

Citation: Heise, N.V.; Major, D.; Hoenke, S.; Kozubek, M.; Serbian, I.; Csuk, R. Rhodamine 101 Conjugates of Triterpenoic Amides Are of Comparable Cytotoxicity as Their Rhodamine B Analogs. *Molecules* 2022, 27, 2220. https://doi.org/10.3390/molecules27072220

Academic Editors: Imtiaz Khan and Sumera Zaib

Received: 11 March 2022
Accepted: 26 March 2022
Published: 29 March 2022

Publisher's Note: MDPI stays neutral with regard to jurisdictional claims in published maps and institutional affiliations.

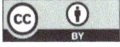

Copyright: © 2022 by the authors. Licensee MDPI, Basel, Switzerland. This article is an open access article distributed under the terms and conditions of the Creative Commons Attribution (CC BY) license (https://creativecommons.org/licenses/by/4.0/).

Abstract: Pentacyclic triterpenoic acids (betulinic, oleanolic, ursolic, and platanic acid) were selected and subjected to acetylation followed by the formation of amides derived from either piperazine or homopiperazine. These amides were coupled with either rhodamine B or rhodamine 101. All of these compounds were screened for their cytotoxic activity in SRB assays. As a result, the cytotoxicity of the parent acids was low but increased slightly upon their acetylation while a significant increase in cytotoxicity was observed for piperazinyl and homopiperazinyl amides. A tremendous improvement in cytotoxicity was observed; however, for the rhodamine B and rhodamine 101 conjugates, and compound **27**, an ursolic acid derived homopiperazinyl amide holding a rhodamine 101 residue showed an $EC_{50} = 0.05$ µM for A2780 ovarian cancer cells while being less cytotoxic for non-malignant fibroblasts. To date, the rhodamine 101 derivatives presented here are the first examples of triterpene derivatives holding a rhodamine residue different from rhodamine B.

Keywords: triterpenoic acid; ursolic acid; oleanolic acid; betulinic acid; rhodamine B; rhodamine 101; cytotoxicity

1. Introduction

Despite significant progress, cancer therapy still falls short of the expectations placed in it many years ago [1,2]. The prognosis for a complete cure is very good for some types of cancer, but still poor for many others, especially when regular screening is taken into account. The high cost of therapy [3–5] is often offset especially for cancers that are difficult to treat by only a slight increase in life expectancy and, at the same time, a significantly reduced quality of life. Thus, the survival rate [6] for testicular cancer is approximately 98% while for pancreatic cancer it is about 1%. The main reason for the reduced quality of life and, thus, a reduced compliance by the affected patients is more or less often insufficient selectivity of the chemotherapeutic agents used. As a consequence, there has been no lack of attempts to improve the efficacy but also to reduce the side effects caused by antitumor drugs (such as weight loss, hair loss, etc.). Furthermore, many different strategies have been tested for a successful drug targeting of tumors—whereby the real problem is usually not the solid primary tumor but the metastases that have already formed and spread throughout the body. These attempts [7] included the use of micelles [8], antibodies [9], liposomes [10], polymers but also of drug-loaded nanoparticles [7].

Although first described several years ago, so-called mitocans (i.e., mitochondria targeting anticancer drugs) [11–16] are currently experiencing a scientific renaissance. Mitocans, which specifically induce a programmed cell death in tumor cells, can be considered as one of the most innovative therapeutic approaches of drug targeting of the "next generation". In the past, we could already show with some examples that compounds derived from pentacyclic triterpenes (such as ursolic, oleanolic, betulinic, platanic, glycyrrhetinic, β-boswellic, tormentic, euspaphic, or asiatic acid) exhibit high cytotoxicity, and can act as mitocans [17–22]. These mitocans might cause either membrane permeabilization but also the opening of the mitochondrial permeability pore [16,17]. However, the deactivation of mitochondrial enzymes cannot completely be ruled out [17].

This cytotoxicity (but also to some extent their pronounced tumor/non-tumor cell selectivity) seems to depend on many parameters. On the one hand, this concerns a dependence on the type of terpene (Figure 1) used: compounds derived from dehydroabietylamine [23] were—by and large—less cytotoxic than those with a pentacyclic triterpenoid backbone [17]. Amides at position C-28 were mostly more active than the analogous esters [22], whereas a direct attachment of a rhodamine B moiety to the triterpenoid backbone resulted in compounds of significantly lowered selectivity [17]. Therefore, the use of a suitable spacer is of crucial importance. Furthermore, triterpene/rhodamine B hybrids holding an ethylenediamine spacer [20] were significantly less active than those with a piperazine spacer; in some cases, the use of a homopiperazine spacer [17] proved successful. However, the presence of a distal cationic center alone is not sufficient for achieving good cytotoxic activity [17,24–26]. Only special delocalized lipophilic cations are useful for a successful mitochondria-targeted chemotherapy. Thereby, quaternary ammonium salts [24] but also malachite green-derived compounds [27] proved to be significantly less cytotoxic than their rhodamine B analogs [17]. Furthermore, the presence of a rhodamine residue is of crucial importance, which is why we decided to extend our studies to rhodamine B and other rhodamines, and to investigate especially the synthesis and cytotoxic activity of (homo)-piperazinyl-spaced triterpenes holding a rhodamine 101 residue in more detail, and to compare their cytotoxic activity with those carrying a rhodamine B unit.

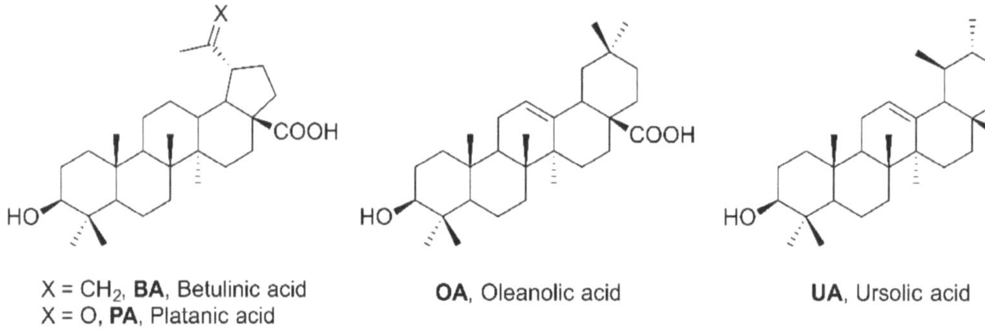

X = CH$_2$, **BA**, Betulinic acid
X = O, **PA**, Platanic acid

OA, Oleanolic acid

UA, Ursolic acid

Figure 1. Structure of betulinic acid (**BA**), platanic acid (**PA**), oleanolic acid (**OA**), and **UA** (ursolic acid).

2. Results

Acetylation (Scheme 1) of betulinic (**BA**, Figure 1), oleanolic (**OA**), ursolic (**UA**), and platanic (**PA**) acid gave well known acetates **1–4**; their carboxyl group was activated with oxalyl chloride followed by the addition of either piperazine or homopiperazine to furnish amides **5–8** and **9–12**, respectively. Activation of rhodamine B or rhodamine 101 with oxalyl chloride and reaction with amides **5–12** furnished piperazine/rhodamine B derived conjugates **13–16** and **17–20** as well as rhodamine 101 derived hybrids **21–24** and **25–28**, respectively. All of these conjugates were violet in color, hence, indicating the presence of an intact cationic rhodamine moiety. This is regarded as a prerequisite for obtaining high cytotoxicity due to interaction with the mitochondrial membrane(s).

The cytotoxicity of the compounds was determined in sulforhodamine B (SRB) assays employing several human tumor cell lines (A375, HT29, MCF-7, A2780, FaDu) as well as two non-malignant cell lines (NIH 3T3, HEK293). The results from these assays are summarized in Tables 1–4.

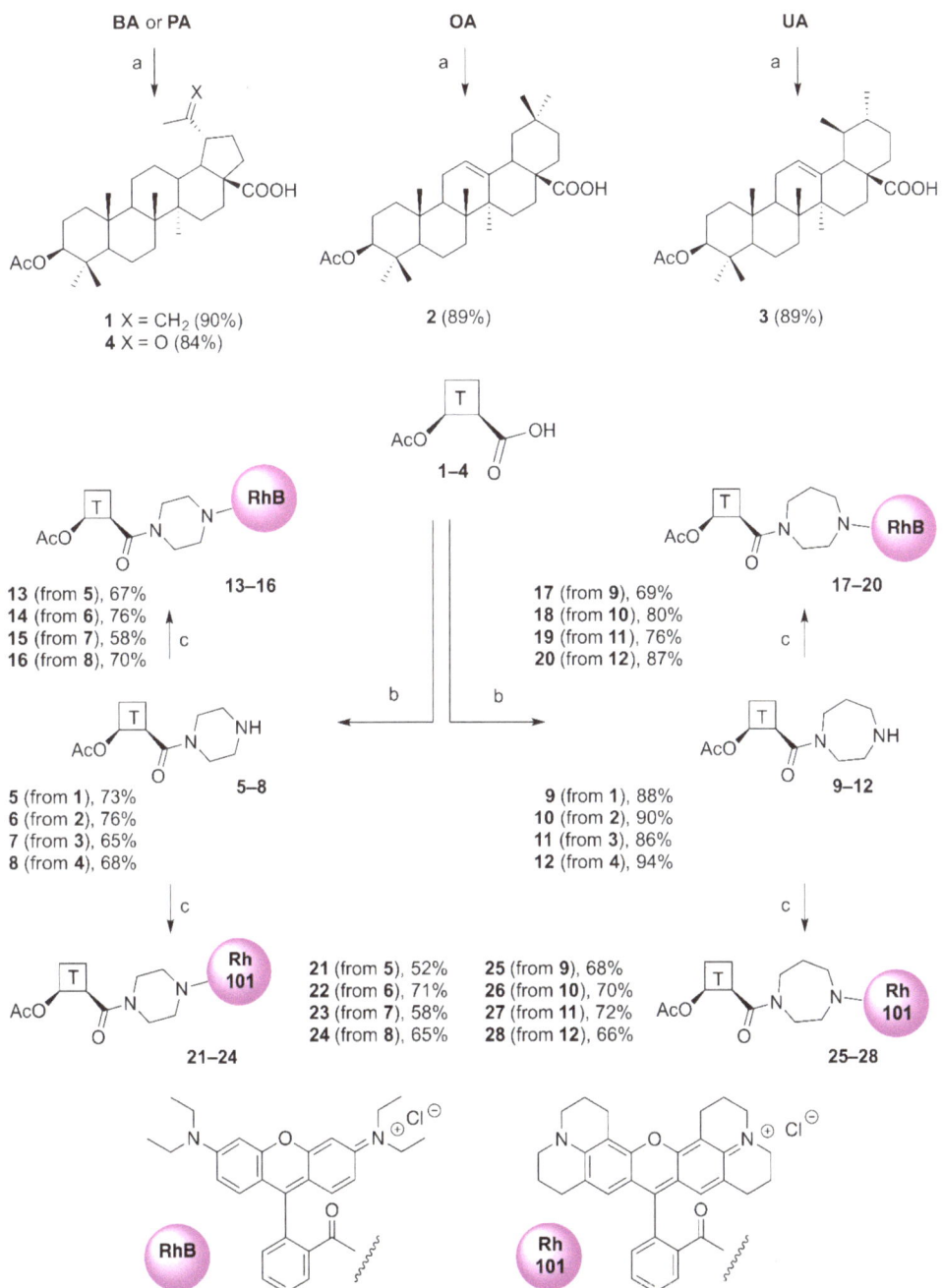

Scheme 1. Reactions and conditions: (a) Ac$_2$O, NEt$_3$, DMAP (cat.), DCM, 20 °C, 1 d; (b) (COCl)$_2$, DMF (cat.), DCM, then DCM (homo)piperazine, 20 °C, 1 h; (c) rhodamine B or rhodamine 101, (COCl)$_2$, NEt$_3$, DMAP (cat.), DCM, 20 °C, 1 d; T—triterpenoic acid; OA—oleanolic acid; UA—ursolic acid; BA—betulinic acid; PA—platanic acid; Rh B—rhodamine B; Rh 101—rhodamine 101.

Table 1. Cytotoxicity of parent compounds **BA**, **OA**, **UA**, and **PA** as well as of their corresponding acetates **1–4** (EC_{50}-values in μM from SRB-assays) after 72 h of treatment; the values are averaged from three independent experiments performed each in triplicate, confidence interval CI = 95%; mean ± standard mean error); n.d. not determined; doxorubicin (**DX**) was used as a positive control. Cell lines: malignant: A375 (melanoma), HT29 (colon adenocarcinoma), MCF-7 (breast adenocarcinoma), A2780 (ovarian carcinoma), FaDu (hypopharyngeal carcinoma); non-malignant: NIH 3T3 (fibroblasts).

Compound	A375	HT29	MCF-7	A2780	FaDu	NIH 3T3
BA	17.7 ± 0.4	14.4 ± 2.3	10.2 ± 1.2	8.8 ± 0.9	13.7 ± 0.9	16.1 ± 1.4
OA	>30	>30	>30	>30	>30	>30
UA	15.4 ± 1.0	10.6 ± 0.7	12.7 ± 0.1	11.7 ± 0.6	18.2 ± 1.7	13.1 ± 1.1
PA	>30	>30	>30	>30	>30	>30
1	19.2 ± 1.7	21.3 ± 2.0	11.0 ± 0.5	18.3 ± 0.5	7.2 ± 1.2	>30
2	13.0 ± 1.1	20.5 ± 1.7	12.9 ± 1.9	9.4 ± 0.5	11.8 ± 0.9	17.5 ± 1.5
3	11.4 ± 1.4	17.3 ± 1.5	12.1 ± 1.2	8.3 ± 0.9	10.7 ± 0.8	16.4 ± 1.7
4	>30	>30	>30	>30	>30	>30
DX	n.d.	0.9 ± 0.2	1.1 ± 0.3	0.02 ± 0.01	1.7 ± 0.3	0.06 ± 0.03

Table 2. Cytotoxicity of 3-O-acetylated triterpenoic amides **5–8** (piperazinyl amimides) and **9–12** (homopiperazinyl amides) (EC_{50}-values in μM from SRB-assays) after 72 h of treatment; the values are averaged from three independent experiments performed each in triplicate, confidence interval CI = 95%; mean ± standard mean error); n.d. not determined; n.s. not soluble; doxorubicin (**DX**) was used as a positive control. Cell lines: malignant: A375 (melanoma), HT29 (colon adenocarcinoma), MCF-7 (breast adenocarcinoma), A2780 (ovarian carcinoma); non-malignant: NIH 3T3 (fibroblasts).

Compound	A375	HT29	MCF-7	A2780	NIH 3T3
5	1.5 ± 0.3	1.0 ± 0.1	1.4 ± 0.1	1.9 ± 0.1	0.9 ± 0.1
6	1.4 ± 0.2	1.3 ± 0.1	1.7 ± 0.2	1.7 ± 0.1	1.7 ± 0.1
7	2.0 ± 0.4	1.9 ± 0.3	1.7 ± 0.2	2.1 ± 0.1	2.1 ± 0.1
8	1.9 ± 0.4	3.9 ± 0.2	2.7 ± 0.3	2.6 ± 0.4	1.3 ± 0.1
9	18.7 ± 1.6	5.1 ± 1.1	10.7 ± 1.0	12.0 ± 0.6	18.7 ± 1.6
10	1.9 ± 0.9	1.9 ± 0.1	1.6 ± 0.1	2.2 ± 0.1	1.8 ± 0.2
11	3.2 ± 0.2	2.0 ± 0.1	2.4 ± 0.1	2.9 ± 0.24	0.9 ± 0.1
12	0.9 ± 0.1	2.3 ± 0.2	1.8 ± 0.2	1.6 ± 0.1	0.6 ± 0.1
DX	n.d.	0.9 ± 0.2	1.1 ± 0.3	0.02 ± 0.01	1.7 ± 0.3

Table 3. Cytotoxicity of 3-O-acetylated triterpenoic amides holding a distal rhodamine B unit **13–20** (EC_{50}-values in μM from SRB-assays) after 72 h of treatment; the values are averaged from three independent experiments performed each in triplicate, confidence interval CI = 95%; mean ± standard mean error); n.d. not determined; n.s. not soluble; doxorubicin (**DX**) was used as a positive control. Cell lines: malignant: A375 (melanoma), HT29 (colon adenocarcinoma), MCF-7 (breast adenocarcinoma), A2780 (ovarian carcinoma); non-malignant: NIH 3T3 (fibroblasts).

Compound	A375	HT29	MCF-7	A2780	NIH 3T3
13	0.09 ± 0.01	0.151 ± 0.022	0.081 ± 0.005	0.050 ± 0.004	0.208 ± 0.034
14	0.09 ± 0.01	0.091 ± 0.010	0.062 ± 0.004	0.032 ± 0.001	0.137 ± 0.006
15	0.04 ± 0.02	0.083 ± 0.007	0.075 ± 0.005	0.038 ± 0.002	0.137 ± 0.009
16	0.08 ± 0.03	0.099 ± 0.016	0.070 ± 0.002	0.036 ± 0.001	0.171 ± 0.006
17	0.76 ± 0.09	0.28 ± 0.01	0.22 ± 0.02	0.22 ± 0.01	0.33 ± 0.07
18	0.04 ± 0.01	0.04 ± 0.01	0.03 ± 0.004	0.02 ± 0.003	0.14 ± 0.02
19	0.51 ± 0.05	0.50 ± 0.07	0.39 ± 0.04	0.45 ± 0.03	0.40 ± 0.03
20	0.24 ± 0.017	0.30 ± 0.027	0.15 ± 0.050	0.12 ± 0.018	0.34 ± 0.056
DX	n.d.	0.9 ± 0.2	1.1 ± 0.3	0.02 ± 0.01	1.7 ± 0.3

Table 4. Cytotoxicity of 3-O-acetylated triterpenoic amides holding a distal rhodamine 101 unit **13–20** (EC_{50}-values in µM from SRB-assays) after 72 h of treatment; the values are averaged from three independent experiments performed each in triplicate, confidence interval CI = 95%; mean ± standard mean error); n.d. not determined; n.s. not soluble; doxorubicin (**DX**) was used as a positive control. Cell lines: malignant: A375 (melanoma), HT29 (colon adenocarcinoma), MCF-7 (breast adenocarcinoma), A2780 (ovarian carcinoma), HeLa (cervical cancer); non-malignant: NIH 3T3 (fibroblasts), HEK293 (human embryonic kidney).

Compound	A375	HT29	MCF7	A2780	HeLa	NIH 3T3	HEK293
21	0.14 ± 0.02	0.36 ± 0.06	0.21 ± 0.03	0.09 ± 0.01	0.12 ± 0.03	0.56 ± 0.07	0.05 ± 0.05
22	0.15 ± 0.01	0.25 ± 0.03	0.23 ± 0.02	0.11 ± 0.01	0.20 ± 0.05	0.36 ± 0.05	0.07 ± 0.02
23	0.16 ± 0.02	0.21 ± 0.07	0.16 ± 0.03	0.08 ± 0.02	0.12 ± 0.02	0.37 ± 0.05	0.04 ± 0.01
24	0.25 ± 0.04	0.26 ± 0.04	0.17 ± 0.02	0.17 ± 0.03	0.21 ± 0.02	0.26 ± 0.04	0.10 ± 0.04
25	0.17 ± 0.05	0.43 ± 0.08	0.22 ± 0.04	0.19 ± 0.04	0.27 ± 0.14	0.56 ± 0.07	0.12 ± 0.04
26	0.07 ± 0.01	0.13 ± 0.03	0.12 ± 0.03	0.07 ± 0.03	0.10 ± 0.05	0.26 ± 0.05	0.05 ± 0.01
27	0.06 ± 0.04	0.08 ± 0.02	0.08 ± 0.03	0.05 ± 0.02	0.09 ± 0.06	0.24 ± 0.03	0.04 ± 0.01
28	0.20 ± 0.03	0.35 ± 0.05	0.20 ± 0.05	0.17 ± 0.04	0.31 ± 0.15	0.39 ± 0.05	0.12 ± 0.03
DX	n.d.	0.9 ± 0.2	1.1 ± 0.3	0.02 ± 0.01	n.d.	1.7 ± 0.3	n.d.

Table 1 shows the results from the SRB assays for the parent compounds and their acetates. Except for **BA** and **UA**, all other triterpenoids held EC_{50} values > 30 µM (cut-off of the assay) for the cancer cell lines but also for the non-malignant fibroblasts NIH 3T3. Acetates **1–4** showed slightly improved cytotoxicity (except **PA** derived **4**); by-and-large, EC_{50} values between 7.2 µM (**1** for FaDu cells) and 21.3 (**1** for A375 cells) were observed. Highest cytotoxicity was found for **1** and FaDu cells, for **2** with respect to A2780 and for **3** also with A2780 cells, respectively. Interestingly, **PA** derived acetate **4** was not cytotoxic at all within the limits of the assay.

Significant improvement was observed for the piperazinyl amides (Table 2), and EC_{50} values between 1.00 (**5** for HT29) and 3.86 (for **PA** derived **8** and HT29 cells) were determined. Except for the latter, all EC_{50} values were smaller than 3 µM. While **5** was cytotoxic with an EC_{50} = 1.5 µM for A375 cells, its homopiperazinyl analog **9** was significantly less active (EC_{50} = 18.7 µM). However, by-and-large, the cytotoxicity of the homopiperazinyl derivatives **9–12** was of the same order as that of the piperazinyl analogs **5–8**.

A dramatic improvement of cytotoxicity, however, was observed for the piperazinyl and homopiperazinyl spaced triterpenoic acid–rhodamine B conjugates **13–20** (Table 3).

Thereby, all of the compounds showed high cytotoxicity for all human tumor cell lines; EC_{50} values ranged from EC_{50} = 0.02 µM (compound **18** and A2780 cells) to EC_{50} = 0.76 µM (compound **17** and A375 cells). Thus, the former compound was as cytotoxic as standard doxorubicin.

Previously, we have shown the high cytotoxicity of several rhodamine B conjugates. Hence, it became of interest to investigate whether this high cytotoxicity is limited to rhodamine B conjugates or can also be found in conjugates holding a rhodamine 101 scaffold. As a result (Table 4), conjugates holding either a piperazinyl or homopiperazinyl spacer were only slightly less cytotoxic than those holding a rhodamine B moiety.

Interestingly enough, in this series of compounds, **UA** derived **27** (carrying a homopiperazine spacer and a rhodamine 101 residue) held the highest cytotoxicity, and the EC_{50} values for this compound were as low as EC_{50} = 0.05 µM (A2780 cells). Cytotoxicity for non-malignant fibroblasts NIH 3T3 were approximately five times lower for both rhodamine scaffolds. Extra staining experiments of A375 cells (acridine orange (AO), Hoechst 33342, rhodamine 123 (Figure 2)) showed **26** to act as a mitocan.

A summary of the hitherto known structural prerequisites to obtain pentacyclic triterpenoids of high cytotoxicity is depicted in Figure 3.

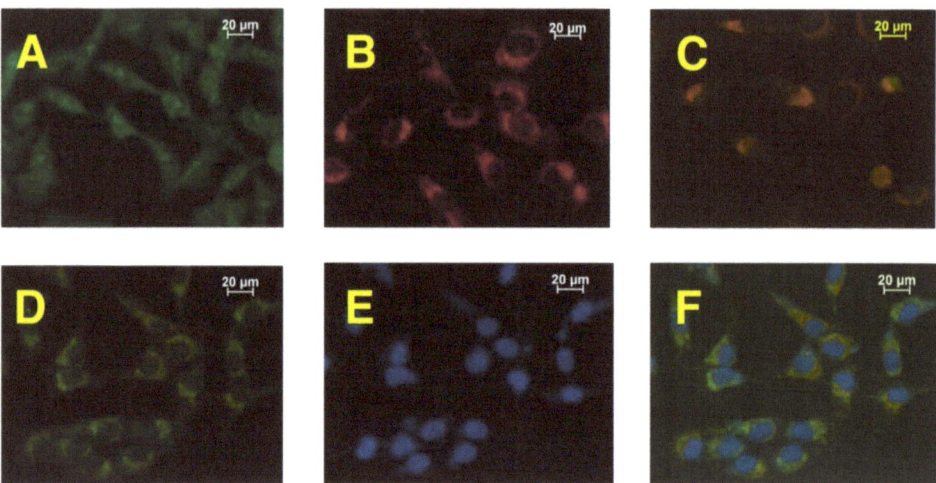

Figure 2. Staining experiments: A375 cells, 24 h; (**A**) control (AO); (**B**) in the presence of **26**; (**C**) merged (AO, **26**); (**D**) control (AO); (**E**) Hoechst 33,342 staining; (**F**) merged (Hoechst 33,342).

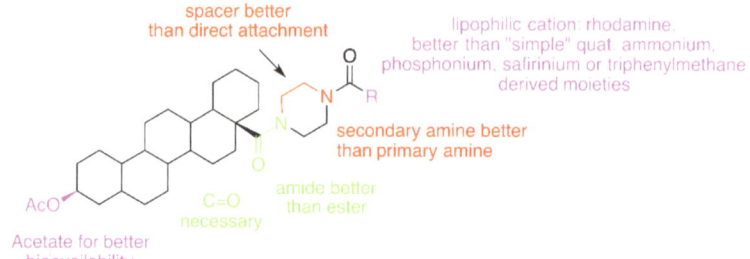

Figure 3. Hitherto known SAR parameters for obtaining pentacyclic triterpenoids of high cytotoxicity.

3. Conclusions

Four representative pentacyclic triterpenoic acids (**BA**, **OA**, **UA**, and **PA**) were selected for a systematic evaluation of cytotoxic derivatives. As a result—and as exemplified for A2780 cancer cells—the cytotoxicity of the parent acids is low but increased slightly upon their acetylation. A significant increase in cytotoxicity was observed when acetates **1–4** were transformed into their piperazinyl amides **5–8**. For the latter, compounds EC_{50} values between EC_{50} = 2.6 to 1.7 µM have been determined. The same trend was observed for the homopiperazinyl derivatives **9–12**. Interestingly, betulinic acid derived **9** (EC_{50} = 12.0 µM) was significantly less cytotoxic than its piperazinyl derivative **5** (EC_{50} = 1.9 µM). A tremendous improvement in cytotoxicity was observed, however, for the rhodamine conjugates, and EC_{50} values between EC_{50} = 0.05–0.032 µM were observed for the piperazinyl rhodamine B conjugates. The corresponding piperazinyl rhodamine 101 conjugates were of comparable bioactivity (EC_{50} = 0.09–0.17 µM). A similar trend was observed for the homopiperazinyl rhodamine conjugates, and EC_{50} = 0.02–0.45 µM (for rhodamine B derived **17–20**) and EC_{50} = 0.05–0.19 µM (for rhodamine 101 derived **25–28**) were determined. Thus, it can be concluded that an optimal combination of pentacyclic triterpene, a suitable spacer and a lipophilic cationic residue must be found to achieve good cytotoxic activity. It was shown that both piperazinyl and homopiperazinyl spacers are equally suitable to serve as anchors for the binding of either rhodamine B or rhodamine

101. Furthermore, the conjugates derived from either rhodamine B or rhodamine 101 are of comparable cytotoxicity.

4. Experimental

NMR spectra were recorded using the Varian spectrometers (Darmstadt, Germany) DD2 and VNMRS (400 and 500 MHz, respectively). MS spectra were taken on a Advion expression^L CMS mass spectrometer (Ithaca, NY, USA); positive ion polarity mode, solvent: methanol, solvent flow: 0.2 mL/min, spray voltage: 5.17 kV, source voltage: 77 V, APCI corona discharge: 4.2 µA, capillary temperature: 250 °C, capillary voltage: 180 V, sheath gas: N_2). Thin-layer chromatography was performed on pre-coated silica gel plates supplied by Macherey-Nagel (Düren, Germany). IR spectra were recorded on a Spectrum 1000 FT-IR-spectrometer from Perkin Elmer (Rodgau, Germany). The UV/Vis-spectra were recorded on a Lambda 14 spectrometer from Perkin Elmer (Rodgau, Germany); optical rotations were measured at 20 °C using a JASCO-P2000 instrument (JASCO Germany GmbH, Pfungstadt, Germany) The melting points were determined using the Leica hot stage microscope Galen III (Leica Biosystems, Nussloch, Germany) and are uncorrected. The solvents were dried according to usual procedures. Microanalyses were performed with an Elementar Vario EL (CHNS) instrument (Elementar Analysensysteme GmbH, Elementar-Straße 1, D-63505, Langenselbold, Germany).

4.1. General Procedure for the Synthesis of Acetates 1–4 (GPA)

To a solution of the triterpenoic acid (**OA**, **UA**, **BA**, **PA**, 1 equiv.) in dry DCM, acetic anhydride (3 equiv.), triethylamine (3 equiv.), and DMAP (cat.) were added, and the mixture was stirred at 20 °C for 1 day. Usual aqueous work-up followed by re-crystallization from ethanol furnished products **1–4**.

4.2. 3β-Acetyloxy-lup-20(29)-en-28-oic Acid (1)

Following GPA, compound **1** (4.90 g, 90%) was obtained from **BA** as a colorless solid; R_f = 0.59 (n-hexane/ethyl acetate, 4:1); m.p. 277–279 °C (lit.: [28] 277–278 °C); $[\alpha]_D$ = +20.7° (c 0.42, CHCl$_3$) [(lit.: [29] $[\alpha]_D$ = +20.7° (c 0.42, CHCl$_3$)]; MS (ESI, MeOH): m/z 487.1 (32%, [M − H]$^-$, 995.0 (100%, [2M − H]$^-$, 1018.6 (29% [2M − 2H + Na]$^-$).

4.3. 3β-Acetyloxy-olean-12-en-oic Acid (2)

Following GPA, compound **2** (2.45 g, 89%) was obtained from **OA** as a colorless solid; R_f = 0.72 (toluene/ethyl acetate/heptane/formic acid, 80:26:10:5); m.p. 286–289 °C (lit.: [30] 264–265 °C); $[\alpha]_D$ = +69.4° (c 0.30, CHCl$_3$) [(lit.: [31] $[\alpha]_D$ = +74.0° (c 1.0, CHCl$_3$)]; MS (ESI, MeOH): m/z 499.4 ([100%, M + H]$^+$), 516.3 (36%, [M + NH$_4$]$^+$, 521.5 [35%, [M + Na]$^+$.

4.4. 3β-Acetyloxy-urs-12-en-oic Acid (3)

Following GPA, compound **3** (2.41 g, 89%) was obtained from **UA** as a colorless solid; R_f = 0.57 (n-hexane/ethyl acetate, 3:1); m. p. 281–283 °C (lit.: [32] 280 °C); $[\alpha]_D$ = +66.5° (c 0.42, CHCl$_3$) [lit.: [33] $[\alpha]_D$ = +63.5° (c 0.5, CHCl$_3$)]; MS (ESI, MeOH): m/z 499.3 (17%, [M + H]$^+$), 521.2 (31%, [M + H]$^+$), 1019.4 (100%, [2M + Na]$^+$).

4.5. 3β-Acetyloxy-20-oxo-30-norlupan-28-oic Acid (4)

Following GPA, compound **4** (6.9 g, 84%) was obtained from **PA** as a colorless solid; R_f = 0.50 (toluene/ethyl acetate/heptane/formic acid, 80:26:10.5); m.p. 265–268 °C (lit.: [34] 252–255 °C); $[\alpha]_D$ = −9.4° (c 0.32, CHCl$_3$) [(lit.: [34] $[\alpha]_D$ = −9.5° (c 0.5, CHCl$_3$)]; MS (ESI, MeOH): m/z 999.5 (100%, [2M − H]$^-$).

4.6. General Procedure for the Synthesis of Acetylated (homo)piperazinyl Amides 5–12 (GPB)

To a solution of the acetylated triterpenoic acid **1–4** (1 equiv.) in dry DCM, DMF (cat.) and oxalyl chloride (4 equiv.) were added followed by the addition of (homo)piperazine

(4 equiv.). After stirring for 1h at 20 °C followed by usual aqueous work-up and column chromatography, products **5–12** were obtained.

4.7. 3β-Acetyloxy-28-(1-piperazinyl)-lup-20(29)en-28-one (**5**)

Following GPB from **1** (2.5 g, 5 mmol) and piperazine (1.6 g, 20.0 mmol), compound **5** (2.07 g, 73%) was obtained as a colorless solid; R_f = 0.40 (SiO$_2$, CHCl$_3$/MeOH, 9:1); m.p. = 166–173 °C (lit.: [35] 162–167 °C); $[\alpha]_D$ = −1.4° (c 0.21, MeOH), [lit.: [35] $[\alpha]_D$ = −1.8° (c 0.32, MeOH); MS (ESI, MeOH): m/z (%) = 567.3 ([100%, M + H]$^+$).

4.8. 3β-Acetyloxy-28-(1-piperazinyl)-olean-12-en-28-one (**6**)

Following GPB from **2** (2.5 g, 5.0 mmol) and piperazine (1.6 g, 29 mmol), **6** (2.16 g, 76%) was obtained as a colorless solid; R_f = 0.40 (SiO$_2$, CHCl$_3$/MeOH, 9:1); m.p. = 172–175 °C (lit.: [35] 173–175 °C); $[\alpha]_D$ = +23.4° (c 0.18, CHCl$_3$), [lit.: [35] $[\alpha]_D$ = +26.6° (c 0.35, MeOH); MS (ESI, MeOH): m/z (%) = 567.4 (100%, [M + H]$^+$).

4.9. 3β-Acetyloxy-28-(1-piperazinyl)-urs-12-en-28-one (**7**)

Following GPB from **3** (2.5 g, 5.0 mmol) and piperazine (1.6 g, 20.0 mmol), **7** (1.84 g, 65%) was obtained as a colorless solid; R_f = 0.40 (SiO$_2$, CHCl$_3$/MeOH, 9:1); m.p. = 187–190 °C (lit.: [35] 187–188 °C); $[\alpha]_D$ = +25.1° (c 0.24, MeOH), [lit.: [35] $[\alpha]_D$ = +24.5° (c 0.29, MeOH); MS (ESI, MeOH): m/z (%) = 567.4 (100%, [M + H]$^+$).

4.10. 3β-Acetyloxy-28-(1-piperazinyl)-30-norlupane-20,28-dione (**8**)

Following GPB from **4** (2.5 g, 5.0 mmol) and piperazine (1.6 g, 20.0 mmol), **17** (1.93 g, 68%) was obtained as a colorless solid; R_f = 0.40 (SiO$_2$, CHCl$_3$/MeOH, 9:1); m.p. = 127–130 °C (lit.: [20] 115–125 °C); $[\alpha]_D$ = −20.3° (c 0.13, CHCl$_3$); MS (ESI, MeOH): m/z (%) = 569.3 (100%, [M + H]$^+$).

4.11. 3β-Acetyloxy-28-(1-homopiperazinyl)-lup-20(29)en-28-one (**9**)

Following GPB from **1** (1.0 g, 2.02 mmol) and homopiperazine (9.8 g, 8.0 mmol), **9** (1.02 g, 88%) was obtained as a colorless solid; R_f = 0.4 (SiO$_2$, CHCl$_3$/MeOH, 9:1); m.p. 190–193°C (lit.: [21] 196–199 °C); $[\alpha]_D$ = +107.6° (c 0.20, CHCl$_3$), [lit.: [21] $[\alpha]_D$ = +109.8° (c 0.38, CHCl$_3$); MS (ESI, MeOH): m/z (%) = 581.4 (100%, [M + H]$^+$).

4.12. 3β-Acetyloxy-28-(1-homopiperazinyl)-olean-12-en-28-one (**10**)

Following GPB from **2** (1.0 g, 2.02 mmol) and homopiperazine (0.8 g, 8.0 mmol), **10** (1.4 g, 90%) was obtained as a colorless solid; R_f = 0.4 (SiO$_2$, CHCl$_3$/MeOH, 9:1); m.p. 182–185 °C (lit.: [21] 187–190 °C); $[\alpha]_D$ = 12.4° (c 0.14, CHCl$_3$), [lit.: [21] $[\alpha]_D$ = +9.9° (c 0.35, CHCl$_3$); MS (ESI, MeOH): m/z = 581.4 (100%, [M + H]$^+$).

4.13. 3β-Acetyloxy28-(1-homopierazinyl)-urs-12-en-28-one (**11**)

Following GPB from **3** (1.0 g, 2.02 mmol) and homopiperazine (0.8 g, 8.0 mmol), **11** (1.1 g, 86%) was obtained as a colorless solid; R_f = 0.4 (SiO$_2$, CHCl$_3$/MeOH, 9:1); m.p. 171–175 °C (lit.: [21] 178–180 °C); $[\alpha]_D$ = +27.0° (c 0.21, CHCl$_3$), [lit.: [21] $[\alpha]_D$ = +29.7° (c 0.34, CHCl$_3$); MS (ESI, MeOH): m/z = 581.4 (100%, [M + H]$^+$, 100%).

4.14. 3β-Acetyloxy-28-(1-homopiperazinyl)-30-norlupane-20,28-dione (**12**)

Following GPB from **4** (1.0 g, 2.02 mmol) and homopiperazine (0.8 g, 8.0 mmol), **12** (1.1 g, 94%) was obtained as a colorless solid; R_f = 0.4 (SiO$_2$, CHCl$_3$/MeOH, 9:1); m.p. 162–165 °C; $[\alpha]_D$ = −29.2° (c 0.16, CHCl$_3$); IR (ATR): ν = 2941m, 2866w, 1732m, 1708m, 1622m, 1464m, 1453m, 1408m, 1367m, 1244vs, 1191m, 1149m, 1133m, 1109w, 1026m, 979m, 947w, 934w, 900w, 750s, 665m, 610w, 557m, 506m, 455w, 410w cm^{-1}; ^{1}H NMR (400 MHz, CDCl$_3$): δ = 4.44 (dd, J = 10.5, 5.5 Hz, 1H, 3-H), 3.89–3.60 (m, 4H, 33-H), 3.40–3.09 (m, 5H, 19-H, 33-H), 2.62 (td, J = 12.1, 4.1 Hz, 1H, 13-H), 2.25 (s, 2H, 35-H), 2.17 (s, 3H, 29-H), 2.14–2.06 (m, 2H, 16-H$_a$ + 18-H), 2.02 (s, 3H, 32-H), 1.97–1.84 (m, 2H, 21-H$_a$ + 22-H$_a$),

1.68–1.14 (m, 15H + 1-H$_a$ + 2-H + 6-H$_a$ + 6-H$_b$ + 7-H + 9-H + 11-H$_a$ + 11-H$_b$ + 15-H + 16-H$_b$ + 21-H$_b$ + 22-H$_b$), 1.06–0.98 (m, 2H, 12-H), 0.96 (s, 4H, 1-H$_b$ + 27-H), 0.89 (s, 3H, 26-H), 0.82 (s, 3H, 24-H), 0.82 (s, 3H, 25-H), 0.81 (s, 3H, 23-H), 0.79–0.74 (m, 1H, 5-H) ppm; ^{13}C NMR (101 MHz, CDCl$_3$): δ = 213.0 (C-20), 175.0 (C-28), 171.2 (C-31), 81.0 (C-3), 55.4 (C-5), 54.9 (C-17), 52.6 (C-18), 50.6 (C-9), 49.9 (C-19), 46.6 (C-33 + C-34), 41.8 (C-14), 40.6 (C-8), 38.3 (C-1), 37.8 (C-4), 37.1 (C-10), 36.0 (C-13), 35.7 (C-22), 34.1 (C-7), 31.7 (C-16), 30.3 (C-29), 29.9 (C-15), 28.6 (C-21), 27.9 (C-24), 27.3 (C-12), 25.7 (C-35), 23.6 (C-2), 21.3 (C-32), 21.1 (C-11), 18.1 (C-6), 16.4 (C-23), 16.2 (C-25), 15.9 (C-26), 14.7 (C-27) ppm; MS (ESI, MeOH): m/z = 583.3 (100%, [M + H]$^+$; analysis calcd for C$_{36}$H$_{58}$N$_2$O$_4$ (582.87): C 74.18, H 10.03, N 4.81; found: C 73.95, H 10.34, N 4.63.

4.15. General Procedure for the Synthesis of the Rhodamine Conjugates 13–28 (GPC)

To a solution of the respective rhodamine (1.15 eq.) in dry DCM at 0 °C, DMF (cat.) and oxalyl chloride (4 eq.) were added (vide supra). This acid chloride was slowly added to the solution of the respective triterpene (1 eq. in DCM) in the presence of triethylamine (1 eq.). After stirring for 1 day at 20 °C, aqueous work-up was carried out as usual and the residue was purified by column chromatography.

4.16. 9-[2-[[4-(3β-Acetyloxy-28-oxo-lup-20(29)en-28-yl)-1-piperazinyl]carbonyl]phenyl]-3,6-bis(diethylamino)-xanthylium chloride (13)

Following GPC from **5** (180 mg, 0.32 mmol) and rhodamine B, **13** (220 mg, 67%) was obtained as a pink solid; R$_f$ = 0.39 (SiO$_2$, CHCl$_3$/MeOH, 9:1); m.p. 247–252 °C (lit.: [20] m.p. 246–250 °C); MS (ESI, MeOH): m/z = 991.6 (100%, [M − Cl]$^+$).

4.17. 9-[2-[[4-(3β-Acetyloxy-28-oxo-olean-12-en-28-yl)-1-piperazinyl]carbonyl]phenyl]-3,6-bis(diethylamino)-xanthylium chloride (14)

Following GPC from **6** (180 mg, 0.32 mmol) and rhodamine B, **14** (250 mg, 76%) was obtained as a pink solid; R$_f$ = 0.40 (SiO$_2$, CHCl$_3$/MeOH, 9:1); m.p. 246–252 °C (lit.: [20] 245–248 °C); MS (ESI, MeOH): m/z = 991.9 (100%, [M − Cl]$^+$).

4.18. 9-[2-[[4-(3β-Acetyloxy-28-oxo-ursan-12-en-28-yl)-1-piperazinyl]carbonyl]phenyl]-3,6-bis(diethylamino)-xanthylium chloride (15)

Following GPC from **7** (180 mg, 0.32 mmol) and rhodamine B, **15** (190 mg, 58%) was obtained as a pink solid; R$_f$ = 0.40 (SiO$_2$, CHCl$_3$/MeOH, 9:1); m.p. 245–251 °C (lit.: [20] 243–245 °C); MS (ESI, MeOH): m/z = 991.7 (100%, [M − Cl]$^+$).

4.19. 9-[2-[[4-(3β-Acetyloxy-20,28-dioxo-30-norlupan-28-yl)-1-piperazinyl]carbonyl]phenyl]-3,6-bis(diethylamino)-xanthylium chloride (16)

Following GPC from **8** (180 mg, 0.32 mmol) and rhodamine B, **16** (230 mg, 70%) was obtained as a pink solid; R$_f$ = 0.37 (SiO$_2$, CHCl$_3$/MeOH, 9:1); m.p. 247–254 °C (lit.: [20] 235–243 °C); MS (ESI, MeOH): m/z = 993.7 (100%, [M − Cl]$^+$).

4.20. 9-[2-[[4-(3β-Acetyloxy-28-oxo-30-norlupan-28-yl)-1-homopiperazinyl]carbonyl]phenyl]-3,6-bis(diethylamino)-xanthylium chloride (17)

Following GPC from **9** (260 mg, 0.32 mmol) and rhodamine B, **17** (229 mg, 69%) was obtained as a pink solid; R$_f$ = 0.50 (SiO$_2$, MeCN/CH$_2$Cl$_2$/H$_2$O, 10:1:1); m.p. 261–266 °C (lit.: [21] 256–260 °C); MS (ESI, MeOH): m/z = 1005.7 (100%, [M − Cl]$^+$).

4.21. 9-[2-[[4-(3β-Acetyloxy-28-oxo-olean-12-en-28-yl]-1-homopiperazinyl]carbonyl]phenyl]-3,6-bis(diethylamino)-xanthylium chloride (**18**)

Following GPC from **10** (270 mg, 0.32 mmol) and rhodamine B, **18** (267 mg, 80%) was obtained as a pink solid; R_f = 0.52 (SiO$_2$, MeCN/CH$_2$Cl$_2$/H$_2$O, 10:1:1); m.p. 235–241 °C (lit.: [21] 238–245 °C); MS (ESI, MeOH): m/z = 1005.8 (100%, [M − Cl]$^+$).

4.22. 9-[2-[[4-(3β-Acetyloxy-28-oxo-urs-12-en-28-yl]-1-homopiperazinyl]carbonyl]phenyl]-3,6-bis(diethylamino)-xanthylium chloride (**19**)

Following GPC from **11** (270 mg, 0.32 mmol) and rhodamine B, **19** (253 mg, 76%) was obtained as a pink solid; R_f = 0.51 (SiO$_2$, MeCN/CH$_2$Cl$_2$/H$_2$O, 10:1:1); m.p. 238–246 °C (lit.: [21] 238–245 °C); MS (ESI, MeOH): m/z = 1005.7 (100%, [M − Cl]$^+$).

4.23. 9-[2-[[4-(3β-Acetyloxy-20,28-dioxo-30-norlupan-28-yl)-1-homopiperazinyl]carbonyl]phenyl]-3,6-bis(diethylamino)-xanthylium chloride (**20**)

Following GPC from **10** (125 mg, 0.21 mmol) and rhodamine B, **18** (190 mg, 87%); was obtained as a pink solid; m.p. 248–250 °C (decomp.); R_f = 0.30 (SiO$_2$, CHCl$_3$/MeOH, 9:1); UV-Vis (CHCl$_3$): λ_{max} (log ε) = 562 nm (5.05); IR (ATR): ν = 2937w, 1730w, 1585s, 1466m, 1411m, 1334s, 1273m, 1244m, 1178m, 1131m, 1072m, 977w, 920w, 822w, 746m, 683m cm^{-1}; ^{1}H NMR (500 MHz, CDCl$_3$): δ = 7.66–7.57 (*m*, 2H, 42-H, 43-H), 7.42–7.36 (*m*, 1H, 40-H), 7.31–7.27 (*m*, 1H, 41-H), 7.25–7.15 (*m*, 2H, 50-H), 6.99–6.83 (*m*, 2H, 49-H), 6.79–6.68 (*m*, 2H, 47-H), 4.40 (*dd*, *J* = 10.4, 5.6 Hz, 1H, 3-H), 3.85–3.31 (*m*, 16H, 32-H, 33-H, 34-H, 36-H, 51-H), 3.27–3.12 (*m*, 1H, 13-H), 2.72–2.57 (*m*, 1H, 19-H), 2.11 (*s*, 3H, 29-H), 2.18–2.06 (*m*, 1H, 16-H$_a$), 1.98 (*s*, 3H, 31-H), 1.96 (*s*, 1H, 18-H), 1.95–0.97 (*m*, 21H, 22-H$_a$, 21-H$_a$, 35-H, 1-H$_a$, 2-H, 16-H$_b$, 21-H$_b$, 6-H, 22-H$_b$, 11-H$_a$, 7-H, 11-H$_b$, 9-H, 15-H, 12-H), 1.32–1.26 (*m*, 12H, 52-H), 0.92 (*s*, 3H, 27-H), 0.89 (*s*, 3H, 24-H), 0.94–0.86 (*m*, 1H, 1-H$_b$), 0.79 (*s*, 9H, 23-H, 25-H, 26-H), 0.73 (*s*, 1H, 5-H$_b$) ppm; ^{13}C NMR (126 MHz, CDCl$_3$): δ = 212.8 (C-20), 174.7 (C-28), 170.7 (30 C-), 168.3 (C-37), 157.5 (C-48), 157.5 (C-44), 155.4 C- (46), 136.5 (C-38) 135.9 (C-39), 132.1 (C-50), 130.1 (C-41), 129.6 (C-42), 129.4 (C-43), 126.3 (C-40), 113.9 (C-49), 113.4 (C-45), 96.2 (C-47), 80.7 (C-3), 55.3 (C-5), 54.7 (C-17), 52.7 (C-18), 50.4 (C-9), 50.0 (C-19), 46.0 (C-51), 41.6 (C-14), 40.4 (C-8), 38.2 (C-1), 37.6 (C-4), 36.9 (C-10), 35.8 (C-13), 35.3 (C-22), 34.1 (C-7), 31.7 (C-35), 31.2 (C-16), 30.0 (C-29), 29.7 (C-15), 28.7 (C-21), 27.7 (C-23), 27.2 (C-12), 23.5 (C-2), 21.1 (C-31), 21.0 (C-11), 18.0 (C-6), 16.3 (C-25), 16.1 (C-26), 16.0 (C-24), 14.4 (C-27), 12.5 (C-52). ppm; MS (ESI, MeOH): m/z 1007 (100%, [M]$^+$); analysis calculated for C$_{64}$H$_{85}$ClN$_4$O$_6$ (1041.84): C 73.78, H 8.22, N 5.38; found: C 73.55, H 8.41, N 5.19.

4.24. 3β-Acetyloxy-28-[4-[3-(2,3,6,7,12,13,16,17-octahydro-1H,5H,11H,15H-pyrido[3,2,1-ij]pyrido[1″,2″,3″:1′,8′]quinolino[6′,5′:5,6]pyrano[2,3-f]quinolin-4-ium-9-yl)benzoyl]piperazine-1-yl]-28-oxo-lup-20(29)-en chloride (**21**)

Following GPC from **5** (0.25 g, 0.44 mmol) and rhodamine 101 (0.25 g, 0.51 mmol), **21** (0.24 g, 52%) was obtained as a pink colored solid; R_f = 0.4 (SiO$_2$, CHCl$_3$/MeOH, 9:1); m.p. >300 °C; IR (ATR): ν = 3400w, 2939w, 2862w, 1728w, 1630m, 1595m, 1542w, 1493m, 1434m, 1360m, 1294vs, 1267s, 1248s, 1195s, 1182s, 1099s, 1058m, 1003m, 978m, 896w, 827w, 772m, 747m, 637m, 560m, 506m, 421s cm^{-1}; ^{1}H NMR (400 MHz, CDCl$_3$): δ = 7.67 (*dd*, *J* = 5.7, 3.3 Hz, 2H, 37-H, 39-H), 7.53–7.48 (*m*, 1H, 38-H), 7.31 (*dd*, *J* = 5.7, 3.2 Hz, 1H, 40-H), 6.68 (*d*, *J* = 6.0 Hz, 2H, 48-H), 4.68 (*s*, 1H, 29-H$_a$), 4.56 (*s*, 1H, 29-H$_b$), 4.44 (*dd*, *J* = 10.2, 5.9 Hz, 1H, 3-H), 3.60–3.48 (*m*, 4H, 49-H), 3.48–3.40 (*m*, 4H, 52-H), 3.40–3.31 (*m*, 8H, 33-H + 34-H), 3.04–2.97 (*m*, 4H, 54-H), 2.91 (*dt*, *J* = 11.9, 6.1 Hz, 1H, 19-H), 2.81–2.74 (*m*, 1H, 13-H), 2.74–2.60 (*m*, 4H, 51-H), 2.14–2.04 (*m*, 4H, 53-H), 2.02 (*s*, 3H, 32-H), 1.98–1.91 (*m*, 4H, 50-H), 1.77 (*q*, *J* = 33.5, 10.4 Hz, 4H, 12-H + 16-H$_a$ + 22-H$_a$), 1.65 (*s*, 3H, 30-H), 1.63–1.44 (*m*, 8H, 1-H + 2-H + 6-H$_a$ + 11-H + 16-H$_b$ + 18-H), 1.44–1.08 (*m*, 10H, 6-H$_b$ + 7-H + 9-H + 15-H + 21-H + 22-H$_b$), 0.92 (*s*, 3H, 27-H), 0.88 (*s*, 3H, 26-H), 0.82 (*s*, 6H, 23-H + 24-H), 0.81 (*s*, 3H, 25-H), 0.77 (*s*, 1H, 5-H) ppm; ^{13}C NMR (101 MHz, CDCl$_3$): δ = 174.1 (C-28), 171.0 (C-31), 167.9 (C-35), 162.7 (C-20), 152.0 (C-43), 151.2 (C-44), 150.9 (C-46), 134.8 (C-41), 131.8 (C-36),

130.7 (C-40), 130.2 (C-39), 129.7 (C-37), 127.5 (C-38), 126.5 (C-48), 123.6 (C-45), 123.6 (C-45), 113.2 (C-42), 109.4 (C-29), 105.4 (C-47), 80.9 (C-3), 55.5 (C-5), 54.6 (C-17), 52.5 (C-18), 51.0 (C-49), 50.7 (C-9), 50.5 (C-52,), 45.7 (C-19), 41.9 (C-14), 40.6 (C-8), 38.4 (C-1), 37.8 (C-4), 37.1 (C-10), 36.9 (C-13), 35.8 (C-22), 34.3 (C-7), 32.5 (C-16), 31.2 (C-21), 29.8 (C-15), 27.9 (C-24), 27.7 (C-51), 25.5 (C-12), 23.7 (C-2), 21.3 (C-32), 20.6 (C-11, C-50), 19.9 (C-54), 19.6 (C-53), 19.5 (C-30), 18.1 (C-6), 16.5 (C-23), 16.2 (C-25), 16.1 (C-26), 14.6 (C-27) ppm; MS (ESI, MeOH): m/z = 1039.3 (100%, [M − Cl]$^+$); analysis calculated for C$_{68}$H$_{87}$N$_4$O$_5$Cl (1075.92): C 75.91, H 8.15, N 5.21; found: C 75.77, H 8.36, N 5.05.

4.25. 3β-Acetyloxy-28-[4-[3-(2,3,6,7,12,13,16,17-octahydro-1H,5H,11H,15H-pyrido[3,2,1-ij]pyrido[1",2",3":1',8']quinolino[6',5':5,6]pyrano[2,3-f]quinolin-4-ium-9-yl)benzoyl]piperazine-1-yl]-28-oxoolean-12-en chloride (**22**)

Following GPC from **6** (0.25 g, 0.44 mmol) and rhodamine 101 (0.25 g, 0.51 mmol), **22** (0.33 g, 71%) was obtained as a pink solid; R$_f$ = 0.4 (SiO$_2$, CHCl$_3$/MeOH, 9:1); m.p. >300 °C; IR (ATR): ν = 3398w, 2941w, 2859w, 1728w, 1631m, 1594s, 1543w, 1494s, 1458m, 1435m, 1361m, 1295Vs, 1267s, 1248s, 1196s, 1182s, 1100s, 1077m, 1035m, 1002m, 897w, 862w, 773w, 733m, 640m, 560m, 498m, 421s cm^{-1}; ^{1}H NMR (500 MHz, CDCl$_3$) δ = 7.70–7.66 (m, 2H, 37-H, 39-H), 7.53–7.49 (m, 1H, 38-H), 7.34–7.30 (m, 1H, 40-H), 6.67 (d, J = 7.5 Hz, 2H, 48-H), 5.23 (t, J = 3.5 Hz, 1H, 12-H), 4.48 (dd, J = 9.9, 6.0 Hz, 1H, 3-H), 3.63–3.51 (m, 4H, 49-H), 3.52–3.40 (m, 4H, 52-H), 3.39–3.29 (m, 8H, 33-H + 34-H), 3.09–3 (m, 4H, 54-H), 3.00–2.96 (m, 1H, 18-H), 2.76–2.62 (m, 4H, 51-H), 2.15–2.07 (m, 5H, 16-H$_a$ + 53-H), 2.04 (s, 3H, 32-H), 2.01–1.91 (m, 4H, 50-H), 1.89–1.81 (m, 1H, 11-H), 1.71–1.48 (m, 10H, 1-H$_a$ + 2-H + 6-H$_a$ + 7-H + 9-H + 15-H$_a$ + 16-H$_b$ + 19-H$_a$), 1.48–1.13 (m, 7H, 6-H$_b$ + 19-H$_b$ + 21-H + 22-H$_a$ + 22-H$_b$), 1.11 (s, 3H, 27-H), 1.08–0.94 (m, 2H, 1-H$_b$ + 15-H$_b$), 0.91 (s, 3H, 25-H), 0.89 (s, 3H, 29-H), 0.88 (s, 3H, 30-H), 0.86 (s, 3H, 24-H), 0.85 (s, 3H, 23-H), 0.82 (s, 1H, 5-H), 0.66 (s, 3H, 26-H) ppm; ^{13}C NMR (126 MHz, CDCl$_3$): δ = 176.4 (C-28), 171.0 (C-31), 167.8 (C-35), 152.8 (C-43), 152.0 (C-44), 152.0 (C-44), 151.3 (C-46), 151.2 (C-46), 144.4 (C-13), 134.8 (C-41), 131.8 (C-36), 130.8 (C-40), 130.2 (C-39), 129.7 (C-37), 127.4 (C-36), 126.5 (C-48), 126.5 (C-48), 123.6 (C-45), 123.5 (C-45), 121.7 (C-12), 113.3 (C-42), 105.5 (C-47), 105.5 (C-47), 80.8 (C-3), 55.3 (C-5), 51.0 (C-49, 49), 50.6 (C-52), 47.6 (C-9, 33, 34), 47.5 (C-17), 46.2 (C-19), 43.5 (C-18), 41.8 (C-14), 39.1 (C-8), 38.0 (C-1), 37.7 (C-4), 37.0 (C-10), 33.9 (C-21), 32.9 (C-30), 32.8 (C-22), 30.3 (C-20), 30.0 (C-7), 28.0 (C-24), 27.8 (C-15), 27.7 (C-51), 25.9 (C-27), 24.0 (C-29), 23.5 (C-2), 23.3 (C-11), 22.5 (C-16), 21.3 (C-32), 20.6 (C-50), 19.9 (C-54), 19.7 (C-53), 18.2 (C-6), 16.9 (C-26), 16.7 (C-23), 15.4 (C-25) ppm; MS (ESI, MeOH): m/z = 1039.3 (100%, [M − Cl]$^+$); analysis calculated for C$_{68}$H$_{87}$N$_4$O$_5$Cl (1075.64): C 75.91, H 8.15, N 5.21; found: C 75.72, H 8.29, N 5.01.

4.26. 3β-Acetyloxy-28-[4-[3-(2,3,6,7,12,13,16,17-octahydro-1H,5H,11H,15H-pyrido[3,2,1-ij]pyrido[1",2",3":1',8']quinolino[6',5':5,6]pyrano[2,3-f]quinolin-4-ium-9-yl)benzoyl]piperazine-1-yl]-28-oxo-urs-12-en chloride (**23**)

Following GPC from **7** (0.25 g, 0.44 mmol) and rhodamine 101 (0.25 g, 0.51 mmol), **23** (0.27 g, 58%) was obtained as a pink solid; R$_f$ = 0.4 (SiO$_2$, CHCl$_3$/MeOH, 9:1); m.p. >300 °C; IR (ATR): ν = 3392w, 2926w, 2867w, 1728w, 1626m, 1594s, 1542w, 1493s, 1457m, 1435m, 1361m, 1294vs, 1266s, 1246s, 1196s, 1181s, 1099s, 1035m, 1004m, 897w, 863w, 773m, 732m, 653m, 561m, 420s cm^{-1}; ^{1}H NMR (500 MHz, CDCl$_3$): δ = 7.71–7.65 (m, 2H, 37-H, 39-H), 7.54–7.48 (m, 1H, 38-H), 7.34–7.30 (m, 1H, 40-H), 6.67 (d, J = 4.7 Hz, 2H, 48-H), 5.17 (s, 1H, 12-H), 4.48 (dd, J = 10.4, 5.5 Hz, 1H, 3-H), 3.56 (dt, J = 17.2, 6.1 Hz, 4H, 49-H), 3.51–3.41 (m, 4H, 52-H), 3.33 (s, 8H, 33-H + 34-H), 3.02 (q, J = 6.0 Hz, 4H, 54-H), 2.68 (ddt, J = 22.7, 15.6, 7.3 Hz, 4H, 51-H), 2.39–2.32 (m, 1H, 18-H), 2.15–2.06 (m, 4H, 53-H), 2.04 (s, 3H, 32-H), 1.99–1.94 (m, 4H, 50-H), 1.91–1.87 (m, 1H + 11-H$_a$), 1.79–1.57 (m, 7H + 1-H$_a$ + 2-H + 11-H$_b$ + 16-H + 22-H$_a$), 1.56–1.40 (m, 5H, 6-H$_a$ + 7-H$_a$ + 9-H + 21-H$_a$ + 22-H$_b$), 1.40–1.20 (m, 4H, 6-H$_b$ + 7-H$_b$ + 19-H + 21-H$_b$), 1.05 (s, 6H, 1-H$_b$ + 15-H + 27-H), 0.99–0.95 (m, 1H, 20-H), 0.93 (s, 3H, 30-H), 0.91 (s, 3H, 25-H), 0.86 (s, 3H, 24-H), 0.86 (s, 3H, 26-H), 0.84 (s, 3H, 29-H), 0.81–0.80 (m, 1H, 5-H), 0.67 (s, 3H, 23-H) ppm; ^{13}C NMR (126 MHz, CDCl$_3$): δ = 174.8

(C-28), 171.0 (C-31), 167.8 (C-35), 152.8 (C-46), 152.0 (C-43), 151.3 (C-44), 151.2 (C-44), 134.8 (C-41), 130.8 (C-40), 130.2 (C-37), 129.8 (C-39), 127.5 (C-38), 126.5 (C-48), 125.2 (C-12), 123.6, 123.5 (C-45), 113.2 (C-42), 105.5 (C-47), 105.5 (C-47), 80.8 (C-3), 55.3 (C-5, 18), 51.0 (C-49), 50.6 (C-52), 48.6 (C-17), 47.5 (C-9, C-33, C-34), 42.1 (C-14), 39.8 (C-19), 39.4 (C-8), 38.7 (C-20), 34.4 (C-22), 32.9 (C-7), 30.4 (C-21), 28.1 (C-15), 28.1 (C-24), 27.7 (C-51), 27.7 (C-51), 23.5 (C-2, 16, 27), 23.3 (C-11), 21.3 (C-30), 21.2 (C-32), 20.6 (C-50), 19.9 (C-54), 19.7 (C-53), 18.2 (C-6), 17.4 (C-29), 16.9 (C-26), 16.7 (C-23), 15.5 (C-25) ppm; MS (ESI, MeOH): m/z = 1039.4 ([M − Cl]$^+$, 100%); analysis calculated for $C_{68}H_{87}N_4O_5Cl$ (1075.64): C 75.91, H 8.15, N 5.21; found: C 75.64, H 8.29, N 4.96.

4.27. 3β-Acetyloxy-28-[4-[3-(2,3,6,7,12,13,16,17-octahydro-1H,5H,11H,15H-pyrido[3,2,1-ij]pyrido[1",2",3":1',8']quinolino[6',5':5,6]pyrano[2,3-f]quinolin-4-ium-9-yl)benzoyl]piperazine-1-yl]-20,28-dioxo-30-norlupan-12-en chloride (**24**)

Following GPC from **8** (0.25 g, 0.44 mmol) and rhodamine 101 (0.25 g, 0.51 mmol), **24** (0.30 g, 65%) was obtained as a pink solid; R_f = 0.4 (SiO$_2$, CHCl$_3$/MeOH, 9:1); m.p. >300 °C; IR (ATR): ν = 3396w, 2940w, 2863w, 1727w, 1627m, 1594s, 1543w, 1493s, 1459m, 1446m, 1439m, 1419m, 1361m, 1295Vs, 1267s, 1195s, 1182s, 1099s, 1035m, 1004m, 979m, 897w, 863w, 773m, 732m, 561m, 505m, 420s cm^{-1}; ^{1}H NMR (500 MHz, CDCl$_3$): δ = 7.70–7.67 (m, 2H, 37-H, 39-H), 7.53–7.49 (m, 1H, 38-H), 7.33–7.30 (m, 1H, 40-H), 6.66 (d, J = 6.8 Hz, 2H, 48-H), 4.44 (dd, J = 10.9, 5.2 Hz, 1H, 3-H), 3.62–3.51 (m, 4H, 49-H), 3.51–3.43 (m, 4H, 52-H), 3.43–3.29 (m, 8H, 33-H + 34-H), 3.15 (td, J = 11.1, 3.1 Hz, 1H, 19-H), 3.06–2.98 (m, 4H, 54-H), 2.78–2.63 (m, 4H, 51-H), 2.58 (td, J = 12.1, 3.8 Hz, 1H, 13-H), 2.14 (s, 3H, 29-H), 2.13–2.08 (m, 4H, 53-H), 2.08–2.04 (m, 1H, 18-H), 2.02 (s, 3H, 32-H), 1.97 (q, J = 6.9 Hz, 5H, 16-H$_a$ + 50-H), 1.88–1.80 (m, 2H, 21-H$_a$ + 22-H$_a$), 1.67–1.54 (m, 4H, 1-H$_a$ + 2-H + 16-H$_b$), 1.54–0.98 (m, 14H, 6-H$_a$ + 6-H$_b$ + 7-H + 9-H + 11-H$_a$ + 11-H$_b$ + 12-H + 15-H + 21-H$_b$ + 22-H$_b$), 0.95 (s, 4H, 1-H$_b$ + 27-H), 0.87 (s, 3H, 26-H), 0.82 (s, 3H, 24-H), 0.82 (s, 3H, 25-H), 0.81 (s, 3H, 23-H), 0.79–0.75 (m, 1H, 5-H) ppm; ^{13}C NMR (126 MHz, CDCl$_3$) δ = 212.6 (C-20), 173.9 (C-28), 170.9 (C-31), 167.8 (C-35), 152.8 (C-43), 152.0 (C-44), 152.0 (C-44), 151.3 (C-46), 151.2 (C-46), 134.7 (C-41), 131.9 (C-36), 130.8 (C-40), 130.3 (C-39), 129.7 (C-37), 127.4 (C-38), 126.5 (C-48), 123.6 (C-45), 123.5 (C-45), 113.2 (C-42), 105.5 (C-47), 55.4 (C-5), 54.5 (C-17), 52.5 (C-18), 51.0 (C-49), 51.0 (C-49), 50.6 (C-52), 50.6 (C-52), 50.5 (C-9), 50.0 (C-19), 41.7 (C-14), 40.5 (C-8), 38.3 (C-1), 37.8 (C-4), 37.1 (C-10), 35.9 (C-13), 35.6 (C-22), 34.2 (C-7), 32.0 (C-16), 30.2 (C-29), 29.8 (C-15), 28.7 (C-21), 27.9 (C-24), 27.7 (C-51), 27.4 (C-12), 23.6 (C-2), 21.3 (C-32), 21.1 (C-11), 20.6 (C-50), 19.9 (C-54), 19.7 (C-53), 18.1 (C-6), 16.5 (C-23), 16.2 (C-25), 16.0 (C-26), 14.6 (C-27) ppm; MS (ESI, MeOH): m/z = 1041.3 ([M − Cl]$^+$, 100%); analysis calculated for $C_{67}H_{85}N_4O_6Cl$ (1077.89): C 74.66, H 7.95, N 5.20; found: C 74.50, H 8.14, N 5.03.

4.28. 3β-Acetyloxy-28-[4-[3-(2,3,6,7,12,13,16,17-octahydro-1H,5H,11H,15H-pyrido[3,2,1-ij]pyrido[1",2",3":1',8']quinolino[6',5':5,6]pyrano[2,3-f]quinolin-4-ium-9-yl)benzoyl]homopiperazine-1-yl]-28-oxo-lup-20(29)-en chloride (**25**)

Following GPC from **9** (0.35 g, 0.60 mmol) and rhodamine 101 (0.25 g, 0.51 mmol), **25** (0.37 g, 68%) was obtained as a pink solid; R_f = 0.4 (SiO$_2$, CHCl$_3$/MeOH, 9:1); m.p. >300 °C; IR (ATR): ν = 2940w, 2865w, 1730w, 1624m, 1595s, 1542w, 1493s, 1459m, 1376m, 1361m, 1294vs, 1268s, 1247m, 1196s, 1180s, 1098s, 1035m, 1018m, 978m, 895w, 772w, 747m, 622m, 421s cm^{-1}; ^{1}H NMR (400 MHz, CDCl$_3$): δ = 7.63–7.51 (m, 2H, 37-H, 39-H), 7.41 (t, J = 9.2 Hz, 1H, 38-H), 7.21 (d, J = 7.4 Hz, 1H, 40-H), 6.68 (dd, J = 26.0, 20.3 Hz, 2H, 48-H), 4.70 (d, J = 18.2 Hz, 1H, 29-H$_a$), 4.55 (d, J = 17.7 Hz, 1H, 29-H$_b$), 4.45–4.38 (m, 1H, 3-H), 3.85–3.62 (m, 4H, 33-H), 3.55–3.45 (m, 8H, 49-H + 52-H), 3.44–3.24 (m, 4H, 34-H), 3.08–2.91 (m, 5H, 19-H + 54-H), 2.89–2.80 (m, 1H, 13-H), 2.78–2.59 (m, 4H), 2.07 (s, 7H, 16-H$_a$ + 53-H + 55-H), 1.99 (s, 3H, 32-H), 1.93 (s, 4H, 50-H), 1.83 (d, J = 4.6 Hz, 2H, 21-H$_a$ + 22-H$_a$), 1.66 (s, 2H, 12-H), 1.62 (s, 3H, 30-H), 1.55 (dd, J = 22.6, 11.1 Hz, 3H, 1-H + 2-H), 1.50–1.40 (m, 3H, 6-H$_a$ + 16-H$_b$ + 18-H), 1.40–1.30 (m, 5H, 7-H + 11-H$_a$ + 21-H$_b$ + 22-H$_b$), 1.30–1.04 (m, 5H, 6-H$_b$ + 9-H + 11-H$_b$ + 15-H$_a$ + 15-H$_b$), 0.93–0.89 (m, 5H, 1-H + 12-H + 27-H), 0.88 (s, 3H, 26-H),

0.82–0.78 (m, 9H, 23-H + 24-H + 25-H), 0.77–0.72 (m, 1H, 5-H) ppm; ^{13}C NMR (126 MHz, CDCl$_3$): δ = 175.5 (C-28), 170.9 (C-31), 168.9 (C-35), 152.8, 152.0 (C-43), 151.9 (C-43), 151.3 (C-44), 151.3 (C-44), 151.2 (C-20), 151.1 (C-46), 136.0 (C-41), 131.1 (C-36), 130.5 (C-40), 129.8 (C-39), 129.5 (C-37), 127.6 (C-38), 126.6 (C-48), 126.4 (C-48), 123.4 (C-45), 123.4 (C-45), 112.9 (C-42), 109.4 (C-29), 105.4 (C-47), 105.3 (C-47), 80.9 (C-3), 55.5 (C-5), 54.8 (C-17), 52.7 (C-18), 51.0 (C-49), 50.5 (C-52), 46.1 (C-33 + 34), 45.9 (C-19), 41.9 (C-14), 40.7 (C-8), 38.4 (C-1), 37.8 (C-4), 37.1 (C-10), 36.8 (C-13), 36.0 (C-22), 34.3 (C-7), 32.3 (C-16), 31.5 (C-21), 29.9 (C-15), 28.9 (C-55), 27.9 (C-24), 27.5 (C-51), 25.5 (C-12), 23.6 (C-2), 21.3 (C-32), 21.1 (C-11), 20.6 (C-50), 19.9 (C-54), 19.7 (C-53), 19.5 (C-30), 18.2 (C-6), 16.4 (C-23), 16.2 (C-25), 16.1 (C-26), 14.6 (C-27) ppm; MS (ESI, MeOH): m/z = 1052.9 ([M − Cl]$^+$, 100%); analysis calculated for C$_{69}$H$_{89}$N$_4$O$_5$Cl (1089.94): C 76.04, H 8.23, N 5.14; found: C 75.76, H 8.31, N 5.02.

4.29. 3β-Acetyloxy-28-[4-[3-(2,3,6,7,12,13,16,17-octahydro-1H,5H,11H,15H-pyrido[3,2,1-ij] pyrido[1″,2″,3″:1′,8′]quinolino[6′,5′:5,6]pyrano[2,3-f]quinolin-4-ium-9-yl)benzoyl]homopiperazine-1-yl]-28-oxo-olean-12-en chloride (**26**)

Following GPC from **10** (0.25 g, 0.60 mmol) and rhodamine 101 (0.25 g, 0.51 mmol), **26** (0.38 g, 70%) was obtained as a pink solid; R$_f$ = 0.4 (SiO$_2$, CHCl$_3$/MeOH, 9:1); m.p. > 300 °C; IR (ATR): ν = 3369vw, 2942w, 2863w, 1729w, 1623m, 1595s, 1543w, 1493s, 1459m, 1361m, 1294vs, 1268s, 1246s, 1195s, 1180s, 1150m, 1098s, 1035m, 985m, 896w, 862w, 771m, 746m, 622m, 575w, 560w, 498m, 421s cm^{-1}; ^{1}H NMR (400 MHz, CDCl$_3$): δ = 7.63–7.58 (m, 2H, 37-H + 39-H), 7.55–7.50 (m, 1H, 38-H), 7.23–7.17 (m, 1H, 40-H), 6.72–6.60 (m, 2H, 48-H), 5.25–5.21 (m, 1H, 12-H), 4.45 (t, J = 7.8 Hz, 1H, 3-H), 3.95–3.60 (m, 4H, 33-H + 34-H), 3.58–3.43 (m, 8H, 49-H + 52-H), 3.41–3.11 (m, 4H, 34-H), 3.06 (s, 1H, 18-H), 3.03–2.95 (m, 4H, 54-H), 2.74–2.61 (m, 4H, 51-H), 2.14–2.02 (m, 7H, 16-H$_a$ + 53-H + 55-H), 2.00 (s, 3H, 32-H), 1.94 (dq, J = 11.1, 5.3 Hz, 4H, 50-H), 1.88–1.79 (m, 2H + 11-H), 1.71–1.41 (m, 10H, 1-H$_a$ + 2-H + 6-H$_a$ + 7-H + 9-H + 15-H$_a$ + 16-H$_b$ + 19-H$_a$), 1.41–1.26 (m, 3H, 6-H$_b$, 21 + 22-H$_a$), 1.26–1.12 (m, 3H, 19-H$_b$ + 22-H$_b$), 1.09 (s, 3H, 27-H), 1.06–0.96 (m, 2H, 1-H$_b$ + 15-H$_b$), 0.94 (s, 3H, 29-H), 0.88 (d, J = 2.0 Hz, 6H, 25-H + 30-H), 0.82 (s, 3H, 24-H), 0.81 (s, 3H, 23-H), 0.79–0.76 (m, 1H, 5-H), 0.66 (s, 3H, 26-H) ppm; ^{13}C NMR (101 MHz, CDCl$_3$): δ = 176.1 (C-28), 171.0 (C-31), 169.0 (C-35), 152.8 (C-43), 152.0 (C-44), 151.9 (C-44), 151.3 (C-46), 151.2 (C-46), 144.8 (C-13), 136.0 (C-41), 130.4 (C-40), 129.9 (C-39), 129.5 (C-37), 127.5 (C-36), 126.5 (C-48), 126.2 (C-48), 123.6 (C-45), 123.5 (C-45), 121.4 (C-12), 113.3 (C-42), 105.5 (C-47), 105.4 (C-47), 80.9 (C-3), 55.3, 51.0 (C-49), 50.5 (C-52), 47.7 (C-17), 47.6 (C-9), 47.6 (C-33 + 34), 46.6 (C-19), 43.5 (C-18), 42.0 (C-14), 39.0 (C-8), 38.0 (C-1), 37.7 (C-4), 37.0 (C-10), 34.0 (C-21), 32.9 (C-30), 32.7 (C-22), 30.5 (C-7), 30.3 (C-20, C-55), 28.0 (C-24), 27.8 (C-15), 27.6 (C-51), 25.9 (C-27), 24.2 (C-29), 23.5 (C-2), 23.3 (C-11), 22.5 (C-16), 21.3 (C-32), 20.6 (C-50), 19.9 (C-54), 19.7 (C-53), 19.6 (C-53), 18.2 (C-6), 17.0 (C-26), 16.6 (C-23), 15.4 (C-25) ppm; MS (ESI, MeOH): m/z = 1053.0 (100%, [M − Cl]$^+$); analysis calculated for C$_{69}$H$_{89}$N$_4$O$_5$Cl (1089.94): C 76.04, H 8.23, N 5.14; found: C 75.81, H 8.40, N 4.86.

4.30. 3β-Acetyloxy-28-[4-[3-(2,3,6,7,12,13,16,17-octahydro-1H,5H,11H,15H-pyrido[3,2,1-ij]pyrido[1″,2″,3″:1′,8′]quinolino[6′,5′:5,6]pyrano[2,3-f]quinolin-4-ium-9-yl)benzoyl]homopiperazine-1-yl]-28-oxo-urs-12-en chloride (**27**)

Following GPC from **11** (0.35 g, 0.60 mmol) and rhodamine 101 (0.25 g, 0.51 mmol), **27** (0.39 g, 72%) was obtained as a pink solid; R$_f$ = 0.4 (SiO$_2$, CHCl$_3$/MeOH, 9:1); m.p. >300 °C; IR (ATR): ν = 2934w, 2866w, 1730w, 1622w, 1594w, 1543w, 1493w, 1459w, 1435w, 1376w, 1361w, 1293w, 1268w, 1246w, 1195w, 1180w, 1143w, 1098w, 1035w, 985w, 966w, 941w, 896w, 862w, 772w, 744w, 715w, 661w, 622w, 574w, 560w, 496w cm^{-1}; ^{1}H NMR (400 MHz, CDCl$_3$): δ = 7.59 (dd, J = 5.7, 3.3 Hz, 2H, 37-H + 39-H), 7.43–7.34 (m, 1H, 38-H), 7.22 (dd, J = 5.7, 3.3 Hz, 1H, 40-H), 6.61 (d, J = 24.5 Hz, 2H, 48-H), 5.18–5.11 (m, 1H-H), 4.44 (dd, J = 11.0, 5.2 Hz, 1H, 3-H), 4.08–3.66 (m, 4H, 34-H), 3.59–3.41 (m, 8H, 49-H + 52-H), 3.38–3.07 (m, 4H, 33-H), 3.02–2.93 (m, 4H, 54-H), 2.67 (h, J = 9.5, 8.8 Hz, 4H, 51-H), 2.45–2.34 (m, 1H, 18-H), 2.11–2.03 (m, 4H, 55-H + 53-H), 2.00 (s, 3H, 32-H), 1.96–1.81 (m, 6H, 11-H + 50-H),

1.79–1.52 (m, 7H, 1-H$_a$ + 2-H + 16-H + 22-H), 1.44 (dt, J = 14.3, 7.8 Hz, 4H, 6-H$_a$ + 7-H$_a$ + 9-H + 21-H$_a$), 1.37–1.11 (m, 4H, 6-H$_b$ + 7-H$_b$ + 19-H + 21-H$_b$), 1.01 (d, J = 11.5 Hz, 6H, 1-H$_b$ + 15-H + 27-H), 0.92 (s, 1H, 20-H), 0.88 (s, 6H, 25-H + 30-H), 0.81 (s, 6H, 24-H + 29-H), 0.80 (s, 3H, 23-H), 0.75 (s, 1H, 5-H), 0.66 (s, 3H, 26-H) ppm; ^{13}C NMR (126 MHz, CDCl$_3$): δ = 176.4 (C-28), 170.9 (C-31), 168.1 (C-35), 152.9 (C-46), 151.9 (C-43), 151.3 (C-44), 138.7 (C-13), 135.7 (C-41), 131.4 (C-36), 130.4 (C-40), 129.8, 129.6 (C-37), 129.5 (C-39), 127.5 (C-38), 126.8 (C-48), 125.0 (C-12), 123.7 (C-45), 113.3 (C-42), 105.3 (C-47), 105.1 (C-47), 80.9 (C-3), 55.3 (C-5, 18), 51.0 (C-49), 50.5 (C-52), 48.8 (C-17), 47.5 (C-9, 33, 34), 42.8 (C-14), 39.3 (C-8, 19), 38.7 (C-20), 38.2 (C-1), 37.6 (C-4), 36.9 (C-10), 34.4 (C-22), 32.9 (C-7), 30.4 (C-21), 30.3 (C-55), 28.0 (C-15, 24), 27.6 (C-51), 27.5 (C-51), 23.5 (C-2, 16, 27), 23.2 (C-11), 21.3 (C-30), 21.2 (C-32), 20.6 (C-50), 20.6 (C-50), 19.9 (C-54), 19.7 (C-53), 19.6 (C-53), 18.1, 17.4 (C-29), 17.0 (C-26), 16.7 (C-23), 15.5 (C-25) ppm; MS (ESI, MeOH): m/z = 1053.1 (100%, [M − Cl]$^+$); analysis calculated for C$_{69}$H$_{89}$N$_4$O$_5$Cl (1089.94): C 76.04, H 8.23, N 5.14; found: C 75.76, H 8.51, N 4.97.

4.31. 3β-Acetyloxy-28-[4-[3-(2,3,6,7,12,13,16,17-octahydro-1H,5H,11H,15H-pyrido[3,2,1-ij]pyrido[1″,2″,3″:1′,8′]quinolino[6′,5′:5,6]pyrano [2,3-f]quinolin-4-ium-9-yl)benzoyl]homopiperazine-1-yl]-20,28-dioxo-30-norlupan-12-en chloride (**28**)

Following GPC from **12** (0.35 g, 0.60 mmol) and rhodamine 101 (0.25 g, 0.51 mmol), **28** (0.35 g, 66%) was obtained as a pink solid; R_f = 0.4 (SiO$_2$, CHCl$_3$/MeOH, 9:1); m.p. > 300 °C; IR (ATR): ν = 3383vw, 2940w, 2863w, 1731w, 1623m, 1594s, 1542w, 1493s, 1459m, 1436m, 1376m, 1361m, 1294vs, 1268s, 1247m, 1195s, 1180s, 1143m, 1099s, 1075m, 1035m, 1018m, 978w, 897w, 862w, 746m, 623w, 561m, 506m, 421s cm^{-1}; ^{1}H NMR (500 MHz, CDCl$_3$): δ = 7.63–7.57 (m, 2H, 37-H + 39-H), 7.41 (d, J = 23.5 Hz, 1H, 38-H), 7.29–7.21 (m, 1H, 40-H), 6.67 (dd, J = 27.4, 18.9 Hz, 2H, 48-H), 4.42 (dt, J = 10.6, 5.4 Hz, 1H, 3-H), 3.93–3.58 (m, 4H, 33-H), 3.58–3.40 (m, 8H, 49-H, 52-H), 3.40–3.08 (m, 5H, 19-H, 34-H), 3.06–2.91 (m, 4H, 54-H), 2.70 (d, J = 27.3 Hz, 5H, 13-H + 51-H), 2.12 (s, 3H, 29-H), 2.10–2.02 (m, 7H, 16-H$_a$ + 53-H + 55-H), 2.00 (s, 4H, 18-H + 32-H), 1.98–1.88 (m, 5H, 22-H$_a$ + 50-H), 1.87–1.80 (m, 1H, 21-H$_a$), 1.66–1.52 (m, 4H, 1-H + 16-H$_b$), 1.45 (q, J = 16.9, 12.1 Hz, 3H, 6-H$_a$ + 21-H$_b$ + 22-H$_b$), 1.39–1.30 (m, 5H, 6-H$_b$ + 7-H + 11-H$_a$ + 12-H$_a$), 1.29–1.19 (m, 4H, 9-H + 11-H$_b$ + 15-H), 0.95–0.93 (m, 2H, 1-H + 12-H$_b$), 0.91 (s, 6H, 26-H + 27-H), 0.83–0.78 (m, 9H, 23-H + 24-H + 25-H), 0.76–0.72 (m, 1H, 5-H) ppm; ^{13}C NMR (126 MHz, CDCl$_3$): δ = 213.0 (C-20), 174.5 (C-28), 170.9 (C-31), 168.9 (C-35), 152.6 (C-43), 151.9 (C-44), 151.3 (C-46), 136.1 (C-41), 131.1 (C-36), 130.5 (C-40), 129.8 (C-39), 129.5 (C-37), 127.5 (C-38), 126.7 (C-48), 126.2 (C-48), 123.7 (C-45), 123.5 (C-45), 112.9 (C-42), 105.3 (C-47), 80.9 (C-3), 55.5 (C-5), 54.9 (C-17), 52.8 (C-18), 51.0 (C-49), 50.6 (C-9), 50.5 (C-52), 50.2 (C-19), 48.0 (C-33 + 34), 41.8 (C-14), 40.6 (C-8), 38.4 (C-1), 37.8 (C-4), 37.1 (C-10), 36.0 (C-13), 35.6 (C-22), 34.2 (C-7), 31.9 (C-16), 30.2 (C-29), 29.9 (C-15), 29.6 (C-55), 28.9 (C-21), 27.9 (C-24), 27.6 (C-51), 27.6 (C-51), 27.3 (C-12), 23.6 (C-2), 21.3 (C-32), 21.2 (C-11), 20.6 (C-50), 19.9 (C-54), 19.7 (C-53), 19.6 (C-53), 18.2 (C-6), 16.5 (C-23), 16.2 (C-25), 16.1 (C-26), 14.7 (C-27) ppm; MS (ESI, MeOH): m/z = 1055.0 (100%, [M − Cl]$^+$); analysis calcd for C$_{68}$H$_{87}$N$_4$O$_6$Cl (1091.92): C 74.80, H 8.03, N 5.13; found: C 74.61, H 8.27, N 4.95.

4.32. Cytotoxicity Assay (SRB)

The cell lines were obtained from Department of Oncology (Martin-Luther-University Halle Wittenberg; they were bought from ATCC; A 375 (CRL-1619), HT29 (HTB-38), MCF7 (HTM-22), A2780 (HTP-77), FaDu (HTP-43), NIH 3T3 (CRL-1658), HEK-293 (CRL-1573)). Cultures were maintained as monolayers in RPMI 1640 medium with L-glutamine (Capricorn Scientific GmbH, Ebsdorfergrund, Germany) supplemented with 10% heat inactivated fetal bovine serum (Sigma-Aldrich Chemie GmbH, Steinheim, Germany) and penicillin/streptomycin (1%, Capricorn Scientific GmbH, Ebsdorfergrund, Germany) at 37 °C in a humidified atmosphere with 5% CO$_2$. The cytotoxicity of the compounds was evaluated using the sulforhodamine-B (Kiton-Red S, ABCR) micro culture colorimetric assay using confluent cells in 96-well plates with the seeding of the cells on day 0 applying appropriate cell densities to prevent confluence of the cells during the period of the experiment. On day 1, the cells were treated with six different concentrations (1, 3, 7, 12, 20, and 30 µM);

thereby, the final concentration of DMSO was always <0.5%, generally regarded as non-toxic to the cells. On day 4, the supernatant medium was discarded; the cells were fixed with 10% trichloroacetic acid. After another day at 4 °C, the cells were washed in a strip washer and dyed with the SRB solution (100 µL, 0.4% in 1% acetic acid) for about 20 min to be followed by washing of the plates (four times, 1% acetic acid) and air-drying overnight. Furthermore, tris base solution (200 µL, 10 mM) was added to each well and absorbance was measured at λ = 570 nm employing a reader (96 wells, Tecan Spectra, Crailsheim, Germany). The EC_{50} values were averaged from three independent experiments performed each in triplicate calculated from semi logarithmic dose response curves applying a non-linear four-parameter Hills-slope equation (GraphPad Prism5; variables top and bottom were set to 100 and 0, respectively).

4.33. Acridine Orange (AO) Staining

On the first day, A375 cells were counted and seeded 1×10^5 in a Petri dish (diameter 4 cm) with coverslips (22 mm × 22 mm) in 2 mL medium. After 24 h, the medium was removed, and treatment was performed with 2 mL of new medium (control) and 2 mL each of 2 times the EC_{50} concentration of compounds **27**. After 24 h, the medium was removed from the samples, the coverslip was rinsed with 1 mL of PBS (with Ca^{2+} and Mg^{2+}), placed on a slide containing 20 µL of AO solution (2.5 µg/mL in PBS), and measured directly on the fluorescence microscope.

4.34. Hoechst 33,3342 and Rhodamine 123 Staining

On day 1, A375 cells were counted and seeded 1×10^5 in a Petri dish (diameter 4 cm) with coverslips (22 mm × 22 mm) in 2 mL medium. After 24 h, the medium was removed, and treatment was performed with 1 mL of new medium containing 1 µL of compound **27** (0.08 mM solution). After another 24 h, additional treatment was performed with 1 µL rhodamine (1 mg/mL in EtOH) and 2 µL Hoechst 33342 (100 µg/mL in DMSO) for (at least) 30 min. The medium was then removed, rinsed once with PBS (with Ca^{2+} and Mg^{2+}), placed on a slide containing 20 µL PBS (with Ca^{2+} and Mg^{2+}), and measured directly on the fluorescence microscope.

Author Contributions: Conceptualization, R.C.; validation, R.C., N.V.H. and M.K.; investigation, N.V.H., S.H. and M.K.; writing—original draft preparation, R.C.; writing—review and editing, N.V.H., D.M., S.H., M.K., I.S. and R.C. All authors have read and agreed to the published version of the manuscript.

Funding: This research received no external funding.

Institutional Review Board Statement: Not applicable.

Informed Consent Statement: Not applicable.

Data Availability Statement: The data presented in this study are available on request from the corresponding author.

Acknowledgments: We like to thank D. Ströhl, Y. Schiller and S. Ludwig for the NMR spectra and the late R. Kluge as well as T. Schmidt for recording numerous MS spectra; IR spectra, micro-analyses and optical rotations were measured by M. Schneider. The cell lines were provided by Th. Müller (Dept. Oncology, Martin-Luther-University Halle-Wittenberg).

Conflicts of Interest: The authors declare no conflict of interest.

Sample Availability: Samples of the compounds are available from the authors.

References

1. Gambardella, V.; Fleitas, T.; Tarazona, N.; Papaccio, F.; Huerta, M.; Rosello, S.; Gimeno-Valiente, F.; Roda, D.; Cervantes, A. Precision Medicine to Treat Advanced Gastroesophageal Adenocarcinoma: A Work in Progress. *J. Clin. Med.* **2020**, *9*, 3049. [CrossRef]
2. Gambardella, V.; Tarazona, N.; Cejalvo, J.M.; Lombardi, P.; Huerta, M.; Rosello, S.; Fleitas, T.; Roda, D.; Cervantes, A. Personalized Medicine: Recent Progress in Cancer Therapy. *Cancers* **2020**, *12*, 1009. [CrossRef] [PubMed]
3. Hofmarcher, T.; Lindgren, P.; Wilking, N.; Jonsson, B. The cost of cancer in Europe 2018. *Eur. J. Cancer* **2020**, *129*, 41–49. [CrossRef]
4. Wilking, N.; Brådvik, G.; Lindgren, P.; Svedman, C.; Jönsson, B.; Hofmarcher, T. A comparative study on costs of cancer and access to medicines in Europe. *Ann. Oncol.* **2020**, *31*, S1197. [CrossRef]
5. Wilking, N.E.; Brådvik, G.; Lindgren, P.; Svedman, C.; Jönsson, B.; Hofmarcher, T. A comparative study on costs of cancer and access to medicines in Europe. *J. Clin. Oncol.* **2020**, *38*, e19051. [CrossRef]
6. Nuffieldtrust. Available online: https://www.nuffieldtrust.org.uk/resource/cancer-survival-rates (accessed on 28 March 2020).
7. Lammers, T.; Kiessling, F.; Hennink, W.E.; Storm, G. Drug targeting to tumors: Principles, pitfalls and (pre-) clinical progress. *J. Control. Release* **2012**, *161*, 175–187. [CrossRef]
8. Klochkov, S.G.; Neganova, M.E.; Nikolenko, V.N.; Chen, K.; Somasundaram, S.G.; Kirkland, C.E.; Aliev, G. Implications of nanotechnology for the treatment of cancer: Recent advances. *Semin. Cancer Biol.* **2021**, *69*, 190–199. [PubMed]
9. Schrama, D.; Reisfeld, R.A.; Becker, J.C. Antibody targeted drugs as cancer therapeutics. *Nat. Rev. Drug Discov.* **2006**, *5*, 147–159. [CrossRef]
10. Moosavian, S.A.; Bianconi, V.; Pirro, M.; Sahebkar, A. Challenges and pitfalls in the development of liposomal delivery systems for cancer therapy. *Semin. Cancer Biol.* **2021**, *69*, 337–348. [CrossRef]
11. Chiu, H.Y.; Tay, E.X.Y.; Ong, D.S.T.; Taneja, R. Mitochondrial Dysfunction at the Center of Cancer Therapy. *Antioxid. Redox Signal.* **2020**, *32*, 309–330. [CrossRef] [PubMed]
12. Dong, L.F.; Gopalan, V.; Holland, O.; Neuzil, J. Mitocans Revisited: Mitochondrial Targeting as Efficient Anti-Cancer Therapy. *Int. J. Mol. Sci.* **2020**, *21*, 7941. [CrossRef]
13. Fialova, J.L.; Raudenska, M.; Jakubek, M.; Kejik, Z.; Martasek, P.; Babula, P.; Matkowski, A.; Filipensky, P.; Masarik, M. Novel Mitochondria-targeted Drugs for Cancer Therapy. *Mini-Rev. Med. Chem.* **2021**, *21*, 816–832. [CrossRef]
14. Macasoi, I.; Mioc, A.; Mioc, M.; Racoviceanu, R.; Soica, I.; Cheveresan, A.; Dehelean, C.; Dumitrascu, V. Targeting Mitochondria through the Use of Mitocans as Emerging Anticancer Agents. *Curr. Med. Chem.* **2020**, *27*, 5730–5757. [CrossRef] [PubMed]
15. Mani, S.; Swargiary, G.; Singh, K.K. Natural Agents Targeting Mitochondria in Cancer. *Int. J. Mol. Sci.* **2020**, *21*, 6992. [CrossRef]
16. Nguyen, C.; Pandey, S. Exploiting Mitochondrial Vulnerabilities to Trigger Apoptosis Selectively in Cancer Cells. *Cancers* **2019**, *11*, 916. [CrossRef]
17. Hoenke, S.; Serbian, I.; Deigner, H.P.; Csuk, R. Mitocanic Di- and Triterpenoid Rhodamine B Conjugates. *Molecules* **2020**, *25*, 5443. [CrossRef] [PubMed]
18. Kahnt, M.; Wiemann, J.; Fischer, L.; Sommerwerk, S.; Csuk, R. Transformation of asiatic acid into a mitocanic, bimodal-acting rhodamine B conjugate of nanomolar cytotoxicity. *Eur. J. Med. Chem.* **2018**, *159*, 143–148. [CrossRef]
19. Serbian, I.; Hoenke, S.; Csuk, R. Synthesis of some steroidal mitocans of nanomolar cytotoxicity acting by apoptosis. *Eur. J. Med. Chem.* **2020**, *199*, 112425. [CrossRef] [PubMed]
20. Sommerwerk, S.; Heller, L.; Kerzig, C.; Kramell, A.E.; Csuk, R. Rhodamine B conjugates of triterpenoic acids are cytotoxic mitocans even at nanomolar concentrations. *Eur. J. Med. Chem.* **2017**, *127*, 1–9. [CrossRef]
21. Wolfram, R.K.; Fischer, L.; Kluge, R.; Strohl, D.; Al-Harrasi, A.; Csuk, R. Homopiperazine-rhodamine B adducts of triterpenoic acids are strong mitocans. *Eur. J. Med. Chem.* **2018**, *155*, 869–879. [CrossRef] [PubMed]
22. Wolfram, R.K.; Heller, L.; Csuk, R. Targeting mitochondria: Esters of rhodamine B with triterpenoids are mitocanic triggers of apoptosis. *Eur. J. Med. Chem.* **2018**, *152*, 21–30. [CrossRef]
23. Wiemann, J.; Al-Harrasi, A.; Csuk, R. Cytotoxic Dehydroabietylamine Derived Compounds. *Anti-Cancer Agents Med. Chem.* **2020**, *20*, 1756–1767. [CrossRef]
24. Brandes, B.; Koch, L.; Hoenke, S.; Deigner, H.P.; Csuk, R. The presence of a cationic center is not alone decisive for the cytotoxicity of triterpene carboxylic acid amides. *Steroids* **2020**, *163*, 108713. [CrossRef] [PubMed]
25. Heise, N.; Hoenke, S.; Simon, V.; Deigner, H.P.; Al-Harrasi, A.; Csuk, R. Type and position of linkage govern the cytotoxicity of oleanolic acid rhodamine B hybrids. *Steroids* **2021**, *172*, 108876. [CrossRef]
26. Hoenke, S.; Christoph, M.A.; Friedrich, S.; Heise, N.; Brandes, B.; Deigner, H.P.; Al-Harrasi, A.; Csuk, R. The Presence of a Cyclohexyldiamine Moiety Confers Cytotoxicity to Pentacyclic Triterpenoids. *Molecules* **2021**, *26*, 2102. [CrossRef]
27. Friedrich, S.; Serbian, I.; Hoenke, S.; Wolfram, R.K.; Csuk, R. Synthesis and cytotoxic evaluation of malachite green derived oleanolic and ursolic acid piperazineamides. *Med. Chem. Res.* **2020**, *29*, 926–933. [CrossRef]
28. Urban, M.; Sarek, J.; Klinot, J.; Korinkova, G.; Hajduch, M. Synthesis of A-Seco Derivatives of Betulinic Acid with Cytotoxic Activity. *J. Nat. Prod.* **2004**, *67*, 1100–1105. [CrossRef]
29. Thibeault, D.; Gauthier, C.; Legault, J.; Bouchard, J.; Dufour, P.; Pichette, A. Synthesis and structure-activity relationship study of cytotoxic germanicane- and lupane-type 3β-O-monodesmosidic saponins starting from betulin. *Bioorg. Med. Chem.* **2007**, *15*, 6144–6157. [CrossRef] [PubMed]

30. Ruzicka, L.; Hofmann, K. Polyterpenes and polyterpenoids. C. Transpositions in the rings A and E of oleanolic acid. Carbon skeleton of pentacyclic triterpenes. *Helv. Chim. Acta* **1936**, *19*, 114–128. [CrossRef]
31. Topcu, G.; Altiner, E.N.; Gozcu, S.; Halfon, B.; Aydogmus, Z.; Pezzuto, J.M.; Zhou, B.-N.; Kingston, D.G.I. Studies on Di- and triterpenoids from Salvia staminea with cytotoxic activity. *Planta Med.* **2003**, *69*, 464–467.
32. Corbett, R.E.; McDowell, M.A. Extractives from the New Zealand Myrtaceae. III. Triterpene acids from the bark of Leptospermum scoparium. *J. Chem. Soc.* **1958**, 3715–3716. [CrossRef]
33. Taketa, A.T.C.; Breitmaier, E.; Schenkel, E.P. Triterpenes and triterpenoidal glycosides from the fruits of Ilex paraguariensis (Mate). *J. Braz. Chem. Soc.* **2004**, *15*, 205–211. [CrossRef]
34. Vystrcil, A.; Budesinsky, M. Triterpenes. XVI. Unusual epimerization of the C-19 acetyl group in 20-oxo-30-norlupane derivatives. *Collect. Czech. Chem. Commun.* **1970**, *35*, 295–311. [CrossRef]
35. Brandes, B.; Hoenke, S.; Fischer, L.; Csuk, R. Design, synthesis and cytotoxicity of BODIPY FL labelled triterpenoids. *Eur. J. Med. Chem.* **2020**, *185*, 111858. [CrossRef] [PubMed]

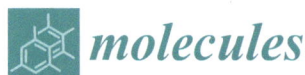

Article

Virtual Screening, Synthesis and Biological Evaluation of *Streptococcus mutans* Mediated Biofilm Inhibitors

Lubna Atta [1], Ruqaiya Khalil [2], Khalid Mohammed Khan [1,3], Moatter Zehra [2], Faiza Saleem [1], Mohammad Nur-e-Alam [4] and Zaheer Ul-Haq [1,2,*]

[1] H. E. J. Research Institute of Chemistry, International Center for Chemical and Biological Sciences, University of Karachi, Karachi 75270, Pakistan; lubnaatta05@gmail.com (L.A.); khalid.khan@iccs.edu (K.M.K.); faizasaleem632@gmail.com (F.S.)
[2] Dr. Panjwani Center for Molecular Medicine and Drug Research, International Center for Chemical and Biological Sciences, University of Karachi, Karachi 75270, Pakistan; ruqaiyakhalil@gmail.com (R.K.); moatterzehra10@yahoo.com (M.Z.)
[3] Department of Clinical Pharmacy, Institute for Research and Medical Consultations (IRMC), Imam Abdulrahman Bin Faisal University, P.O. Box 31441, Dammam 31441, Saudi Arabia
[4] Department of Pharmacognosy, College of Pharmacy, King Saud University, P.O. Box 2457, Riyadh 11451, Saudi Arabia; mohnalam@ksu.edu.sa
* Correspondence: zaheer.qasmi@iccs.edu; Tel.: +92-21-99261672

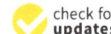

Citation: Atta, L.; Khalil, R.; Khan, K.M.; Zehra, M.; Saleem, F.; Nur-e-Alam, M.; Ul-Haq, Z. Virtual Screening, Synthesis and Biological Evaluation of *Streptococcus mutans* Mediated Biofilm Inhibitors. *Molecules* 2022, 27, 1455. https://doi.org/10.3390/molecules27041455

Academic Editors: Imtiaz Khan and Sumera Zaib

Received: 31 December 2021
Accepted: 18 February 2022
Published: 21 February 2022

Publisher's Note: MDPI stays neutral with regard to jurisdictional claims in published maps and institutional affiliations.

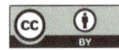

Copyright: © 2022 by the authors. Licensee MDPI, Basel, Switzerland. This article is an open access article distributed under the terms and conditions of the Creative Commons Attribution (CC BY) license (https://creativecommons.org/licenses/by/4.0/).

Abstract: Dental caries, a global oral health concern, is a biofilm-mediated disease. Streptococcus mutans, the most prevalent oral microbiota, produces extracellular enzymes, including glycosyltransferases responsible for sucrose polymerization. In bacterial communities, the biofilm matrix confers resistance to host immune responses and antibiotics. Thus, in cases of chronic dental caries, inhibiting bacterial biofilm assembly should prevent demineralization of tooth enamel, thereby preventing tooth decay. A high throughput screening was performed in the present study to identify small molecule inhibitors of *S. mutans* glycosyltransferases. Multiple pharmacophore models were developed, validated with multiple datasets, and used for virtual screening against large chemical databases. Over 3000 drug-like hits were obtained that were analyzed to explore their binding mode. Finally, six compounds that showed good binding affinities were further analyzed for ADME (absorption, distribution, metabolism, and excretion) properties. The obtained in silico hits were evaluated for in vitro biofilm formation. The compounds displayed excellent antibiofilm activities with minimum inhibitory concentration (MIC) values of 15.26–250 μg/mL.

Keywords: dental caries; biofilm; glucosyltransferases; virtual screening; antibiofilm; antimicrobial ADMET profiling

1. Introduction

Dental caries is one of the major health concerns in both developing and industrialized countries [1]. It is a biofilm-mediated disease attributed to dysbiosis in the oral microbiome [2]. The oral environment is influenced by several factors, primarily diet and host immune competence, promoting the virulence and adhesion of pathogenic microorganisms [3,4]. The prime agent associated with dental caries is *Streptococcus mutans*, which produces organic acids, exhibits acid tolerance mechanisms, and produces extracellular enzyme glucosyltransferases which produce complex sticky glucans [5]. These glucans serve as binding sites for the attachment of other microorganisms, producing a biofilm. The bacteria associated with the biofilm are resistant to host defense, mechanical and oxidative stress, and antibiotics [6]. Microbes within the mature biofilms produce copious amounts of acids, mainly lactic acid, and propionic acid, causing demineralization of the tooth surfaces and eventually dental caries [7].

Several different approaches have been developed to prevent dental caries such as mechanical methods, effective use of fluoride, and sugar substitutes (xylitol) in extreme conditions [8–10]. Natural products such as polyphenols, catechins, cranberry constituents, and other plant analogs exhibit antibiofilm activity [11–14]. However, the non-selective antimicrobial activity presented by these compounds results in further dysbiosis. Recently, targeted antimicrobials have been developed to eliminate *S. mutans* with a minimal effect on normal microbiota [15]. The microorganisms in the biofilm assembly have become more resistant to antibiotics and host defense systems, so there is a need for new therapeutic agents with minimal toxicity and more bioavailability.

The formation of dental biofilm initiates with the attachment of microorganisms on the tooth surface. The microorganism produces extracellular exopolysaccharides (EPS) which provide binding sites to other microorganisms and result in complex biofilm formation [16]. *S. mutans* is an essential contributor to the production of the extracellular matrix. It produces three types of glucosyltransferases (Gtfs): GtfB, GtfC, and GtfD. The GtfB and GtfC are mutansucrases that produce mainly insoluble glucan with (α 1–3) glycosidic linkages from sucrose. GtfD is a dextransucrase that produces soluble glucans with (α1–6) linkages. All Gtfs comprises three functional regions: N-terminal variable junction region, C-terminal glucan-binding region, and ahighly conserved catalytic region in the middle, which is essential for the glucan synthesis [17–19]. The crystal structure of GtfC provides crucial insights for drug design and development of the new Gtf inhibitors [20]. The secondary structure of GtfC comprises four separate domains: A, B, C, and IV (Figure 1). The ligand-binding domain lies in domain A (comprising residues of both sub-domains A1, and A2), while the calcium-binding domain is the interface of domains A and B. The presence and orientation of calcium is significant for enzymatic activity [21,22].

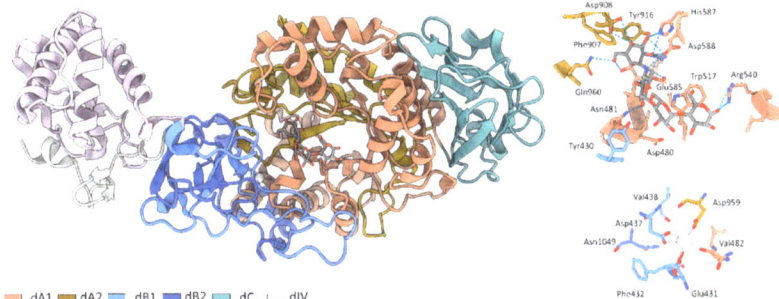

Figure 1. Structure of *S. mutans* glycosyltransferase (PDB: 3AIC), showing all the four domains (A, B, C and IV). Insets represents the molecular co-ordination of calcium ion (grey sphere) and acarbose (grey sticks). Hydrogen bonds between acarbose and the surrounding amino acids are presented as blue dashed lines.

In the present study, pharmacophore modeling approaches, mainly ligand-based, have been implemented to identify the potential hits to inhibit biofilm formation. The multiple pharmacophore models were generated and are utilized for the screening of an in-house compound database. The molecular docking analysis of identified virtual hits was performed. The virtual hits show interactions with crucial residues of the protein. ADMET properties display a low percent of human absorption, molecular weight (250–500), and water solubility (−3.50–5.10). Further, the antibiofilm activity of the compounds was also investigated against *S. mutans* ATCC: 25175 strains. The virtual hits displayed modest antibiofilm activity against *S. mutans*.

2. Results and Discussion

Dental caries is a multifunctional disorder in which different oral microbiomes, predominantly *S. mutans*, interact with dietary sugars to produce cariogenic plaques. The available treatments to combat dental caries are non-selective, board-spectrum, and cause dysbiosis, which in severe cases lead to oral cancers. The present study was carried out to identify, synthesize, and characterize novel small molecule selective inhibitors targeting *S. mutans* glucosyltransferase.

2.1. Virtual Screening

For virtual screening, a series of ligand-based pharmacophore models were developed using the features of the training set. The models were developed using different combinations of shared pharmacophoric features of the training compounds i.e., 5-o-caffeoyl shikimic acid and p-coumaric acid (model 1), eckol and epicatechin (model 2), and apigenin and caffeic acid (model 3). The three models presented different pharmacophoric features, resulting in scaffold hopping and chemical diversity. For instance, model 1 comprises four features: two hydrogen bond acceptors (HBA) and one hydrogen bond donor (HBD), and one hydrophobic (Figure 2). Model 2 exhibits four features: one hydrophobic, two hydrogen bond acceptors, and one hydrogen bond donor. In the case of model 3, there were no hydrophobic characteristics, and the selected features included two hydrogen bond donors and two hydrogen bond acceptors.

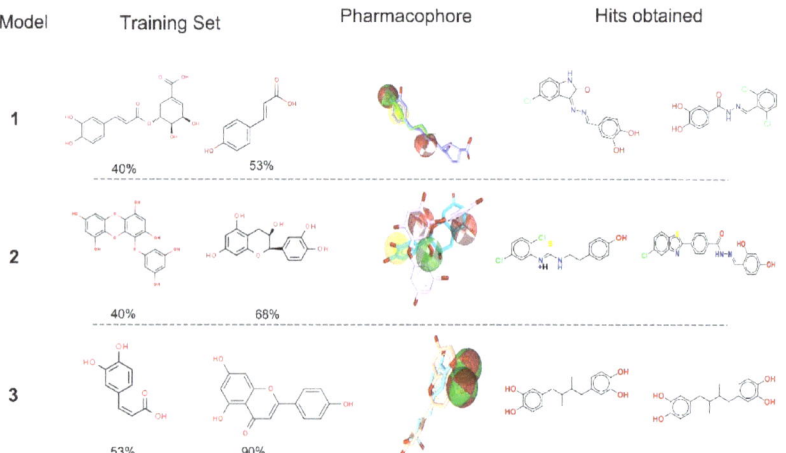

Figure 2. Chemical structures of the training set employed for pharmacophore modelling, and the top-ranked hits from each model.

The three selected models were subjected to vigorous testing using a dataset of reported inhibitors, negative controls, and decoys. Further, the sensitivity and selectivity of the models were accessed. The sensitivity and specificity of model 1, model 2, and model 3 was 0.6, 0.7, and 0.7, respectively (Table 1). The retrieval rate of the active compounds from the training datasets was quite encouraging, so these optimized models were recruited for the screening of an in-house dataset of drug-like compounds.

Table 1. Validation hit rate of the generated pharmacophore models.

Model	Actives	In-Actives	Decoys	Sensitivity
Model 1 (5-O-caffeoyl shikimic acid + p-coumaric acid)	16	2	100	0.6
Model 2 (Eckol + Epicatechin)	17	1	81	0.7
Model 3 (Apigenin and Caffeic acid)	16	1	75	0.7

Model 1, model 2, and model 3 retrieved 2043, 1730 and 2180 hits, respectively. In total, 5953 virtual hits were obtained from these multiple pharmacophore models. To find the possible drug candidates, Lipinski's rule of five (Ro5) was applied, which resulted in 3059 unique drug-like hits. The pharmacophore-based virtual screening resulted in 3059 unique hits. The resultant hits were then subjected to docking studies using the crystal structure of *S. mutans* glycosyltransferase. Prior to the docking studies, the benchmarking of the docking software was performed. Based on the RMSD values between the coordinates of the cognate ligand and the simulated pose (Table S2 Supplementary Materials), MOE-dock was selected for the docking of the identified virtual hits from the preceding step.

For the identification of potential drug like compounds, PLIF analysis was performed after molecular docking to analyze the interaction patterns of the compounds with the active site of glucosyltransferases (Figure S1 Supplementary Materials). The active site of glycosyltransferase comprises several charged and polar residues, including Asp480, Glu515, Trp517, His587, Asp588, Asp593, Asn862, Asp909, and Asn914. The complementarity of the active site is reflected in the presence of polar and heterocycles in the identified hits. The scaffolds selected by models 1 and 2 include different classes of heterocyclic compounds indole and hydrazide (A3898, A3566, A4554, and A6996). Model 3 identified two hits, A13419 and A4554, a carbothioamide and indole, respectively. The final six compounds were selected based on their good interaction with the crucial residues of protein. The 2D structure of the selected hits (n = 6) and the interaction pattern in static mode are presented in Figure 2 and Table 2, respectively.

Table 2. ADMET properties and results of the microbiological assays of the selected hits.

Code	ADMET Properties				Biological Activity			
	Molecular Weight (g/mol)	Lipophilicity (Qplog Po/W)	Water Solubility (PlogS)	Oral Absorption	MIC [1] (µg/mL)	MBC [2] (µg/mL)	MBIC [3] (µg/mL)	Biofilm Inhibition (%)
A3566	315	1.86	−3.68	Low	15.62	n.d.	3.91	71.86
A3898	325	1.95	−4.6	High	250.00	250.00	250.00	86.50
A4554	341	3.01	−5.09	High	125.00	n.d.	125.00	87.55
A6996	423	2.94	−5.74	Low	-	-	-	-
A12324	302	2.38	−4.5	High	250.00	n.d.	250.00	88.58
A13419	227	1.22	−1.43	Low	250.00	n.d.	250.00	88.57

[1] Minimum Inhibitory Concentration, [2] Minimum Bactericidal Concentration, [3] Minimum Biofilm Inhibitory Concentration, n.d. Not Determined.

All six hits exhibited hydrogen bonds with Asn862 and Asn914 in the active site. Further, A3898 also mediated hydrophobic interactions with Tyr430 and Asp480 (Figure 3A). A3566 extends hydrophobic contacts with the indole ring of Trp517 and His587 (Figure 3B). Hit A6996 shows hydrophobic interaction with Tyr430 and Trp517. Moreover, A6996 establishes a hydrogen bond with the carbonyl moiety of Asp909. Nitrogen moiety in the aliphatic chain forms a hydrogen bond with Glu515 (Figure 3C). The amide moiety of A4554 is involved in hydrogen bond interactions with Asn481 and Glu515. The compound also shows hydrophobic interactions with Trp517 (Figure 3D). The hits obtained from model 3 include A13419 and A12324. A12324 exhibits hydrogen bonds with His587, Asp588, and Asp593 (Figure 3E). A13419 also forms a hydrogen bond with Arg475, Glu515, His587, and Asp909 (Figure 3F).

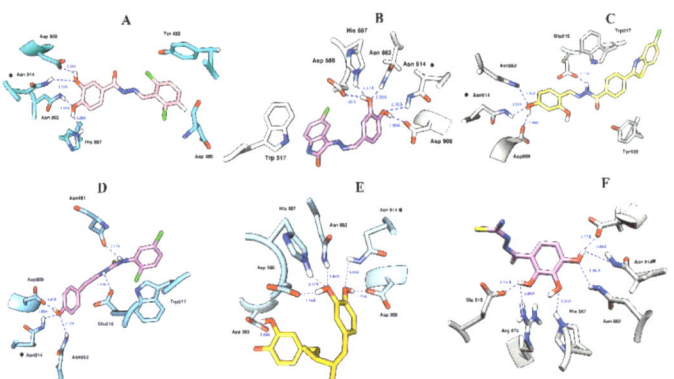

Figure 3. The 3D interactions of the selected hits (**A**) A3898 (pink), (**B**) A3566 (purple), (**C**) A6996 (yellow), (**D**) A4554 (purple), (**E**) A12324 (gold), (**F**) A13419 (plum).

2.2. ADMET Profiling

Pharmacokinetic profiles of selected hits were predicted by SwissADME. The molecular weight of the selected hit varied from 227–423 (g/mol), Plog values were in the range of 1.22–3.01 and water solubility varied from −1.43–5.74, respectively (Table 2). The compounds A12324, A38989, and A3566 were found to exhibit decent oral bioavailability (Table 2 and Figure 4). A4554 could permeate the blood–brain barrier, which is not desirable in the current context. Except for A12324 (a substrate of PGP, PGP+), none of the compounds are P-glycoprotein (PGP) binders, that is, the intestinal absorption of these compounds is not compromised by the activity of p-glycoprotein efflux pumps located in the intestinal lumina. Further, Protox-II server was employed to evaluate organ toxicity (hepatotoxicity) and oral toxicity of the selected hits. All the compounds were found to be non-cytotoxic and safe for oral consumption.

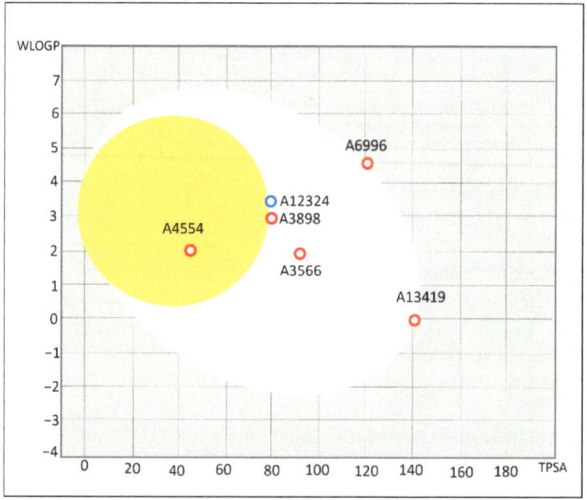

Figure 4. Predicted human intestinal (HIA), and P-glycoprotein efflux (P-gp) inhibition of the selected hits. The compounds lying in the egg-white region could be absorbed by the human intestinal lumen (HIA permeable), and those in the yolk can also permeate the blood–brain barrier. The compounds with blue spots are substrates of P-glycoprotein, while non-substrates are presented as red spots. The visual was obtained from SwissADME webserver.

2.3. Antimicrobial and Biofilm Inhibition

The selected compounds were then evaluated for the antibiofilm activity against *S. mutans* strains (ATCC: 25175). All compounds displayed modest biofilm activity against *S. mutans*. The compound A3566 showed the most promising antimicrobial and antibiofilm properties against the targeted pathogen with MIC of 15.62 µg/mL (Table 2).

The biofilm inhibition observed in the crystal violet assay was further consolidated by light microscopy analysis. The untreated well of *S. mutans* showed intact biofilm densely stained with crystal violet (Figure 5A). When *S. mutans* was treated with A3566 at MIC (4 µg/mL) concentration, the biofilm formation was reduced to almost 80%, whereas, at sub-MIC (2 µg/mL) level almost 50% of the biofilm was reduced (Figure 5B,C). The microscopic evaluation further complemented the biofilm-inhibiting potential of A3566 against *S. mutans*.

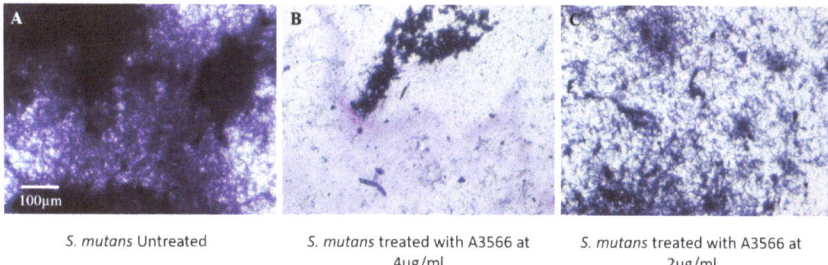

S. mutans Untreated   S. mutans treated with A3566 at 4µg/ml   S. mutans treated with A3566 at 2µg/ml

Figure 5. Biofilm inhibition potential of LN 3566 against *S. mutans*. (**A**) Untreated control, (**B**) treated with A3566 at 4 µg/mL, (**C**) treated with LN 3566 at 2 µg/mL. Images were captured using a Nikon TE2000 inverted microscope with 200× total magnification.

3. Materials and Methods

3.1. Pharmacophore-Based Virtual Screening

We curated a database of compounds with inhibitory activity reported against glycosyltransferases through literature searches. The curated database consisted of structurally diverse chemical scaffolds (Table S1 Supplementary Materials) including quinazoline, flavonoids, and polyphenols [11,18,23,24]. To validate the hypothesis, and to reduce the instances of false-positive hits, a database of reported inactive compounds [25,26] ($n = 9$, Table S2 Supplementary Materials), and a decoy database was also curated. A total of 1695 decoys were generated using DUDE web server [27]. For lead identification, an in-house dataset comprising 14,500 compounds of both synthetic and natural origins was used.

All the chemical structures (excluding decoys) were sketched using ChemDraw Ultra Bio version 9.0 [28]. In the case of decoys, the chemical structures were obtained from the DUDE web server in SDF format which was converted to MOL2 format using Obabel [29]. The compound libraries were then exported to MOE 2019 [30] software to assign partial charges chemical ionization, protonation, the addition of missing hydrogen atoms using Protonate 3D algorithm [31] followed by minimization under MMFF94x force field [32] with a gradient value of 0.1 kcal/molA^2.

3.2. Pharmacophore Generation and Validation

The pharmacophore models were constructed using LigandScout 4.4 [33]. For every compound in the training set, thirty different conformations were generated using OMEGA [34]. Different functional groups of the compounds were recruited to generate a series of pharmacophore models mapping the shared features of the training set. Different combinations of compounds were aligned to generate shared feature pharmacophore. The developed models were then subjected to screening for initial validation. The sensitivity and selectivity of different models were then assessed. The models with optimum matrices were employed to screen the database.

3.3. Preparation and Screening of Database

For hit identification, we employed an in-house database comprising 14,500 diverse compounds, of both natural and synthetic origin. All compounds were prepared for screening using the protocol mentioned above. For virtual screening, the 'idbgen' in LigandScout was used to convert the database into LigandScout specific multi-conformation database (ldb), which can store multiple conformations of each compound. After the removal of duplicates, the databases were screened with generated pharmacophore models to identify the potential hits. The identified virtual hits were filtered with the Lipinski rule of five [35] to identify the drug-like compounds. The potential hits obtained after the Lipinski filter were analyzed for their binding mode with molecular docking.

3.4. Molecular Docking

The binding energy of each compound was calculated using molecular docking [36,37]. Initially, a redocking experiment was conducted to establish the efficiency of the docking protocol to reproduce the crystal pose. Coordinates of glucansucrase Streptococcus mutans were obtained from the RSCB protein data bank (PDB ID:3AIC) [38]. The structure was imported in MOE and was subjected to the 'protein preparation' module for the addition of missing atoms, assignment of partial charges (using AMBER99), and protonation (using Protonate 3D algorithm). For ligand placement and scoring, the triangle matcher algorithm and London-dG scoring function were used. The docking site was designated using the coordinates of the cognate ligands (AC1 and GLC). For each compound, a single top-ranked pose was retrieved, and binding energy was recorded.

Furthermore, to analyze the protein–ligand contact profile, the protein–ligand interaction fingerprint (PLIF) module in MOE was used. PLIP [39] analysis helps to identify the key residues of the respective protein which was responsible for binding with the ligand. PLIP provides detail of seven different interactions (hydrogen bonds, hydrophobic contacts, pi-stacking, pi-cation interactions, salt bridges, water bridges, and halogen bonds. The compounds exhibiting contacts with crucial residues were selected for hit optimization.

3.5. ADMET Profiling

The ADMET profiles of the identified compounds were evaluated with the help of the SwissADME web server [40,41].

3.6. General Procedure for the Synthesis of Compounds

The identified hits were then synthesized to perform the biochemical assays against the biofilm.

A3566: In the first step, hydrazone was prepared by refluxing a mixture of 5-chloroisatin (1 g) and hydrazine hydrate (10 mL). Then, hydrazone so prepared (1 mmol) and 3,4-dihydroxybenzaldehyde (1 mmol) in methanol were reacted together under reflux for 3 h. TLC was used for monitoring the proceeding of reaction. After reaction completion, crystalline powder of Schiff base was collected, washed with methanol, and dried. Recrystallization from methanol afforded pure crystals. The structure was confirmed by using ^{1}HNMR, and EI-MS.

Yield: 69%; ^{1}H NMR: (300 MHz, DMSO-d_6): 10.9 (s, 1H, N–H), 9.6 (s, 1H, O–H), 8.57 (s, 1H, –N=CH), 7.4 (s, 1H, H-4), 7.38 (d, 1H, $J_{6,7}$ = 7.5 Hz, H-6), 7.25 (d, 1H, $J_{6',5'}$ = 7.8 Hz, H-6'), 7.1 (s, 1H, H-2'), 6.9 (d, 1H, $J_{5',6'}$ = 7.8 Hz, H-5'), 6.86 (d, 1H, $J_{7,6}$ = 7.5 Hz, H-7); EI MS: m/z (rel. abund.%), 315 (M$^+$, 5), 287 (100), 180 (32), 152 (85), 109 (36), 63 (40).

A3898: (E)-N'-(2,6-dichlorobenzylidene)-3,4-dihydroxybenzohydrazide was synthesized by treating an equimolar amount of 2,6-dichlorobenzaldehyde with 3,4-dihydroxybenzohydrazide in a suitable amount of DMF and stirring the reaction mixture overnight at room temperature. Progress of the reaction was monitored by thin-layer chromatography (TLC). After completion, the reaction mixture was poured in ice water to precipitate out the final product, which was filtered and washed with hot ethanol to afford the pure product. The compound was characterized by ^{1}HNMR and EI-MS analysis.

Yield: 97%; ^{1}H-NMR (300 MHz, DMSO-d_6); 11.83 (s, 1H, NH), 9.27 (s, 2H, OH), 8.59 (s, 1H, N=C-H), 7.56 (d, 2H, $J_{3',4'-5'-4'}$ = 6 Hz, H-3′, H-5′), 7.45 (dd, 1H, $J_{4'-3'-4'-5'}$ = 7.5 Hz, H-4′), 7.39 (dd, 2H, $J_{6,2-2,6}$ = 1.8 Hz, H-6, H-2), 6.82 (d, 1H, $J_{5,6}$ = 8.1 Hz, H-5); EI MS m/z (% rel. Abund.); 324 (M$^+$, 90), 256 (57), 152 (47), 136 (100), 120 (65), 109 (58), 81 (24), 44 (11).

A4554: In the first step, 2,3,4-trihydroxy benzaldehyde (10 mmol) and thiosemicarbazide (10 mmol) were taken in ethanol (50 mL) into a 250 mL round-bottomed flask with a few drops of glacial acetic acid. The reaction mixture was refluxed for 4 h. Precipitates of the product appeared in the reaction mixture. Progress of the reaction was monitored by thin-layer chromatography (TLC). After completion, precipitates were filtered and washed with 10 mL cold ethanol to afford the pure product in good yield. In the second step, thiosemicarbazone intermediate (0.5 mmol), 3,4-dichlorophenacyl bromide (0.5 mmol), and triethylamine (0.5 mmol) were taken in ethanol into a 100 mL round-bottomed flask and refluxed for 3 h. Progress of the reaction was monitored by the thin layer chromatography (TLC). Precipitates appeared in the reaction mixture which was filtered and washed with 5 mL cold ethanol to afford the pure products. The compound was characterized by spectroscopic analysis.

Yield: 75%; ^{1}H-NMR (400 MHz, DMSO-d_6): δ 11.99 (s, 1H, NH), 9.63 (s, 1H, OH), 9.46 (s, 1H, OH), 8.48 (s, 1H, OH), 8.18 (s, 1H, H-C=N), 8.065 (d, $J_{2'',6''}$ = 1.6Hz, 1H, H-2″), 7.83 (dd, $J_{6'',2''}$ = 1.6 Hz, $J_{6'',5''}$ = 8.4 Hz, 1H, H-6″), 7.66 (d, $J_{5'',6''}$ = 8.4 Hz, 1H, H-5″), 7.50 (s, 1H, H-5′), 6.88 (d, $J_{6,5}$ = 8.8 Hz, 1H, H-6), 6.39 (d, $J_{5,6}$ = 8.4 Hz, 1H, H-5); EI MS: m/z (rel. abund.%); 394 (M$^+$, 100), 396 (M^{+2}, 64), 324 (17), 285 (35), 190 (28), 81 (24).

A6996: Synthesis and characterization of the compound published previously [42].

A13419: 2,3,4-Trihydroxy benzaldehyde (1 mmol) and thiosemicarbazide (1 mmol) were taken in ethanol (5 mL) into a 100 mL round-bottomed flask and acidified with a few drops of glacial acetic acid. The reaction mixture was refluxed for 4 h. Precipitates of the product appeared in the reaction mixture. Progress of the reaction was monitored by thin-layer chromatography (TLC). After completion, precipitates were filtered and washed with 10 mL cold ethanol to afford the pure (E)-2-(2,3,4-trihydroxybenzylidene)hydrazine-1-carbothioamide product in good yield.

Yield 78%; ^{1}H-NMR (300 MHz, DMSO-d_6): 11.16 (s, 1H, NH), 9.48 (br s, 1H, OH), 8.94 (br s, 1H, OH), 8.40 (br s, 1H, NH2), 8.20 (s, 1H, –HC=N–), 7.93 (br s, 1H, OH), 7.72 (br s, 1H, NH2), 7.11 (d, 1H, J = 8.4 Hz, phH), 6.32 (d, 1H, J = 8.4 Hz, phH). MS (ESI): m/z (rel. abund.%), 228 (M^{+1})

A12334 [43]: This is a commercially available compound and was obtained from a local market.

3.7. Antimicrobial and Biofilm Inhibition Studies

Streptococcus mutans (ATCC: 25175) strains were used for in vitro assessment of antimicrobial and antibiofilm activities of the hit compounds. S. mutans was grown and passed using heart infusion broth (Oxoid, UK) supplemented with 1% sucrose. The strains were grown aerobically at 37 °C for 24 h.

The minimum inhibitory concentration of the selected compounds was evaluated using the micro broth dilution method as described previously [44]. Briefly, compounds were two-fold serially diluted in the range of 500 to 1 μg/mL. S. mutans (5 × 10^5 cells/mL) were inoculated in each except negative control. The eleventh and twelfth wells served as positive (media plus S. mutans) and negative (only media) controls. The plate was incubated overnight at 37 °C. The following day, the lowest concentration of the compound inhibiting bacterial growth was recorded as the minimum inhibitory concentration (MIC). The minimum bactericidal concentration (MBC) was evaluated by plating the optically clear well to a new fresh media plate. The lowest concentration that inhibited bacterial growth was recorded as MBC. The biofilm-inhibiting potential of the compounds was evaluated using the crystal violet staining method [45]. The following equation is used for the calculation of % biofilm inhibition.

$$\%\text{biofilm inhibition} = \{(\text{O.D. in control} - \text{O.D. of test})/\text{O.D. in control}\} \times 100$$

The biofilm inhibition was further complemented with light microscopic observation after staining with crystal violet as described previously [44]. Briefly, *S. mutans* was treated with A3566 at inhibitory and sub-inhibitory concentrations. After incubation, the wells were washed and heat-fixed. Biofilm mass was stained with 0.1% crystal violet for 20 min. After staining, the excess dye was removed and plates were dried. Images of biofilm structure were visualized under Nikon TE2000 inverted microscope (Nikon, Tokyo, Japan) at 200× total magnification.

4. Conclusions

In this study, in silico strategies and microbiological assays/bioassays were employed to identify small molecules that target glycosyltransferases from *S mutans*. A virtual screening based on pharmacophores followed by intermolecular interaction profiling produced six hits. These hits exhibited high binding affinity, due to a combination of hydrophobic interactions and electrostatic interactions with key target residues. Additionally, these compounds displayed excellent antibiofilm activity when tested due to their good pharmacokinetic profile as predicted by SwissADME. The results highlighted the potential of the identified hits as candidates for in vivo testing, which in the future may serve as the basis for the development of new, effective, and potent derivatives for the treatment of dental caries.

5. Prospects and Limitations

As a result of the limited number and diversity of compounds reported in the study, one of its intrinsic limitations is the small training set. Thus, the pharmacophore hits may not represent the full range of possible ligands with similar properties. Another limitation comes from the adoption of the antibacterial and bio-film inhibition assay as a surrogate for in vitro glycosyltransferase inhibitory assay. Future studies employing larger datasets and more exhaustive methods are required to explore available chemical space and identify potent inhibitors of *S. mutans* glycosyltransferase.

Supplementary Materials: The following supporting information can be downloaded online. Table S1: Training dataset collected from literature, Table S2: Structures of the inactive compounds obtained from literature, Table S3: Benchmarking results using RMSD between simulated and cognate poses, and Table S4: Results of the cytotoxicity prediction of the compounds using Pro Tox -11 webserver, Figure S1: PLIF analysis of the virtual hits.

Author Contributions: Conceptualization, Z.U.-H.; methodology, L.A.; software, M.N.-e.-A.; validation, L.A., Z.U.-H. and M.Z.; formal analysis, L.A. and F.S.; investigation, L.A., R.K. and F.S.; resources, Z.U.-H. and M.N.-e.-A.; data curation, L.A.; writing—original draft preparation, L.A. and R.K.; writing—review and editing, Z.U.-H., R.K. and K.M.K.; visualization, L.A.; supervision, Z.U.-H. and K.M.K.; project administration, Z.U.-H.; funding acquisition, Z.U.-H. and M.N.-e.-A. All authors have read and agreed to the published version of the manuscript.

Funding: This research received no external funding.

Institutional Review Board Statement: Not Applicable.

Informed Consent Statement: Not Applicable.

Data Availability Statement: Data are available from authors on request.

Acknowledgments: The authors extend their appreciation to Ayaz Ahmed for his kind support in the execution of microscopy, and biological activity.

Conflicts of Interest: The authors declare no conflict of interest.

Sample Availability: Samples of the compounds are available from the authors.

References

1. Hujoel, P.P.; Hujoel, M.L.A.; Kotsakis, G.A. Personal oral hygiene and dental caries: A systematic review of randomised controlled trials. *Gerodontology* **2018**, *35*, 282–289. [CrossRef] [PubMed]
2. Tanner, A.C.R.; Kressirer, C.A.; Rothmiller, S.; Johansson, I.; Chalmers, N.I. The Caries Microbiome: Implications for Reversing Dysbiosis. *Adv. Dent. Res.* **2018**, *29*, 78–85. [CrossRef] [PubMed]
3. Reibel, J. Tobacco and Oral Diseases. *Med. Princ. Pract.* **2003**, *12*, 22–32. [CrossRef] [PubMed]
4. Hu, J.; Jiang, W.; Lin, X.; Zhu, H.; Zhou, N.; Chen, Y.; Wu, W.; Zhang, D.; Chen, H. Dental Caries Status and Caries Risk Factors in Students Ages 12–14 Years in Zhejiang, China. *Med. Sci. Monit.* **2018**, *24*, 3670–3678. [CrossRef] [PubMed]
5. María Alejandra, B.; Mariano Daniel, O. Virulence Factors of Streptococcus mutans Related to Dental Caries. In *Staphylococcus and Streptococcus*; Intech Open: Cordoba, Argentina, 2020.
6. Gebreyohannes, G.; Nyerere, A.; Bii, C.; Sbhatu, D.B. Challenges of intervention, treatment, and antibiotic resistance of biofilm-forming microorganisms. *Heliyon* **2019**, *5*, e02192. [CrossRef]
7. Bowen, W.H.; Koo, H. Biology of Streptococcus mutans-Derived Glucosyltransferases: Role in Extracellular Matrix Formation of Cariogenic Biofilms. *Caries Res.* **2011**, *45*, 69–86. [CrossRef]
8. Chen, X.; Daliri, E.B.-M.; Kim, N.; Kim, J.-R.; Yoo, D.; Oh, D.-H. Microbial etiology and prevention of dental caries: Exploiting natural products to inhibit cariogenic biofilms. *J. Pathog.* **2020**, *9*, 569. [CrossRef]
9. Horst, J.A.; Tanzer, J.M.; Milgrom, P.M. Fluorides and Other Preventive Strategies for Tooth Decay. *Dent. Clin. N. Am.* **2018**, *62*, 207–234. [CrossRef]
10. Gupta, P.; Gupta, N.; Pawar, A.P.; Birajdar, S.S.; Natt, A.S.; Singh, H.P. Role of Sugar and Sugar Substitutes in Dental Caries: A Review. *ISRN Dent.* **2013**, *2013*, 1–5. [CrossRef]
11. Sakanaka, S.; Okada, Y. Inhibitory Effects of Green Tea Polyphenols on the Production of a Virulence Factor of the Periodontal-Disease-Causing Anaerobic Bacterium Porphyromonas gingivalis. *J. Agric. Food Chem.* **2004**, *52*, 1688–1692. [CrossRef]
12. Xu, X.; Zhou, X.D.; Wu, C.D. Tea catechin epigallocatechin gallate inhibits Streptococcus mutans biofilm formation by suppressing gtf genes. *Arch. Oral Biol.* **2012**, *57*, 678–683. [CrossRef] [PubMed]
13. Koo, H.; Duarte, S.; Murata, R.M.; Scott-Anne, K.; Gregoire, S.; Watson, G.E.; Singh, A.P.; Vorsa, N. Influence of Cranberry Proanthocyanidins on Formation of Biofilms by *Streptococcus mutans* on Saliva-Coated Apatitic Surface and on Dental Caries Development in vivo. *Caries Res.* **2010**, *44*, 116–126. [CrossRef] [PubMed]
14. Koh, C.-L.; Sam, C.-K.; Yin, W.-F.; Tan, L.; Krishnan, T.; Chong, Y.; Chan, K.-G. Plant-Derived Natural Products as Sources of Anti-Quorum Sensing Compounds. *Sensors* **2013**, *13*, 6217–6228. [CrossRef]
15. Ren, Z.; Cui, T.; Zeng, J.; Chen, L.; Zhang, W.; Xu, X.; Cheng, L.; Li, M.; Li, J.; Zhou, X.; et al. Molecule Targeting Glucosyltransferase Inhibits Streptococcus mutans Biofilm Formation and Virulence. *Antimicrob. Agents Chemother.* **2016**, *60*, 126–135. [CrossRef] [PubMed]
16. Featherstone, J.D.B. Dental caries: A dynamic disease process. *Aust. Dent. J.* **2008**, *53*, 286–291. [CrossRef] [PubMed]
17. Lemos, J.A.; Palmer, S.R.; Zeng, L.; Wen, Z.T.; Kajfasz, J.K.; Freires, I.A.; Abranches, J.; Brady, L.J. The Biology of Streptococcus mutans. *Microbiol. Spectr.* **2019**, *7*, GPP3–GPP0051. [CrossRef] [PubMed]
18. Ren, Z.; Chen, L.; Li, J.; Li, Y. Inhibition ofStreptococcus mutanspolysaccharide synthesis by molecules targeting glycosyltransferase activity. *J. Oral Microbiol.* **2016**, *8*, 31095. [CrossRef]
19. Argimón, S.; Alekseyenko, A.V.; DeSalle, R.; Caufield, P.W. Phylogenetic Analysis of Glucosyltransferases and Implications for the Coevolution of Mutans Streptococci with Their Mammalian Hosts. *PLoS ONE* **2013**, *8*, e56305. [CrossRef]
20. Ito, K.; Ito, S.; Shimamura, T.; Weyand, S.; Kawarasaki, Y.; Misaka, T.; Abe, K.; Kobayashi, T.; Cameron, A.D.; Iwata, S. Crystal Structure of Glucansucrase from the Dental Caries Pathogen Streptococcus mutans. *J. Mol. Biol.* **2011**, *408*, 177–186. [CrossRef]
21. Leemhuis, H.; Pijning, T.; Dobruchowska, J.M.; van Leeuwen, S.S.; Kralj, S.; Dijkstra, B.W.; Dijkhuizen, L. Glucansucrases: Three-dimensional structures, reactions, mechanism, α-glucan analysis and their implications in biotechnology and food applications. *J. Biotechnol.* **2013**, *163*, 250–272. [CrossRef]
22. Vujicic-Zagar, A.; Pijning, T.; Kralj, S.; Lopez, C.A.; Eeuwema, W.; Dijkhuizen, L.; Dijkstra, B.W. Crystal structure of a 117 kDa glucansucrase fragment provides insight into evolution and product specificity of GH70 enzymes. *Proc. Natl. Acad. Sci. USA* **2010**, *107*, 21406–21411. [CrossRef] [PubMed]
23. Kim, Y.; Jang, S.-J.; Kim, H.-R.; Kim, S.-B. Deodorizing, antimicrobial and glucosyltransferase inhibitory activities of polyphenolics from biosource. *Korean J. Chem. Eng.* **2017**, *34*, 1400–1404. [CrossRef]
24. Yanagida, A.; Kanda, T.; Tanabe, M.; Matsudaira, F.; Oliveira Cordeiro, J.G. Inhibitory Effects of Apple Polyphenols and Related Compounds on Cariogenic Factors of Mutans Streptococci. *J. Agric. Food Chem.* **2000**, *48*, 5666–5671. [CrossRef] [PubMed]
25. Nijampatnam, B.; Zhang, H.; Cai, X.; Michalek, S.M.; Wu, H.; Velu, S.E. Inhibition of Streptococcus mutans Biofilms by the Natural Stilbene Piceatannol Through the Inhibition of Glucosyltransferases. *ACS Omega* **2018**, *3*, 8378–8385. [CrossRef]
26. Nijampatnam, B.; Casals, L.; Zheng, R.; Wu, H.; Velu, S.E. Hydroxychalcone inhibitors of Streptococcus mutans glucosyl transferases and biofilms as potential anticaries agents. *Bioorg. Med. Chem. Lett.* **2016**, *26*, 3508–3513. [CrossRef]
27. Mysinger, M.M.; Carchia, M.; Irwin, J.J.; Shoichet, B.K. Directory of Useful Decoys, Enhanced (DUD-E): Better Ligands and Decoys for Better Benchmarking. *J. Med. Chem.* **2012**, *55*, 6582–6594. [CrossRef]

28. Cousins, K.R. ChemDraw Ultra 9.0. CambridgeSoft, 100 CambridgePark Drive, Cambridge, MA 02140. www.cambridgesoft.com. See Web site for pricing options. *J. Am. Chem. Soc.* **2005**, *127*, 4115–4116. [CrossRef]
29. O'Boyle, N.M.; Banck, M.; James, C.A.; Morley, C.; Vandermeersch, T.; Hutchison, G.R. Open Babel: An open chemical toolbox. *J. Cheminform.* **2011**, *3*, 33. [CrossRef]
30. *Molecular Operating Environment (MOE)*; 2019.01; Chemical Computing Group ULC: Montreal, QC, Canada, 2020.
31. Labute, P. Protonate 3D: Assignment of ionization states and hydrogen coordinates to macromolecular structures. *Proteins Struct. Funct. Bioinform.* **2008**, *75*, 187–205. [CrossRef]
32. Halgren, T.A. Merck molecular force field. I. Basis, form, scope, parameterization, and performance of MMFF94. *J. Comput. Chem.* **1996**, *17*, 490–519. [CrossRef]
33. Wolber, G.; Langer, T. LigandScout: 3-D Pharmacophores Derived from Protein-Bound Lingands and Their Use as Virtual Screening Filters. *ChemInform* **2005**, *45*, 160–169. [CrossRef]
34. *OpenEye Scientific Software*; OpenEye: Santa Fe, NM, USA, 2017. Available online: http://www.eyesopen.com (accessed on 30 December 2021).
35. Benet, L.Z.; Hosey, C.M.; Ursu, O.; Oprea, T.I. BDDCS, the Rule of 5 and drugability. *Adv. Drug Deliv. Rev.* **2016**, *101*, 89–98. [CrossRef] [PubMed]
36. Morris, G.M.; Lim-Wilby, M. Molecular Docking. In *Methods in Molecular Biology*; Humana Press: Totowa, NJ, USA, 2008; pp. 365–382.
37. Trott, O.; Olson, A.J. AutoDock Vina: Improving the speed and accuracy of docking with a new scoring function, efficient optimization, and multithreading. *J. Comput. Chem.* **2010**, *31*, 455–461. [CrossRef] [PubMed]
38. Berman, H.M.; Battistuz, T.; Bhat, T.N.; Bluhm, W.F.; Bourne, P.E.; Burkhardt, K.; Feng, Z.; Gilliland, G.L.; Iype, L.; Jain, S.; et al. The Protein Data Bank. *Acta Crystallogr. Sect. D Biol. Crystallogr.* **2002**, *58*, 899–907. [CrossRef] [PubMed]
39. Salentin, S.; Schreiber, S.; Haupt, V.J.; Adasme, M.F.; Schroeder, M. PLIP: Fully automated protein–ligand interaction profiler. *Nucleic Acids Res.* **2015**, *43*, W443–W447. [CrossRef]
40. Daina, A.; Michielin, O.; Zoete, V. SwissADME: A free web tool to evaluate pharmacokinetics, drug-likeness and medicinal chemistry friendliness of small molecules. *Sci. Rep.* **2017**, *7*, 42717. [CrossRef]
41. Daina, A.; Zoete, V. A BOILED-Egg To Predict Gastrointestinal Absorption and Brain Penetration of Small Molecules. *ChemMedChem* **2016**, *11*, 1117–1121. [CrossRef]
42. Taha, M.; Arbin, M.; Ahmat, N.; Imran, S.; Rahim, F. Synthesis: Small library of hybrid scaffolds of benzothiazole having hydrazone and evaluation of their β-glucuronidase activity. *Bioorg. Chem.* **2018**, *77*, 47–55. [CrossRef]
43. Moridani, M.Y.; Siraki, A.; Chevaldina, T.; Scobie, H.; O'Brien, P.J. Quantitative structure toxicity relationships for catechols in isolated rat hepatocytes. *Chem.-Biol. Interact.* **2004**, *147*, 297–307. [CrossRef] [PubMed]
44. Arshia; Khan, A.K.; Khan, K.M.; Ahmed, A.; Taha, M.; Perveen, S. Antibiofilm potential of synthetic 2-amino-5-chlorobenzophenone Schiff bases and its confirmation through fluorescence microscopy. *Microb. Pathog.* **2017**, *110*, 497–506. [CrossRef]
45. Ahmed, D.; Anwar, A.; Khan, A.K.; Ahmed, A.; Shah, M.R.; Khan, N.A. Size selectivity in antibiofilm activity of 3-(diphenylphosphino)propanoic acid coated gold nanomaterials against Gram-positive Staphylococcus aureus and Streptococcus mutans. *AMB Express* **2017**, *7*, 210. [CrossRef] [PubMed]

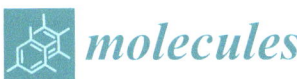

Article

Design, Synthesis and Molecular Docking Study of Novel 3-Phenyl-β-Alanine-Based Oxadiazole Analogues as Potent Carbonic Anhydrase II Inhibitors

Kashif Rafiq [1,2], Najeeb Ur Rehman [1,*], Sobia Ahsan Halim [1], Majid Khan [1,3], Ajmal Khan [1] and Ahmed Al-Harrasi [1,*]

[1] Natural and Medical Sciences Research Center, University of Nizwa, P.O Box 33, Birkat Al Mauz, Nizwa 616, Oman; kashifrafiq@unizwa.edu.om (K.R.); sobia_halim@unizwa.edu.om (S.A.H.); majidk166@yahoo.com (M.K.); ajmalkhan@unizwa.edu.om (A.K.)
[2] Department of Chemistry, Abdul Wali Khan University Mardan, Mardan 23200, Pakistan
[3] H. E. J. Research Institute of Chemistry, International Center for Chemical and Biological Sciences, University of Karachi, Karachi 75270, Pakistan
* Correspondence: najeeb@unizwa.edu.om (N.U.R.); aharrasi@unizwa.edu.om (A.A.-H.); Tel.: +968-2544-6328 (A.A.-H.); Fax: +968-2544-6612 (A.A.-H.)

Abstract: Carbonic anhydrase-II (CA-II) is strongly related with gastric, glaucoma, tumors, malignant brain, renal and pancreatic carcinomas and is mainly involved in the regulation of the bicarbonate concentration in the eyes. With an aim to develop novel heterocyclic hybrids as potent enzyme inhibitors, we synthesized a series of twelve novel 3-phenyl-β-alanine 1,3,4-oxadiazole hybrids (**4a–l**), characterized by ^{1}H- and ^{13}C-NMR with the support of HRESIMS, and evaluated for their inhibitory activity against CA-II. The CA-II inhibition results clearly indicated that the 3-phenyl-β-alanine 1,3,4-oxadiazole derivatives **4a–l** exhibited selective inhibition against CA-II. All the compounds (except **4d**) exhibited good to moderate CA-II inhibitory activities with IC$_{50}$ value in range of 12.1 to 53.6 µM. Among all the compounds, **4a** (12.1 ± 0.86 µM), **4c** (13.8 ± 0.64 µM), **4b** (19.1 ± 0.88 µM) and **4h** (20.7 ± 1.13 µM) are the most active hybrids against carbonic CA-II. Moreover, molecular docking was performed to understand the putative binding mode of the active compounds. The docking results indicates that these compounds block the biological activity of CA-II by nicely fitting at the entrance of the active site of CA-II. These compounds specifically mediating hydrogen bonding with Thr199, Thr200, Gln92 of CA-II.

Keywords: 3-phenyl-β-alanine 1,3,4-oxadiazole hybrids; carbonic anhydrase-II; α-glucosidase; structure-activity relationship; molecular docking

1. Introduction

Carbonic anhydrases (CAs, EC 4.2.1.1) are a class of well-studied metalloenzymes widely distributed in living organisms [1]. These are strongly involved in regulating cell homeostasis, intracellular pH, fluid secretion, ion transport and biosynthetic reactions by catalyzing the reversible hydration of carbon dioxide (CO$_2$) to bicarbonate ion (HCO^{3-}) and proton (H$^+$) [2–7]. This simple reaction is crucial for many physiological mechanisms including electrolyte secretion, acid-base tuning, tumorigenesis, respiration, bone resorption, calcification and biosynthesis of important molecules such as glucose, urea, and lipids [8,9]. These enzymes are common in almost all organisms from simple to complex [10,11]. The extracellular pH in tumors is more acidic than intracellular pH [11]. To generate the pH gradient between the extracellular and intracellular compartments, tumor cells express ion transport proteins and CA enzymes [12–14]. The CA-II is expressed in malignant brain tumors [15–17], renal cancer cell lines, and gastric and pancreatic carcinomas [15,17]. CA-II has also been used since long time for the treatment of glaucoma, epilepsy, leukemia, and cystic fibrosis [18,19]. It is remarkable that ubiquitous hCA-I and II are the main off-target isoforms because these are involved in many physiological and biochemical processes [20]. Due to the key role of this enzyme in several diseases, its inhibition is considered therapeutically important.

Oxadiazoles are heterocyclic compounds which have a diversity of useful biological effects including antibacterial [21], antifungal [22], analgesic [23], anti-inflammatory [24], antiviral [25], anticancer [26], antihypertensive [27], anticonvulsant [28] and anti-diabetic [29]. 1,3,4-Oxadiazole nucleus is present in the molecules of drugs such as: furamizole (antibacterial), tiodazosin (an α-1 adrenergic antagonist), nesapidil (antihypertensive), raltegravir (antiretroviral), and zibotentan (anticancer) (Figure 1) [30]. The most commonly used synthetic route for the synthesis of 1,3,4-oxadiazoles includes the reactions of acid hydrazides with acid chlorides, carboxaldehyde, carboxylic acids and cyclization of the formed acylhydrazines using a dehydrating agent, such as phosphorous pentaoxide, thionyl chloride, or phosphorous oxychloride [31]. On the other hand, 1,3,4-oxadiazoles are thermally stable and neutral heteroaromatic compounds containing two nitrogens and one oxygen atom, affects the pharmacokinetic and physicochemical properties of the compounds in which it is present [32]. It makes diverse noncovalent interactions with various active sites of enzymes and receptors in biological systems and, thus display versatile pharmacological activities like anti-inflammatory [33], antidepressant [34], anti-proliferative [35], analgesic [36] and antiviral effect [32,37,38].

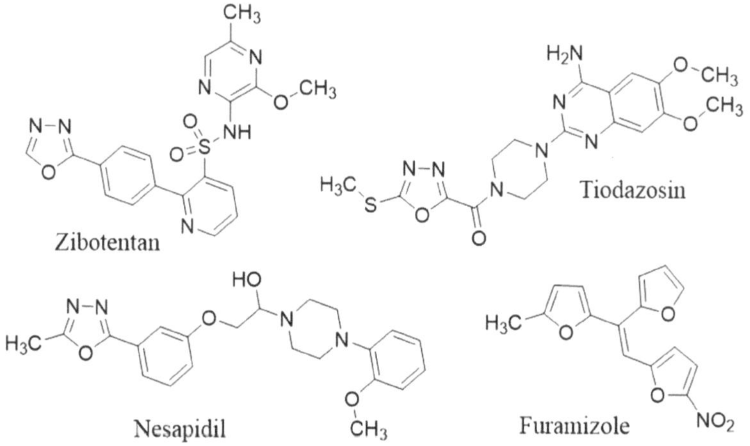

Figure 1. Some reported 1,3,4-oxadiazole derivative drugs.

Previously, Vats et al. have synthesized novel 4-functionalized 1,5-diaryl-1,2,3-triazoles containing benzenesulfonamide moiety as carbonic anhydrase I, II, IV and IX inhibitors [39], while novel benzenesulfonamides bearing 1,2,3-triazole linked hydroxy trifluoromethylpyrazolines and hydrazones as selective carbonic anhydrase isoforms IX and XII inhibitors were reported by Sharma et al. [40]. Similarly, Kumar et al. described that the synthesis of novel benzenesulfonamide containing 1,2,3-triazoles [41] and benzenesulphonamide-bearing 1,4,5-trisubstituted-1,2,3-triazoles [42] showed potent inhibition against human carbonic anhydrase isoforms I, II, IV and IX inhibitors. Bianco et al. have successfully been synthesized N-acylbenzenesulphonamide dihydro-1,3,4-oxadiazole hybrids against hCA IX and XII [43]. Recently, Sharma et al. have reported the novel benzenesulfonamides incorporating 1,3,4-oxadiazole hybrids as potent inhibitor of carbonic anhydrase I, II, IX, and XII isoenzymes [44], while Swain et al., have efficiently been synthesized have efficiently been synthesized benzenesulphonamide based 1,3,4-oxadiazoles as selective carbonic anhydrase XIII inhibitors [45]. Our group recently reported a novel class of CAs inhibitors belonging to the 1H-1,2,3-triazole derivatives [46,47].

Our focus was on the identification of novel drug-like compounds against CA-II enzyme to combat CA-II related disorders. Keeping in mind the importance of these scaffolds in the present work, we designed and synthesized a series of novel 3-phenyl-β-alanine 1,3,4-oxadiazole hybrids **4a–l** with the oxadiazole ring offering an important pharmacophore. With the hope to obtain an effective carbonic anhydrase II enzyme inhibitors, we planned to synthesize new compounds, characterized by spectroscopic techniques including ^{1}H-, ^{13}C-NMR and HRMS, and to explore their carbonic anhydrase enzyme inhibition. Later, computational docking method was applied to investigate the mode of binding of these compounds in the active site of CA-II.

2. Results and Discussion

2.1. Chemistry

The interest in finding an effective carbonic anhydrase II enzyme inhibitor has been increased in recent decades, especially with the exploring of possible relationships between carbonic anhydrase II and cancer [48–50]. CA is present in human (h) with sixteen (16) different isoforms identified from hCA I-hCA XV. All these isoforms are widely dispersed in different tissues/organs and are associated with a range of pivotal physiological activities. Due to their involvement in various physiological roles, inhibitors of different human isoforms of CA have found clinical applications for the treatment of various diseases including glaucoma, retinopathy, epilepsy, hemolytic anemia, and obesity [51]. However, clinically used inhibitors of CA (acetazolamide, brinzolamide, dorzolamide, etc.) are not selective causing the undesirable side effects. Recently we have investigated the interaction of CA-II isozymes with several types of natural and synthetic compounds [46,47,52,53]. Furthermore, 1,3,4-oxadiazole derivatives were found to be strong inhibitors against carbonic anhydrase II enzyme [39–42,44]. Inspired by these advances, we sought to investigate the application of this reagent in oxadiazole synthesis.

Molecular iodine plays an important role in organic synthesis, owing to its commercial availability, low cost, and low toxicity [54,55]. Recently, it has been successfully employed to synthesize indole derivatives [56,57] and oxazoles [58–60]. Compound **1** was synthesized through esterification of 3-phenyl-β-alanine in methanol (MeOH) by adding thionyl chloride, followed by protection of the amino group as tert-butyloxycarbonyl (Boc), which is then treated with hydrazine in the presence of MeOH at room temperature Scheme 1).

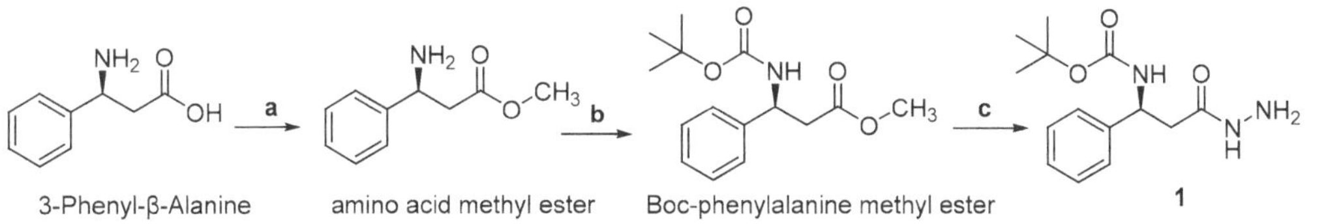

Scheme 1. Reagents and conditions: (**a**) SOCl$_2$, MeOH, 0 °C, overnight; (**b**) NaCO$_3$, H$_2$O, Boc, EtOAc (**c**) NH$_2$NH$_2$.H$_2$O, MeOH, rt, 24 h (**1**).

Our investigation started with the cyclization of 3-phenyl-β-alanine hydrazones **3a–l** to the corresponding 1,3,4-oxadiazole **4a–l**. The synthesis and NMR data of the substrates **3a–l** were already reported by our group. These compounds were prepared via the condensation of different benzaldehyde moieties **2a–l** (0.6 mmol, 1.2 equiv.) with phenylalanine hydrazide (**1**, 0.5 mmol, 1 equiv.) in ethanol at refluxing temperature in 90% yield [52] (Scheme 2). The oxidative cyclization of **3a–l** to **4a–l** was achieved by utilizing molecular iodine in the presence of potassium carbonate (1.8 mmol, 3 equiv.) and DMSO (2 mL) which is the most effective media (solvent) for this conversion at 100 °C. The structures of the resulting compounds were confirmed by ^{1}H-, IR, and ^{13}C-NMR spectroscopy as well as mass spectrometry (HRESIMS).

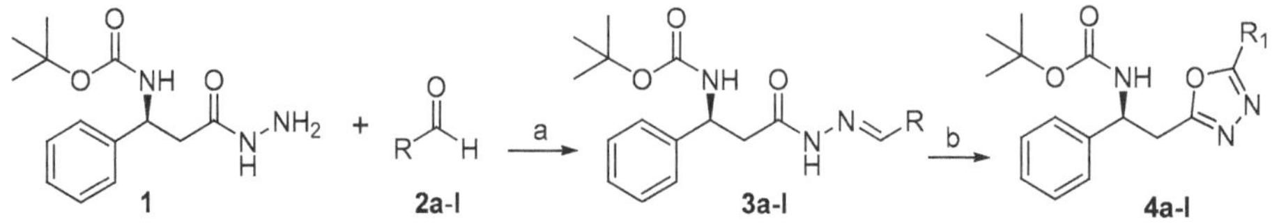

Scheme 2. Reagents and conditions: (**a**) EtOH, 80 °C, Reflux overnight, (**3a–l**, 90%); (**b**) K_2CO_3, DMSO, 100 °C, Reflux overnight (**4a–l**).

2.2. Carbonic Anhydrase-II Enzyme Inhibition and Structural-Activity Relationship

All the synthetic compounds reported herein, and standard carbonic anhydrase inhibitor acetazolamide were assessed for their inhibition properties towards the relevant recombinant human carbonic anhydrase-II using the colorimetric method. Most of the synthesized compounds strongly inhibited CA-II enzyme ranging from 12.1 to 53.6 µM. Among all, compounds **4a** (12.1 ± 0.86 µM), **4c** (13.8 ± 0.64 µM), **4i** (18.1 ± 1.31 µM), **4b** (19.1 ± 0.88 µM) and **4h** (20.7 ± 1.13 µM) were found to be the best CA-II inhibitors, while compounds **4g** (21.5 ± 0.99 µM), **4k** (22.4 ± 1.32 µM), **4f** (25.1 ± 1.04 µM), and **4e** (26.6 ± 0.80 µM) demonstrated moderate activity (Table 1). Compared to standard (acetazolamide), compound **4l** (53.6 ± 0.96 µM) was found to be weak inhibitor against CA-II among all derivatives.

Table 1. Carbonic anhydrase-II activity of the compounds **4a–l**.

Compounds	R	% Inhibition	$IC_{50} \pm SEM$ (µM)
4a	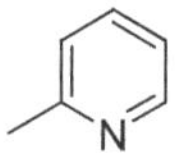 2a (pyridine)	96.2	12.1 ± 0.86
4b	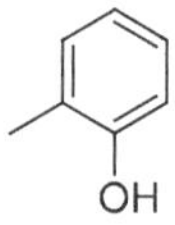 2b (2-hydroxyphenyl)	93.5	19.1 ± 0.88
4c	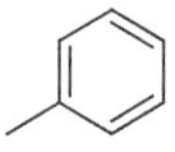 2c (phenyl)	95.5	13.8 ± 0.64
4d	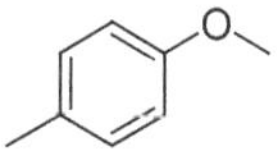 2d (4-methoxyphenyl)	29.0	N/A
4e	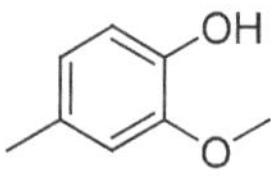 2e (hydroxy-methoxyphenyl)	97.3	26.6 ± 0.80
4f	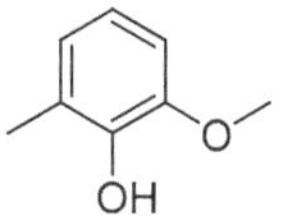 2f (methoxy-hydroxyphenyl)	93.8	25.1 ± 1.04
4g	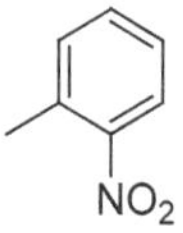 2g (2-nitrophenyl)	79.5	21.5 ± 0.99

Table 1. Cont.

Compounds	R	% Inhibition	IC$_{50}$ ± SEM (µM)
4h	2h (4-NO$_2$-phenyl)	94.6	20.7 ± 1.13
4i	2i (4-OH-phenyl)	58.0	18.1 ± 1.31
4j	2j (dimethoxyphenyl)	96.7	26.6 ± 1.47
4k	2k (dimethoxy-methylphenyl)	87.8	22.4 ± 1.43
4l	2l (4-Cl-phenyl)	67.6	53.6 ± 0.96
Standard	Acetazolamide	84.6	18.2 ± 1.43

N/A = Not active, SEM = Standard error mean.

Comparing compound **4i** with **4b**, the higher activity of the **4i** may be possible due to the presence of -OH group at para position of phenyl ring. A comparison between 4g with **4h** revealed a slight decrease in inhibition of **4g**, which is likely due to the presence of nitro group (electron-withdrawing substituent) at ortho position of the phenyl ring. This suggests that the inhibitory activity of CA-II enzyme could be possibly increased with an electron-withdrawing substituent at para position of the phenyl ring. A slight change in activities between **4j** and **4k** as well as **4e** and **4f** was observed. The higher inhibition of **4k** and **4f** could be accounted for the arrangements of functional groups attached to the phenyl ring. Compound **4a** (IC$_{50}$ = 12.1 µM) exerted a stronger inhibition than other compounds in the series, which is possibly due to the presence of pyridine ring instead of phenyl. Similarly, a higher inhibition of compound **4c** is observed when compared with compounds **4d** and **4l** which is probably due to the absence of electron withdrawing groups at para position of the phenyl ring.

2.3. Molecular Docking Results

All the active compounds were docked at the active site of CA-II (PDB code: 3HS4) to predict the best possible binding modes of each active compound through molecular docking. The standard drug, acetazolamide binds at the active site and mediates several interactions including ionic interactions with Zn ion, hydrogen bonding with the side chains of His94, His96, Thr199 and Thr200 within the active pocket of CA-II. The binding mode of acetazolamide is shown in Figure 2. Several active compounds, including **4a**, **4c** and **4i**, exhibited CA-II inhibitory activity (in range of 12.1 to 18.1 µM) higher than the standard drug. The binding mode of the most active compound **4a** depict that the carbamate moiety of the compound is involved in binding with the active site residues. Whereas oxadiazol ring and its substituted R group (pyridinyl ring) resided at the entrance of the active site. Moreover, the carbamate substituted phenyl ring was also fitted neatly in the groove near the active site entrance. The carbamate moiety of the compound mediated multiple H-bonding interaction with the amino group of Thr199 and Thr200, and side chain of Thr200. Moreover, the side chain of Gln92 also provides H-bond to the oxadiazole ring of the compound. We observed that the compound does not interact with the Zn ion in the active site, however, by interacting with several active site residues through H-bonds, and complete blockage of active site entrance, **4a** inhibits the function of CA-II. Similar orientation was observed for compound **4c** (the second highest active inhibitor), **4i** and **4b**, however, carbamate moiety of these compounds interacted with the amino group and the side chain of Thr200. Additionally, -OH group at the substituted hydroxyl phenyl ring of **4b** mediated H-bonding with the side chain of Gln92. The docked conformation of **4h** was completely like the binding mode of **4b**, the carbonyl oxygen of **4h** binds with the amino group of Thr200, however, the oxadiazol and the substituted nitrophenyl rings did not interact with the surrounding residues. Interestingly, the carbamate and the oxadiazol ring of **4g** do not interact with the surrounding residues, while its methoxy oxygen interacted with the amino group of Thr199 through H-bond. The substituted nitrophenyl rings of compounds **4h** and **4g** were found to be surface exposed. Similarly, the carbamate oxygen of **4k** and **4f** and oxadiazol ring of **4f** formed H-bonds with the amino nitrogen of Thr200, and side chain of Gln92, respectively. The binding mode of compounds **4e** and **4j** demonstrated that the carbamate nitrogen of **4e** interacted with a water molecule in the vicinity of active site, while the substituted R group mediated π-π interaction with the phenyl ring of Phe131, whereas the carbonyl oxygen of **4j** accepted H-bond with the amino group of Thr199. The least active compound of this series, **4l** only mediates bidentate interaction with the amino nitrogen and side chain -OH of Thr200 through its carbamate moiety. The binding interactions of each compound within the active site of CA-II are tabulated in Table 2. The docked view of the most active compound **4a** is presented in Figure 2.

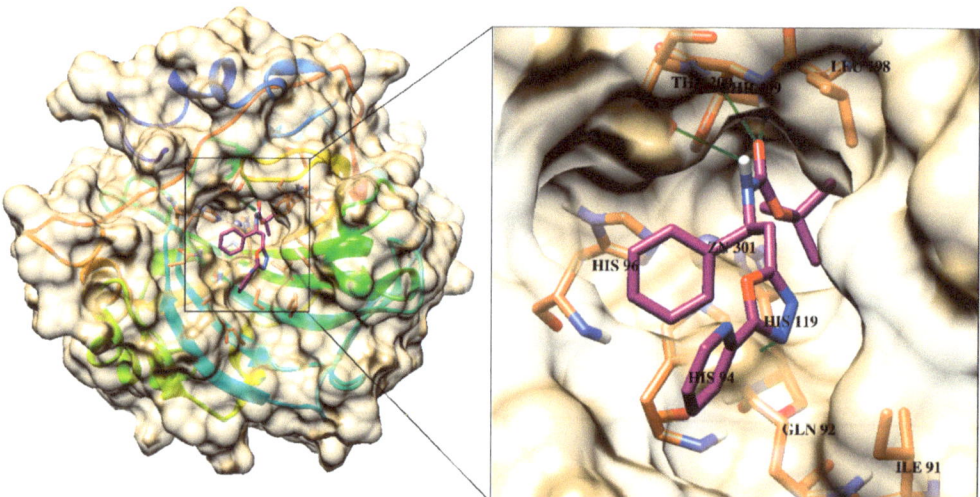

Figure 2. The binding mode of most active compound **4a** is shown in the active site of CA-II. The ligand is presented in magenta stick model, 3D-structure of CA-II is shown in surface model, interacting residues are depicted in coral stick model and H-bonds are presented in green lines.

The pharmacokinetic properties of the active compounds were predicted through BOILED- Egg model of SwissADME [61]. In the BOILED-Egg analysis, all the compounds showed high gastro-intestinal absorption, while none of the compounds exhibited blood brain barrier permeability. Moreover, all the compounds followed Lipinski rule of five drug-likeness criteria, and no PAIN alerts. In addition, accept **4a**, all the compounds were found as non-substrate for P-glycoprotein (Table 3). The predicted ADMET profile of the compounds suggest that these compounds could act as beneficial inhibitor of CA-II.

Table 2. Molecular docking results of active inhibitors.

Compounds	Score (kcal/mol)	Interactions			
		Ligand Atom	Receptor Atom	Bond Type	Distance (Å)
4a	−8.96	O25	N-THR199	HBA	1.87
		O25	N-THR200	HBA	2.37
		6-ring	HOH-1247	π-H	3.53
4c	−8.2	N22	OG1-THR200	HBD	1.97
		O25	N-THR200	HBA	2.39
4i	−8.05	N22	OG1-THR200	HBD	2.95
		O25	N-THR200	HBA	2.61
4b	−7.88	O25	N-THR200	HBA	2.26
		O25	OG1-THR 200	HBA	1.80
		6-ring	O-HOH1247	π-H	3.46
4h	−7.63	O25	OG1-THR200	HBA	2.23
4g	−7.68	O26	N-THR199	HBA	1.87
4k	−7.80	O25	OG1-THR200	HBA	2.11
4f	−7.10	O21	NE2-GLN92	HBA	2.97
		O25	N-THR200	HBA	2.21
4e	−7.09	N22	O-HOH1191	HBD	1.99
		6-ring	6-ring-PHE131	π-π	3.01
4j	−7.10	O25	N-THR199	HBA	2.20
4l	−6.23	N22	OG1-THR200	HBD	1.82
		O25	N-THR200	HBA	2.08

HBA = Hydrogen bond acceptor, HBD = Hydrogen bond donor.

Table 3. The pharmacokinetic profile of active inhibitors.

Molecule	NRB	HBA	HBD	TPSA	iLOGP	GIA	BBBP	PgpS	Lipinski V	PAINS Alerts
4a	8	6	1	90.14	3	High	No	Yes	0	0
4b	8	6	2	97.48	3.34	High	No	No	0	0
4c	8	5	1	77.25	3.54	High	No	No	0	0
4e	9	7	2	106.71	3.56	High	No	No	0	0
4f	9	7	2	106.71	3.45	High	No	No	0	0
4g	9	7	1	123.07	2.96	High	No	No	0	0
4h	9	7	1	123.07	3.11	High	No	No	0	0
4i	8	6	2	97.48	3.15	High	No	No	0	0
4j	10	7	1	95.71	3.81	High	No	No	0	0
4k	10	7	1	95.71	3.64	High	No	No	0	0
4l	8	5	1	77.25	3.75	High	No	No	0	0
AZM	3	6	1	178.33	0	Low	No	No	0	0

NRB = Number of rotatable bonds, HBA = H-bond acceptors, HBD = H-bond donors, TPSA = Topological polar surface area, GIA = Gastrointestinal absorption, BBBP = Blood brain barrier permeant, PgpS = P glycoprotein substrate, Lipinski V = Violation of lipinski rule of 5.

3. Material and Methods

3.1. General Instrumentation

All reagents were purchased from Sigma-Aldrich Chemical Company (St. Louis, MO, USA). Solvents used for chemical reactions were purified and dried by standard procedures. Melting point was determined using digital melting point apparatus SMP10 (Stuart[TM], Cole-Parmer, Beacon Rd, Stone, Staffordshire, ST15 OSA, UK). Infrared (IR) spectra were recorded on an ATR-Tensor 37 attenuated total reflectance spectrometer (Bruker, Ettlingen, Baden-Württemberg, Germany) in the range from 400 to 4000 cm^{-1}. High-resolution electrospray ionization mass spectrometry (HR-ESI-MS, Agilent technologies, 6530, Q-TOF

LC/MS, Agilent, country of origin USA/EU, made in Singapore) was used for the determination of compound masses. The ^{1}H- (600 MHz) and ^{13}C- (150 MHz) NMR spectra were recorded on Bruker (Zürich, Switzerland) nuclear magnetic resonance spectrometers using the solvent peak as internal reference (CDCl$_3$, δH: 7.26; δC: 77.2–76.8; DMSO, δH: 2.49; δC: 40.0–39.1). The following abbreviations were used to explain for NMR signals as s = singlet, d = doublet, dd = doublet of doublet, t = triplet, m = multiplet, J = coupling constant. Chemical shifts are expressed in parts per million (δ) values and coupling constants (J) are given in Hertz (Hz). All reactions were monitored by Thin-Layer-Chromatography (TLC, Merck, Darmstadt, Germany) using pre-coated aluminum sheets (silica gel 60 F$_{254}$). TLC plates were visualized under the UV light at 254 and 366 nm and by spraying with the ninhydrin reagent. Solvents for chromatography were of technical grade and distilled prior to use.

3.2. General Procedure for the Synthesis 3-phenyl-β-alanine-1,3,4-Oxadiazoles Derivatives

3-Phenyl-β-alanine (10 mmol, 1.65 g) was used as a starting material for the synthesis of Boc-3-phenyl-β-alanine hydrazide (**1**). Esterification of the carboxylate group was done by the slow addition of thionyl chloride (15 mmol, 2.1 mL) to a solution of methanol (20 mL) containing 3-phenyl-β-alanine at 0 °C. The reaction solution was stirred for overnight (24 h.) at room temperature, while the completion of the reaction was carefully monitored by TLC for ensuring that all amount of amino acid changed to ester. After reaction completion, the solvent (MeOH) was evaporated under vacuum and the resultant product was filtered.

In the second step, amino acid methyl ester (9.8 mmol, 1.75 g) was added to a solution of anhydrous Na$_2$CO$_3$ (1.2 g, 12 mmol) and H$_2$O (40 mL) in a 100 mL RB flask. Then, di-*tert*-butyl dicarbonate (Boc anhydride, 10 mmol, 2.1 g) was dissolved in EtOAc (20 mL), added to that solution and the reaction was allowed to stir for 24 h at room temperature. The progress of the reaction was continuously observed by TLC. When the reaction was completed, the pH was adjusted to 5.5 with oxalic acid and then the desired product was extracted with an organic solvent (EtOAc). The solvent was dried over anhydrous MgSO$_4$ and evaporated under reduced pressure to obtain the corresponding Boc-phenylalanine methyl ester (91%).

In the third step, hydrazine monohydrate (2 mL, 32 mmol) was added to a solution of methanol (20 mL) containing Boc-phenylalanine methyl ester (9.1 mmol, 2.5 g) and stirred under room temperature for 24 h to afford phenylalanine hydrazide (**1**). The reaction mixture was thoroughly checked by TLC. After reaction completion, the solvent was evaporated under reduced pressure and the product tert-butyl (S)-(3-hydrazinyl-3-oxo-1-phenylpropyl) carbamate (**1**, yield 89%) was washed with methanol. White powder; Yield: 86%; m-p. 187–190 °C; FT-IR (solid, cm^{-1}): 3318, 1694, 1664, and 1580, 1362, 1260, 1160, and 1092; ^{1}H-NMR (CDCl$_3$): δ 8.54 (1H, s, NH), 7.30 (1H, C NH), 4.88 (?H, NH-NH$_2$), 7.11–7.28 (5H, m), 4.97 (CH-NH), 2.93–3.14 (2H, CH$_2$), 1.36 (9H, s); ^{13}C-NMR (CDCl$_3$): δ 28.3, 38.5, 55.2, 79.7, 126.0, 126.6, 126.7, 128.0, 128.5, 155.3, 143.2, 155.9, 177.3; HRMS (ESI+) *m/z*: 302.1477 [M + Na]$^+$.

In the fourth step, a solution of aldehyde (0.6 mmol) added to a stirred solution of **1** (0.5 mmol) in EtOH (5 mL) at room temperature for 24 h. The progress of the reaction was monitored with TLC system of EtOAc/*n*-hexane (3:7). After completion of the reaction, the product (**3**) was filtered, washed with *n*-hexane for removing any excess of aldehyde. The resulting residue was redissolved in DMSO (2 mL), followed by addition of potassium carbonate (3 mmol) and iodine (1.2 mmol) in sequence. The reaction mixture was stirred at 100 °C until the conversion was complete (1–4 h, monitored by TLC,). After being cooled to room temperature, it was treated with 5% Na$_2$S$_2$O$_3$ (20 mL), extracted with EtOAc (10 mL, three times). The combined organic layer was washed with brine (10 mL × 1), dried over anhydrous sodium sulfate, and concentrated. The given residue was purified through preparative thin layer chromatography (TLC) using a mobile phase of EtOAc and *n*-hexane (3:7) to afford the desired oxadiazoles. All compounds were obtained in fare yields ranging from 57 to 64%. The structures of all compounds were established by HRMS, ^{1}H- and ^{13}C-NMR and same procedure was use for the synthesis of other compounds.

3.2.1. Tert-Butyl (S)-(1-phenyl-2-(5-(pyridin-2-yl)-1,3,4-oxadiazol-2-yl) ethyl) carbamate (**4a**)

White solid powder; Yield: 57%; FTIR (solid, cm^{-1}): 3320, 1690, 1666, and 1585, 1365, 1264, 1160, and 1094; ^{1}H-NMR (CDCl$_3$): δ 8.76 (1H), 8.18 (1H), 7.86 (1H), 7.45 (1H), 7.25–7.10 (5H, m), 5.40 (1H, NH), 5.19 (1H, CH), 3.22, 3.35 (2H), 1.37 (9H, s); ^{13}C-NMR (CDCl$_3$): δ 28.2, 39.9, 48.5, 80.4, 123.2, 126.0, 127.2, 128.7, 129.4, 135.2, 137.3, 143.3, 150.3, 164.2, 167.1; HRMS (ESI$^+$) m/z: 366.1756 [M + H]$^+$.

3.2.2. Tert-Butyl (S)-(2-(5-(2-hydroxyphenyl)-1,3,4-oxadiazol-2-yl)-1-phenylethyl) carbamate (**4b**)

Solid powder; Yield: 56%; FTIR (solid, cm^{-1}): 3318, 1689, 1670, and 1594, 1445, 1375, 1340, 1302 and 1160; ^{1}H-NMR (CDCl$_3$): δ 10.86 (1H, OH, s), 8.15 (1H), 7.65 (1H), 7.42 (1H), 7.30 (1H), 7.25–6.72 (5H, m), 5.36 (1H, NH), 5.09 (1H, CH), 3.29, 3.28 (2H), 1.41 (9H, s); ^{13}C-NMR (CDCl$_3$): δ 28.2, 39.8, 48.6, 81.2, 86.8, 109.5, 119.9, 121.5, 124.9, 126.8, 127.5, 128.7, 128.9, 129.3, 133.8, 134.7, 143.3, 154.8, 157.7, 165.8; HRMS (ESI$^+$) m/z: 382.1814 [M + H]$^+$.

3.2.3. Tert-Butyl(S)-(1-phenyl-2-(5-phenyl-1,3,4-oxadiazol-2-yl)ethyl) carbamate (**4c**)

Pale yellow Color; Yield: 58%; FTIR (solid, cm^{-1}): 3336, 1710, 1668, 1608, 1375, 1335, 1290 and 1080; ^{1}H-NMR (CDCl$_3$, 600 MHz): δ 7.88–7.39 (5H, m), 7.22–7.07 (5H, m), 5.47 (1H, NH), 5.25 (1H, CH), 3.23, 3.20 (2H), 1.33 (9H, s); ^{13}C-NMR (150 MHz, CDCl$_3$): δ 28.2, 29.6, 48.5, 80.3, 123.6, 126.8, 127.1, 128.6, 129.0, 132.9, 131.7, 135.6, 154.9, 164.9, 166.2; HRMS (ESI$^+$) m/z: 366.1948 [M + H]$^+$.

3.2.4. Tert-Butyl(S)-(2-(5-(4-methoxyphenyl)-1,3,4-oxadiazol-2-yl)-1-phenylethyl) carbamate (**4d**)

White solid powder; Yield: 57%; FTIR (solid, cm^{-1}): 3324, 1704, 1672, 1602, 1452, 1370, 1268, 1160, and 1020; ^{1}H-NMR (CDCl$_3$): δ 7.81 (1H), 7.80 (1H), 6.90 (1H), 6.89 (1H), 7.24–7.07 (5H, m), 5.47 (1H, NH), 5.22 (1H, CH), 3.78 (3H, CH$_3$), 3.23,3.17 (2H), 1.32 (9H, s); ^{13}C-NMR (CDCl$_3$): δ 28.2, 29.6, 48.5, 55.4, 114.4, 116.0, 127.1, 128.6, 129.3, 135.6, 154.9, 162.3, 164.8, 165.6; HRMS (ESI$^+$) m/z: 396.1960 [M + H]$^+$.

3.2.5. Tert-Butyl(S)-(2-(5-(4-hydroxy-3-methoxyphenyl)-1,3,4-oxadiazol-2-yl)-1-phenylethyl) carbamate (**4e**)

Yellow powder; Yield: 56%; FTIR (solid, cm^{-1}): 3333, 1696, 1668, 1590, 1450, 1370, 1252, 1160, 1030; ^{1}H-NMR (CDCl$_3$): δ 9.80 (1H, OH, s), 7.63 (1H), 7.51 (1H), 7.25–7.11 (5H, m), 6.87 (1H), 5.43 (1H, NH), 5.31 (1H, CH), 4.44 (3H, OCH$_3$), 3.94,3.86 (2H), 1.38 (9H, s); ^{13}C-NMR (CDCl$_3$): δ 28.2, 34.4, 38.5, 48.6, 40.9, 52.5, 56.1, 107.7, 109.5, 119.9, 121.5, 124.9, 126.8, 128.7, 129.3, 136.5, 145.0, 155.3, 167.8, 190.8; HRMS (ESI$^+$) m/z: 436.2279 [M + H]$^+$.

3.2.6. Tert-Butyl(S)-(2-(5-(2-hydroxy-3-methoxyphenyl)-1,3,4-oxadiazol-2-yl)-1-phenylethyl) carbamate (**4f**)

Crystalline powder; Yield: 61%; FTIR (solid, cm^{-1}): 3320, 1690, 1664, 1594, 1450, 1405, 1358, 1257, 1164, and 1090; ^{1}H-NMR (CDCl$_3$, 600 MHz): δ 9.90 (1H, OH, s), 8.17 (1H), 7.93 (1H), 7.29–7.10 (5H, m), 6.85 (1H), 5.27 (1H, NH), 4.45 (1H, CH), 3.91 (3H, OCH3), 3.91,3.87 (2H), 1.37 (9H, s); 13C-NMR (150 MHz, CDCl$_3$): δ 28.2, 34.4, 38.1, 56.3, 113.7, 114.2, 117.5, 119.5, 121.4, 124.5, 126.9, 128.4, 129.5, 136.3, 145.6, 151.1, 155.9, 167.4, 172.8, 196.6; HRMS (ESI$^+$) m/z: 436.1883 [M + H]$^+$.

3.2.7. Tert-Butyl(S)-(2-(5-(2-nitrophenyl)-1,3,4-oxadiazol-2-yl)-1-phenylethyl) carbamate (**4g**)

Yellow powder; Yield: 56%; FTIR (solid, cm^{-1}): 3310, 1703, 1666, 1614, 1455, 1346, 1324, 1236, 1059; ^{1}H-NMR (CDCl$_3$): δ 8.05 (1H), 7.87 (1H), 7.67 (1H), 7.71 (1H), 7.29–7.13 (5H, m), 5.34 (1H, NH), 5.13 (1H, CH), 3.30,3.18 (2H), 1.38 (9H, s); ^{13}C-NMR (CDCl$_3$): δ 28.2,

39.8, 48.4, 118.7, 124.8, 127.3, 128.7, 129.4, 131.9, 132.6, 133.3, 135.0, 148.1, 154.8, 161.8, 167.3; HRMS (ESI⁺) *m*/*z*: 411.1694 [M + H]⁺.

3.2.8. Tert-Butyl(S)-(2-(5-(4-nitrophenyl)-1,3,4-oxadiazol-2-yl)-1-phenylethyl) carbamate (**4h**)

Light yellow powder; Yield: 61%; FTIR (solid, cm⁻¹): 3322, 1701, 1664, 1610, 1430, 1365, 1345, 1208, and 1163; ¹H-NMR (CDCl₃): δ 8.38 (1H), 8.37 (1H), 8.17 (1H), 8.16 (1H), 7.32–7.17 (5H, m), 5.41 (1H, NH), 5.20 (1H, CH), 3.34,3.33 (2H), 1.45 (9H, s); ¹³C-NMR (CDCl₃): δ 28.2, 29.7, 40.0, 48.6, 124.3, 124.5, 126.9, 127.4, 127.8, 128.8, 129.0, 129.1, 129.3, 135.1, 149.7, 154.8, 163.2, 167.4; HRMS (ESI⁺) *m*/*z*: 411.1705 [M + H]⁺.

3.2.9. Tert-Butyl (S)-(2-(5-(4-hydroxyphenyl)-1,3,4-oxadiazol-2-yl)-1-phenylethyl) carbamate (**4i**)

White solid powder; Yield: 59%; FTIR (solid, cm⁻¹): 3330, 1705, 1668, and 1608; ¹H-NMR (CDCl₃): δ 7.78 (1H), 7.77 (1H), 7.26 (1H), 7.20 (1H), 7.12–6.86 (5H, m), 5.30 (1H, NH), 5.16 (1H, CH), 3.29,3.24 (2H), 1.38 (9H, s); ¹³C-NMR (CDCl₃): δ 28.2, 29.3, 29.7, 29.7, 31.9, 40.0, 48.5, 80.7, 116.0, 116.1, 127.2, 128.7, 128.9, 129.4, 135.4, 158.9, 164.9, 165.5; HRMS (ESI⁺) *m*/*z*: 382.1463 [M + H]⁺.

3.2.10. Tert-Butyl (S)-(2-(5-(3,4-dimethoxyphenyl)-1,3,4-oxadiazol-2-yl)-1-phenylethyl) carbamate (**4j**)

White amorphous powder; Yield: 64%; FTIR (solid, cm⁻¹): 3326, 1701, 1670, 1595, 1420, 1370, 1336, 1252, 1208, and 1143; ¹H-NMR (CDCl₃): δ 7.50 (1H), 7.49 (1H), 7.45 (1H), 7.27–7.12 (5H, m), 6.90 (1H), 5.32 (1H, NH), 5.18 (1H, CH), 3.92 (6H, OCH₃), 3.27,3.26 (2H), 1.40 (9H, s); ¹³C-NMR (CDCl3): δ 28.3, 40.1, 48.5, 56.0, 56.1, 80.5, 109.5, 111.1, 116.2, 120.4, 127.2, 128.6, 129.4, 135.5, 149.3, 152.1, 164.9, 165.7; HRMS (ESI⁺) *m*/*z*: 426.2066 [M + H]⁺.

3.2.11. Tert-Butyl (S)-(2-(5-(2,5-dimethoxyphenyl)-1,3,4-oxadiazol-2-yl)-1-phenylethyl) carbamate (**4k**)

Colorless solid; Yield: 61%; FTIR (solid, cm⁻¹): 3328, 1711, 1667, 1602, 1524, 1342, 1272, 1228, 1155, and 1066; ¹H-NMR (CDCl₃): δ 7.30 (1H), 7.24–7.11 (5H, m), 7.03 (1H), 6.96 (1H), 5.36 (1H, NH), 5.22 (1H, CH), 3.86,3.78 (6H, OCH₃), 3.30,3.27 (2H), 1.40 (9H, s); ¹³C-NMR (CDCl₃): δ 28.3, 40.0, 48.5, 56.0, 56.6, 60.4, 80.3, 113.1, 113.7, 114.5, 119.4, 127.1, 128.6, 129.4, 135.5, 152.3, 153.4, 163.6, 165.8; HRMS (ESI⁺) *m*/*z*: 426.2065 [M + H]⁺.

3.2.12. Tert-Butyl (S)-(2-(5-(4-chlorophenyl)-1,3,4-oxadiazol-2-yl)-1-phenylethyl) carbamate (**4l**)

White powder; Yield: 57%; FTIR (solid, cm⁻¹): 3350, 1698, 1663, and 1603, 1532, 1336, 1266, 1224, 1172, and 1066; ¹H-NMR (CDCl₃): δ 7.88 (1H), 7.87 (1H), 7.45 (1H), 7.44 (1H), 7.27–7.12 (5H, m), 5.32 (1H, NH), 5.16 (1H, CH), 3.28,3.27 (2H), 1.40 (9H, s); ¹³C-NMR (CDCl₃): δ 28.2, 29.7, 39.9, 48.6, 80.6, 122.2, 127.3, 128.2, 128.7, 129.3, 129.4, 135.3, 138.1, 154.8; HRMS (ESI⁺) *m*/*z*: 400.1467 [M + H]⁺.

3.3. Carbonic Anhydrase II Inhibition Assay

A total reaction volume of 200 µL containing 20 µL of the synthetic compounds **4a–l** prepared in DMSO, followed by the addition of 140 µL of the HEPES-tris buffer, 20 µL of purified bovine erythrocyte CA-II (0.15 mg/mL) prepared in buffer, and 20 µL of a solution of 4-nitrophenyl acetate [36,44]. 20 µL of tested compounds were incubated with the enzyme carbonic anhydrase II (EC 4.2.1.1) for 15 min in 96-well flat bottom plate. The rate of product formation was monitored with the addition of 20 µL of 4-NPA as substrate, prepared in ethanol at the final concentration of 0.7 mM at 25 °C for 30 min with regular intervals of 1 min, by using spectrophotometer (xMark™ Microplate, Bio-Rad, Hercules, CA, USA). HEPES-tris was used as a buffer for the reaction at the final concentration of 20 mM at pH 7.4.

3.4. Molecular Docking

Docking was conducted on Molecular Operating Environment [45] using X-ray crystal structure of human carbonic anhydrase II complexed with acetazolamide (PDB code: 3HS4, resolution: 1.10 Å) [62]. The docking performance of MOE was tested previously [36,44] by re-docking experiment which shows that MOE is efficient in docking of CA-II inhibitors. In the re-docking, the X-ray conformation of acetazolamide was re-docked at its cognate binding site, where it was docked with RMSD = 0.61 Å. The re-docked conformation is shown in Figure S37. The protein file was prepared for docking by QuickPrep module of MOE which adds missing hydrogen atoms on residues and calculate partial charges using pre-defined force field (we applied Amber10:EHT force field). The two-dimensional (2D-) structures of ligands were prepared by ChemDraw, later converted into 3D-form by MOE using WASH module of MOE which adds hydrogen atoms and partial charges on ligands. Subsequently, the 3D-structure of each compound was minimized until the gradient was reached to 0.1RMS kcal/mol/Å. After the preparation of protein and ligand files, docking was performed by Triangle Matcher docking algorithm and London dG scoring function. Thirty docked conformation of each ligand was saved, and the best docked orientation was selected based on the docking score and binding interactions. The pharmacokinetic profile of the active hits was predicted through SwissADME server using BOILED-Egg model [61,63].

4. Conclusions

In summary, a series of twelve new 3-phenyl-β-alanine 1,3,4-oxadiazoles **4a–l** have been synthesized and CA-II were performed in vitro. From all derivatives, compounds **4a** (12.1 µM) and **4c** (13.8 µM) exhibited the most potent activity against CA-II enzyme. In addition, structure-activity relationship of the active compounds has been established. When the results were compared, it was observed that these molecules show more effective inhibition than the standard inhibitor. Based on molecular docking strategy, we observed the mode of binding interaction of the active hits with the active site residues of CA-II, which suggests that the compounds mainly interact with the Thr199 and Thr200, thus inhibit the activity of CA-II. Based on these results, we suggest that these molecules can be used against CA-II related diseases.

Supplementary Materials: The following supporting information can be downloaded, Figures S1–S36: ^{1}H- (CDCl$_3$, 600 MHz), ^{13}C-NMR and HRESIMS of the compounds **4a–l**, Figure S37: The re-docked orientation of acetazolamide.

Author Contributions: K.R. synthesized the compounds. N.U.R. performed structural elucidation and wrote original draft of the manuscript. A.K. and M.K., performed carbonic anhydrase II inhibition. S.A.H. conducted in silico studies. A.A.-H. supervised the project and assisted in reviewing and editing the manuscript. All authors have read and agreed to the published version of the manuscript.

Funding: The authors are thankful to The Oman Research Council (TRC) through the funded Research Grant Program (BFP/RGP/CBS/21/002).

Institutional Review Board Statement: Not applicable.

Informed Consent Statement: Not applicable.

Data Availability Statement: The spectroscopic data is available in the supporting information to the researchers.

Acknowledgments: The authors are thankful to the University of Nizwa for the generous support to this project. We are also grateful to the analytical and technical staffs of the University for assistance.

Conflicts of Interest: The authors declare no conflict of interest.

Sample Availability: The data presented in this study is available in the Supplementary Material.

References

1. Payaz, D.Ü.; Küçükbay, F.Z.; Küçükbay, H.; Angeli, A.; Supuran, C.T. Synthesis carbonic anhydrase enzyme inhibition and antioxidant activity of novel benzothiazole derivatives incorporating glycine, methionine, alanine, and phenylalanine moieties. *J. Enzym. Inhib. Med. Chem.* **2019**, *1*, 343–349. [CrossRef] [PubMed]
2. Akocak, S.; Lolak, N.; Nocentini, A.; Karakoc, G.; Tufan, A.; Supuran, C.T. Synthesis and biological evaluation of novel aromatic and heterocyclic bis-sulfonamide Schiff bases as carbonic anhydrase I, II, VII and IX inhibitors. *Bioorganic Med. Chem.* **2017**, *12*, 3093–3097. [CrossRef] [PubMed]
3. D'Ascenzio, M.; Guglielmi, P.; Carradori, S.; Secci, D.; Florio, R.; Mollica, A.; Ceruso, M.; Akdemir, A.; Sobolev, A.P.; Supuran, C.T. Open saccharin-based secondary sulfonamides as potent and selective inhibitors of cancer-related carbonic anhydrase IX and XII isoforms. *J. Enzym. Inhib. Med. Chem.* **2017**, *1*, 51–59. [CrossRef] [PubMed]
4. Gokcen, T.; Gulcin, I.; Ozturk, T.; Goren, A.C. A class of sulfonamides as carbonic anhydrase I and II inhibitors. *J. Enzym. Inhib. Med. Chem.* **2016**, *2*, 180–188. [CrossRef] [PubMed]
5. Gul, H.I.; Mete, E.; Taslimi, P.; Gulcin, I.; Supuran, C.T. Synthesis, carbonic anhydrase I and II inhibition studies of the 1,3,5-trisubstituted-pyrazolines. *J. Enzym. Inhib. Med. Chem.* **2017**, *1*, 189–192. [CrossRef] [PubMed]
6. Ibrahim, D.A.; Lasheen, D.S.; Zaky, M.Y.; Ibrahim, A.W.; Vullo, D.; Ceruso, M.; Supuran, C.T.; Abou El Ella, D.A. Design and synthesis of benzothiazole-6-sulfonamides acting as highly potent inhibitors of carbonic anhydrase isoforms I, II, IX and XII. *Bioorganic Med. Chem.* **2015**, *15*, 4989–4999. [CrossRef] [PubMed]
7. Sağlık, B.N.; Cevik, U.A.; Osmaniye, D.; Levent, S.; Çavuşoğlu, B.K.; Demir, Y.; Ilgın, S.; Özkay, Y.; Koparal, A.S.; Beydemir, Ş. Synthesis, molecular docking analysis and carbonic anhydrase I-II inhibitory evaluation of new sulfonamide derivatives. *Bioorganic Chem.* **2019**, *91*, 103153. [CrossRef]
8. Angeli, A.; Ferraroni, M.; Supuran, C.T. Famotidine, an antiulcer agent, strongly inhibits Helicobacter pylori and human carbonic anhydrases. *ACS Med. Chem. Lett.* **2018**, *10*, 1035–1038. [CrossRef]
9. Khloya, P.; Celik, G.; Vullo, D.; Supuran, C.T.; Sharma, P.K. 4-Functionalized 1,3-diarylpyrazoles bearing benzenesulfonamide moiety as selective potent inhibitors of the tumor associated carbonic anhydrase isoforms IX and XII. *Eur. J. Med. Chem.* **2014**, *76*, 284–290. [CrossRef]
10. Aggarwal, M.; Boone, C.D.; Kondeti, B.; McKenna, R. Structural annotation of human carbonic anhydrases. *J. Enzym. Inhib. Med. Chem.* **2013**, *2*, 267–277. [CrossRef]
11. Supuran, C.T. Carbonic anhydrases-an overview. *Curr. Pharm. Des.* **2008**, *7*, 603–614. [CrossRef] [PubMed]
12. Lee, A.H.; Tannock, I.F. Heterogeneity of intracellular pH and of mechanisms that regulate intracellular pH in populations of cultured cells. *Cancer Res.* **1998**, *9*, 1901–1908.
13. Montcourrier, P.; Silver, I.; Farnoud, R.; Bird, I.; Rochefort, H. Breast cancer cells have a high capacity to acidify extracellular milieu by a dual mechanism. *Clin. Exp. Metastasis* **1997**, *4*, 382–392. [CrossRef]
14. Webb, S.; Sherratt, J.; Fish, R. Mathematical modelling of tumor acidity: Regulation of intracellular pH. *J. Theor. Biol.* **1999**, *2*, 237–250. [CrossRef] [PubMed]
15. Frazier, M.L.; Lilly, B.J.; Wu, E.F.; Ota, T.; Hewett-Emmett, D. Carbonic anhydrase II gene expression in cell lines from human pancreatic adenocarcinoma. *Pancreas* **1990**, *5*, 507–514. [CrossRef]
16. Parkkila, A.-K.; Herva, R.; Parkkila, S.; Rajaniemi, H. Immunohistochemical demonstration of human carbonic anhydrase isoenzyme II in brain tumours. *Histochem. J.* **1995**, *12*, 974–982. [CrossRef]
17. Parkkila, S.; Rajaniemi, H.; Parkkila, A.-K.; Kivelä, J.; Waheed, A.; Pastoreková, S.; Pastorek, J.; Sly, W.S. Carbonic anhydrase inhibitor suppresses invasion of renal cancer cells in vitro. *Proc. Natl. Acad. Sci. USA* **2000**, *5*, 2220–2224. [CrossRef]
18. Achal, V.; Pan, X. Characterization of urease and carbonic anhydrase producing bacteria and their role in calcite precipitation. *Curr. Microbiol.* **2011**, *3*, 894–902. [CrossRef]
19. Şentürk, M.; Gülçin, İ.; Beydemir, Ş.; Küfrevioğlu, Ö.İ.; Supuran, C.T. In vitro inhibition of human carbonic anhydrase I and II isozymes with natural phenolic compounds. *Chem. Biol. Drug Des.* **2011**, *6*, 494–499. [CrossRef]
20. Supuran, C.T. Structure and function of carbonic anhydrases. *Biochem. J.* **2016**, *14*, 2023–2032. [CrossRef]
21. Desai, N.; Dodiya, A.M.; Rajpara, K.M.; Rupala, Y.M. Synthesis and antimicrobial screening of 1,3,4-oxadiazole and clubbed thiophene derivatives. *J. Saudi Chem. Soc.* **2014**, *3*, 255–261. [CrossRef]
22. Wani, M.Y.; Ahmad, A.; Shiekh, R.A.; Al-Ghamdi, K.J.; Sobral, A.J. Imidazole clubbed 1,3,4-oxadiazole derivatives as potential antifungal agents. *Bioorganic Med. Chem.* **2015**, *15*, 4172–4180. [CrossRef] [PubMed]
23. Dewangan, D.; Verma, V.S.; Nakhate, K.T.; Tripathi, D.K.; Kashyap, P.; Dhongade, H. Synthesis, characterization, and screening for analgesic and anti-inflammatory activities of new 1,3,4-oxadiazole derivatives linked to quinazolin-4-one ring. *Med. Chem. Res.* **2016**, *10*, 2143–2154. [CrossRef]
24. Singh, A.K.; Lohani, M.; Parthsarthy, R. Synthesis, characterization and anti-inflammatory activity of some 1,3,4-oxadiazole derivatives. *Iran. J. Pharm. Res. IJPR* **2013**, *2*, 319.
25. Gan, X.; Hu, D.; Chen, Z.; Wang, Y.; Song, B. Synthesis and antiviral evaluation of novel 1,3,4-oxadiazole/thiadiazole-chalcone conjugates. *Bioorganic Med. Chem. Lett.* **2017**, *18*, 4298–4301. [CrossRef] [PubMed]
26. Abdo, N.Y.M.; Kamel, M.M. Synthesis and anticancer evaluation of 1,3,4-oxadiazoles, 1,3,4-thiadiazoles, 1,2,4-triazoles and Mannich bases. *Chem. Pharm. Bull.* **2015**, *5*, 369–376. [CrossRef]

27. Schlecker, R.; Thieme, P.C. The synthesis of antihypertensive 3-(1,3,4-oxadiazol-2-yl) phenoxypropanolahines. *Tetrahedron* **1988**, *11*, 3289–3294. [CrossRef]
28. Tabatabai, S.A.; Lashkari, S.B.; Zarrindast, M.R.; Gholibeikian, M.; Shafiee, A. Design, synthesis and anticonvulsant activity of 2-(2-phenoxy) phenyl-1,3,4-oxadiazole derivatives. *Iran. J. Pharm. Res. IJPR* **2013**, *12*, 105.
29. Shyma, P.; Balakrishna, K.; Peethambar, K.; Vijesh, M. Synthesis, characterization, antidiabetic and antioxidant activity of 1,3,4-oxadiazole derivatives bearing 6-methyl pyridine moiety. *Der Pharma. Chem.* **2015**, *12*, 137–145.
30. Musmade, D.; Pattan, S.; Manjunath, S.Y. Oxadiazole a nucleus with versatile biological behavior. *Int. J. Pharm. Chem.* **2015**, *1*, 11–20.
31. Sengupta, P.; Mal, M.; Mandal, S.; Singh, J.; Maity, T.K. Evaluation of antibacterial and antifungal activity of some 1,3,4 oxadiazoles. *Iran. J. Pharmacol. Ther.* **2008**, *2*, 165–167.
32. Glomb, T.; Szymankiewicz, K.; Świątek, P. Anti-cancer activity of derivatives of 1,3,4-oxadiazole. *Molecules* **2018**, *12*, 3361. [CrossRef] [PubMed]
33. Abd-Ellah, H.S.; Abdel-Aziz, M.; Shoman, M.E.; Beshr, E.A.; Kaoud, T.; Ahmed, A.-S.F. New 1,3,4-oxadiazole/oxime hybrids: Design, synthesis, anti-inflammatory, COX inhibitory activities and ulcerogenic liability. *Bioorganic Chem.* **2017**, *74*, 15–29. [CrossRef] [PubMed]
34. Tantray, M.A.; Khan, I.; Hamid, H.; Alam, M.S.; Dhulap, A.; Kalam, A. Synthesis of benzimidazole-linked-1,3,4-oxadiazole carboxamides as GSK-3β inhibitors with in vivo antidepressant activity. *Bioorganic Chem.* **2018**, *77*, 393–401. [CrossRef]
35. Yadagiri, B.; Gurrala, S.; Bantu, R.; Nagarapu, L.; Polepalli, S.; Srujana, G.; Jain, N. Synthesis and evaluation of benzosuberone embedded with 1,3,4-oxadiazole, 1,3,4-thiadiazole and 1,2,4-triazole moieties as new potential anti proliferative agents. *Bioorganic Med. Chem. Lett.* **2015**, *10*, 2220–2224. [CrossRef]
36. Manjunatha, K.; Poojary, B.; Lobo, P.L.; Fernandes, J.; Kumari, N.S. Synthesis and biological evaluation of some 1,3,4-oxadiazole derivatives. *Eur. J. Med. Chem.* **2010**, *11*, 5225–5233. [CrossRef]
37. Hajimahdi, Z.; Zarghi, A.; Zabihollahi, R.; Aghasadeghi, M. Synthesis, biological evaluation, and molecular modeling studies of new 1,3,4-oxadiazole-and 1,3,4-thiadiazole-substituted 4-oxo-4 H-pyrido [1, 2-a] pyrimidines as anti-HIV-1 agents. *Med. Chem. Res.* **2013**, *5*, 2467–2475. [CrossRef]
38. Xu, W.-M.; Li, S.-Z.; He, M.; Yang, S.; Li, X.-Y.; Li, P. Synthesis and bioactivities of novel thioether/sulfone derivatives containing 1,2,3-thiadiazole and 1,3,4-oxadiazole/thiadiazole moiety. *Bioorganic Med. Chem. Lett.* **2013**, *21*, 5821–5824. [CrossRef]
39. Vats, L.; Sharma, V.; Angeli, A.; Kumar, R.; Supuran, C.T.; Sharma, P.K. Synthesis of novel 4-functionalized 1,5-diaryl-1,2,3-triazoles containing benzenesulfonamide moiety as carbonic anhydrase I, II, IV and IX inhibitors. *Eur. J. Med. Chem.* **2018**, *150*, 678–686. [CrossRef]
40. Sharma, V.; Kumar, R.; Bua, S.; Supuran, C.T.; Sharma, P.K. Synthesis of novel benzenesulfonamide bearing 1,2,3-triazole linked hydroxy-trifluoromethylpyrazolines and hydrazones as selective carbonic anhydrase isoforms IX and XII inhibitors. *Bioorganic Chem.* **2019**, *85*, 198–208. [CrossRef]
41. Kumar, R.; Vats, L.; Bua, S.; Supuran, C.T.; Sharma, P.K. Design and synthesis of novel benzenesulfonamide containing 1,2,3-triazoles as potent human carbonic anhydrase isoforms I, II, IV and IX inhibitors. *Eur. J. Med. Chem.* **2018**, *155*, 545–551. [CrossRef] [PubMed]
42. Kumar, R.; Sharma, V.; Bua, S.; Supuran, C.T.; Sharma, P.K. Synthesis and biological evaluation of benzenesulphonamide-bearing 1,4,5-trisubstituted-1,2,3-triazoles possessing human carbonic anhydrase I, II, IV, and IX inhibitory activity. *J. Enzym. Inhib. Med. Chem.* **2017**, *1*, 1187–1194. [CrossRef] [PubMed]
43. Bianco, G.; Meleddu, R.; Distinto, S.; Cottiglia, F.; Gaspari, M.; Melis, C.; Corona, A.; Angius, R.; Angeli, A.; Taverna, D. N-Acylbenzenesulfonamide dihydro-1,3,4-oxadiazole hybrids: Seeking selectivity toward carbonic anhydrase isoforms. *ACS Med. Chem. Lett.* **2017**, *8*, 792–796. [CrossRef] [PubMed]
44. Sharma, V.; Kumar, R.; Angeli, A.; Supuran, C.T.; Sharma, P.K. Tail approach synthesis of novel benzenesulfonamides incorporating 1,3,4-oxadiazole hybrids as potent inhibitor of carbonic anhydrase I, II, IX, and XII isoenzymes. *Eur. J. Med. Chem.* **2020**, *193*, 112219. [CrossRef]
45. Swain, B.; Singh, P.; Angeli, A.; Aashritha, K.; Nagesh, N.; Supuran, C.T.; Arifuddin, M. 3-Functionalised benzenesulphonamide based 1,3,4-oxadiazoles as selective carbonic anhydrase XIII inhibitors: Design, synthesis and biological evaluation. *Bioorganic Med. Chem. Lett.* **2021**, *37*, 127856. [CrossRef]
46. Avula, S.K.; Rehman, N.U.; Khan, M.; Halim, S.A.; Khan, A.; Rafiq, K.; Csuk, R.; Das, B.; Al-Harrasi, A. New synthetic 1H-1,2,3-triazole derivatives of 3-O-acetyl-β-boswellic acid and 3-O-acetyl-11-keto-β-boswellic acid from Boswellia sacra inhibit carbonic anhydrase II in vitro. *Med. Chem. Res.* **2021**, *6*, 1185–1198. [CrossRef]
47. Avula, S.K.; Khan, M.; Halim, S.A.; Khan, A.; Al-Riyami, S.A.; Csuk, R.; Das, B.; Al-Harrasi, A. Synthesis of new 1H-1,2,3-triazole analogs in aqueous medium via "click" chemistry: A novel class of potential carbonic anhydrase-II inhibitors. *Front. Chem.* **2021**, *9*, 642614. [CrossRef]
48. von Neubeck, B.; Gondi, G.; Riganti, C.; Pan, C.; Parra Damas, A.; Scherb, H.; Ertürk, A.; Zeidler, R. An inhibitory antibody targeting carbonic anhydrase XII abrogates chemoresistance and significantly reduces lung metastases in an orthotopic breast cancer model in vivo. *Int. J. Cancer* **2018**, *8*, 2065–2075. [CrossRef]
49. Angeli, A.; Trallori, E.; Carta, F.; Di Cesare Mannelli, L.; Ghelardini, C.; Supuran, C.T. Heterocoumarins are selective carbonic anhydrase IX and XII inhibitors with cytotoxic effects against cancer cells lines. *ACS Med. Chem. Lett.* **2018**, *9*, 947–951. [CrossRef]

50. Vullo, D.; Innocenti, A.; Nishimori, I.; Pastorek, J.R.; Scozzafava, A.; Pastoreková, S.; Supuran, C.T. Carbonic anhydrase inhibitors. Inhibition of the transmembrane isozyme XII with sulfonamides—a new target for the design of antitumor and antiglaucoma drugs? *Bioorganic Med. Chem. Lett.* **2005**, *4*, 963–969. [CrossRef]
51. Kumar, S.; Rulhania, S.; Jaswal, S.; Monga, V. Recent advances in the medicinal chemistry of carbonic anhydrase inhibitors. *Eur. J. Med. Chem.* **2021**, *209*, 112923. [CrossRef] [PubMed]
52. Rafiq, K.; Khan, M.; Muhammed, N.; Khan, A.; Rehman, N.U.; Al-Yahyaei, B.E.M.; Khiat, M.; Halim, S.A.; Shah, Z.; Csuk, R. New amino acid clubbed Schiff bases inhibit carbonic anhydrase II, α-glucosidase, and urease enzymes: In silico and in vitro. *Med. Chem. Res.* **2021**, *3*, 712–728. [CrossRef]
53. Ur Rehman, N.; Halim, S.A.; Khan, M.; Hussain, H.; Yar Khan, H.; Khan, A.; Abbas, G.; Rafiq, K.; Al-Harrasi, A. Antiproliferative and carbonic anhydrase II inhibitory potential of chemical constituents from Lycium shawii and aloe vera: Evidence from in silico target fishing and in vitro testing. *Pharmaceuticals* **2020**, *5*, 94. [CrossRef] [PubMed]
54. Banerjee, A.K.; Vera, W.; Mora, H.; Laya, M.S.; Bedoya, L.; Cabrera, E.V. Iodine in organic synthesis. *J. Sci. Ind. Res.* **2006**, *65*, 299–308. [CrossRef]
55. Ren, Y.-M.; Cai, C.; Yang, R.-C. Molecular iodine-catalyzed multicomponent reactions: An efficient catalyst for organic synthesis. *RSC Adv.* **2013**, *20*, 7182–7204. [CrossRef]
56. Gao, W.-C.; Jiang, S.; Wang, R.-L.; Zhang, C. Iodine-mediated intramolecular amination of ketones: The synthesis of 2-acylindoles and 2-acylindolines by tuning N-protecting groups. *Chem. Commun.* **2013**, *43*, 4890–4892. [CrossRef] [PubMed]
57. He, Z.; Li, H.; Li, Z. Iodine-Mediated Synthesis of 3 H-Indoles via Intramolecular Cyclization of Enamines. *J. Org. Chem.* **2010**, *13*, 4636–4639. [CrossRef]
58. Jiang, H.; Huang, H.; Cao, H.; Qi, C. TBHP/I2-mediated domino oxidative cyclization for one-pot synthesis of polysubstituted oxazoles. *Org. Lett.* **2010**, *23*, 5561–5563. [CrossRef]
59. Wan, C.; Gao, L.; Wang, Q.; Zhang, J.; Wang, Z. Simple and efficient preparation of 2,5-disubstituted oxazoles via a metal-free-catalyzed cascade cyclization. *Org. Lett.* **2010**, *17*, 3902–3905. [CrossRef]
60. Wan, C.; Zhang, J.; Wang, S.; Fan, J.; Wang, Z. Facile synthesis of polysubstituted oxazoles via a copper-catalyzed tandem oxidative cyclization. *Org. Lett.* **2010**, *10*, 2338–2341. [CrossRef]
61. Daina, A.; Michielin, O.; Zoete, V. SwissADME: A free web tool to evaluate pharmacokinetics, drug-likeness and medicinal chemistry friendliness of small molecules. *Sci. Rep.* **2017**, *1*, 42717. [CrossRef] [PubMed]
62. Sippel, K.H.; Robbins, A.H.; Domsic, J.; Genis, C.; Agbandje-McKenna, M.; McKenna, R. High-resolution structure of human carbonic anhydrase II complexed with acetazolamide reveals insights into inhibitor drug design. *Acta Crystallogr. Sect. F Struct. Biol. Cryst. Commun.* **2009**, *10*, 992–995. [CrossRef] [PubMed]
63. Daina, A.; Zoete, V. A boiled-egg to predict gastrointestinal absorption and brain penetration of small molecules. *ChemMedChem* **2016**, *11*, 1117. [CrossRef] [PubMed]

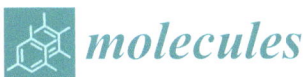

Article

Approach for the Design of Covalent Protein Kinase Inhibitors via Focused Deep Generative Modeling

Atsushi Yoshimori [1,†], Filip Miljković [2,†] and Jürgen Bajorath [2,*]

[1] Institute for Theoretical Medicine Inc., 26-1, Muraoka-Higashi 2-Chome, Fujisawa 251-0012, Japan; yoshimori@itmol.com
[2] Department of Life Science Informatics and Data Science, B-IT, LIMES Program Unit Chemical Biology and Medicinal Chemistry, Rheinische Friedrich-Wilhelms-Universität, Friedrich-Hirzebruch-Allee 6, D-53115 Bonn, Germany; miljkovi@bit.uni-bonn.de
* Correspondence: bajorath@bit.uni-bonn.de; Tel.: +49-228-736-9100
† These authors contributed equally to this work.

Abstract: Deep machine learning is expanding the conceptual framework and capacity of computational compound design, enabling new applications through generative modeling. We have explored the systematic design of covalent protein kinase inhibitors by learning from kinome-relevant chemical space, followed by focusing on an exemplary kinase of interest. Covalent inhibitors experience a renaissance in drug discovery, especially for targeting protein kinases. However, computational design of this class of inhibitors has thus far only been little investigated. To this end, we have devised a computational approach combining fragment-based design and deep generative modeling augmented by three-dimensional pharmacophore screening. This approach is thought to be particularly relevant for medicinal chemistry applications because it combines knowledge-based elements with deep learning and is chemically intuitive. As an exemplary application, we report for Bruton's tyrosine kinase (BTK), a major drug target for the treatment of inflammatory diseases and leukemia, the generation of novel candidate inhibitors with a specific chemically reactive group for covalent modification, requiring only little target-specific compound information to guide the design efforts. Newly generated compounds include known inhibitors and characteristic substructures and many novel candidates, thus lending credence to the computational approach, which is readily applicable to other targets.

Keywords: deep machine learning; generative modeling; kinase inhibitor design; Bruton's tyrosine kinase; covalent inhibitors

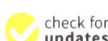

Citation: Yoshimori, A.; Miljković, F.; Bajorath, J. Approach for the Design of Covalent Protein Kinase Inhibitors via Focused Deep Generative Modeling. *Molecules* **2022**, *27*, 570. https://doi.org/10.3390/molecules27020570

Academic Editor: Keykavous Parang

Received: 21 December 2021
Accepted: 15 January 2022
Published: 17 January 2022

Publisher's Note: MDPI stays neutral with regard to jurisdictional claims in published maps and institutional affiliations.

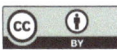

Copyright: © 2022 by the authors. Licensee MDPI, Basel, Switzerland. This article is an open access article distributed under the terms and conditions of the Creative Commons Attribution (CC BY) license (https://creativecommons.org/licenses/by/4.0/).

1. Introduction

Increasing interest in artificial intelligence methods is impacting computer-aided drug design and widening its scope [1]. Generative modeling is among the new approaches enabled through the application of deep neural network architectures [1–4]. It aims to produce novel chemical entities through deep learning from existing chemical matter, either by generally expanding biologically relevant chemical space through the generation of novel virtual libraries or by focusing on compounds with specific biological activities [2–4]. Although generative modeling is intensely investigated at present, reports of practical applications impacting medicinal chemistry are still rare [1]. This is typically the case for newly introduced (computational and experimental) methodologies, which will require time until they mature and measurably contribute to the practical drug design and medicinal chemistry programs.

So far, most drug design efforts have concentrated on generating reversible noncovalent inhibitors of target proteins, a hallmark of small-molecule drug discovery. In contrast, covalent inhibitors have experienced comparatively little interest, especially in the era of molecular and structure-based approaches [5]. Most covalent inhibitors permanently disable biological targets and ultimately lead to their degradation. Hence, covalent inhibitors are often associated with unfavorable pharmacological properties and undesired side effects, due to the non-selective inhibition of targets. However, these views have partly changed over the past decade as potential advantages of covalent inhibitors have increasingly been realized if unique or only weakly conserved residues important for the activity of given targets can be modified [5,6], leading to so-called targeted covalent inhibitors (TCIs) [6]. Often quoted favorable properties of TCIs include, among others, a high degree of target occupancy, long physiological half-life and ensuing high efficacy, or potential decoupling of pharmacodynamic and pharmacokinetic effects [5,6].

For the generation of reactive groups in TCIs that form covalent bonds to side-chain atoms of cysteine, lysine, or tyrosine residues, often termed chemical "warheads", a variety of chemical reactions are applicable [6]. In addition, to facilitate non-permanent inhibition by TCIs, chemistry is also available to achieve covalent-reversible inhibition, which balances advantages of non-covalent as well as covalent interference with given targets [6].

Protein kinase inhibition is not only one of the major focal points of contemporary drug discovery efforts [7] but also a growth area for covalent inhibition. This is the case because most non-covalent kinase inhibitors developed thus far target the highly conserved ATP cofactor binding site in the catalytic kinase domain, giving rise to potential off-target promiscuity [7,8]. Accordingly, in kinase drug discovery, covalent inhibition is also considered as a mechanism to render the inhibitor selective for confined subsets of kinases having free cysteine residues in the active site region that are only little conserved across the human kinome [8].

A representative and instructive example is provided by Bruton's tyrosine kinase (BTK) [9], which belongs to the TEC (gene) family of non-receptor tyrosine kinases [10]. TEC kinases are expressed in hematopoietic, kidney, and liver cells and implicated in T-helper-cell activation through participation in cytokine receptor-dependent signaling pathways [10]. Hence, this kinase family includes therapeutic targets for the treatment of inflammatory diseases and leukemia, with BTK being the most intensely studied member and a major drug target [11]. For BTK, a variety of non-covalent as well as covalent inhibitors have been reported over the years [12]. Importantly, BTK is a primary target of the marketed covalent drug ibrutinib [13], depicted in Figure 1. Ibrutinib contains an acrylamide warhead acting as a Michael acceptor in the formation of a covalent bond with the thiol group of a cysteine residue in the active site of BTK (Cys481).

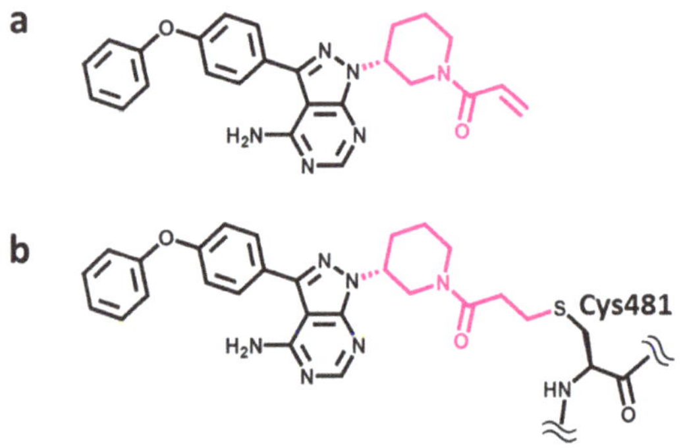

Figure 1. Structure of ibrutinib. The covalent drug ibrutinib contains an acrylamide warhead, colored magenta in (**a**), which forms a covalent bond to the thiol group of a Cys481 in BTK, shown in (**b**).

In this work, we have addressed the question of whether novel covalent inhibitors of BTK could be designed via deep generative modeling by focusing on ibrutinib as a template and its interactions with BTK. To our knowledge, herein, we introduce the first generative design strategy for covalent enzyme inhibitors and report a number of new BTK candidate compounds for follow-up investigations in medicinal chemistry.

2. Results and Discussion

2.1. Selected Covalent BTK Inhibitors

We aimed to design covalent BTK inhibitors containing an acrylamide/Michael acceptor warhead, for which the drug ibrutinib served as a template [13], as shown in Figure 1a. The warhead reacts with the SH-group of cysteine residues, forming a covalent bond (Figure 1b). Hence, kinases having a free cysteine within or in the vicinity of the active site (including the cofactor and substrate binding site) might be inhibited by such compounds. However, this is only possible if the warhead can reach the thiol group of cysteine residues and be accommodated in the binding site, which might be prevented, for example, by steric hindrance or other chemical incompatibilities. This offers opportunities to render covalent inhibitors target-selective by modifying the remaining non-reactive parts of their structure to fit into a given binding site. In any event, this specific mode of covalent inhibition principally limits potential kinase targets to a subset of kinases having a free cysteine in the active site region. BTK contains a free cysteine in the F2 subsite (αD-1 position) in the front region of the ATP cofactor binding site, the location of which is shared by a total of 12 human kinases (plus isoforms) [8].

2.2. Inhibitor Distribution

We searched ChEMBL [14] for covalent BTK inhibitors containing the piperidine-based Michael acceptor warhead of ibrutinib, for which high-confidence activity data were available, and identified a total of 34 such inhibitors, shown in Supplementary Figure S1. We then searched ChEMBL for covalent inhibitors of other kinases having the same warhead and identified such inhibitors for a total of 20 kinases, with 1–35 inhibitors per kinase, as reported in Table 1. These included several kinases with a cysteine at the position corresponding to BTK but also others with a free cysteine at a different position. Eighteen of the 20 kinases were found to share varying numbers of inhibitors with BTK. Among these was erbB1 with 35 inhibitors. For BTK and erbB1, most inhibitors belonging to this class were available, with 34 and 35 compounds, respectively. BTK and erbB1 have a free cysteine at corresponding positions in their structure, but only share one covalent inhibitor with the piperidine-based Michael acceptor warhead (Table 1), hence indicating the potential for selective covalent inhibition of related kinases. We also found that 7 of the 34 BTK inhibitors were promiscuous on the basis of high-confidence activity data, i.e., they were active against two or more kinases. Promiscuous inhibitors included ibrutinib, reported to be active against a total of 11 targets. The remaining 27 inhibitors were active against BTK. Data available for ibrutinib, which represents an extensively investigated drug, might provide a realistic estimate for the degree of selectivity that can be expected for this class of inhibitors, although other BTK inhibitors containing this warhead might be more selective than ibrutinib, given their steric and chemical features.

2.3. Artificial Intelligence-Assisted Inhibitor Design

New BTK candidate inhibitors were designed using the DeepSARM, which combines the SAR matrix (SARM) data structure with deep learning and generative modeling [15]. The methodology is detailed in the Supplementary Methods. The underlying principles are as follows: From a given compound dataset, the SARM approach extracts all structurally related analogue series and organizes these series in matrices reminiscent of R-group tables, as shown in Supplementary Figure S2a. This is facilitated by applying a dual-compound fragmentation scheme yielding core structure fragments (Keys) and substituents (Values). In the first round, compounds are fragmented, yielding a Key 1 and Value 1 fragment, and in the second round, the Key 1 fragments from the first fragmentation, yielding a Key 2 and Value 2 fragment. This fragmentation scheme identifies all compounds and core structures that are only distinguished by a chemical change at a single site. Accordingly, each qualifying Key 2 fragment represents a series of analogues with structural modifications at a single site and each SARM contains a subset of structurally closely related series with core fragments distinguished by a structural change at a given site. As such, cells in the SARM represent individual dataset compounds and empty cells represent currently unexplored combinations of Key 1 and Value 1 fragments, providing candidate compounds for series expansion (Supplementary Figure S2a).

Table 1. Reported are inhibitors from ChEMBL containing the piperidine-based Michael acceptor warhead with activity against different kinases and their overlap with BTK inhibitors. Kinases with a free cysteine residue at a position corresponding to BTK are given in bold. # stands for Number.

Protein Kinase	# of Inhibitors with Warhead	# of BTK Inhibitors with Warhead
Epidermal growth factor receptor erbB1	35	1
Tyrosine-protein kinase BTK	34	34
Tyrosine-protein kinase JAK1	9	5
Tyrosine-protein kinase JAK3	8	6
Tyrosine-protein kinase JAK2	7	4
Receptor protein-tyrosine kinase erbB-4	4	3
Tyrosine-protein kinase ITK/TSK	4	2
Tyrosine-protein kinase TYK2	4	4
Receptor protein-tyrosine kinase erbB-2	3	2
Tyrosine-protein kinase BLK	3	3
Tyrosine-protein kinase BMX	3	2
Tyrosine-protein kinase TEC	2	1
Fibroblast growth factor receptor 1	2	0
Fibroblast growth factor receptor 2	2	1
Tyrosine-protein kinase TXK	2	2
Tyrosine-protein kinase receptor RET	1	1
Dual specificity mitogen-activated protein kinase kinase 1	1	1
Tyrosine-protein kinase SRC	1	0
Tyrosine-protein kinase Lyn	1	1
Tyrosine-protein kinase LCK	1	1

Based upon this hierarchical decomposition scheme and the ensuing SARM data structure, a compound design strategy can be implemented to explore combinations of novel fragments as follows: Combinations of Key 2 and Value 2 fragments yield Key 1, i.e., complete core structures, of novel compounds. If the resulting core structures are combined with newly generated Value 1 fragments, new compounds are obtained. For ibrutinib, the corresponding ([Key 2 − Value 2] − Value 1) fragment assembly is illustrated in Figure 2a and a candidate compound containing two novel (Key 2, Value 1) fragments in Figure 2b. Importantly, for the design of covalent BTK inhibitors attempted herein, Value 2 fragments completing the inhibitor core structure are required to contain the invariant warhead.

Following this general design approach, new Key 2, Value 2, and Value 1 fragments are required to obtain new compounds. The generation of Key 2, Value 2, and Value 1 is facilitated using DeepSARM. To further expand the close-in analogue design space provided by SARM, DeepSARM is composed of three sequence-to-sequence (Seq2Seq) models representing an encoder–decoder framework for learning the corresponding structural fragments and generating new ones. These Seq2Seq models represent a recurrent neural network architecture successfully used in natural language processing to transform a sequence of characters into another (hence the name). The Seq2Seq models in DeepSARM are also termed Key, Value 2, and Value 1 Generator, respectively. The DeepSARM architecture is illustrated in Supplementary Figure S2b. To expand the compound design space, DeepSARM is first pre-trained on a large set of compounds (for instance, a collection of kinase inhibitors across the human kinome) and then fine-tuned on a smaller compound set (such as known inhibitors of a specific kinase target). The generation of a SARM with compounds composed of new fragments from DeepSARM is illustrated in Supplementary Figure S2c.

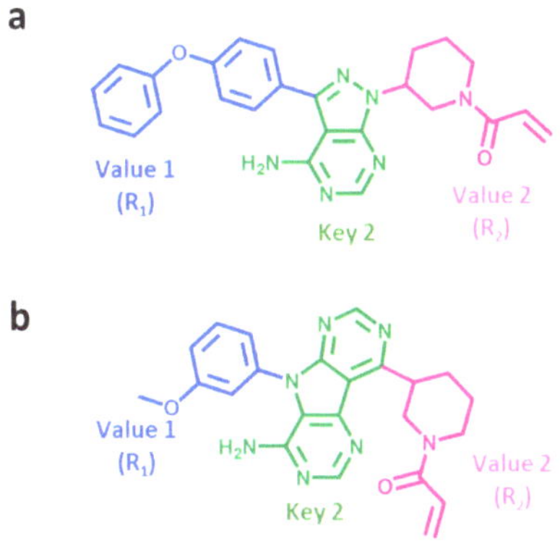

Figure 2. Key 2, Value 2, and Value 1 fragment assembly. Shown is the DeepSARM fragment composition of (**a**) ibrutinib and (**b**) a candidate compound. Key 2, Value 2 (R_2), and Value 1 (R_1) are displayed in green, magenta, and blue, respectively.

DeepSARM fragment design via Seq2Seq models is guided by cumulative log-likelihood scores from the Seq2Seq models (see the Supplementary Methods). Given the derivation of this scoring function, small scores close to 0 are obtained for compounds whose structural fragments are similar to known inhibitors or identical and large scores approaching 1 for compounds with novel fragments not contained in the training data. Hence, increasing log-likelihood scores indicate the structural novelty of candidate compounds.

2.4. BTK Inhibitor Design

DeepSARM was pre-trained with 45,441 kinase inhibitors from the Kinase SARfari collection of ChEMBL [14] and then fine-tuned using the 34 covalent BTK inhibitors with the piperidine-based Michael acceptor warhead depicted in Supplementary Figure S1. Hence, only a small set of inhibitors was used for fine-tuning of the generative model.

2.4.1. Key 2 Structures

First, Key 2 fragments were generated, representing the major substructure of the inhibitor scaffold, and evaluated using an ibrutinib core structure-based pharmacophore model based upon the ibrutinib-BTK X-ray complex structure (see Section 3), as illustrated in Figure 3a. Accordingly, from 50,000 initially sampled Key 2 structures, 59 Key 2 fragments passing the rotational bond filter and the pharmacophore filter were selected, and 18 of these fragments were prioritized that closely matched the pharmacophore, depicted in Figure 3b. These structures included a variety of modifications of the ibrutinib Key 2, including the introduction or replacement of ring heteroatoms and, interestingly, tricyclic Key 2 variants. These findings confirmed the ability of DeepSARM to generate a considerable spectrum of scaffold modifications compared to the original core structures of BTK inhibitors used for fine-tuning.

We then encoded only the cyclic structures of Key 2 fragments of newly designed BTK inhibitors for substructure searching in ChEMBL or only kinase and BTK inhibitors with available high-confidence activity data. As reported in Table 2, 6 of the 18 Key 2 fragments were not detected in ChEMBL. Moreover, 8 and 14 Key 2 fragments were novel in all kinase inhibitors or only BTK inhibitors, respectively, while the remaining structures were already available. These findings confirmed the ability of DeepSARM to regenerate known inhibitory structural motifs and generate novel structures, hence providing a variety of plausible hinge-binding motifs for covalent BTK inhibitors and lending further credence to the design approach.

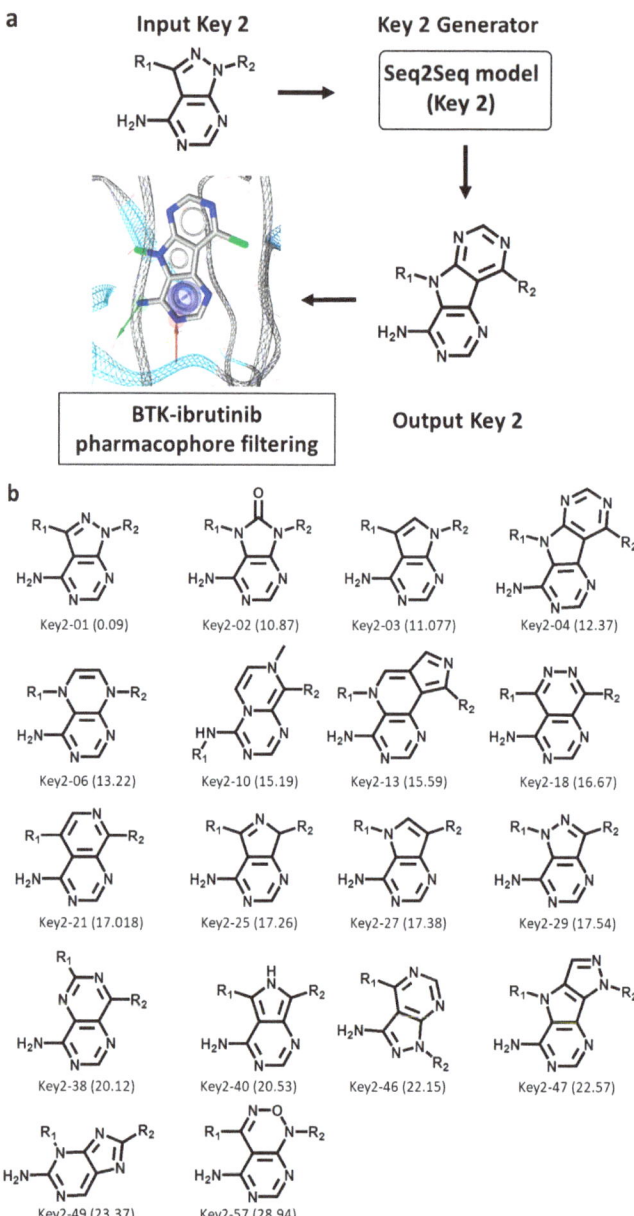

Figure 3. Generation of new Key 2 fragments. (**a**) The computational workflow for generating Key 2 fragments using the Seq2Seq model (Key 2) and pharmacophore filtering. In the lower left image, pharmacophore features including hydrogen bond donor, hydrogen bond acceptor, and aromatic groups are shown as a green arrow, red arrow, and blue circle, respectively. (**b**) The structure of 18 newly generated Key 2 fragments. Below each structure, the identification number and log-likelihood score (in parentheses) are provided.

Table 2. Reported are the numbers of cyclic Key 2 substructures from newly designed BTK inhibitors detected in different sets of ChEMBL compounds with high-confidence activity data. Key 2 fragments not detected in any ChEMBL compounds are shown in bold. # stands for Number.

Key 2 Fragments	# of Covalent BTK Inhibitors	# of All BTK Inhibitors	# of Kinase Inhibitors	# of All ChEMBL Compounds
Key2-01	24	110	1021	2463
Key2-02	1	10	33	97
Key2-03	1	63	2239	2799
Key2-04	0	0	1	1
Key2-06	0	0	0	0
Key2-10	0	0	0	0
Key2-13	0	0	0	0
Key2-18	0	0	0	82
Key2-21	0	0	227	342
Key2-25	0	0	0	0
Key2-27	0	0	153	769
Key2-29	0	0	25	471
Key2-38	0	0	0	81
Key2-40	0	0	3	61
Key2-46	24	110	1021	2463
Key2-47	0	0	0	0
Key2-49	0	0	2	76
Key2-57	0	0	0	0
Σ inhibitors in datasets	34	963	56,288	272,896

2.4.2. Value 2 and Value 1 Structures

On the basis of the Key 2-01 prioritized by pharmacophore fitting, Value 2 fragments were generated and filtered for the presence of the invariant warhead, as illustrated in Figure 4a. A total of 10,000 Value 2 fragments were sampled, 7 of which were found to contain the warhead, as shown in Figure 4b. Thus, these findings confirmed the ability of DeepSARM modeling to reproduce the desired warhead. Moreover, similar to the observations made for Key 2 structures, these Value 2 fragments displayed modifications of the ring moiety attached to Michael acceptor group.

The selected Key 2 and Value 2 fragments were then combined to obtain Key 1 structures used as input for the generation of Value 1 fragments according to Supplementary Figure S2b. For each Key 1, 2000 Value 1 fragments were sampled and the top 100 Value 1 fragments with the lowest log-likelihood score (similar to known inhibitors) were selected for the generation of candidate compounds according to Supplementary Figure S2c. Value 1 fragments generated from [Key 2-01 — Value 2] fragments are shown in Supplementary Figure S3. Since Value 1 fragments represent substituents in newly assembled candidate compounds, preference was given here to fragments similar to those in known BTK inhibitors.

2.4.3. Candidate Compounds

Next, we characterized the generated candidate inhibitors. For each of the 18 prioritized Key 2 structures, a 7 × 100 [Value 2 × Value 1] SARM-like matrix was generated in which matrix cells represented unique ([Key 2 — Value 2] — Value 1) combinations (candidate compounds) color-coded by cumulative DeepSARM log-likelihood scores, as shown in Figure 5. From the top left to the bottom right in Figure 5, matrices are arranged in the order of increasing scores, indicating increasing structural novelty compared to compounds used for fine-tuning (vide supra). As can be seen, for prioritized Key 2 fragments, compounds with varying structural novelty were obtained—an interesting finding.

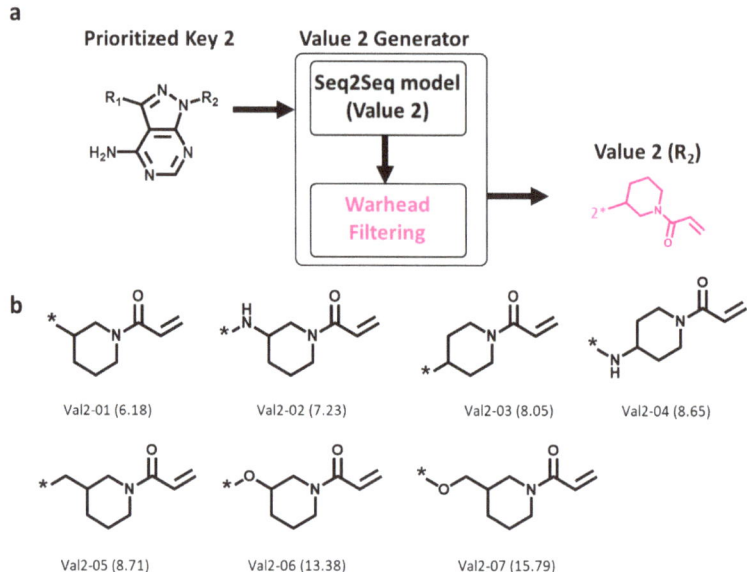

Figure 4. Generation of Value 2 fragments. (**a**) Workflow for generating Value 2 fragments using the Seq2Seq model (Value 2) and warhead filtering, and (**b**) new Value 2 fragments. Below each structure, the identification number and log-likelihood score (in parentheses) are provided. * indicates the fragment attachment point.

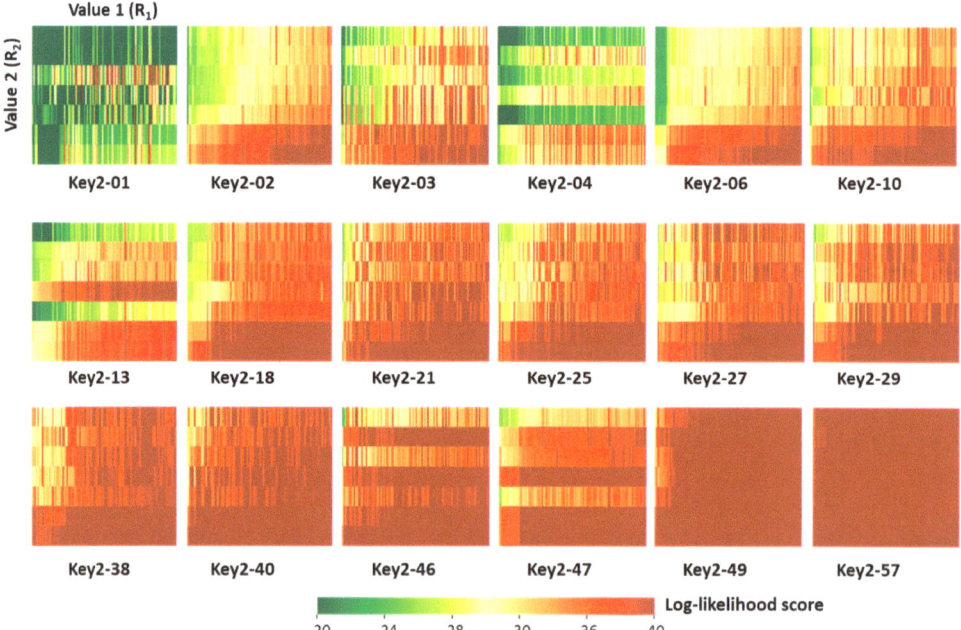

Figure 5. [Value 2 × Value 1] matrix for each of the 18 prioritized Key 2 fragments. The matrix cells represented unique ([Key 2 − Value 2] − Value 1) combinations (candidate compounds) color-coded by cumulative log-likelihood scores.

The candidate inhibitors were then subjected to pharmacophore fitting using a compound-based pharmacophore model (see the Section 3) to prioritize compounds for follow-up analysis. Supplementary Figure S4 shows a Key 2-based matrix representation according to Figure 5 color-coded by pharmacophore score. With the exception of compounds containing Key 2-10, all matrices revealed small subsets of candidate compounds closely fitting the ibrutinib-BTK pharmacophore, while 34 different inhibitors were used for fine-tuning. Importantly, the number of compounds passing the pharmacophore filter did not inversely correlate with the structural novelty of the fragments forming the candidate compounds. For example, compounds containing Key 2-57 displayed the overall highest structural novelty but were also among the Key 2-based compound subsets most frequently matching the pharmacophore. Figure 6 shows a superposition of a candidate inhibitor containing Key 2-21 passing the pharmacophore filter onto the crystallographic binding mode of ibrutinib, and Supplementary Figure S5 shows examples of hypothetical complexes of BTK with candidate inhibitors obtained by pharmacophore fitting, indicating plausible binding modes.

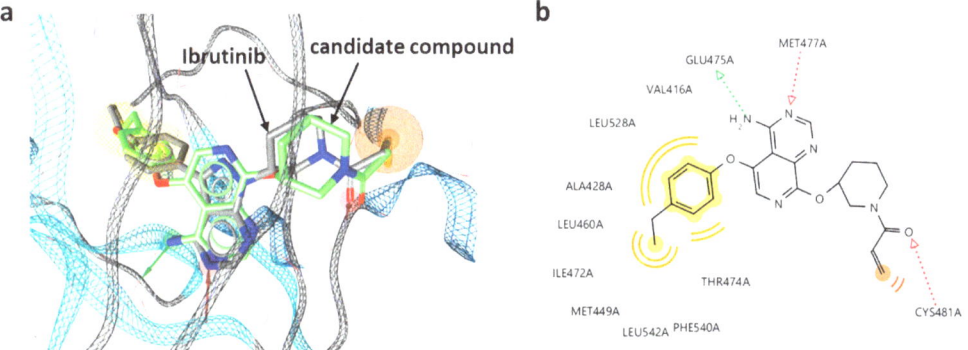

Figure 6. Hypothetical complexes of candidate inhibitors from DeepSARM and BTK. (**a**) Superposition of a candidate inhibitor containing Key 2-21 onto the crystallographic binding mode of ibrutinib. Pharmacophore features including two hydrogen bond acceptors, one hydrogen bond donor, one residue bonding point, and two optional hydrophobic features are represented as red arrows, green arrow, and orange/yellow sphere, respectively. (**b**) A corresponding diagram of candidate inhibitor–BTK interactions is shown.

These three compounds are representative candidates for further consideration. In all three cases, the acrylamide warhead is closely aligned with the targeted Cys481 residue (the carbonyl oxygen of the acrylamide warhead is positioned in hydrogen bonding distance to the thiol group). In addition, the differently substituted phenyl moieties in these compounds closely fit into a hydrophobic pocket in the active site of BTK distant from the reactive group, which further stabilizes binding. Importantly, the three candidate inhibitors contain different Key 2 structures, including two bicyclic cores (Key 2-21, with two fused six-membered rings; Key 2-49, fused six- and five-membered rings) and a tricyclic core (Key 2-04). Despite these chemically significant differences, these core fragments in these compounds are similarly positioned, including the tricyclic core, and interact with the same BTK residues (Glu475 and Met477). Thus, the putative binding modes closely resemble the experimental structure of ibrutinib and are plausible. The comparison of these candidate compounds suggests that there is a variety of opportunities for further chemical optimization.

Finally, the set of 1491 candidate compounds from DeepSARM passing the ibrutinib-BTK pharmacophore filter was compared to the 106 unique compounds with the piperidine-based Michael acceptor warhead contained in the high-confidence activity data subset of ChEMBL (Table 1). Only seven candidate compounds were contained in ChEMBL, revealing that the vast majority of BTK inhibitor candidates from DeepSARM represented new compounds. Corroborating insights were obtained by principal component analysis (PCA) of kinome inhibitor chemical space including DeepSARM candidate inhibitors (see the Section 3). As shown in Supplementary Figure S6, most of the known covalent BTK inhibitors containing the piperidine-based Michael acceptor warhead mapped to a peripheral region of kinome inhibitor space, while other BTK inhibitors were widely distributed over this space. Newly designed candidate compounds predominantly populated the region outlined by covalent BTK inhibitors used for fine-tuning, hence reflecting the desired focusing effect, and also further extended the kinome inhibitor space in this region with many new candidate compounds. Both focusing on known active compounds and generating chemical novelties around them were central aspects of the inhibitor design strategy reported herein.

3. Materials and Methods

3.1. DeepSARM Training

For pre-training of Seq2Seq models for Key 2, Value 2, and Value 1 generation, the number of epochs was set to 30, 10, and 30, respectively. For fine-tuning of Seq2Seq models for Key 2, Value 2, and Value 1, epochs were set to 50, 500, and 500, respectively. For all 3 models, the batch size was set to 64 and compound datasets were divided into training and validation sets (9:1) for pre-training and fine-tuning. Scripts for model derivation were written in Python and the Seq2Seq models were built using keras [16] (with 256-dimensional latent LSTM encoding space). Details of the DeepSARM architecture are provided as Supplementary Methods.

3.2. Fragment Generation Using DeepSARM

The Seq2Seq model (Key 2) was used to generate the Key 2 fragment, and the SMILES string [17] representing the ibrutinib Key 2 ("Nc1ncnc2c1c([At])nn2[*:1]") (Figure 2a) was used as the input Key 2 fragment (where [At] and [*:1] are designated attachment points of Value 1 and Value 2, respectively). For sampling of 50,000 Key 2 fragments, the temperature factor was set to 2.0. Key 2 fragments without rotational bonds were selected. Value 2 fragments were generated from the Seq2Seq model (Value 2) using the ibrutinib Key 2 as the input fragment. For sampling of 10,000 Value 2 fragments, the temperature factor was set to 2.0. Value 2 fragments found to contain the piperidine-based Michael acceptor warhead were selected. Value 1 fragments were then generated with the Seq2Seq model (Value 1) using Key 1 fragments (assembled from Key 2 and Value 2 fragments) as the input. For each Key 1 fragment, 2000 Value 1 fragments were sampled, setting the temperature factor to 1.5.

3.3. Pharmacophore Modeling

For Key 2 fragment and candidate compound selection, two pharmacophore models were constructed from the co-crystal structure of ibrutinib bound to BTK (PDB [18] ID: 5p9j) using LigandScout 4.4 [19]. Both pharmacophore models were derived using an ensemble of exclusion volume spheres calculated based upon the X-ray structure of the ibrutinib-BTK complex.

To construct a pharmacophore model for Key 2 selection, three pharmacophore features were defined for the ibrutinib Key 2 fragments: aromatic, hydrogen bond acceptor, and hydrogen bond donor. In the X-ray structure, two hydrogen bonds were formed between the ibrutinib Key 2 and the hinge region of BTK (involving residues Glu475 and Met477). The pharmacophore model is shown in Figure 3a. The 'idbgen' module of LigandScout 4.4 was used for conformer generation of the 59 Key 2 fragments from the Seq2Seq model (Key 2). After conformer generation with default parameter settings, pharmacophore fitting was carried out setting the LigandScout scoring function to 'Relative Pharmacophore-Fit' and the conformation match mode to 'BEST'.

For the selection of candidate compounds, a pharmacophore model with six pharmacophore features was derived, including two hydrogen bond acceptors, one hydrogen bond donor, one residue bonding point, and two optional hydrophobic features. The pharmacophore model is shown in Figure 6a. The residue bonding point feature is located in the vicinity of Cys481, which reacts with the warheads of covalent BTK inhibitors. After conformer generation using the 'idbgen' module with 'icon-best' parameter settings, pharmacophore fitting was carried out using 'Relative Pharmacophore-Fit' and setting the conformation match mode to 'BEST'.

3.4. Principal Component Analysis

The 1491 DeepSARM candidate compounds were combined with the high-confidence kinase inhibitor data subset from ChEMBL and subjected to PCA. A total of 56,288 kinase inhibitors were compared to DeepSARM candidates, including 34 BTK covalent inhibitors, 929 other BTK inhibitors, and 55,325 inhibitors of other human kinases. For PCA, compounds were represented using extended-connectivity fingerprints [20] with bond diameter six (ECFP6) hashed to 2048-bit vectors. The first two principal components were used for generating a PCA plot.

4. Conclusions

In this work, we have introduced a computational approach for the design of covalent kinase inhibitors that combines fragment- and structure-based design components with deep generative modeling learning. As an exemplary application, the design of covalent BTK inhibitors containing an invariant piperidine-based acrylamide warhead was presented. Only limited information about specifically active known compounds was sufficient to effectively guide the design, reproduce a desired chemical warhead, as well as characteristic inhibitor substructures, and generate many novel candidate compounds. On the basis of the X-ray structure of the ibrutinib-BTK complex, candidate inhibitors were found to display meaningful chemical features and plausible binding modes. As demonstrated herein, the fragment-based design component of DeepSARM is well-suited for retaining chemical groups essential for covalent inhibition and embedding them into different structural environments inferred by deep learning from structures of kinase inhibitors. As presented in our proof-of-concept study, the approach for covalent inhibitor design is easily applicable to other targets and chemical warheads. For BTK, the exemplary kinase target investigated herein, nearly 1500 candidate inhibitors were obtained meeting the design constraints. As a part of our study, this set of candidate compounds (and the 34 BTK inhibitors used for fine-tuning) has been made freely available as an open-access deposition on the Zenodo platform [21] as a resource for medicinal chemistry applications on BTK and other TEC kinases.

Supplementary Materials: The following supporting information can be downloaded online. Figure S1: Covalent BTK inhibitors with an acrylamide warhead; Figure S2: SAR matrix generation using DeepSARM; Figure S3: Value 1 fragments from DeepSARM for BTK inhibitor design; Figure S4: Key 2-based Value 1 × Value 2 matrices color-coded on the basis of pharmacophore scores; Figure S5: Hypothetical complexes of candidate inhibitors from DeepSARM with BTK; Figure S6: Principal component analysis of kinome inhibitor space. Supplementary Methods.

Author Contributions: Conceptualization, A.Y., F.M. and J.B.; methodology, A.Y., F.M. and J.B.; formal analysis, A.Y., F.M. and J.B.; data curation, F.M.; writing—original draft preparation, J.B.; writing—review and editing, A.Y., F.M. and J.B.; supervision, J.B. All authors have read and agreed to the published version of the manuscript.

Funding: This research received no external funding.

Institutional Review Board Statement: Not applicable.

Informed Consent Statement: Not applicable.

Data Availability Statement: Newly designed BTK candidate inhibitors reported in this study are available as an open-access deposition via the following link: https://doi.org/10.5281/zenodo.5848494 (accessed on 14 January 2022).

Conflicts of Interest: The authors declare no conflict of interest.

References

1. Bajorath, J.; Kearnes, S.; Walters, W.P.; Meanwell, N.A.; Georg, G.I.; Wang, S. Artificial Intelligence in Drug Discovery: Into the Great Wide Open. *J. Med. Chem.* **2020**, *63*, 8651–8652. [CrossRef] [PubMed]
2. Segler, M.H.S.; Kogej, T.; Tyrchan, C.; Waller, M.P. Generating Focused Molecule Libraries for Drug Discovery with Recurrent Neural Networks. *ACS Cent. Sci.* **2018**, *4*, 120–131. [CrossRef]
3. Skalic, M.; Jiménez, J.; Sabbadin, D.; De Fabritis, G. Shape-based Generative Modeling for *De Novo* Drug Design. *J. Chem. Inf. Model.* **2019**, *59*, 1205–1214. [CrossRef]
4. Blaschke, T.; Arús-Pous, J.; Chen, H.; Margreitter, C.; Tyrchan, C.; Engkvist, O.; Papadopoulos, K.; Patronov, A. REINVENT 2.0: An AI Tool for De Novo Drug Design. *J. Chem. Inf. Model.* **2020**, *60*, 5918–5922. [CrossRef]
5. Singh, J.; Petter, R.C.; Baillie, T.A.; Whitty, A. The Resurgence of Covalent Drugs. *Nat. Rev. Drug Discov.* **2011**, *10*, 307–317. [CrossRef] [PubMed]
6. Gehringer, M.; Laufer, S.A. Emerging and Re-Emerging Warheads for Targeted Covalent Inhibitors: Applications in Medicinal Chemistry and Chemical Biology. *J. Med. Chem.* **2019**, *62*, 5673–5724. [CrossRef] [PubMed]
7. Attwood, M.M.; Fabbro, D.; Sokolov, A.V.; Knapp, S.; Schiöth, H.B. Trends in Kinase Drug Discovery: Targets, Indications and Inhibitor Design. *Nat. Rev. Drug Discov.* **2021**, *20*, 839–861. [CrossRef] [PubMed]
8. Chaikuad, A.; Koch, P.; Laufer, S.A.; Knapp, S. The Cysteinome of Protein Kinases as a Target in Drug Development. *Angew. Chem. Int. Ed.* **2018**, *57*, 4372–4385. [CrossRef] [PubMed]
9. Mohamed, A.J.; Yu, L.; Bäckesjö, C.-M.; Vargas, L.; Faryal, R.; Aints, A.; Christensson, B.; Berglöf, A.; Vihinen, M.; Nore, B.F.; et al. Bruton's Tyrosine Kinase (BTK): Function, Regulation, and Transformation with Special Emphasis on the PH Domain. *Immunol. Rev.* **2009**, *228*, 58–73. [CrossRef] [PubMed]
10. Berg, L.J.; Finkelstein, L.D.; Lucas, J.A.; Schwartzberg, P.L. TEC Family Kinases in T Lymphocyte Development and Function. *Annu. Rev. Immunol.* **2005**, *23*, 549–600. [CrossRef] [PubMed]
11. Hendriks, R.W.; Yuvaraj, S.; Kil, L.P. Targeting Bruton's Tyrosine Kinase in B Cell Malignancies. *Nat. Rev. Cancer* **2014**, *14*, 219–232. [CrossRef] [PubMed]
12. Liang, C.; Tian, D.; Ren, X.; Ding, S.; Jia, M.; Xin, M.; Thareja, S. The Development of Bruton's Tyrosine Kinase (BTK) Inhibitors from 2012 to 2017. *Eur. J. Med. Chem.* **2018**, *151*, 315–326. [CrossRef] [PubMed]
13. Deeks, E.D. Ibrutinib: A Review in Chronic Lymphocytic Leukemia. *Drugs* **2017**, *77*, 225–236. [CrossRef] [PubMed]
14. Bento, A.P.; Gaulton, A.; Hersey, A.; Bellis, L.J.; Chambers, J.; Davies, M.; Krüger, F.A.; Light, Y.; Mak, L.; McGlinchey, S.; et al. The ChEMBL Bioactivity Database: An Update. *Nucleic Acids Res.* **2014**, *42*, D1083–D1090. [CrossRef] [PubMed]
15. Yoshimori, A.; Bajorath, J. Deep SAR Matrix: SAR Matrix Expansion for Advanced Analog Design Using Deep Learning Architectures. *Future Drug Discov.* **2020**, *2*, FDD36. [CrossRef]
16. Ketkar, N. Introduction to keras. In *Deep Learning with Python*; Apress: Berkeley, CA, USA, 2017; pp. 97–111.
17. Weininger, D. SMILES, a Chemical Language and Information System. 1. Introduction to Methodology and Encoding Rules. *J. Chem. Inf. Comput. Sci.* **1988**, *28*, 31–36. [CrossRef]
18. Berman, H.M.; Westbrook, J.; Feng, Z.; Gilliland, G.; Bhat, T.N.; Weissig, H.; Shindyalov, I.N.; Bourne, P.E. The Protein Data Bank. *Nucleic Acids Res.* **2000**, *28*, 235–242. [CrossRef] [PubMed]
19. Wolber, G.; Langer, T. LigandScout: 3-D Pharmacophores Derived from Protein-Bound Ligands and their Use as Virtual Screening Filters. *J. Chem. Inf. Model.* **2005**, *45*, 160–169. [CrossRef] [PubMed]
20. Rogers, D.; Hahn, M. Extended-Connectivity Fingerprints. *J. Chem. Inf. Model.* **2010**, *50*, 742–754. [CrossRef] [PubMed]
21. Candidate Compounds from the Design of Covalent Bruton's Tyrosine Kinase (BTK) Inhibitors via Focused Deep Generative Modeling. Available online: https://doi.org/10.5281/zenodo.5848494 (accessed on 14 January 2022).

Review

Evaluation of Substituted Pyrazole-Based Kinase Inhibitors in One Decade (2011–2020): Current Status and Future Prospects

Mohammed I. El-Gamal [1,2,3,*], Seyed-Omar Zaraei [2,†], Moustafa M. Madkour [2,†] and Hanan S. Anbar [4,*]

1. Department of Medicinal Chemistry, College of Pharmacy, University of Sharjah, Sharjah 27272, United Arab Emirates
2. Sharjah Institute for Medical Research, University of Sharjah, Sharjah 27272, United Arab Emirates; holor@live.com (S.-O.Z.); moustafatrika22@hotmail.com (M.M.M.)
3. Department of Medicinal Chemistry, Faculty of Pharmacy, University of Mansoura, Mansoura 35516, Egypt
4. Department of Clinical Pharmacy and Pharmacotherapeutics, Dubai Pharmacy College for Girls, Dubai 19099, United Arab Emirates
* Correspondence: drmelgamal2002@gmail.com or malgamal@sharjah.ac.ae (M.I.E.-G.); dr.hanan@dpc.edu (H.S.A.)
† These authors contributed equally to this work.

Abstract: Pyrazole has been recognized as a pharmacologically important privileged scaffold whose derivatives produce almost all types of pharmacological activities and have attracted much attention in the last decades. Of the various pyrazole derivatives reported as potential therapeutic agents, this article focuses on pyrazole-based kinase inhibitors. Pyrazole-possessing kinase inhibitors play a crucial role in various disease areas, especially in many cancer types such as lymphoma, breast cancer, melanoma, cervical cancer, and others in addition to inflammation and neurodegenerative disorders. In this article, we reviewed the structural and biological characteristics of the pyrazole derivatives recently reported as kinase inhibitors and classified them according to their target kinases in a chronological order. We reviewed the reports including pyrazole derivatives as kinase inhibitors published during the past decade (2011–2020).

Keywords: anticancer; anti-inflammatory; kinase inhibitor; neurodegenerative disorders; pyrazole

1. Introduction

Pyrazole derivatives have attracted much attention during the last decades due to their interesting pharmacological properties and manifold applications. They are among the most extensively investigated groups of compounds amid the azole family [1]. The pyrazole ring can provide solutions for pharmacodynamic and pharmacokinetic issues. Vast numbers of pyrazole derivatives exhibit a broad-spectrum of therapeutic effects including anti-bacterial, anti-convulsant, analgesic, antimicrobial, anti-inflammatory, antidiabetic, sedative, antirheumatic, anticancer, and antitubercular activities [2,3].

The phosphorylation reactions were first discovered in glycogen metabolism and glycogen phosphorylase was identified in the 1960s [4]. Since then, kinases have been interesting therapeutic targets due to their involvement in a variety of cellular functions such as metabolism, cell cycle regulation, survival, and differentiation. A protein kinase is an enzyme that phosphorylates other protein substrates by chemically adding the terminal γ-phosphate group of adenosine triphosphate (ATP) to serine, threonine or tyrosine residues. Phosphorylation leads to a conformational change and thereby activates the functionality of the substrate proteins. There are >500 known protein kinases [5]. Indeed, deregulation of kinase function plays a fundamental role in cancer as well as immunological, inflammatory, degenerative, metabolic, cardiovascular and infectious diseases, and here arises the need for kinase inhibitors. Kinase inhibition is an interesting therapeutic avenue but clinical safety of the inhibitors must be considered [6]. There are tens of kinase inhibitors approved for marketing to date [6]: some of them bearing pyrazole moiety such as crizotinib [7], erdafitinib [8], and ruxolitinib [9] (Figure 1).

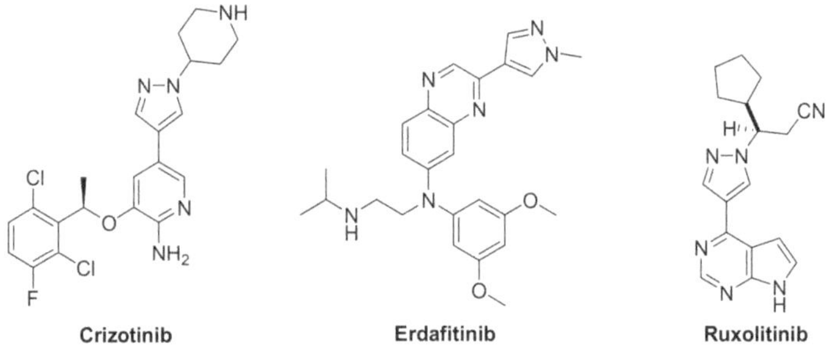

Figure 1. Structures of crizotinib, erdafitinib, and ruxolitinib.

In this article, the recently reported pyrazole-based kinase inhibitors discussed in articles published during the past decade (2011–2020) have been reviewed. They have been classified according to their different kinase targets, and are presented herein according to the alphabetical order of the kinases' names.

2. Pyrazole-Based Akt Kinase Inhibitors
2.1. Compound 1

Akt kinase, which is also named protein kinase B, is a serine-threonine kinase that is involved in PI3K-Akt-mTOR signaling pathway. This pathway is important for cell survival, apoptosis, proliferation, and metabolism. There are three known isozymes of Akt: Akt1, 2, and 3. Akt inhibitors are potential anticancer agents. Compound **1** (Figure 2) is a conformationally restricted analogue of GSK2141795 (uprosertib) (Figure 3), a known pyrazole-based Akt inhibitor. This was done with the aim of optimizing biological activity, selectivity, and metabolic stability. The structure of AT-7867 (Figure 3), another old pyrazole-based Akt inhibitor, inspired that research group to hybridize both structures in order to obtain compound **1** and its analogues. Compound **1** was tested against a 23-kinase panel and it exerted selectivity towards the Akt family. Its IC_{50} value against Akt1 is 61 nM, while the IC_{50} value of GSK2141795 is 18 nM. Western blotting showed that compound **1** decreased the level of phosphorylation of GSK3β in PC-3 cells, a substrate of Akt. In addition, compound **1** reduced the level of p-PRAS40 in LNCaP cells with IC_{50} equal to 30.4 nM, which is more potent than GSK2141795 (IC_{50} = 75.63 nM). Compound **1** demonstrated antiproliferative activity against HCT116 and OVCAR-8 cell lines (IC_{50} = 7.76 and 9.76 µM, respectively). Dichlorophenyl moiety was the best option for the highest biological activity. Any other halogen substitution other than the dichloro led to lower potency [10].

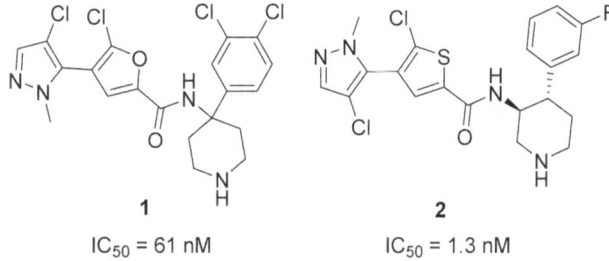

Figure 2. Structures of pyrazole-based Akt inhibitors and their IC_{50} values.

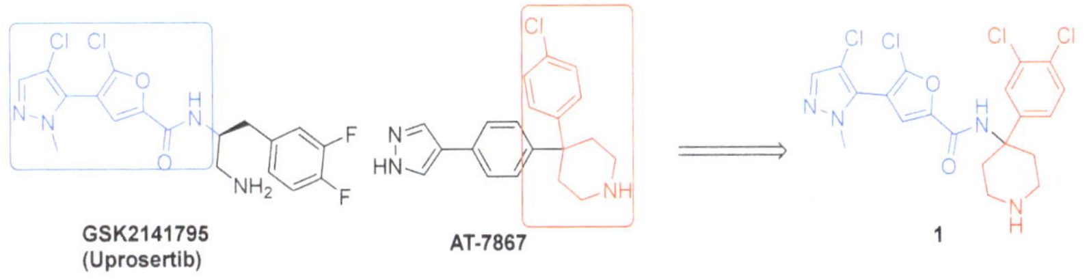

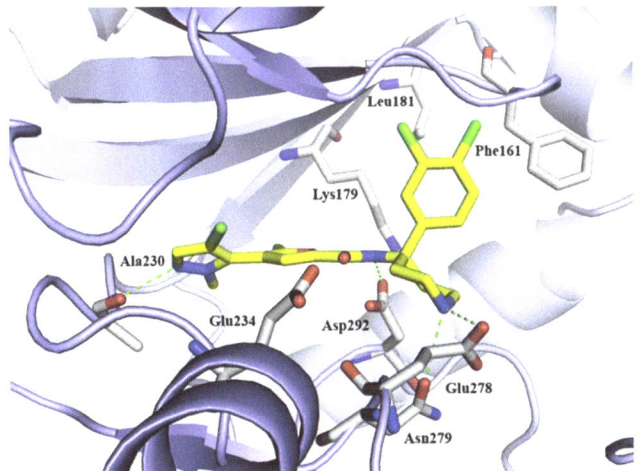

Figure 3. Structures of **G-SK2141795** and **AT-7867** and the hybridization to yield compound **1**.

Docking of compound **1** into the crystal structure of Akt1 showed its position in the ATP binding site (Figure 4). The non-methylated nitrogen of pyrazole ring accepts a hydrogen bond from Ala230 backbone *NH*. The amide hydrogen donates another hydrogen bond to Asp292. In addition, the piperidine *NH* donates two hydrogen bonds to Glu278 and Asn279. Moreover, the dichlorophenyl ring occupies a lipophilic pocket under the P-loop and forms hydrophobic interactions with Phe161 and Leu181 [10].

Figure 4. In silico binding interactions of compound **1** with Akt1 kinase crystal structure [10].

2.2. Compound **2**

Compound **2** (Figure 2) was designed as a rigid analogue of GSK2110183 (afuresertib) (Figure 5). Afuresertib is a pyrazole-based Akt1 kinase inhibitor whose K_i value is 0.08 nM. It possesses a flexible part in its structure, which was constrained in compound **2**. Its IC_{50} value against Akt1 is 1.3 nM. In addition, it showed antiproliferative activity against HCT116 colon cancer cell line (IC_{50} = 0.95 µM, 1.84-fold more potent than uprosertib). Compound **2** induced apoptosis in HCT116 cells and arrested their cell cycle at S phase. More interestingly, compound **2** demonstrated much higher potency over leukemia cell lines. For example, its IC_{50} values against MM1S, CEM-C1, and CCRF-CEM cell lines are 0.002, 0.007, and 0.008 µM, respectively. In the MM1S xenograft model, compound **2** could reduce tumor growth by 42%. Upon oral administration of 10 mg/kg of compound **2** in rats, its oral bioavailability is 52.5%. Moreover, compound **2** had a moderate inhibitory effect on hERG (40% inhibition when tested at 3 µM concentration). The SAR shows that the two chloro and one fluoro atoms in the structure of compound **2** are the best for activity. Replacement of any of them with any other group weakened the potency [11].

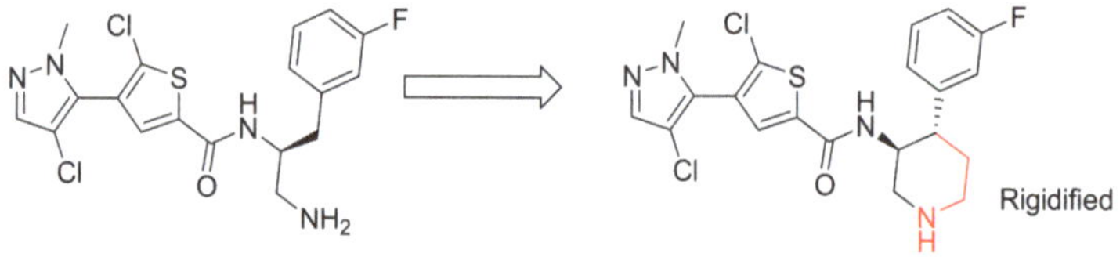

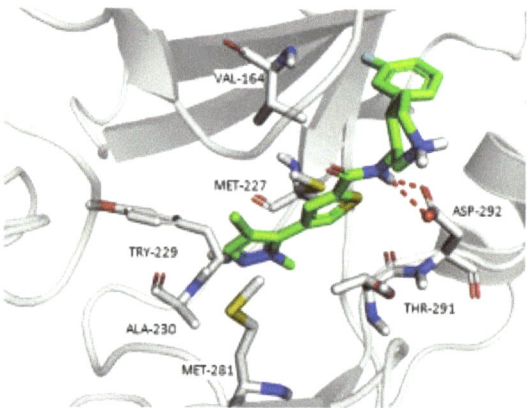

Figure 5. Structures of G-SK2110183 and the rigidification site to yield compound **2**.

The putative binding interactions of compound **2** with Akt1 crystal structure are illustrated in Figure 6. The fluorophenyl ring occupies a hydrophobic pocket and forms hydrophobic interactions with Gly162, Val164, Lys179, and Leu181. In addition, the amide hydrogen donates a hydrogen bond to Asp292 [11].

Figure 6. In silico binding interactions of compound **2** with Akt1 kinase crystal structure [11].

3. Pyrazole-Based ALK Kinase Inhibitors

Compound 3

Inspired by the lack of brain-penetrant ALK inhibitor for elucidation of ALK's role and mechanism in brain functions, Fushimi et al., developed compound **3** (Figure 7) [12]. The development stage started with lead discovery through high-throughput screening to find a potent brain-penetrant ALK inhibitor. The lead possesses imidazo[1,2-*b*]pyridazine scaffolded and with further SAR, compound **A** (Figures 8 and 9), which had a potency comparable to crizotinib but lacked selectivity (potent TrkA inhibition and moderate kinase activity), was developed. To achieve selectivity to ALK over TrkA, a cocrystal structure of compound in ALK's active site was generated. The cocrystal structure indicated an interaction between pyrazole and Glu1197 and Met1199 in the hinge region, the N at position 5 forcing the pyrazole to adopt a conformation optimal for interaction due to a steric clash with hydrogen at position 4 of pyrazole. The interaction between Leu1256 and imidazole ring, the pyridazine ring, and the 2,4-difluorophenyl group stabilized the L shaped confirmation (Figure 9).

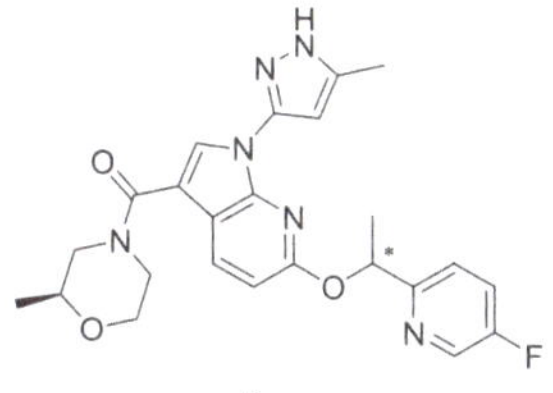

Figure 7. Structure of compound 3.

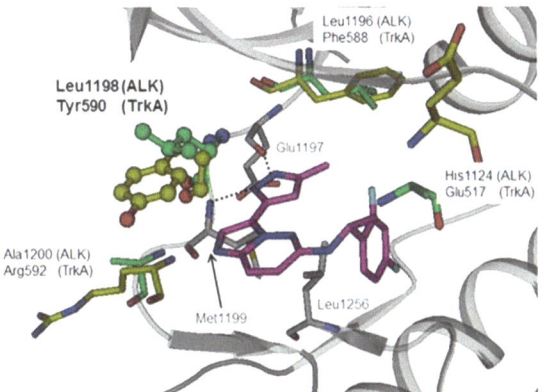

Figure 8. Cocrystal structure of compound **A** bound ALK protein. Different residues in ALK (green) and TrkA (yellow) around compound **A** (magenta) [12].

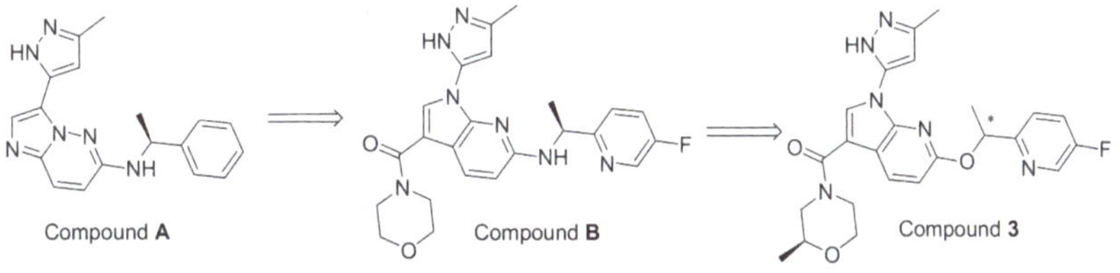

Figure 9. A schematic view of the development of compound 3 and the key changes to structure from the lead compound.

Focusing on Leu1198 in the hinge region of ALK is a key towards selectivity against ALK than TrkA. The corresponding amino acid in TrkA is the bulkier Tyr590, which means narrower binding space. A substituent at position 1 of imidazo[1,2-*b*]pyridazine nucleus would be beneficial to access the Leu1198 region. Since there is no possibility of introducing a substituent, the imidazopyridazine nucleus of compound **A** was replaced with 1*H*-pyrrolo[2,3-*b*]pyridine. Moreover, sulfonyl and carbonyl moieties with varieties of substituents were introduced to position 3 in order to clash with Tyr590 of TrkA and achieve the desired selectivity. The modified series verified the hypothesis and revealed an improvement of selectivity to ALK over TrkA. Compound **B** with morpholinylamide group at position 3 (Figure 9) had an IC$_{50}$ of 2.5 nM against ALK enzymatic assay and 23 nM in ALK cellular assay while having moderate inhibitory activity against TrkA (250 nM). To further develop the lead compound, a cocrystal structure of compound **B** with ALK aligned with TrkA was obtained (Figure 10).

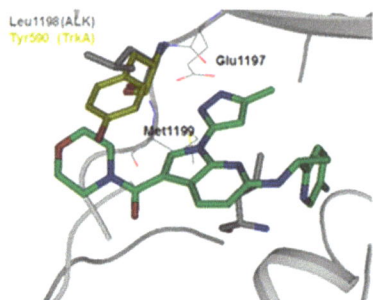

Figure 10. Cocrystal structure of compound **B** in ATP binding site of human ALK protein (gray). The relative position of Tyr590 based on crystal structure is shown in yellow [12].

Although compound **B** achieved the desired activity and selectivity on ALK, it was found that it had a high P-gp efflux (MDR1 BA/AB ratio = 18), most probably due to its increased polarity. Compound **3** has an excellent kinase profile with high selectivity and almost no activity against any kinase except focal adhesion kinase (FAK) at 100 nM (10-fold selectivity towards ALK over FAK). The IC_{50} of compound **3** against ALK kinase in cell-free and cellular kinase assays are 2.9 and 27 nM, respectively. CNS penetration was evaluated in mice and revealed brain concentration and plasma partition coefficient (K_p) values being the highest 1 h post-administration. In addition, plasma protein binding and brain tissue binding calculated as fraction unbound were measured to be 0.08 and 0.017, respectively [12].

4. Pyrazole-Based Apoptosis Signal-Regulating Kinase Inhibitors

Compound 4

Compound **4** (Figure 11) is a pyrazole derivative reported as ASK1 kinase inhibitor. ASK1 regulates both apoptosis and inflammation, and it has been involved in some diseases such as amyotrophic lateral sclerosis (ALS) and multiple sclerosis (MS). To study ASK1 modulation's implication on neurodegenerative diseases, Xin et al., discussed the design and synthesis of ASK1 inhibitors based on a previous work that identified a macrocyclic compound (cell IC_{50} = 95 nM) obtained from the lead compound (IC_{50} = 607 nM, cell IC_{50} > 20 μM) (Figure 12). In this work, modifications on the distal phenyl ring were performed to improve potency of the lead towards ASK1. Docking of the lead into ASK1 revealed that the phenyl ring is placed in the solvent exposed area, and that explains the weak potency of the lead [13].

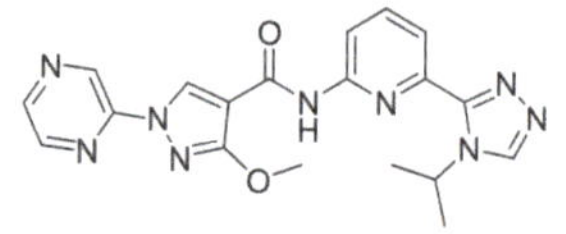

Figure 11. Structure of compound **4**.

Potency was improved by replacing the hydrophobic phenyl ring with a more polar heterocycle such as the five-membered pyrazole. The first analogue, **C** (Figure 13) showed a 20-fold increase in potency compared to the lead compound (IC_{50} = 29 nM) on ASK1. Further investigations led to **D** (Figure 13), the positional isomer of **C**. Compound **D** was superior to **C** cell's assay cell (**D**'s IC_{50} = 6.8 μM vs. **C**'s, cell IC_{50} > 20 μM). To mask the *NH* of amide, substituents were introduced on the pyrazole ring. The modification introduced in **C** induces an important conformational distortion. Introduction of methoxy had a dramatic effect on the potency. Compound **E** (Figure 13) had an IC$_{50}$ of 90 nM on cell assay but had a low in vivo clearance in a rat PK experiment [13].

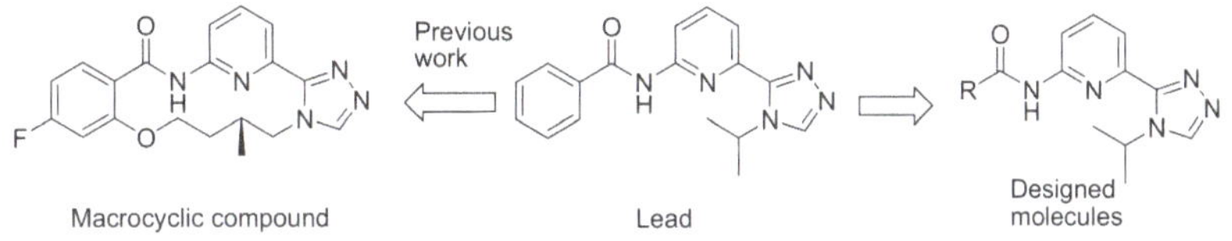

Figure 12. A scheme depicting macrocyclic compound, the lead compound, and a general structure of the target compounds [13].

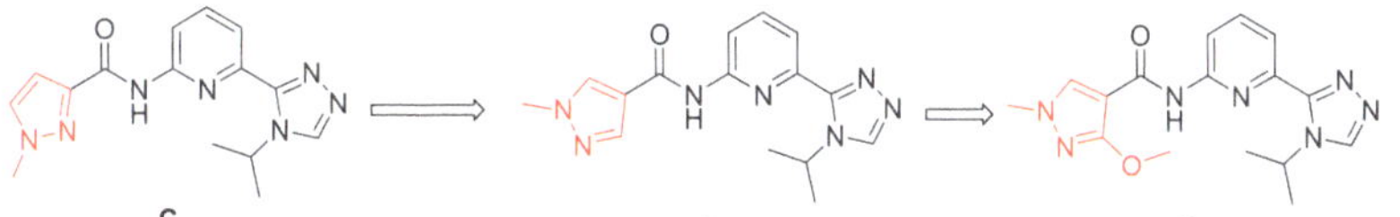

Figure 13. A scheme depicting compounds **C**, **D**, and **E**.

A number of modifications were done to improve the in vivo clearance, such as the macrocyclisation strategy which was employed in previous studies or reduction of the polar surface area (PSA). Results varied from improved potency but high in vivo clearance or high efflux ratio to loss of activity. The research group decided to increase the structural diversity of pyrazole compounds by adding different substituents on N's pyrazole. The N-alkylated pyrazoles exhibited high potency (compound **F**, cell IC$_{50}$ = 12 nM, Figure 14) yet all suffered from a high efflux rate. The N-pyridinyl derivatives showed a low efflux rate and acceptable potency (compound **G**'s IC$_{50}$ = 299 nM, Figure 14). Continuous development and modification to the substituent attached to pyrazole led to the discovery of compound **4** (Figures 11 and 14). It had a good balance of potency (cell IC$_{50}$ = 138 nM) and an efflux rate of 5.0 [13].

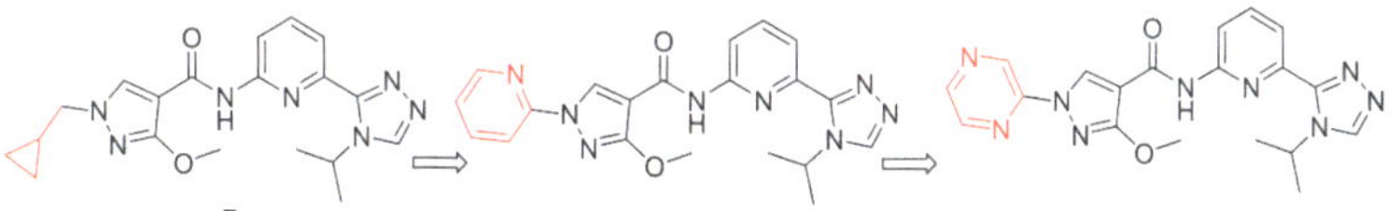

Figure 14. A scheme depicting compounds **F**, **G**, and **4**.

5. Pyrazole-Based Aurora Kinase Inhibitors

5.1. Compound 5

Aurora kinases are serine-threonine kinases that are involved in the mitosis process. Over-expression of Aurora kinases leads to cancer. Compound **5** (Barasertib, AZD1152) (Figure 15) is a highly selective Aurora B kinase inhibitor. Its IC$_{50}$ value against Aurora B is 0.37 nM in a cell-free assay, which is over 3000-fold more selective toward Aurora B than Aurora A [14].

The binding interactions of barasertib with Aurora B were studied by X-ray crystallography (Figure 16). It is reported that the compound occupies the interface between the small and the large lobes [15].

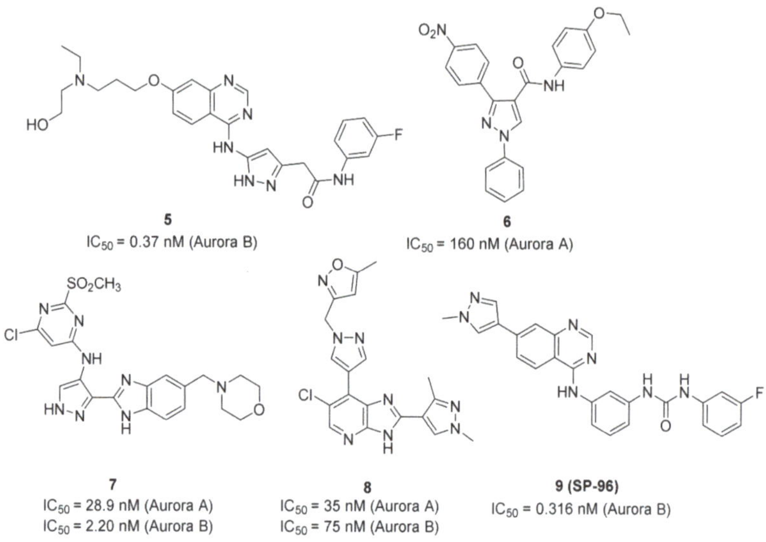

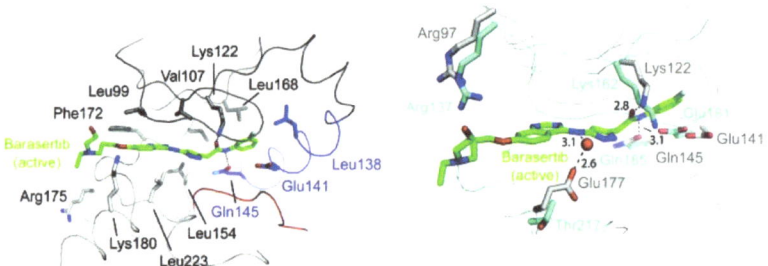

Figure 15. Structures of pyrazole-based Aurora kinase inhibitors and their IC$_{50}$ values.

Figure 16. Binding interactions of compound **5** with Aurora B crystal structure [15].

5.2. Compound 6

Li et al., have reported a series of pyrazole-based Aurora A kinase-inhibiting antiproliferative agents. Compound **6** (Figure 15) is the most promising among them. Its IC$_{50}$ values against HCT116 colon cancer cell line, MCF7 breast cancer cell line, and Aurora kinase are 0.39, 0.46, and 0.16 µM, respectively. SAR study of this series showed that the nitro group is more optimal than hydrogen, methyl, methoxy, or chloro substituent [16]. A quantitative structure-activity relationship (QSAR) study on this series of compounds was carried out. It revealed that inclusion of bulky electron-withdrawing groups at *para* positions (in place of nitro and ethoxy) maximized the inhibitory potency against Aurora A kinase [17].

5.3. Compound 7

A series of pyrazolyl benzimidazole have been reported as antiproliferative agents possessing Aurora A/B kinase inhibitory effect. Compound **7** (Figure 15) is the most potent among this series. Its IC$_{50}$ values against U937 (leukemia), K562 (leukemia), A549 (lung), LoVo (colon), and HT29 (colon) cancer cell lines are 5.106, 5.003, 0.487, 0.789, and 0.381 µM, respectively. In addition, it exerted strong potency against Aurora A and B (IC$_{50}$ = 28.9 and 2.2 nM, respectively). The SAR showed that the morpholino ring is more favorable for activity than *H*, diethylamino, or piperidine. Docking of compound **7** into the crystal structure of Aurora A and B revealed binding into the active site. In the case of Aurora A, the benzimidazole ring forms hydrophobic interactions with a hydrophobic pocket formed by Ala213, Pro214, Leu215, and Gly216, and the hydrogen of *NH* donates a hydrogen bond to backbone amide of Ala213. The morpholino oxygen atom accepts a hydrogen bond from Arg137. In case of Aurora B, the pyrazole ring forms hydrogen bonds with *NH* of Ala173 and backbone carbonyl of Glu171. In addition, the pyrimidine ring forms two hydrogen bonds with backbone *NH* of Lys122. This rationalizes the stronger potency of compound **7** against Aurora B compared to Aurora A [18].

5.4. Compound 8

Compound **8** (Figure 15) is a dual inhibitor of Aurora A/B (IC$_{50}$ = 35 and 75 nM, respectively). However, it is not very selective towards these two kinases. Upon testing at 1 µM concentration against a 105-kinase panel, it demonstrated more than 80% inhibition against 22 kinases. Compound **8** is potent against SW620 and HCT116 colon cancer cell lines (IC$_{50}$ = 0.35 and 0.34 µM, respectively). The methylisoxazole moiety is more optimal than substituted phenyl in terms of potency and stability [19].

5.5. Compound 9

Frag-1 (Figure 17) has been reported as an Aurora B inhibitor with an IC$_{50}$ value of 116 nM. A docking study revealed a non-occupied pocket in front of the amino group (Figure 14). Lakkaniga et al., decided to extend the structure towards this vacant pocket in order to achieve better potency. This recently reported study led to the discovery of SP-96 (compound **9**) (Figures 15 and 17). It is a very potent and selective non-ATP-competitive Aurora B inhibitor (IC$_{50}$ = 0.316 nM). SP-96 is over 2000-fold more selective against Aurora B than FLT3 and KIT. Regarding the terminal fluorophenyl ring, halogen substituents are more tolerated than bulkier substituents. *Meta*-fluoro is more optimal than para or ortho positional isomers. The central phenyl ring in between urea and *NH* should be meta-disubstituted for selectivity against Aurora B. If *para*-disubstituted, the molecule inhibits Aurora B, FLT, and KIT. The pyrazole ring comes at the solvent exposure, which is why polar moiety at this place is more favorable than hydrophobic ones. Furthermore, attachment of a pyrazole ring at position 6 of the quinazoline ring is unfavorable for activity [20].

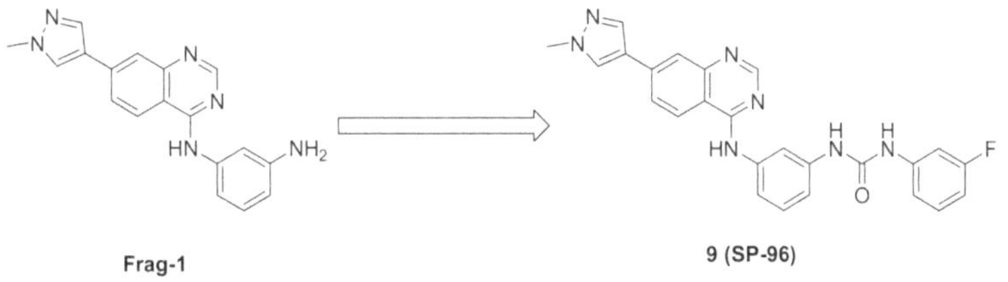

Figure 17. Modification to **Frag-1** to form compound **9** (**SP-96**).

6. Pyrazole-Based BCR-ABL Kinase Inhibitors

6.1. Compound 10

Bcr-Abl inhibition is a potential therapeutic strategy for treatment of chronic myeloid leukemia (CML). Some pyrazole-based inhibitors of Bcr-Abl kinase have been reported in the literature during the last decade. In compound **10** (Figure 18), the diarylamide moiety was quoted from the structures of imatinib and ponatinib (Figure 19), known Bcr-Abl inhibitory anti-leukemia drugs. The IC$_{50}$ values of compound **10** over Bcr-Abl kinase and K562 leukemia cell lines are 14.2 nM and 0.27 µM, respectively. Removal of trifluoromethyl group from its structure significantly decreased the potency [21].

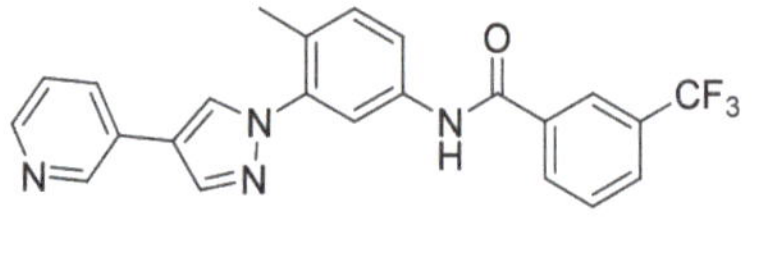

10
IC$_{50}$ = 14.2 nM

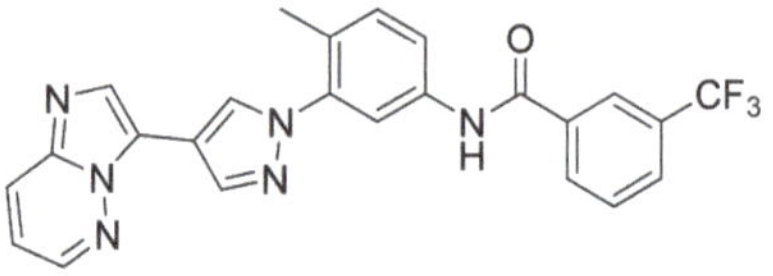

11
IC$_{50}$ = 8.5 nM

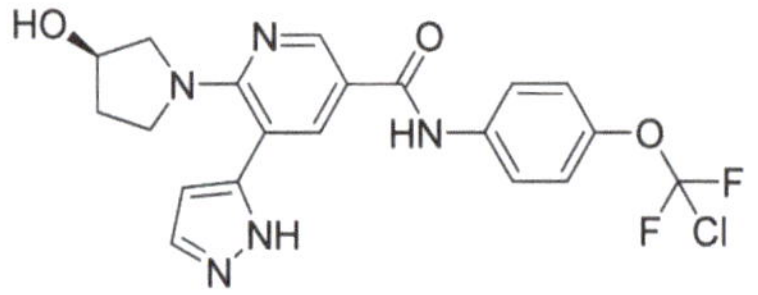

12 (Asciminib, ABL-001)
IC$_{50}$ = 0.5 nM

Figure 18. Structures of pyrazole-based BCR-ABL kinase inhibitors and their IC$_{50}$ values.

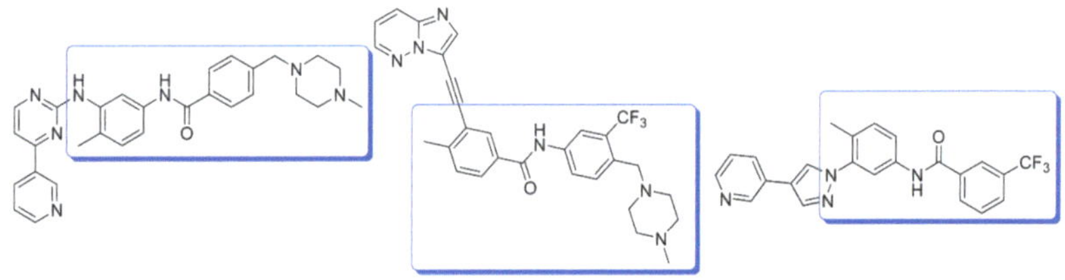

Imatinib

Ponatinib

10

Figure 19. Structures of pyrazole-based BCR-ABL kinase inhibitors and their IC$_{50}$ values.

Docking study of compound **10** into the Bcr-Abl crystal structure was performed to study its binding mode. The pyridine ring is the hinge region-binding moiety of this structure, similar to imatinib. The pyridyl nitrogen accepts a hydrogen bond from Met318. The amide linker forms two more hydrogen bonds with Glu286 and Asp381. Moreover, the pyrazole ring forms pi-pi stacking interaction with Thr315 (Figure 20) [21].

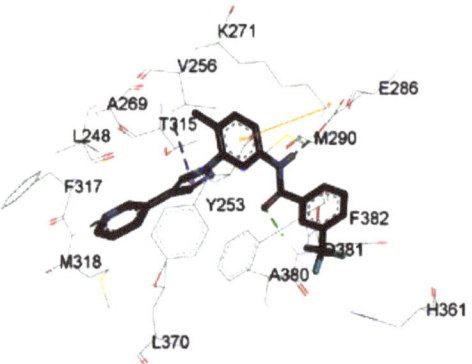

Figure 20. Putative binding mode of compound **10** with Bcr-Abl crystal structure [21].

6.2. Compound 11

The same research group also reported compound **11** (Figure 18) possessing imidazo[1,2-b]pyridazine nucleus as a hinge region binder similar to ponatinib. Instead of the alkyne linker of ponatinib, compound **11** possesses a pyrazole ring similar to compound **10**. The imidazo[1,2-b]pyridazine nucleus was found more favorable for activity against Bcr-Abl kinase than the pyridine ring of compound **10** (Figure 21) [22].

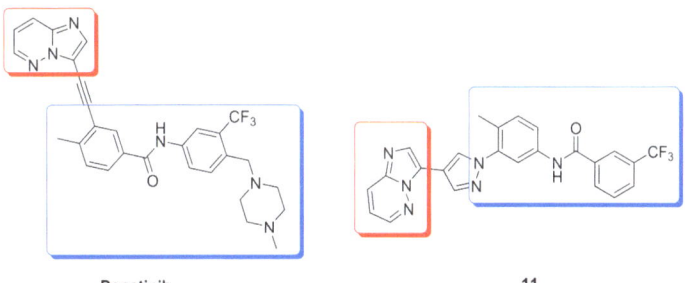

Figure 21. Modifications to ponatinib structure leading to compound **11**.

6.3. Compound 12

Compound **12** (Asciminib, ABL-001) (Figure 18) is a non-ATP competitive inhibitor of Bcr-Abl kinase with a K_d value of 0.5–0.8 nM and an IC_{50} value of 0.5 nM. It is able to inhibit the T315I mutant Bcr-Abl as well (IC_{50} = 25 nM) [23,24]. Asciminib is a clinical candidate currently under clinical trials in patients with CML, alone or in combination with imatinib [25].

An X-ray crystallography study of asciminib cocrystal with Bcr-Abl confirmed that it is an allosteric inhibitor, unlike nilotinib (Figure 22). The pyrazole ring forms a hydrogen bond with backbone carbonyl of Glu481 in addition to a hydrophobic interaction with Thr453. The chlorine atom forms the Van der Waals interaction with Leu448, Val487, and Ile508 [24].

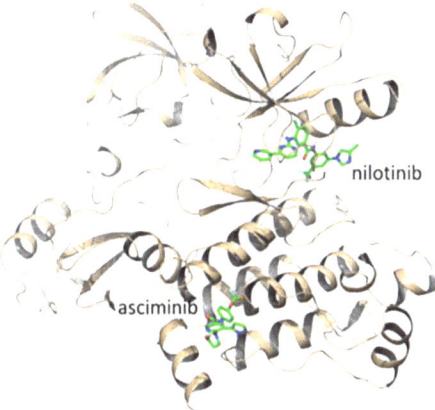

Figure 22. Comparison between the binding sites of asciminib and nilotinib [24].

I502L or V468F mutations of Bcr-Abl kinase can lead to resistance of the leukemia cells to asciminib. Molecular dynamics studies revealed that I502L mutation changes the myristoyl pocket conformation while V468F shifts asciminib outside the myristoyl pocket (Figure 23). These mutations lead to declined binding affinity of the molecule with the kinase [26].

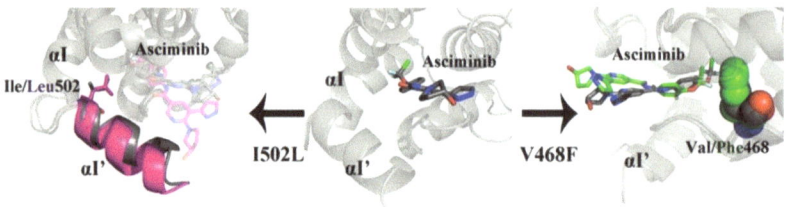

Figure 23. Effects of I502L and V468F mutations of Bcr-Abl kinase on the binding affinity of asciminib [26].

7. Pyrazole-Based Calcium-Dependent Kinase Inhibitors

7.1. Compound 13

Compound **13** (Figure 24) has been reported as an inhibitor of *Plasmodium falciparum* calcium-dependent protein kinase 1 whose IC_{50} value equals 56 nM. This kinase is essential for a parasite's life cycle stages of motility and to invade the red blood cells. Compound **13** showed anti-parasitic activity against *Plasmodium falciparum* with an IC_{50} value of 0.262 µM. The pyrazole ring is inserted in this structure instead of the 6-membered (hetero)aromatic rings to decrease logD and improve aqueous solubility and ADME profile. When incubated with human or mouse liver microsomal enzymes for 30 min, the remaining percentages of compound **13** were 80% and 84%, respectively. The SAR of this compound and its analogues revealed that fluoro is more optimal than cyano, and primary amino on the cyclohexyl ring is more favorable for activity than pyrrolidinyl or piperidinyl [27].

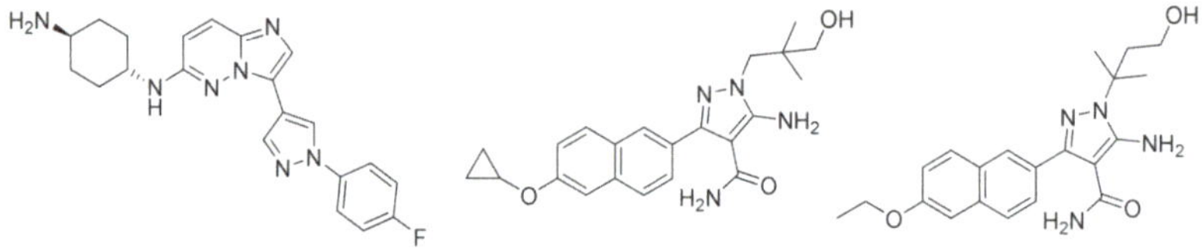

Figure 24. Structures of pyrazole-based calcium dependent kinase inhibitors and their IC_{50} values.

7.2. Compounds 14 and 15

Cryptosporidium parvum is a parasite that causes diarrhea in children all over the world. Its calcium-dependent protein kinase 1 is essential for its invasion and growth. Compounds **14** (BKI 1708) and **15** (BKI 1770) (Figure 24) have been recently reported as inhibitors of that kinase with anti-parasitic activity both in vitro and in vivo. The IC_{50} of both compounds against the kinase are 0.7 and 2.5 nM, respectively. In addition, EC_{50} values against the microbe are 0.41 and 0.51 µM, respectively. The naphthalene ring is more optimal for activity than any other heterocyclic fused bicyclic ring systems. BKI 1708 exerted in vivo efficacy against mouse model of cryptosporiodiosis when administered at 8 mg/kg once daily. It is safe up to 200 mg/kg with no tendency to induce cardiotoxicity. Similarly, BKI 1770 was efficacious at 30 mg/kg but twice daily, safe up to 300 mg/kg, and there is no cardiotoxicity liability [28].

8. Pyrazole-Based Checkpoint Kinase Inhibitors

8.1. Compounds 16 and 17

Checkpoint kinase 2 (Chk2) is involved in DNA damage response pathway. In addition, it is over-expressed by different types of cancer cells as it is essential for their survival. Chk2 inhibition is an avenue for cancer treatment. Galal et al., have reported a series of pyrazole-based Chk2 inhibitors. Compounds **16** and **17** (Figure 25) are examples of the most promising derivatives of that series. Their IC$_{50}$ values against Chk2 in cell-free assay are 48.4 and 17.9 nM, respectively. In general, derivatives possessing amide moiety on the benzimidazole nucleus are more potent than carboxylic acid or nitro analogues. Furthermore, both compounds showed antiproliferative activity against HepG2 (hepatocellular carcinoma), HeLa (cervical), and MCF7 (breast) cancer cell lines but compound **17** is more potent (IC$_{50}$ = 10.8, 11.8, and 10.4 µM, respectively). Both compounds induced cell cycle arrest in MCF7 cells, and both of them exerted synergistic cytotoxicity in vitro and in vivo, in combination with doxorubicin or cisplatin [29].

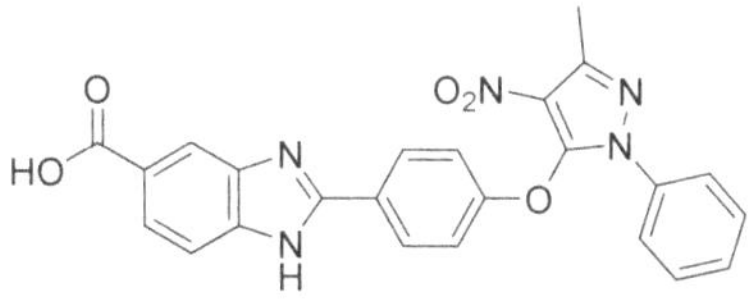

Figure 25. Structures of pyrazole-based checkpoint kinase 2 inhibitors and their IC$_{50}$ values.

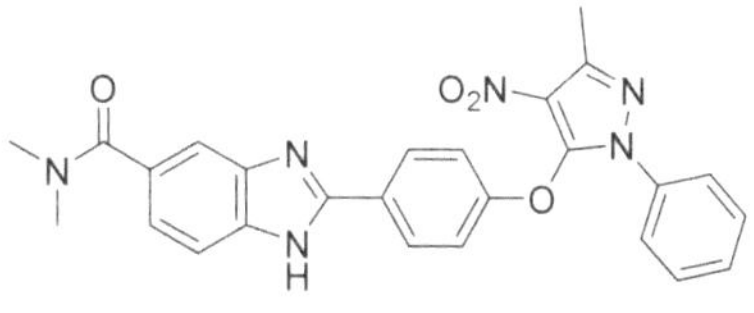

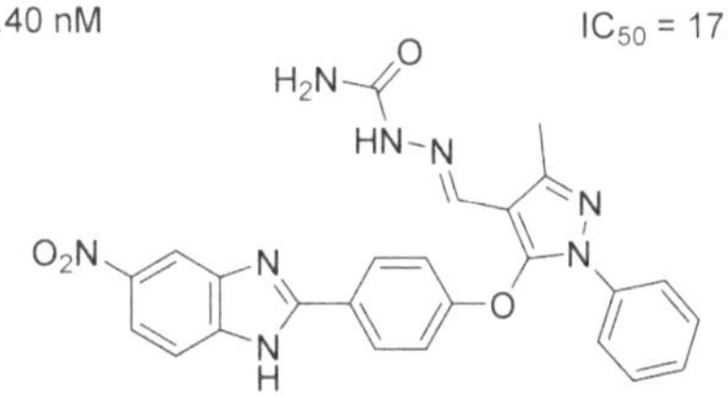

8.2. Compound 18

The same group that published on compounds **16** and **17** reported derivatives of them bearing semicarbazone moiety as inhibitors of Chk2. Compound **18** (Figure 25) is an example of this newer series (IC$_{50}$ against Chk2 = 41.64 nM). It produced modest potency against HepG2, HeLa, and MCF7 cell lines with 2-digit micromolar IC$_{50}$ values. Compound **18** alone arrested S phase of MCF7 cell cycle, while in combination with doxorubicin, it arrested G2/M phase. It exerted synergistic effect in vivo in breast cancer model in combination with doxorubicin [30]. It is noteworthy that the same group reported another series of Chk2 inhibitors possessing cyanopyrimidine instead of the pyrazole core and some of these derivatives showed improved potency [31].

9. Pyrazole-Based Cyclin-Dependent Kinase Inhibitors

9.1. Compound 19

Compound **19** (Figure 26) is an azo-diaminopyrazole derivative designed with similarity to CAN508, an old selective cyclin-dependent kinase (CDK)-9 inhibitor (IC$_{50}$ = 350 nM) (Figure 27). The phenolic moiety of CAN508 was replaced with 4-pyridyl and the *NH* of the pyrazole ring was methylated. This led to alteration of the CDK selectivity profile of the compound. Instead of inhibiting CDK9 like CAN508, compound **19** is a selective CDK4 inhibitor with an IC$_{50}$ value of 420 nM. It is more selective toward CDK4 than CDK1, 2, 7, and 9. *N*-Methylation was found more appropriate than *N*-acylation. Compound **19** was also tested for antiproliferative activity against K562, MCF7, and RPMI-8226 cancer cell lines but exerted modest activity. Its IC$_{50}$ values are 67.4, 37.7, and 50 µM, respectively. It was further investigated for ability to induce apoptosis, and it happened in RPMI-8226 multiple myeloma cell line only [32].

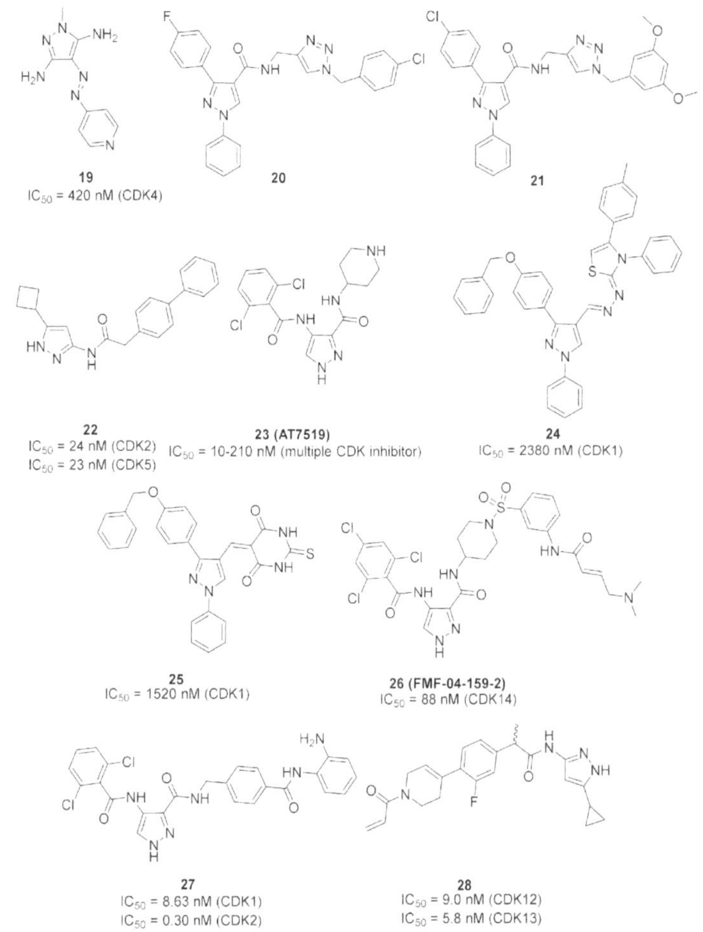

Figure 26. Structures of pyrazole-based CDK inhibitors and their IC$_{50}$ values.

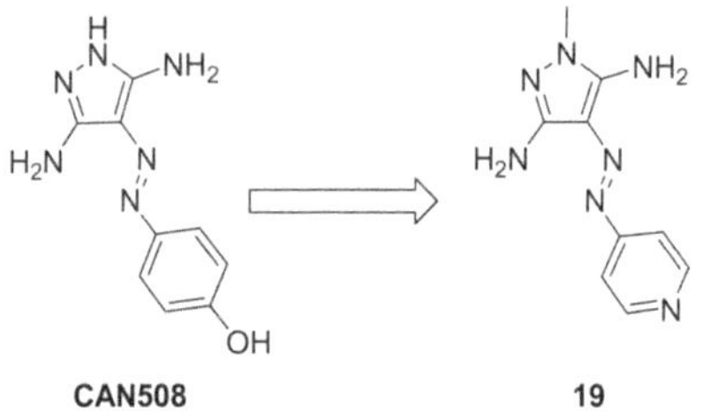

Figure 27. Structure of **CAN508** and the development of compound **19** from it.

9.2. Compounds 20 and 21

Compounds **20** and **21** (Figure 26) are the most promising CDK1-inhibitory antiproliferative agents among a series of pyrazole derivatives. Both compounds exhibited submicromolar IC$_{50}$ values against MCF7 cells (IC$_{50}$ = 0.13 and 0.15 µM, respectively), MIA-PaCa pancreatic cancer cell line (IC$_{50}$ = 0.28 and 0.34 µM, respectively), and HeLa cervical cancer cell line (IC$_{50}$ = 0.21 and 0.73 µM, respectively). The SAR study indicated that when the R1 group is a monohalogen such as fluoro or chloro, the antiproliferative activity is higher than in the case of methoxy. Both compounds **20** and **21** induced cell cycle arrest in MCF7 cell line in G2/M phase in a dose-dependent pattern. Western blotting indicated that both compounds suppressed CDK1 expression in MCF7 cells at 50 and 100 nM concentrations. In particular, compound **21** completely inhibited its expression at 100 nM. In addition, both compounds induced apoptosis in MCF7 cells due to decreased mitochondrial inner membrane potential and increased reactive oxygen species formation [33].

Docking of both compounds **20** and **21** into the crystal structure of CDK1 was carried out (Figure 28). The pyrazole ring of both compounds interacts with Asp86 and Leu135. The N-phenyl ring interacts with Gly11, Glu12, and Gln132. The triazole ring interacts with Ala31, Gly81, and Leu83. In addition, the substituted benzyl ring forms hydrophobic interactions with Thr15, Val18, and Lys33. Moreover, the substituted phenyl moiety attached to position 3 of the pyrazole ring interacts with Ile10, Phe82, Ser84, Met85, and Lys89. The dimethoxy substituents of compound **21** form additional interactions with Asn133 and Leu134 [33].

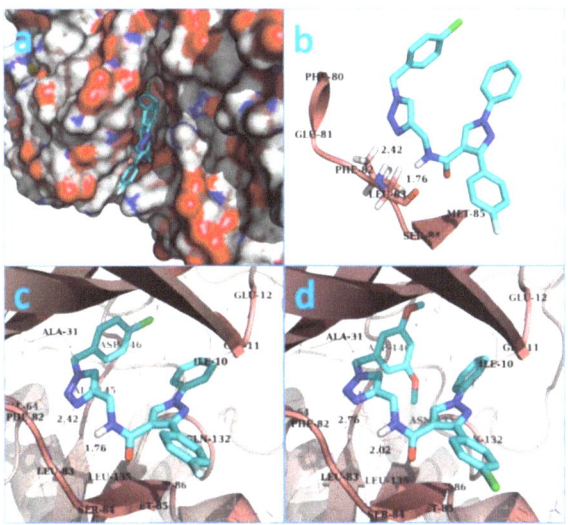

Figure 28. Putative bind interactions of compounds **20** (a–c) and **21** (d) [33].

9.3. Compounds 22 and 23

A series of 3,5-disubstituted pyrazole derivatives were synthesized and tested against pancreatic ductal adenocarcinoma cell lines. Compound **22** (Figure 26) is the most potent among them. It induced apoptosis in MiaPaCa2 cell line through a 3.2-fold increase in caspase-3/7 level. It was further tested for antiproliferative activity against MiaPaCa2 and four other pancreatic ductal adenocarcinoma cell lines, namely AsPC1, BxPC3, SUIT2, and S2-013 after a 3-day incubation period. Its IC_{50} values are 0.247, 0.315, 0.924, 0.209, and 0.192 µM, respectively. AT7518 (**23**) (Figure 26), an old pyrazole-based CDK inhibitor was the positive control in that assay. Its IC_{50} values against the same five cell lines are 0.411, 0.533, 0.640, 0.557, and 2.77 µM, respectively. The SAR study of compound **22** and its derivatives revealed that cyclobutyl is more optimal for activity than hydrogen, methyl, isopropyl, cyclopropyl, cyclopentyl, or phenyl. In addition, the biphenyl moiety is more favorable than naphthalene, ethylenedioxyphenyl, or dimethoxyphenyl. Compound **22** was also tested against a panel of fourteen kinases and exerted preference toward CDK2 and 5 (IC_{50} = 24 and 23 nM, respectively) [34].

It is noteworthy that AT7519 (**23**) is a multi-CDK inhibitory agent that inhibits CDK1, 2, 4, 6, and 9 with IC_{50} values ranging from 10 to 210 nM. It inhibits GSK3β as well with IC_{50} value of 89 nM. It induces apoptosis against different cancer types such as colon cancer and multiple myeloma [35,36].

9.4. Compounds 24 and 25

Compounds **24** and **25** (Figure 26) were reported as potent antiproliferative agents with CDK1 kinase inhibitory effect. They exerted strong potency against three hepatocellular carcinoma (HepG2, Huh7, and SNU-475), one colon cancer (HCT116), and one renal cancer (UO-31) cell lines. The IC_{50} values of compound **24** against these five tested cell lines are 0.05, 0.065, 1.93, 1.68, and 1.85 µM, respectively. In addition, compound **25** exerted IC_{50} values of 0.028, 1.83, 1.70, 0.035, and 2.24 µM, respectively against them. Both compounds inhibited CDK1 but with modest activity (IC_{50} = 2.38 and 1.52 µM, respectively). Moreover, the two compounds stimulated caspase-3 and induced HepG2 cell cycle arrest in G2/M phase [37].

9.5. Compound 26

FMF-04-159-2 (compound **26**) (Figure 26) is an extended analogue of AT7519 (Figure 29) that possesses an α,β-unsaturated carbonyl moiety. That is why it acts as an irreversible inhibitor. It has been reported as an inhibitor of CDK14 kinase, a member of TAIRE subfamily of CDKs that includes CDK15-18, in addition to CDK14. The IC_{50} values of compound **26** against CDK14 in cell-free and whole-cell kinase assays are 88 and 500 nM, respectively. Moreover, it exerted antiproliferative activity against the HCT116 colorectal cancer cell line (IC_{50} = 1.14 µM). Although compound **26** is 8.6-fold less potent than AT7519 on the HCT116 cell line, it possesses the merit of improved potency and selectivity toward CDK14. The authors of this work recommend further structural optimization and investigation in order to optimize the kinase and cellular potency [38].

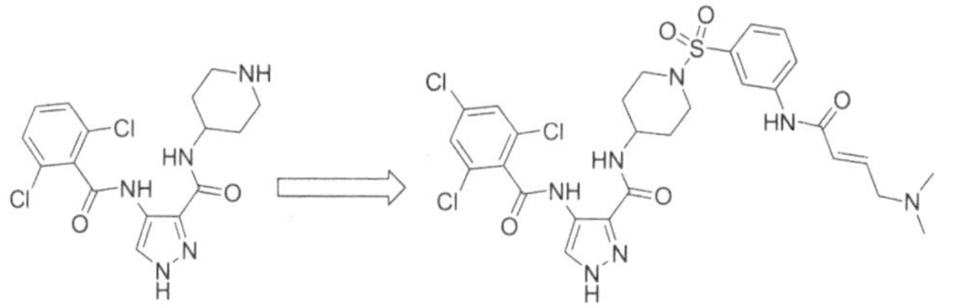

Figure 29. Structure of AT7519 and the development of compound **26** (FMF-04-159-2).

9.6. Compound 27

Compound **27** (Figure 26) has been recently reported as a dual inhibitor of CDK and histone deacetylase (HDAC). Its IC_{50} values against CDK1, CDK2, HDAC1, HDAC2, and HDAC3 are 8.63, 0.30, 6.40, 0.25, and 45.0 nM, respectively. In addition, it exerted high potency against HCT116 colorectal cancer cell line with sub-micromolar IC_{50} value of 0.71 µM. When tested on NIN3T3 normal cells, its IC_{50} value was 4.47 µM. So, its selectivity index is 6.3. The SAR study showed that o-dichlorophenyl moiety is more optimal than other substituents such as fluoro or methoxy. In addition, the aniline motif is the best solvent exposure moiety compared with other polar moieties such as hydroxamic acid. Compound **27** could induce apoptosis and stop the cell cycle of HCT116 at G2/M phase. In an in vivo HCT116 xenograft model in nude mice, compound **27** was intraperitoneally injected once daily for 22 days at doses of 12.5 and 25 mg/kg. It reduced the tumor size by 37% and 51%, respectively. In vivo PK evaluation of compound I following i.p. injection of 20 mg/kg showed the following parameters: $t_{1/2}$ = 2.61 h, T_{max} = 2.00 h, C_{max} = 7570 ng/mL, and bioavailability = 63.6% [39].

Docking of compound **27** into the crystal structure of CDK2 was performed in order to study its binding mode (Figure 30). The NH directly attached to the pyrazole ring forms a hydrogen bond as a donor with Glu81. In addition, the hydrogen atom of the carboxamide moiety attached to pyrazole at position 3 forms another hydrogen bond with

Leu83. Moreover, the aniline NH_2 together with NH next to it forms two hydrogen bonds with His84 [39].

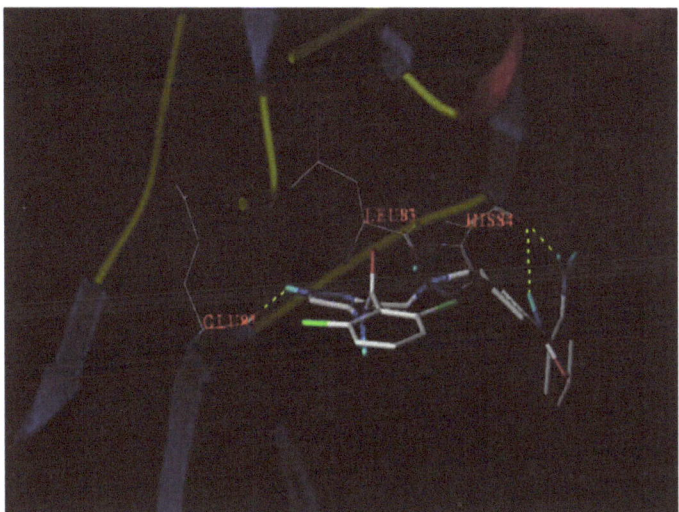

Figure 30. Docking pose of compound **27** into the crystal structure of CDK2 [39].

9.7. Compound 28

Compound **28** (Figure 26) is a patented pyrazole derivative claimed as selective CDK12/13 inhibitor. Its IC_{50} values against CDK12 and 13 are 9 and 5.8 nM, respectively. It is much less potent over CDK7 (IC_{50} = 880 nM). It possesses an α,β-unsaturated carbonyl moiety that is able to act as a covalent binder and irreversibly inhibit the kinases [40].

10. Pyrazole-Based EGFR Kinase Inhibitors

Compound 29

Aiming at an anti-EGFR activity, a series possessing pyrazole scaffold was designed, synthesized, and evaluated. Compound **29** (Figure 31) presented itself as the most promising in the series, demonstrating an antiproliferative effect against MCF-7 breast cancer cell line (IC_{50} = 0.30 µM) and B16-F10 melanoma cell line (IC_{50} = 0.44 µM) tumor cells compared to erlotinib (MCF-7, IC_{50} = 0.08 µM and B16-F10, IC_{50} = 0.12 µM). Further biological evaluation to assess the potential inhibition of autophosphorylation of EGFR and HER-2 kinases using solid-phase ELISA assay was done. Compound **29** showed the highest inhibitory activity with IC_{50} = 0.21 ± 0.05 µM for EGFR and IC_{50} = 1.08 ± 0.15 µM for HER-2 kinases. In comparison, erlotinib demonstrated IC_{50} = 0.03 ± 0.002 µM against EGFR and IC_{50} = 0.14 ± 0.02 µM against HER-2 kinases. In the series, the trend of activity showed a preference towards electron donating groups rather than electron withdrawing ones on the distal phenyl ring as well the phenyl ring directly attached to pyrazole [41].

The molecular docking study of compound **29** with EGFR (Figure 31, left) and HER2 (right) showed compound **29** binding to the ATP binding pocket. In EGFR's molecular docking, compound **29** bonded through hydrophobic interaction, an H-bonding between the methoxy of distal side chain reacted with Lys A721, and the unsubstituted phenyl ring interacted with Leu694 through pi-sigma interaction [41].

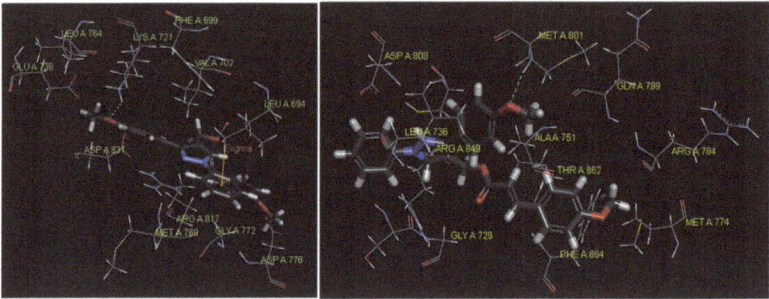

Figure 31. The structure of compound 29 and its IC50 value (**up**). Structure and molecular docking of compound **29** into EGFR (**left**) and HER2 (**right**). The dotted lines = hydrogen bond; yellow line = pi-sigma interactions [41].

11. Pyrazole-Based FGFR Inhibitors

11.1. Compound 30

Fibroblast growth factor receptor (FGFR) 1–4 kinases are over-expressed in different types of tumors. Compound **30** (AZD4547) (Figure 32) is a clinical candidate that possesses pan-FGFR inhibitory effect. It is orally bioavailable, well tolerated in vivo, and has exerted dose-dependent anticancer activity in tumor models [42]. It is currently under investigation in clinical trials in patients with lymphoma, glioma, lung, breast, gastric, and esophageal types of cancer [43].

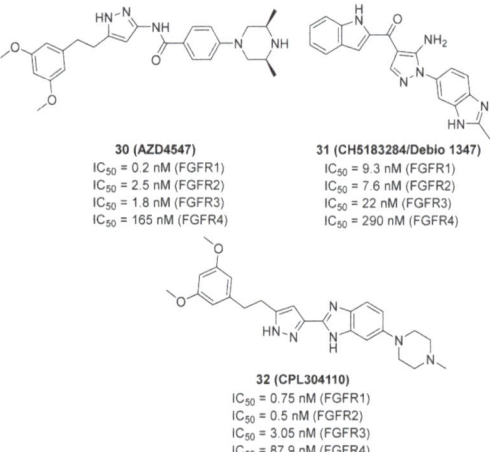

Figure 32. Structures of pyrazole-based FGFR inhibitors and their IC_{50} values.

AZD4547 is a type I inhibitor of FGFR1, i.e., it binds to DFG-in conformation of the kinase. It forms four hydrogen bonds with pyrazole N and NH, amide NH, and methoxy oxygen (Figure 33) [44].

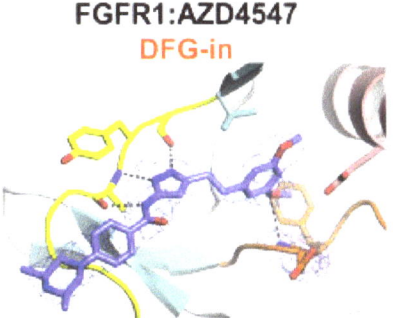

Figure 33. Binding mode of AZD4547 (**30**) with FGFR1 kinase crystal structure [44].

11.2. Compound 31

Compound **31** (CH5183284/Debio 1347) (Figure 32) is a pan-FGFR clinical candidate that was tested in one clinical trial and will be shortly tested in another two clinical trials against breast cancer and other solid tumors [45]. Its IC_{50} values against FGFR-1, -2, -3, and -4 are 9.3, 7.6, 22, and 290 nM, respectively. It is more selective against the FGFR family than the KDR and Src kinases (IC_{50} = 2100 and 5900 nM, respectively). Moreover, it exerted potential antiproliferative activity (IC_{50} values against gastric SNU-16 and colon HCT116 cancer cell lines are 17 nM and 5.9 µM, respectively). Its aqueous solubility equals 29 µg/mL, and its IC_{50} value against hERG is 6.9 µM. In addition, its hit-to-lead design rationale is illustrated in Figure 34 [46].

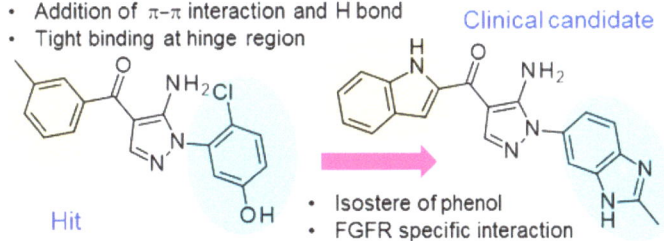

Figure 34. Hit-to-lead rational design of CH5183284 [46].

Docking studies were conducted to understand the binding mode of compound **31** with FGFR1 and to rationalize its selectivity towards FGFR1 instead of KDR and Src. Its binding interactions are illustrated in Figure 35. The benzimidazole nitrogens form hydrogen bonds with E531 and D641. Moreover, the benzimidazole nucleus forms hydrophobic interactions with Val561, I545, and F641. It is more appropriate for activity than phenoxy or indole. The primary amino group donates a hydrogen bond to E562 while the ketone oxygen accepts a hydrogen bond from A564. Compound **31** is less potent against the KDR kinase because the L889 residue disrupts S-pi interaction with the benzimidazole nucleus. Similarly, the T314 and I339 of Src kinase do not interact with the molecule like V561 and V559 of FGFR1 [46].

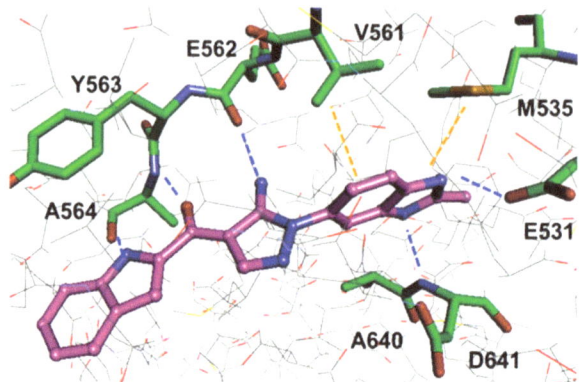

Figure 35. Putative binding mode of compound **31** with FGFR1 crystal structure [46].

11.3. Compound 32

Compound **32** (CPL304110) (Figure 32) is a clinical candidate that has been recently reported as a pan-FGFR inhibitor. Its IC_{50} values against FGFR-1, -2, -3, and -4 are 0.75, 0.5, 3.05, and 87.9 nM, respectively. When tested against a 13-kinase panel, it was selective against FGFR family only. It showed high potency against different cancer cell lines with over-expressed FGFR, and the highest potency was against FGFR-2-amplified SNU-16 gastric cancer cell line (IC_{50} = 85.64 nM). CPL304110 demonstrated an acceptable PK profile, low toxicity, and potent in vivo anticancer activity. Its *N*-methylpiperazinyl moiety is more favorable than morpholino, pyrazole, or urea. Compound **32** is currently under investigation in phase I clinical trials to test its safety in patients with bladder, gastric, or lung cancers [47].

Docking into FGFR-1 crystal structure showed the following interactions: (i) Benzimidazole *NH* donates a hydrogen bond to carbonyl oxygen of Ala564; (ii) Pyrazole *N* accepts a hydrogen bond from *NH* of Ala564; (iii) Pyrazole *NH* donates a hydrogen bond to carbonyl of Glu562; (iv) Methoxy oxygen accepts a hydrogen bond from *NH* of Asp641 in the gatekeeper region; (v) *N*-Methylpiperazinyl is the solvent exposure moiety of this structure [47].

12. Pyrazole-Based IKK Kinase Inhibitors

Compound 33

Curcumin derivatives were designed and synthesized for potential cytotoxic effect by targeting IKKβ, a sub-unit of IKK. The designed derivatives included the introduction of a substituted pyrazole ring to curcumin at methylene carbon. They were tested against the HeLa human cervical cancer cell line with curcumin and paclitaxel as positive controls. Compound **33** (Figure 36) showed an IC_{50} of 14.2 µg/mL which was more potent than curcumin (42.4 µg/mL) but less potent than paclitaxel (4.3 nM/mL). The investigations of the SAR of curcumin derivatives showed the importance of halogen atoms (4-chloro and 4-bromo) on activity and how they increase the activity compared to other derivatives. Derivatives with electron-withdrawing groups in the same position of the halogen were superior to their electron donating counterparts and the unsubstituted phenyl ring. An evaluation of the induction of apoptosis in terms of cleavage of the caspase-3 enzyme was performed. Compound **33** exhibited 69.6% of apoptosis, significantly higher than the 19.9% induced by curcumin [48].

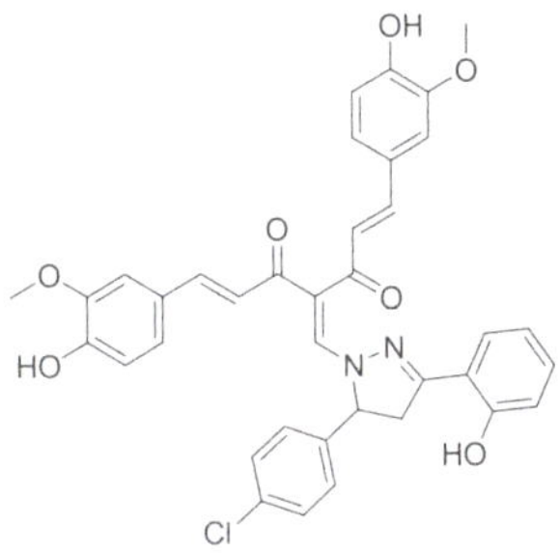

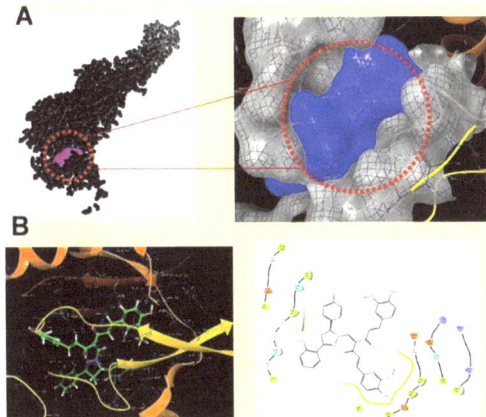

Figure 36. Structure of compound **33**, an IKK kinase inhibitor.

Molecular docking of compound **33** and other derivatives was performed with the crystal structure of IKKβ in the hinge region as the ATP binding site for favorable interactions (Figure 37). The co-crystallized inhibitor KSA was employed as the control ligand. Curcumin interacts with the gatekeeper residue Glu97, forms a hydrogen bond with Asp166, and has several hydrophobic interactions with the activation loop. Most of the designed compounds interacted with Glu97 and Cys99 residues, which was ATP's adenine target during ATP's interaction with the catalytic domain of IKKβ. Compound **33** interacts with Glu97 and Cys99 of the binding pocket of the receptor through the hydroxyl oxygen of curcumin's backbone, while hydroxyl's oxygen at pyrazole accepts hydrogen bonds from Gly24 and Thr23. Carbonyl oxygen of curcumin forms a hydrogen bond interaction with Asn150 [48].

Figure 37. Compound **33**'s molecular docking complex with IKKβ. (**A**) Interaction complex of IKKβ with compound **33** (docking score = −11.874). Next to it the zoomed-in view of the interaction of compound **33** into binding grooves displayed in surface binding view. (**B**) 3D view of compound **33** (ball-stick view) binding mode with key amino acids (cartoon view). The 2D pose view is also shown next to it [48].

13. Pyrazole-Based IRAK Inhibitors

13.1. Compound 34

The interleukin-1 receptor associated kinase 4 (IRAK4) is an intracellular serine-threonine kinase that is an upstream protein for IL-1R/TLR signaling pathway. This family of kinases includes IRAK1, IRAK2, and IRAK-M in addition to IRAK4. Inhibition of IRAK4 is a potential therapeutic target for treatment of inflammation. Compound **34** (Figure 38) has been reported as a potent and selective inhibitor of IRAK4 (IC_{50} = 5 nM).

It was tested at 1 µM concentration against 108 kinases and only the IRAK4 was more than 80% inhibited. Replacement of the methyl group attached to the pyridyl ring with bulkier alkyl substituents decreased the potency. Moreover, replacement of the methyl attached to the piperazine ring with isopropyl or sulfonyl led to poor aqueous solubility. Likewise, replacement of the pyridyl and piperazinyl rings with two phenyl rings decreased aqueous solubility and weakened the potency against IRAK4 (IC_{50} = 690 nM). The aqueous solubility of compound **34** at pH 7 is 156 µM. At the cellular level, compound **34** exerted strong potency (IC_{50} = 83 nM) against the lipopolysaccharide-induced THP1-XBlue cells. It is also orally active in the mice antibody-induced arthritis model and inhibited cytokine release [49].

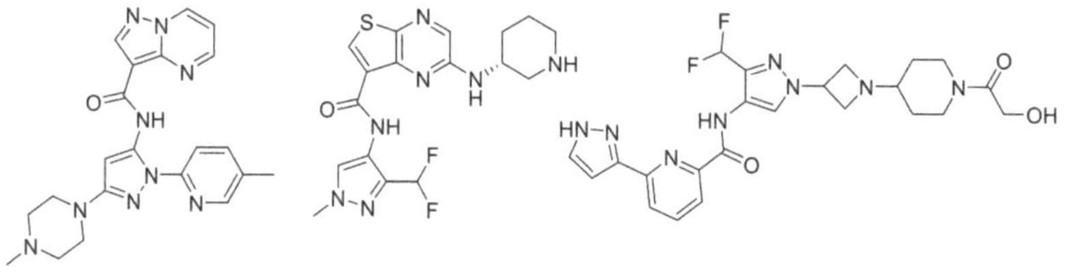

Figure 38. Structures of pyrazole-based IRAK4 inhibitors and their IC_{50} values.

13.2. Compound 35

Compound **35** (Figure 38) has been reported as a potent IRAK4 inhibitor with an IC_{50} value of 0.4 nM. In addition, it exerted cellular activity against human peripheral blood mononuclear cells (hPBMCs) with IC_{50} value = 3 nM. Upon testing in MDCK cells, compound **35** was found to possess good permeability (25×10^{-6} cm/s). Replacement of the thienopyrazine nucleus with pyrazolo[1,5-a]pyrimidine led to a decreased permeability despite higher potency in a cell-free assay against the IRAK4 kinase. On the other hand, replacement of the thienopyrazine nucleus with pyrrolo[2,1-f][1,2,4]triazine or pyrrolo[1,2-b]pyridazine slightly increased the permeability but reduced the potency against IRAK4. Thus compound **35** is the most balanced derivative among these analogues with high potency and permeability [50].

13.3. Compound 36

Compound **36** (Figure 38) is a recently patented compound that possesses an IC_{50} value of 0.51 nM against IRAK4. The series analogues are claimed for treatment of autoimmune diseases, inflammatory disorders, and cancer. Any substitution of the pyrazole NH or any modification of the alcoholic side chain attached to the piperidine ring led to reduced potency against IRAK4 [51].

14. Pyrazole-Based ITK Inhibitors

14.1. Compounds 37 and 38

The Interleukin-2 inducible T-cell kinase (ITK) is a member of the Tec tyrosine kinase family that is a T-cell signaling downstream of the T-cell receptor. Inhibition of ITK can help treat inflammatory disorders such as asthma. A research group at Genentech Inc. has reported the development and optimization of a series of pyrazole-based ITK inhibitors. In the beginning, they reported a series of indazole derivatives out of which compound **37** (Figure 39) is the most potent ITK inhibitor (K_i = 0.1 nM). Compound **37** inhibited the phospholipase C-gamma (PLCγ) kinase with a K_i value of 25 nM. Despite the strong potency of compound **37** against ITK, it suffers from poor PK properties. For example, it is orally unavailable in rats. In addition, it suffers from poor permeability in MDCK (0.3×10^{-6} cm/s). Furthermore, it is not a selective ITK inhibitor. When tested at 0.1 µM concentration over 218 kinases, it exerted more than 70% inhibition of 58 kinases [52]. The group decided to replace indazole with tetrahydroindazole and replaced the pyrazole ring attached to it with geminal dimethyl (compound **38**, GNE-9822, Figure 39) with the aim of improving kinase selectivity and ADME properties (Figure 40). GNE-9822 inhibits ITK with a K_i value of 0.7 nM. In addition, it is much more selective than compound **37**. At 0.1 μM concentration, it showed >70% inhibition of only six out of 286 tested kinases. Moreover, its K_i value against PLCγ equals 55 nM. The enantiomer of compound **38** is much less potent against ITK (K_i = 15 nM) and starts showing inhibitory effects against the Aurora **37** kinase (K_i = 170 nM). The permeability of GNE-9822 in MDCK improved significantly (4.6×10^{-6} cm/s) and oral bioavailability in rat increased to 40% following a 5 mg/kg dose (compared to 0% in the case of compound **37**) [53].

37 Ki = 0.1 nM

38 (GNE-9822) Ki = 0.5 nM

39 (GNE-4997) Ki = 0.09 nM

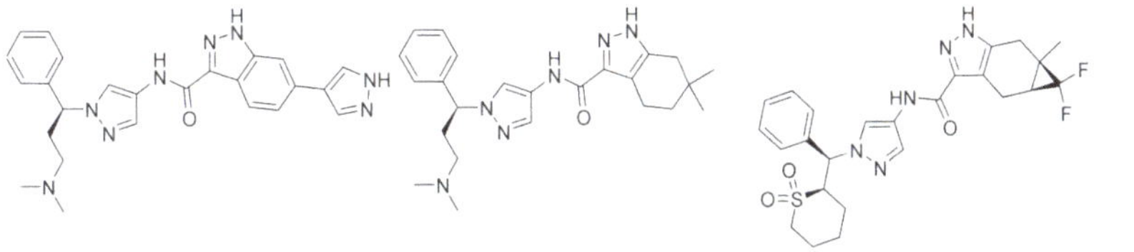

Figure 39. Structures of pyrazole-based ITK inhibitors and their Ki values.

37

38 (GNE-9822)

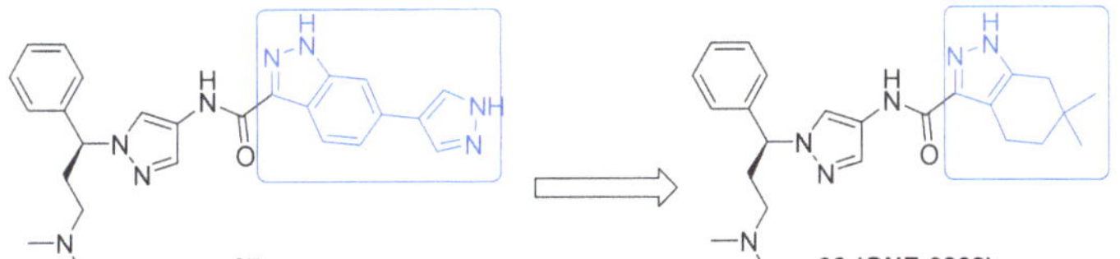

Figure 40. Development of compound **38** (GNE-9822) from compound **37** and the replacement of terminal 6-pyrazoloindazole with dimethyl-tetrahydroindazole.

The real binding mode of GNE-9822 with the ITK kinase was studied by X-ray crystallography (Figure 41). One methyl group attached to the tetrahydroindazole nucleus interacts hydrophobically with Phe435. The benzylic phenyl also forms a hydrophobic interaction with Phe437. In addition, the tetrahydroindazole *NH* donates a hydrogen bond to Glu436 [53].

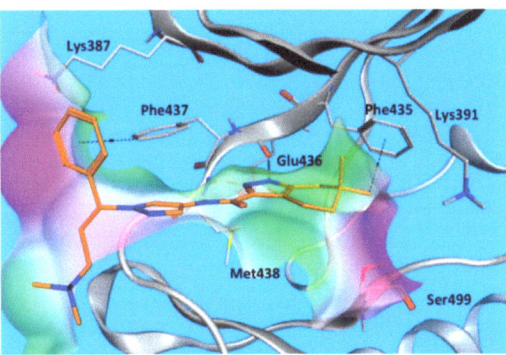

Figure 41. Co-crystal binding interactions of GNE-9822 (compound **38**) with ITK [53].

14.2. Compound **39**

The same group of Genentech Inc. did further structural modification in order to enhance potency and selectivity, and at the same time reduce toxicity. They omitted the basic solubilizing moiety of the last series (dimethylamino-possessing side chain) and replaced it with cyclic sulfone. The less basic molecule **39** (GNE-4997) (Figure 39) exerted less toxicity than GNE-9822 (% inhibition values of hERG at 10 µM concentration are 6.8% and 88%, respectively). In addition, the potency of GNE-4997 against ITK increased significantly to reach a K_i value of 0.09 nM. Furthermore, GNE-4997 could reduce IL-2 and IL-13 production in mice. The 6-membered sulfone ring is optimal for potency against ITK compared to the corresponding 5-membered or open chain sulfone as well as the 6-membered sulfinyl (S=O) [54].

GNE-4997 bound with the ITK kinase cocrystal was studied by X-ray (Figure 42). Its amide hydrogen donates a hydrogen bond to Met438 carbonyl. The pyrazole ring anchors the molecule into the hinge region through the formation of two hydrogen bonds with *NH* of Met438 and carbonyl of Glu436. The cyclic sulfone ring plays a role in orientating the phenyl ring towards Phe437. Lastly, difluoromethylene occupies a hydrophobic pocket near the Phe435 gatekeeper residue [54].

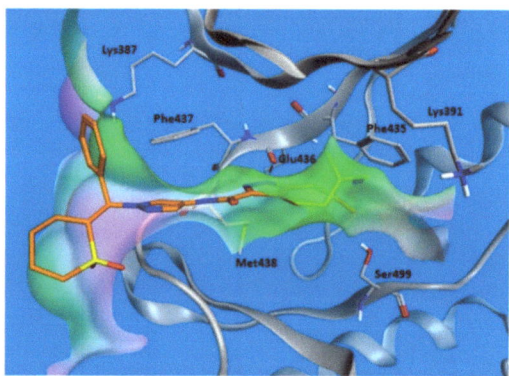

Figure 42. Co-crystal binding interactions of GNE-4997 (compound **39**) with ITK [54].

In conclusion, GNE-4997 possesses several advantages over compounds **37** and **38**. It is a more potent ITK inhibitor, less toxic, with retained kinase selectivity. It may require further optimization in the future to improve its aqueous solubility, which is only 3.9 µM (17.4-fold less than GNE-9822) [54].

15. Pyrazole-Based JAK Inhibitors

15.1. Compounds **40** and **41**

A series of JAK inhibitors were designed and synthesized based on a lead compound from a previous work done by the same research group (Figure 43). Their previous finding showed that substitution on pyrazole's *N* has no effect on activity, so by omitting the substituent on pyrazole's *N*, focusing on the bioisosteric ring replacement of the central pyrimidine ring, and hoping to discover novel compounds with improved activity, three series were developed and compared based on their biological results. The three series were composed of three different central rings—a pyrimdine ring, a quinazoline fused ring and a pyrrolo[2,3-*d*]pyrimidine fused ring. Additional variations to the structures to investigate SAR were sought, such as changing the tether link's length between the phenylamine derivative and the central heterocycle ring and having a different substituent on the distal phenyl ring (Figure 44) [55].

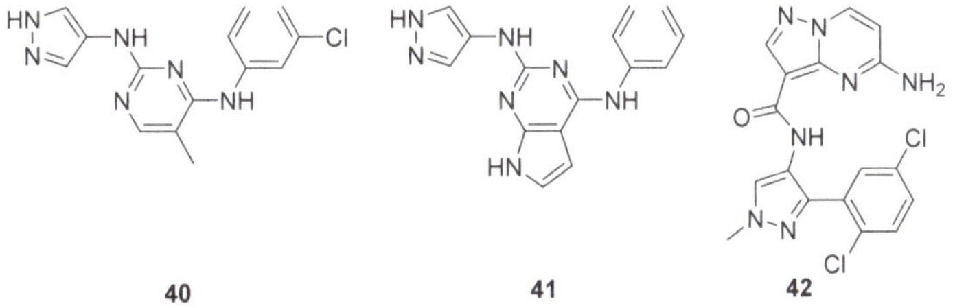

Figure 43. Structures of pyrazole-based JAK inhibitors and their IC_{50}/Ki values.

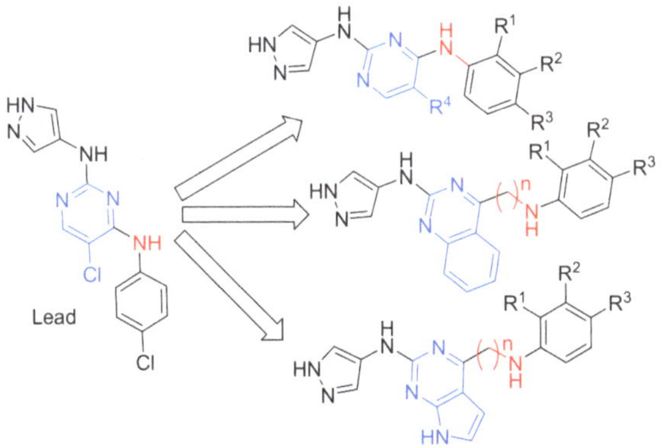

40
IC_{50} = 3.4 nM (JAK1)
IC_{50} = 2.2 nM (JAK2)
IC_{50} = 3.5 nM (JAK3)

41

42
Ki = 2.5 nM (JAK2)

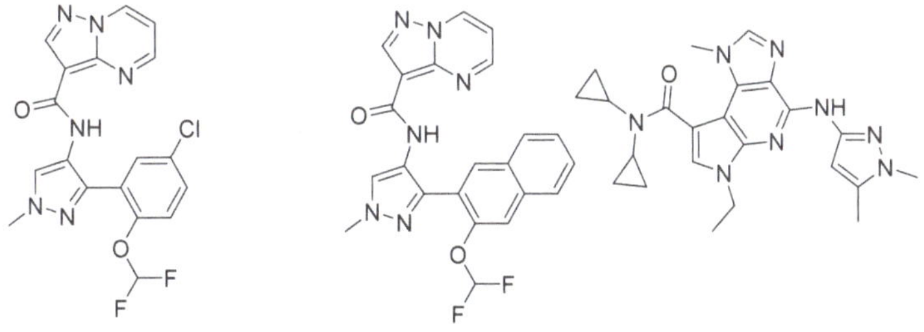

43
Ki = 0.21 nM (JAK1)
Ki = 0.088 nM (JAK2)

44
Ki = 0.31 nM (JAK1)
Ki = 0.14 nM (JAK2)

45 (BMS-911543)
IC_{50} = 75 nM (JAK1)
IC_{50} = 1.1 nM (JAK2)
IC_{50} = 360 nM (JAK3)

Figure 44. Schematic view of general designed compounds synthesized and tested.

The different derivatives were tested in vitro against three JAK subtypes (JAK1,2 and 3) in a kinase assay at different concentrations, screened at 20 nM (as they were interested in activities in the nanomolar range only), and compared to positive control staurosporine (a prototypical ATP-competitive kinase inhibitor; IC_{50}: JAK1 3 nM, JAK2 2 nM, JAK3 1 nM) and Ruxolitinib (an approved JAK inhibitor; inhibition at 20 nM: JAK1 97%, JAK2 99%, JAK3 95%). The quinazoline fused ring lost activity, and pyrrolo[2,3-*d*]pyrimidine had a moderate activity at 20 nM while pyrimidine-based derivatives showed high activity at 20 nM. Compound **40** (Figure 43) inhibited JAK1, 2 and 3 at 20 nM with an inhibition of 88%, 80%, and 79% respectively. The IC_{50} values measured for **40** on JAK1, 2 and 3 were 3.4, 2.2, and 3.5 nM, respectively. Activity dropped upon replacing the Chlorine atom on the pyrimidine ring with hydrogen or fluorine atoms [55].

Next, derivatives were tested against the HEL (human erythroleukemia) cell line since the mutation JH2 pseudokinase domain of the Janus kinase 2 gene (JAK2 V617F) existed in it. Compounds were screened at 5 µM and the results were consistent with the trend seen in the kinase profile. The most active compounds (pyrimidine series and pyrrolo[2,3-b]pyrimidine series) were further tested against human prostate cancer PC-3, human breast cancer MCF-7, human erythroleukemia HEL, human myelogenous leukemia K562, and human lymphoid leukemia MOLT4 cell lines, while having ruxolitinib as the reference standard. Oddly, the pyrimidine series showed high antiproliferative activity against all cell lines tested (e.g., compound **40** IC_{50} against: PC-3 IC_{50} = 1.08 µM, MCF-7 IC_{50} = 1.33 µM, HEL IC_{50} = 1.08 µM, K562 IC_{50} = 0.77 µM, MOLT4 IC_{50} = 1.61 µM), while **41** showed remarkable selectivity to HEL (IC_{50} = 0.35 µM) and K562 (IC_{50} = 0.37 µM) (Figure 43). In addition to that, the compounds were inferior to ruxolitinib in kinase assay yet superior in cell-based assay, suggesting an off-target effect. To screen the off-target activity, two best representative compounds (**40** and **41**) were tested against multiple kinases. Compound **40** had an activity against Flt-3, VEGFR-2, PDGFRα, and TYK2 while **41** showed selectivity to JAK2 and 3 over the other tested kinases. These results explain the reason behind compound **40**′s activity against multiple cell lines and **41**′s activity against HEL and K562 cell lines. Docking of compound **40** in JAK2′s ATP binding pocket revealed the contribution by pyrazoles' nitrogens in H-bonding with Glu930 and Leu932 (Figure 45) [55].

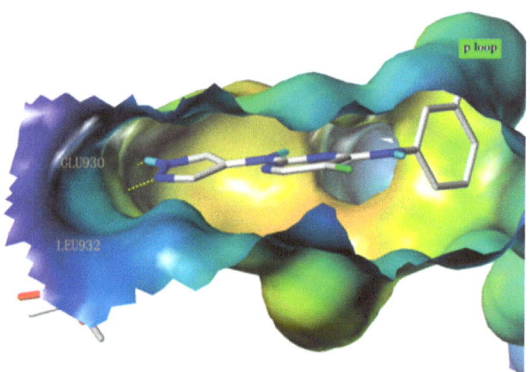

Figure 45. Docking of compound **40** with JAK2 crystal structure [55].

15.2. Compound **42**

Philadelphia (Ph)-negative myeloproliferative disorders are a group of hematological disorders at the pluripotent hematopoietic stem cell level. These disorders include essential thrombocythemia, idiopathic myelofibrosis, and polycythemia vera. Activating mutation in JAK2 has a role in the progression of the disease by activating JAK-STAT signaling pathways [56].

Although a number of clinical candidates that are known small molecule JAK inhibitors for myeloproliferative disorder therapy are being clinically developed, and FDA approval of pan-JAK inhibitor ruxilitinib for the treatment of intermediate or high-risk myelofibrosis has confirmed and validated JAK as a clinical target for myeloproliferative disorders, no selective JAK2 inhibitor has been investigated yet. Ruxilitinib inhibits JAK1 and JAK2 equivalently, while the inhibition of JAK3 and Tyk2 is less pronounced. The JAK2 selective inhibitor will potentially improve the safety index; hence, chronic administration for the treatment of MRDs as well as decreasing the immunosuppressive side effects arising by inhibiting other members of JAK such as JAK1, JAK3, or Tyk2) is required. The degree of selectivity towards JAK2 over JAK1 is still unknown, but the group envisioned at least a 10-fold selectivity towards JAK2 over JAK1 for a potential biological activity [57].

Discovery of the lead compound was achieved through high-throughput screening. The Pyrazolo[1,5-*a*]pyrimidine scaffold showed promising inhibitory activity against JAK2, with a nearly 10-fold selectivity to JAK2 over JAK1 and an even better selectivity against other members. Further lead optimization studies were performed to discover the selective, potent and orally active compound **42** (Figure 43). The lead compound, a 2-amino compound (Figure 46), showed a K_i of 2.5 nM inhibition against JAK2, potent inhibitory activity with an IC_{50} of 131 nM in a JAK2-driven SET2 cell-based assay through measuring the inhibition of pSTAT5, which is a downstream target of JAK2, low potential for reversible inhibition of five major human CYP450 isozymes, good in vitro permeability profile, moderate selectivity (~9–30×) against the other JAK family members and excellent selectivity when tested against a 177-kinase panel. Yet the lead had some limitations, the most important ones being low microsomal stability in five different species and poor thermodynamic aqueous solubility. In vivo pharmacokinetic profiling was done on rats and mice. The lead compound showed low plasma clearances in both mice and rats (3 and 6.8 mL/min/kg, respectively), extremely low V_d in both species (V_{dss} = 0.27 and 0.19 L/kg, respectively), and high plasma protein binding in both species (98.7% and 99.6%, respectively) which explained the low plasma clearance and low volume of distribution. The lead compound also had poor oral bioavailability in mice and rats (8.6% and 1%, respectively), which can be explained by poor aqueous solubility; hence, permeability was efficient. The group's hypothesis for the poor aqueous solubility was due to high crystal packing forces hence multiple aromatic rings (four) and multiple potential hydrogen bond donors (HBDs) and acceptors (HBAs) exist in the structure of the lead compound, and not due to the high hydrophobicity of the compound, since the cLogP was 2.1. The two other lead compounds, the 2-des-amino compound and the 2-methylamino compound (Figure 47), were also investigated to explore the impact of removing HBD on oral bioavailability and other limitations shown by the 2-amino compounds. The 2-des-amino compound showed improved oral exposure compared to the 2-amino compound (F_{oral} = 44% vs. 1%); the improvement might be due to the greater kinetic aqueous solubility of 2-des-amino compared to the 2-amino compound hence both compounds showed similar thermodynamic solubility as well as similar permeability in MDCK cells. The rat plasma clearance and the V_d of the 2-des-amino compound was similar to the 2-amino compound. The activity in both the enzymatic assay against JAK2 and the cellular assay were nearly 10-fold less potent compared to the 2-amino compound. The 2-methylamino compound showed higher free fraction on rat plasma compared to 2-amino compound (1.7% vs. 0.4%), which expectedly showed a high clearance in rat microsomes compared to the 2-amino compound (48 vs. 39 mL/min/kg). The oral bioavailability of the 2-methylamino was higher compared to the 2-amino compound (F_{oral} (%) = 30 vs. 1) which can be explained by the improved kinetic aqueous solubility. The 2-methylamino compound was only 2-fold less potent compared to the 2-amino compound in the JAK2 enzymatic assay (K_i = 5.1 nM) [57].

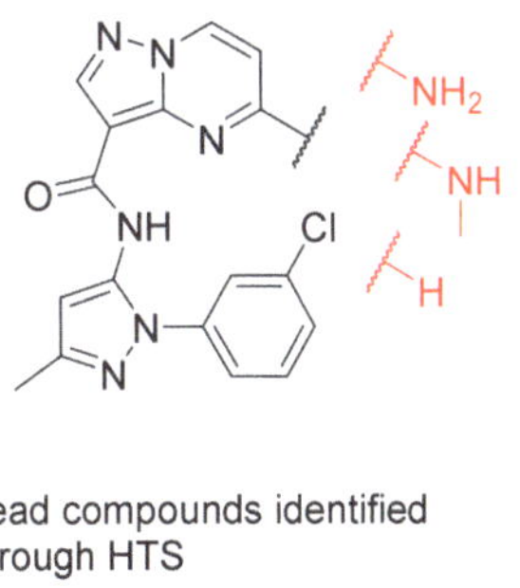

Figure 46. Depicting the structure of Pyrazolo[1,5-a]pyrimidine scaffold lead compounds discovered through HTS.

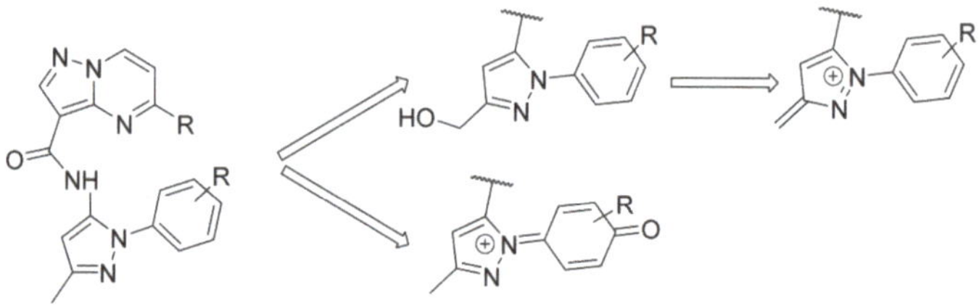

Figure 47. Schematic view of possible active metabolites formed in the 3-methyl-N-arylpyrazole core.

Another limitation predicted by the group and one they decided to work on was the formation of potential reactive metabolites of lead compounds, hence lead compounds showed poor solubility as well as poor human liver microsomal stability. The 3-methyl-N-arylpyrazole center in the lead compound is especially critical in the formation of potential reactive metabolites, so the N-aryl moiety could be oxidized to paraquinoneimine, since the group hypothesized the role an electron rich aryl ring could play in contributing to the poor microsomal stability. In addition to that, the 3-methyl substituent is concerning since it can be oxidized in a two-step fashion into the pyrazoleiminium species through the oxidation of the 3-methylalcohol metabolite (Figure 47) [57].

The 2-des-amino compound's co-crystal structure with JAK2 revealed two bonds of a pyrazolo[1,5-*a*]pyrimidine core and the active sites which were a hydrogen bond between *N1* and Leu932 backbone's *NH*, and a weak, non-classical, yet possible H-bond between *C7'*s *CH* and Glu930 backbone carbonyl (although the distance of H-bond is long (3.4 Å)). The phenyl ring occupies the hydrophobic sugar pocket of the ATP binding site. The amide's carbonyl and *N2* of pyrazole formed H-bond with waters. The sequence homology of JAK1 and JAK2 is quite similar, yet some differences exist and can be targeted to discover a selective inhibitor. The group decided to exploit Asp939 in JAK2 (in close proximity to pyrazole's methyl substituent), which is equivalent to Glu966 in JAK1, in order to improve selectivity between the two isoforms (Figure 48) [57].

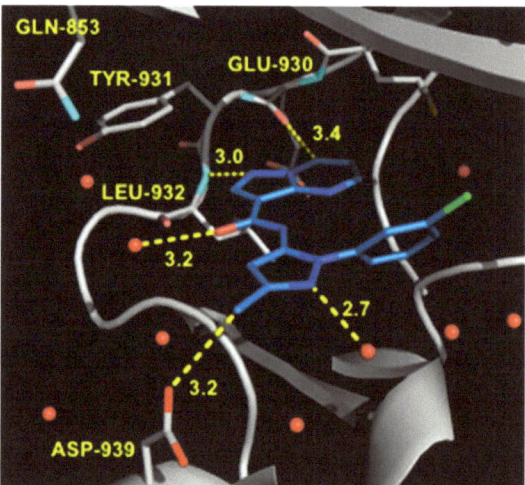

Figure 48. Co-crystal structure of 2-des-amino compound in the active site of the JAK2 kinase domain (2.3 Å). P-loop removed to allow a better view of the key active site interactions. Dashed lines = close contacts between ligand and protein with distances labeled in Å [57].

Bioisosteric replacement of the 3-methyl-N-arylpyrazole moiety of the 2-des-amino compound with various pyridine analogues as well as regioisomers of pyrazole were prepared and tested. In summary, the pyridinyl compounds were active yet not as active as the pyrazoles. The most active compound was compound **A** (Figure 49) with a K_i of 3.2 nM and a selectivity of 8.1-fold towards JAK2 over JAK1, 36.5-fold towards JAK2 over JAK3 and 18.3-fold towards JAK2 over Tyk2. Compound **H**'s activity was superior to the other regioisomer of pyrazole, which can be explained by the high energy required for the amide and pyrazole groups to adopt a coplanar conformation that is caused by the lone pair repulsion of the N2 of pyrazole and lone pair of the amide's oxygen. In addition to that, the binding mode of the 2-des-amino compound showed an interaction between the N2 of pyrazole and water. This interaction is lacking in regioisomeric pyrazole due to the absence of HBA in that position, while compound **H** retains such a position and bonding. The activity of compound **H** is superior to the 2-des-amino compound which might be due to higher polarization of the *CH* bond of N-methyl moiety of compound **H** compared to the C-methyl moiety in the 2-des-amino compound. The improved polarizability might improve bonding between the N-methyl group and Asp939. In terms of acidity, the 2-des-amino compound's methyl is more acidic compared to compound **H** hence resonance stabilization is a factor when it comes to the resulting anion (calculated pKa 40 vs. 43 respectively). Yet the partial positive charge on the N-methyl moiety in compound **H** is greater because of the greater polarization. Rat plasma clearance of compound **H** was similar to that of the 2-des-amino compound (12.5 vs. 13.3 mL/min/kg). Oral bioavailability of compound **H** is higher in comparison to the 2-des-amino compound despite having poor kinetic and thermodynamic solubilities (both around 1 µM). A possible explanation given by the author is that compound **H** precipitated in crystalline form [57].

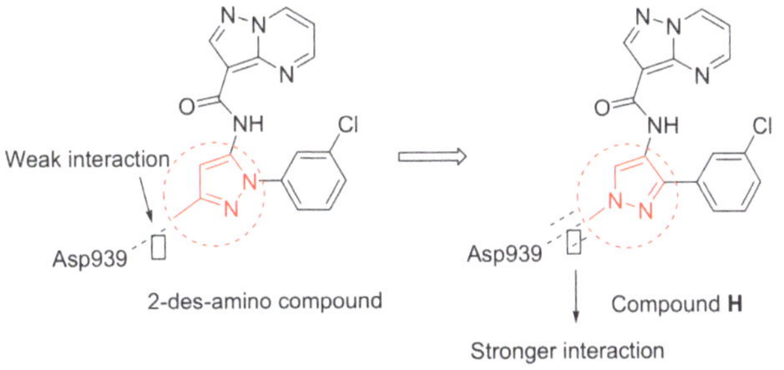

Figure 49. Schematic view of the steps in development and lead optimization.

Compound **H**'s activity persuaded the group to investigate similar modification on the 2-amino lead compound. The modification led to a 2-fold increase in potency, a slight improvement of selectivity towards JAK2 over JAK1, and predictable clearance through rat liver microsomes, yet the oral bioavailability was still low (around 7%). The low oral exposure was explained by the poor kinetic and thermodynamic aqueous solubility. The group decided to replace the N-methyl moiety with various substituents in order to improve solubility and stability against human liver microsomes. Although some physiochemical and pharmacokinetic improvements were discovered, the potency was affected dramatically. The group decided to modify the distal phenyl ring. This modification led to the discovery of **42**. It had a K_i of 0.1 nM against JAK1, <10-fold selectivity over JAK1, JAK3, Tyk2 towards JAK2, an IC_{50} of 7.4 nM against pSTAT5 (in Jak2-driven SET2 cell-based assay), good oral bioavailability (F_{oral}(%) = 63), which can be explained by low plasma clearance and high permeability, hence the solubility was poor and devoid of reversible CYP inhibition for the five major isoforms with only minimal time-dependent inhibition (TDI) of CYP3A4 (TDI IC_{50} = 5.8 µM with a 38% shift in AUC). Compound **42** was selective against a panel of 183 kinases (at 0.01 µM) and only inhibited 5 kinases outside the JAK family [57].

The excellent profile of compound **42** motivated the team to test on a SCID mouse the SET2 xenograft model that is dependent on JAK2 for growth, where the aim is to observe whether compound **42** can knock down the Jak2-mediated phosphorylation of STAT5. Sixty-four percent inhibition of pSTAT5 was observed at the 1-h time point at a dose of 100mg/Kg, and while the plasma concentration of compound **42** decreased, the inhibition of pSTAT5 also decreased [57].

15.3. Compounds 43 and 44

Interleukin-13 (IL-13) is a cytokine implemented in various allergic inflammations, so it can be exploited for the treatment of diseases such as asthma and atopic dermatitis. IL-13 activates three isoforms of JAKs (JAK1, JAK2 and Tyk2), thus inhibiting the JAKs' activity can prove clinically beneficial in the treatment of some allergic inflammation conditions. However, it is unknown which isoform is more important and has a bigger role in mediating the IL-13 effect. In this paper, the Genentech group that worked on compound **42** (Figure 43) explored the possibility of JAK1 inhibition in mediating and controlling the IL-13 effect. The group developed compounds **43** and **44** (Figure 43) through different rounds of SAR analysis. The lead compound was modified first at position 2 and when it was replaced with a different substituent, the most potent compound was compound **43** with the substituent's difluromethoxy moiety (Figure 50) [58].

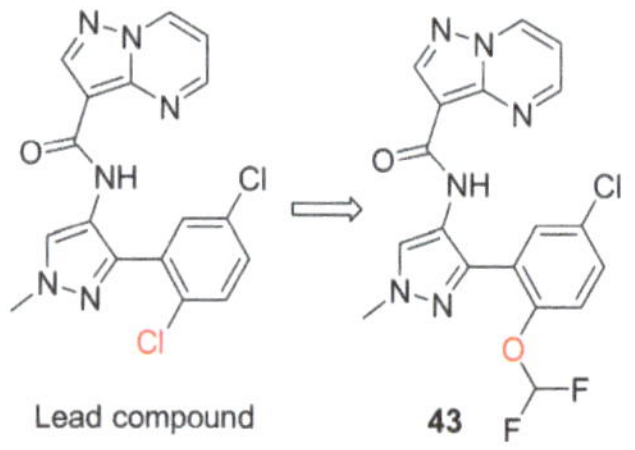

Figure 50. Schematic view the development of **43**.

Compound **43** has a K_i of 0.21 nM against JAK1, K_i of 0.088 nM against JAK2, and exhibited an IC_{50} of 4.7 nM in IL-13 stimulated BEAS-2B cells monitored for pSTAT6 formation in the presence or absence of a JAK inhibitor (IL-13-pSTAT6 cell-based assay). In the X-ray crystal structure, the difluromethoxyphenyl moiety had Van der Waals interactions with Leu1010 and side chain methylene of Ser963. The fluorine atom forms dipolar interactions with the backbone carbonyl carbon of Gly1020. The polarized hydrogen atom of the difluoromethoxy group forms a non-classical hydrogen bond with the backbone carbonyl of Arg1007. The pyrazolopyrimidine core binds to the hinge region (Leu959 and Glu957) and interacts with the gatekeeper Met956 side chain, the N-methyl binds to Glu 966, and the chlorine atom interacts through Van der Waals interaction with the P-loop region (Figure 51) [58].

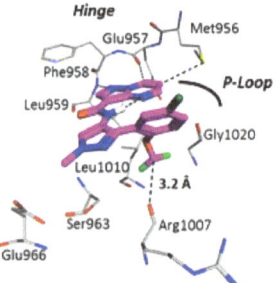

Figure 51. X-ray crystal structures of compound **43** in complex with JAK1 [58].

The next step undertaken was the modification of the heterocyclic tether (pyrazole) with the idea of improving co-planarity between the heterocycle and the amide. This modification led to a loss of activity. The last set of modifications was done to the distal phenyl moiety with a different substituent or by replacing the phenyl ring with other rings, leading to the discovery of compound **44**. Compound **44** had a K_i of 0.31 nM against JAK1, a K_i of 0.14 nM against JAK2, and an IC_{50} of 6.4 nM in the IL-13-pSTAT6 cell-based assay. To test the series' selectivity, a sample compound was screened on a panel of 71 kinases and showed off-target activity against LRRK2 and FYN. The LRRK2 activity is concerning since it has a role in lung toxicity. Both compounds **43** and **44** were 47-fold and 83-fold more selective respectively towards JAK1 over LRRK2. Lastly, the series was tested for its metabolic stability and it exhibited poor to moderate stability against human liver microsomes. This series of compounds showed interesting biological activity and requires further development [58].

15.4. Compound 45

The JAK2-V617F mutation activates JAK/STAT signaling pathway which has a role in the progression of myeloproliferative disorders MPD). Compound **45** (BMS-911543, Figure 43) was developed and discovered to be an inhibitor of JAK2. The group discussed the development from a lead compound which had a 4,5-dimethylthiazole ring instead of the pyrazole of compound **45**. The X-ray crystal structure of the lead compound showed an interaction between the N of pyrazole with the Tyr931 residue through H-bonding. It also showed unfavorable interactions of dimethyl moieties with non-conserved residues in the extended hinge region of other JAK family members, but this unfavorable interaction provided high selectivity which was desirable (Figure 52). The biggest drawback of the thiazole compound was its ADMET profile where it exhibited formation of reactive metabolites across species due to microsomal instability. Thiazole moiety of the lead compound was modified in its substituent or replaced with other heterocylces such as triazole and pyrazole. BMS-911543 was discovered and showed an IC_{50} of 1.1 nM against JAK2, an IC_{50} of 75, 360 and 66 nM on JAK1, JAK3 and Tyk2, respectively. The X-ray crystal structure of BMS-911543 was similar to the lead compound [59].

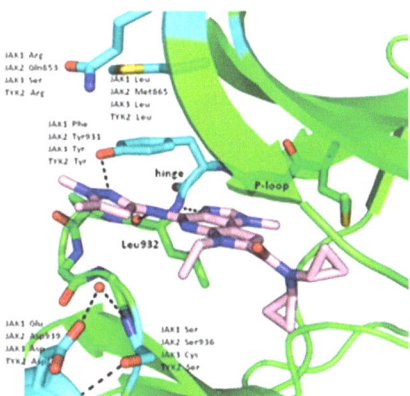

Figure 52. X-ray crystallized BMS-911543 (**45**) bound to the kinase catalytic domain of JAK2; Pick = BMS-911543's Carbon; Green = JAK2's carbon green; Cyan = residues near the C-4 group, which differ in the JAK family; dashed lines = hydrogen bonds [59].

16. Pyrazole-Based JNK Inhibitors

16.1. Compound 46

c-Jun N-terminal kinases (JNK) are MAPKs that play a crucial role in inflammatory disorders. Compound **46** (Figure 53) is the most potent JNK-1 inhibitor among a series of pyrazole carboxamide derivatives (IC$_{50}$ = 2.8 µM). It was tested for in vivo anti-inflammatory activity against carrageenan-induced paw edema model in rats and reduced the paw inflammation by 73.11%, 81.81%, 91.89%, and 66.33% after 1, 2, 3, and 4 h following the injection. The furan ring of compound **46** was the most optimal for activity compared to the substituted phenyl, isoxazole, thiazole, pyridine, naphthalene, benzimidazole, or cyclopropyl. The docking study showed that compound **46** is an ATP-competitive inhibitor of the JNK-1 kinase. Its phenyl ring forms hydrophobic interactions with Val40 and Leu168. The pyrazole *NH* donates a hydrogen bond to the carbonyl backbone of Glu109, and the amide oxygen accepts a hydrogen bond from *NH* of Met111. The pyrazole ring faces Ile32, Leu110, and Val158 hydrophobic residues (Figure 54) [60].

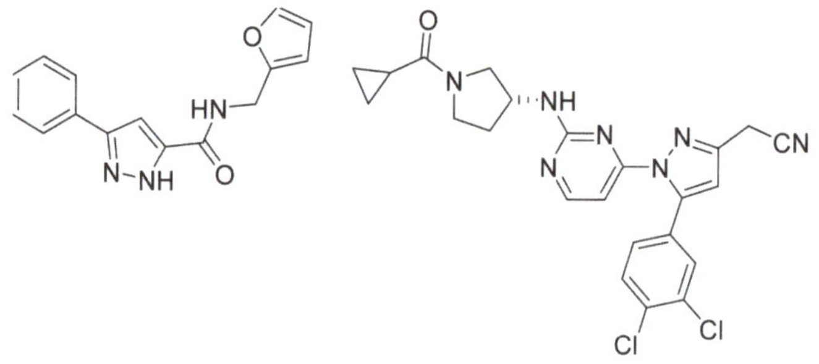

46
IC$_{50}$ = 2800 nM (JNK1)

47
IC$_{50}$ = 227 nM (JNK3)

Figure 53. Structures of pyrazole-based JNK inhibitors and their IC$_{50}$ values.

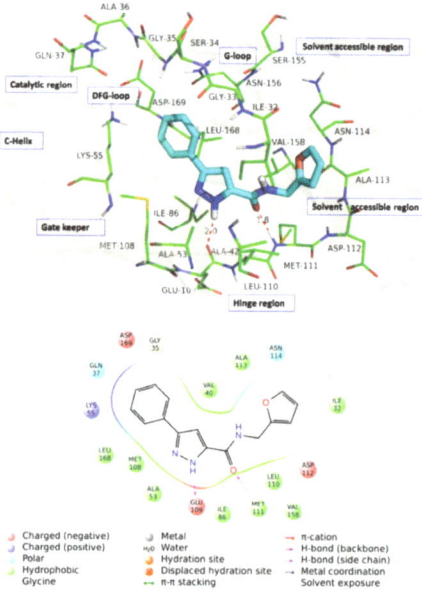

Figure 54. Docking pose and putative binding interactions of compound **46** with JNK-1 kinase crystal structure [60].

16.2. Compound 47

JNK3 is a potential target for neurodegenerative disorder therapy. Compound 47 (Figure 53) is a pyrazole-based selective JNK3 inhibitor whose IC_{50} value against the kinase is 227 nM. It was tested against a 38-kinase panel and was favored over JNK3. The SAR of this series indicated that 3,4-dichlorophenyl is more optimal for JNK3 inhibition than nitrophenyl, naphthyl, or other fused bicyclic rings. In addition, the nitrile group is more favorable than the primary amide. The docking study was carried out and the binding mode is illustrated in Figure 55. The aminopyrimidinyl is the hinge region-binding moiety of this structure. It forms two hydrogen bonds with Met149. The carbonyl oxygen of compound 47 accepts a hydrogen bond from Gln155. In addition, the cyano nitrogen accepts two hydrogen bonds from the backbone and side chain of Asn152. Lastly, the dichlorophenyl ring occupies a hydrophobic pocket and forms hydrophobic interactions. Its meta-chloro atom forms a halogen bond with Lys93 [61].

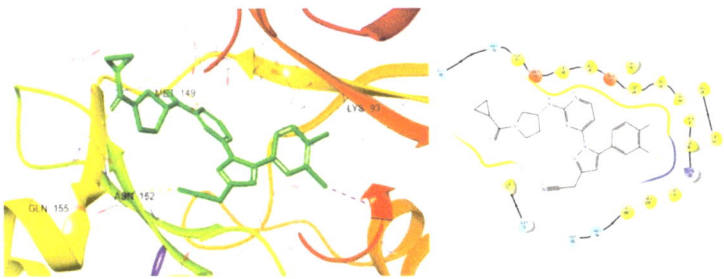

Figure 55. Putative binding mode of compound 47 with JNK3 crystal structure [61].

17. Pyrazole-Based LRRK Inhibitors

17.1. Compounds 48–50

Leucine-rich repeat kinase 2 (LRRK2) is a potential target for treatment of Parkinson's disease. Compounds 49 (GNE-0877) and 50 (GNE-9605) were developed via structural optimization of the solvent-exposed part of the ATP-binding site of compound 48 in order to improve human hepatocyte stability and brain exposure to the molecule, and to decrease the compound's ability to inhibit or induce CYP (Figures 56 and 57). The Ki values of compounds 48–50 against LRRK2 are 9, 0.7, and 2 nM, respectively. In addition, the IC_{50} values of the three compounds against pLRRK2 are 28, 3, and 19 nM, respectively. So the structural modifications done in compounds 49 and 50 led to improved potency. In addition, the brain-to-plasma ratio of compounds 49 and 50 in rats are 0.6 and 0.51, respectively, which is higher than that of compound 48 (0.37). Furthermore, the oral bioavailability of compounds 49 and 50 following 1 mg/kg administration in rats is 35% and 74%, respectively [62].

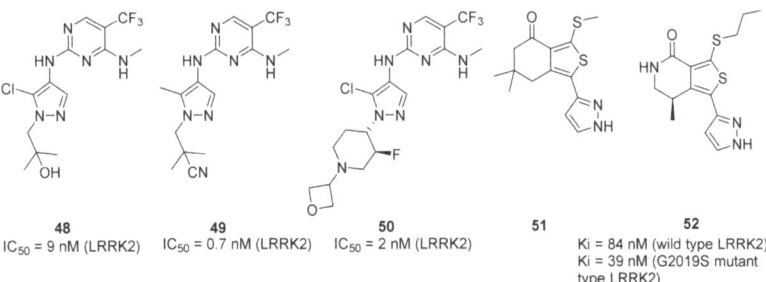

Figure 56. Structures of pyrazole-based LRRK inhibitors and their IC_{50}/Ki values.

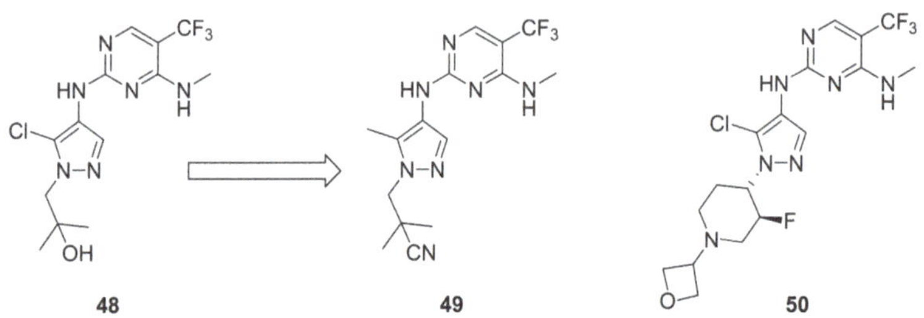

Figure 57. Development of compounds 49 and 50 from structural modification of compound 48.

17.2. Compounds 51 and 52

Compound **51** (Figure 56) was identified through high throughput screening by the Merck company as an inhibitor of LRRK2. Structural optimization via insertion of the lactam led to improved CNS exposure and PK properties. In addition, the *N*-propylthio is more optimal for activity than isopropyl or other alkyl or cycloalkyl substituents attached to sulfur. Moreover, the methyl group attached to the lactam ring with this stereochemistry is the most favorable for activity compared to other alkyl substituents and other orientations (Figure 58). The K_i values of compound **52** (Figure 56) against the wild-type LRRK2 and the G2019S mutant-type LRRK2 kinases are 84 and 39 nM, respectively. Furthermore, the oral bioavailability of compound **52** is 98% after oral administration of 10 mg/kg in rats [63].

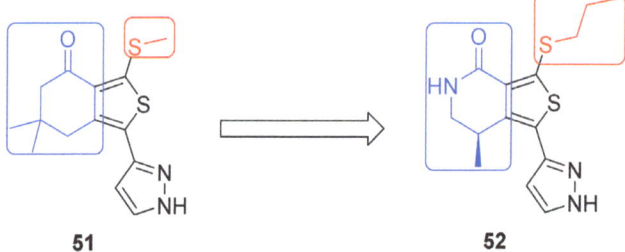

Figure 58. Development of compound **52** from **51** through introduction of amide lactam ring instead of cyclic ketone and extension of methylthio to propylthio.

18. Pyrazole-Based Lsrk Inhibitor

Compound 53

(*S*)-4,5-Dihydro-2,3-pentanedione (commonly known as (*S*)-DPD) is a small signaling molecule that is phosphorylated by LsrK kinase. The resultant phosphor-DPD activates bacterial quorum sensing (QS). Thus, LsrK inhibition can interfere with QS and can help fix the problem of bacterial resistance. A series of 1,3,5-trisubstituted pyrazole derivatives were reported as LsrK inhibitors. Compound **53** (Figure 59) is the most potent among this series but with modest potency (IC_{50} = 119 μM). The SAR study indicates that the pyrazole core is more favorable for LsrK inhibition than pyridine or pyrimidine. Moreover, *N*-methylpyrazole is more optimal than unsubstituted pyrazole or pyrazole-bearing higher alkyl, cycloalkyl, or phenyl at *N1*. Unsubstituted phenyl at position 3 of the pyrazole ring is more optimal compared to substituted phenyl, heteroaryl, or cyclohexyl. The docking of compound **53** into the LsrK crystal structure showed formation of only one hydrogen bond between an oxygen atom with Thr275 (Figure 60) [64,65].

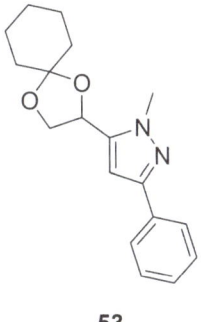

53

Figure 59. Structure of compound **53**, a pyrazole-based Lsrk inhibitor.

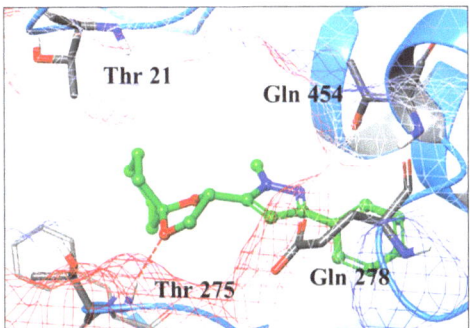

Figure 60. Docking pose of compound **53** into LsrK crystal structure [64,65].

19. Pyrazole-Based MEK/ERK Kinase Inhibitors

19.1. Compound 54

The 1,3,4-triarylpyrazole scaffold was employed in designing a series of diarylureas and diarylamides linkers with different substituents, and a chloro hydroxy or methoxy substituent on the phenyl ring targeting hydrogen bonds in the active site. This series was tested for antiproliferative activity on the A375P melanoma human cell line. The amide linkers had higher potency compared to their urea counterpart, with compound **54** (Figure 61) as the most potent in the series (IC_{50} = 6.7 µM), surpassing the FDA-approved multi-targeted kinase inhibitor sorafenib (IC_{50} = 11.5 µM). To investigate the potential mechanism of action, compound **54** was tested in different concentrations (1, 3, and 5 µM) against the ERK-containing A375P cell lysate and compared with sorafenib. Both compound **54** and sorafenib decreased phosphorylation of ERK1/2 in a dose-dependent pattern [66].

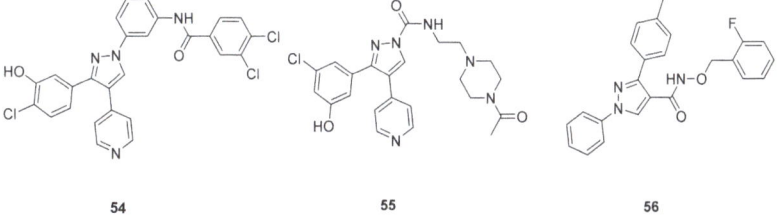

Figure 61. Structures of pyrazole-based MEK/ERK inhibitors.

19.2. Compound 55

Compound **55** (Figure 61) is part of a series consisting of a 3,4-diarylpyrazole center, with a variety of N-alkylcarboxamide chains. The inspiration behind designing and synthesizing this series was to target COX-2 and ERK1/2 simultaneously as suppressing both can have a desirable synergistic antiproliferative activity. Compound **55** exhibited an IC_{50} = 2.7 µM on MDA-MB-435 melanoma cell line. An investigation of the activity in suppressing the MEK/ERK pathway was performed using MEK/ERK-containing A375P cell lysate which was treated with three different concentrations (1, 3, and 10 µM) of test compounds including compound **55** and sorafenib for comparison. Compound **55** at 10 µM suppressed phosphorylation of MEK1/2 (inhibition percentage of 80.6%) and ERK1/2 (inhibition percentage of 87.5%) compared to sorafenib's results (80.7% & 94.9%, respectively) in a dose-dependent manner. To explore the prospect of COX-2 inhibition using an enzyme immunoassay, test compounds including **55** were studied and compared to celecoxib. The best compounds were further tested on COX-1 to determine the selectivity profile between the two enzymes. Compound **55** inhibited COX-2 with IC_{50} = 0.30 µM (celecoxib had an IC_{50} value of 0.29 µM), did not show any inhibition of COX-1 up to 50 µM (also celecoxib) and had a selectivity index of 166.67, which is comparable to celecoxib's selectivity index (172.41). Replacement of the hydroxyl group with methoxy diminished the activity. In addition, N-acetylpiperazinyl is more optimal than the corresponding analogues such as pyrrolidine, piperidine, morpholine, or dialkylamino. Furthermore, hydroxyl and chloro groups *meta* to one another are more favorable for activity than the *ortho*-disubstituted phenyl with the same two groups [67].

19.3. Compound 56

1,3-Diphenyl-N-benzyloxy-1H-pyrazole-4-carboxamide derivatives were synthesized and biologically evaluated. In vitro antiproliferative activity was measured using the MTT assay against three cancer cell lines (HeLa, MCF-7, and A549) and compared to gefitinib. Compound **56** (Figure 61) had the best results on the three cell lines with a GI_{50} of 1.18, 2.11, and 0.26 µM, respectively (gefitinib's results were 1.52 µM, 6.71 µM, 2.86 µM). Moreover, the toxicity of the series was investigated against the human kidney epithelial cell 293T and compound **56** showed a median cytotoxic concentration of 20.57 µM. Further tests to assess MEK inhibition using the recombinant proteins of RAF–MEK–ERK cascade kinase assay revealed that compound **56** had the best activity with an IC_{50} = 91 nM versus an IC_{50} = 89 nM by the positive control U0126. In addition, the phosphorylation level of ERK was measured in a cell-based assay which predictably inhibited the activity of ERK phosphorylation in the B-RAF mutant cell line which showed an IC_{50} of 0.61 µM and had an excellent selectivity profile [68].

Compound **56** was docked into the MEK1 active site to gain an insight of the binding interactions. The 1,3-diphenyl-1H-pyrazole scaffold occupied the ATP binding pocket deeply, showed a good shape complementarity, and exhibited hydrophobic interactions with multiple residues of the ATP binding pocket. On the other end, the chain with the aromatic end had a cation-pi interaction with Lys156 (Figure 62) [68].

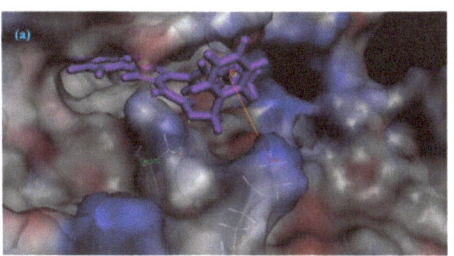
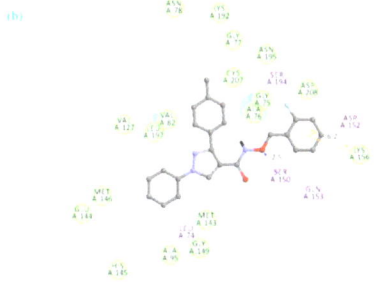

Figure 62. (a) Docking pose of compound **56** into the active site of the MEK1 protein-kinase. Hydrogen bond is illustrated as dashed line. (b) 2D binding mode of compound **56** with MEK1 active site [68].

20. Pyrazole-Based p38α/MAPK14 Kinase Inhibitors

20.1. Compound 57

P38α/MAPK1's role in inflammatory diseases is the control and management of the production of cytokines (tumornecrosis factor-α (TNF-α), interleukin-1 (IL-1), interleukin-6 (IL-6), and interleukin-1b (IL-1b)), thus regulating the downstream signaling that mediates inflammatory response. Inflammatory disorders such as rheumatoid arthritis, inflammatory bowel syndrome, and psoriasis can be managed with p38α /MAPK1 inhibition [69].

Based on that rationale, compound **57** (Figure 63) was discovered when a series of triarylpyrazoles where designed and synthesized as inhibitors of p38α /MAPK1. The series consisted of a pyrazole core, with three aryl arms around it. The phenol was designed as hydroxyl or methoxy derivatives, investigating the hydrophobicity as well as the potential of H-bonding. The *N*-phenyl arm was attached to the halogenated phenyl ring tethered with urea or amide linkers, testing the effect of the length of the tether as well as the possibility of extra H-bonding due to the additional *NH* group in the urea tether compared to amide [69].

The series was tested on a p38α /MAPK1 and a trend was noticed. The methoxy derivatives were superior to the hydroxyl derivatives, hinting at the presence of some hydrophobic pockets that can be accessed by a methoxy moiety. Another trend observed is the amide linker's higher activity compared to that of urea linkers. The different substituent on the terminal phenyl ring also showed intolerability towards bulkier substituents, and trifluoromethyl substituted phenyl rings are better for activity. Compound **57** with an amide linker showed the highest potency in the series (IC_{50} = 22 nM). Further testing on a panel of 40 kinases at 10 µM to determine the selectivity of compound **57** was performed. Compound **57** exerted over 50% inhibition to A-RAF, B-RAF (wild type), B-RAF (V600E), RAF1, c-MET, and p38α and less than 50% on the other 36 kinases. To test the inhibitory activity of compound **57** against the p38α inside the cells, the NanoBRET target engagement assay was performed against the HEK293 cells with MAPK14-NanoLuc®Fusion VectorDNA. Compound **57** showed an EC_{50} of 0.52 µM, which is comparable to dasatinib's 0.47 µM (positive reference), but lower than SB 203580's 0.06 µM (another positive control which is a potent p38α /MAPK1) [69].

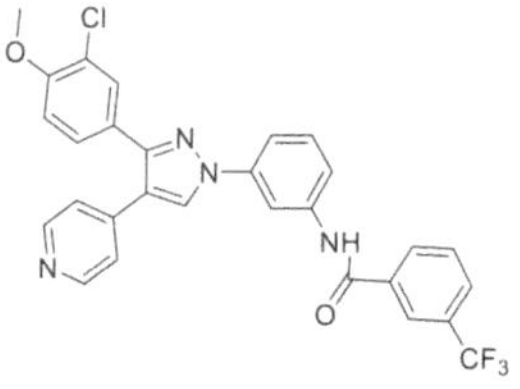

Figure 63. Structures of pyrazole-based p38α/MAPK14 kinase inhibitors and their IC_{50} values.

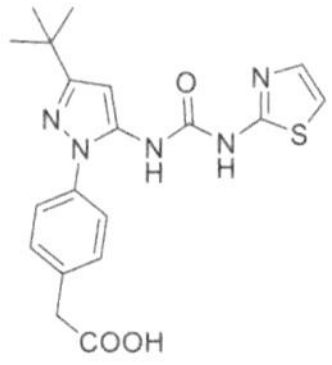

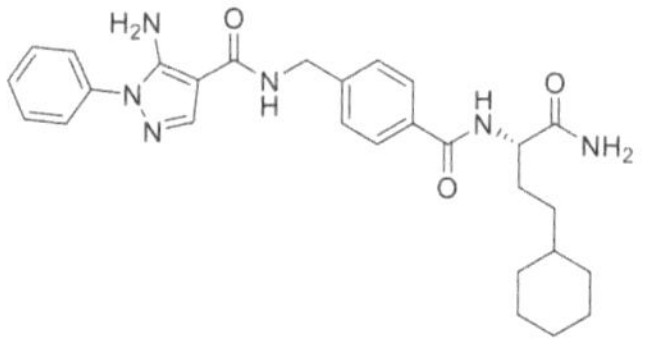

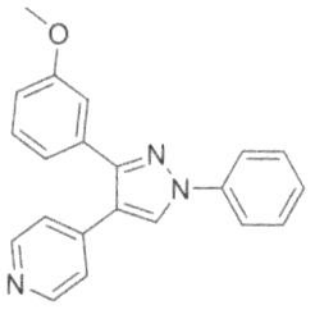

An additional test was performed to confirm the downstream inhibition of TNF-α production in lipopolysaccharide-stimulated THP-1 human cells. Compound **57** inhibited TNF-α production with an IC_{50} of 58 nM while SB 203580 had an IC_{50} of 20 nM. To investigate compound **57**'s properties, it was tested against hERG and showed less potency compared to E-4031, and 23.76 times more selectivity against the HEK293 cells (nanoBRE-Tassay) than hERG. The plasma stability profile of compound **57** was also tested and revealed high stability in both human and rat plasma. Compound **57** was 100% unchanged after 30 min and decreased to 98.4% after 2 h, while procaine was 1.2% after 30 min and 0.2% after 2 h. The in vivo pharmacokinetic (PK) profiling of compound **57** at 10 mg/kg showed 11.32% oral bioavailability and high plasma stability. Lastly, compound **57** showed no gastric ulcerogenicity upon administration of 50 mg/kg once daily for 5 consecutive days in in vivo anti-inflammatory screening using carrageenan-induced paw edema model in rats compared to diclofenac through an intraperitoneal (i.p.) injection [69].

The docking of this series with highly resolved X-ray crystal structures for the human p38α was performed to explain the activity. The docking results revealed that the tether was projected outward of the ATP binding pocket, and the *NH* of amide formed H-bonding with Ser-154 residue while the urea linker failed due to improper alignment. The halogenated phenyl ring at the end of the amide linker showed intolerability to bulky substituents due to the hindrance it exerts on the molecule to enter deep into the kinase active site. The pyridinyl's *N* bonds with Gly-110 and Met-109 in the hinge region. The 3-chloro-4-methoxy motif is buried deep in the kinase active site (Figure 64) [69].

20.2. Compound 58

A series of *N*-pyrazole, *N'*-thiazole-urea derivatives were studied as p38α inhibitory agents. Compound **58** (Figure 63) is the most potent among this series with IC_{50} value of 135 nM against p38α. Despite its high potency against p38α, compound **58** is unable to inhibit in vivo phosphorylation of MK2, a well-known substrate of p38. This is attributed to poor cellular permeability of compound **58** because of the charged carboxylate group. Structural modification of the carboxylic acid group can lead to the optimization of pharmacokinetic and pharmacodynamic properties. The ethyl ester analogue of compound **58** could effectively inhibit phosphorylation of MK2 in HeLa cells with an IC_{50} value of 6 μM but its IC$_{50}$ value against p38α is 639 nM. Further lead optimization can lead to analogues with improved characteristics [70].

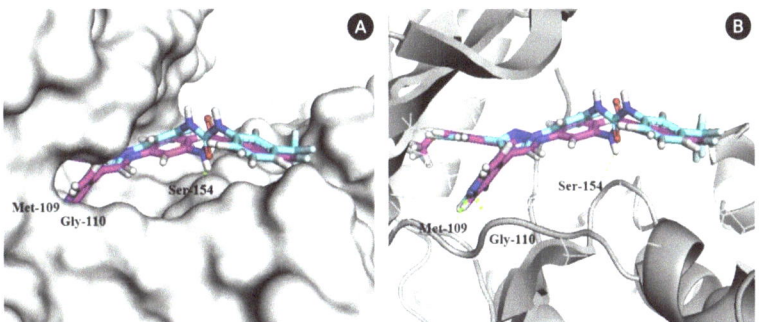

Figure 64. Binding mode of urea and amide derivatives; (**A**) binding mode of a urea compound (one of the compounds in the series, cyan) and **57** (magenta, amide), (**B**) best-docked pose for another two derivatives within the p38α kinase active site. Green dotted lines illustrate hydrogen bonding interactions [69].

20.3. Compound 59

A library of DNA-encoded small molecules was studied for potential inhibitory effect against p38α. Compound **59** (VPC00628, Figure 63) is the most potent and selective molecule identified from 12,600,000 tested compounds. Its IC$_{50}$ against p38α is 7 nM, and it was selected for further studies. Compound **59** is a type II kinase inhibitor that binds to the kinase DFG-out inactive form. Figure 65 illustrates the binding interactions of compound **59** with the DFG-out form of p38α. Pyrazole carboxamide *NH* acts as a hydrogen bond donor with the Thr gatekeeper, the pyrazole ring nitrogen interacts with the hinge region, and the N-phenyl forms a hydrophobic interaction with the P-loop tyrosine. The other part of the structure containing cyclohexyl and bisamide occupies a type-II pocket. When tested at 2 µM concentration against a 99-human kinase panel, it showed preferential selectivity towards p38α and p38β compared to the other 97 tested kinases. In a human monocytic cell line, compound **59** strongly inhibited TNF-α secretion with an IC$_{50}$ value of 46 nM. Replacement of the terminal primary amide with the N-ethyl-N-methyl tertiary amide led to a selective type-II inhibitor of p38α despite weaker potency (IC$_{50}$ = 14 nM). It was tested against a 468-kinase panel at 1 µM concentration and inhibited only thirteen kinases including p38α and p38β (98.5% and 96.6% inhibition, respectively) [71].

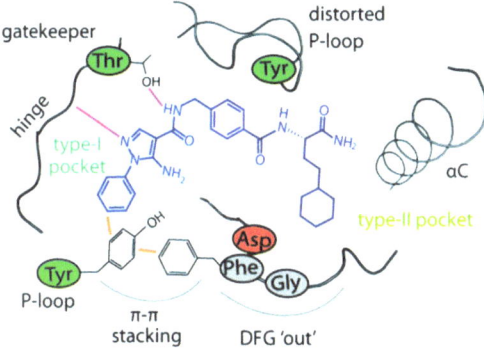

Figure 65. Binding mode of compound **59** with p38α crystal structure [72].

20.4. Compound **60**

Compound **60** (Figure 63) is the most potent inhibitor and antiproliferative agent among a series of 1,3,4-triarylpyrazole derivatives. Upon testing against a 15-kinase panel, it inhibited V600E-B-RAF, C-RAF, FLT3, and P38α/MAPK14. The highest potency was reported against p38α with an IC_{50} of 515 nM. In addition, it exerted potential antiproliferative activity against National Cancer Institute's (NCI) 60 cancer cell line panel, and the three most sensitive cell lines are the RPMI-8226 and K-562 leukemia cell lines in addition to the MDA-MB-468 breast cancer cell line (IC_{50} values equals 1.71, 3.42, and 6.70 µM, respectively). Compound **60** induces apoptosis but not necrosis in the RPMI-8226 leukemia cell line. Replacement of the methoxy group with hydroxyl or any substitution on the pyridyl ring reduced the activity [73].

21. Pyrazole-Based PDK Inhibitors

Compound **61**

Pyruvate dehydrogenase kinase 4 (PDK4) inhibition is a potential avenue for treatment of metabolic disorders such as hyperglycemia and insulin resistance, in addition to cancer and allergies. Ahn et al., have reported a series of pyrazole-possessing anthraquinone derivatives as inhibitors of the PDK4 kinase. Compound **61** (Figure 66) is the most potent PDK4 inhibitor among this series (IC_{50} = 84 nM). Any substitution on the piperidine *NH* or any modification of the ring carbonyl led to diminished activity. Compound **61** could enhance the glucose tolerance in the diet-induced obesity model in mice. In addition, it alleviated the allergic reactions in a passive cutaneous anaphylaxis model in mice. Moreover, it exerted modest antiproliferative activity against some cancer cell lines with 2-digit micromolar IC_{50} values. Compound **61** also demonstrated a weak inhibitory effect against CYP isozymes with 2-digit micromolar range. After oral administration of 10 mg/kg dose of compound **61** to male rats, the oral bioavailability was 63.6%, and t1/2 and t_{max} were 21.6 and 6 h, respectively [74].

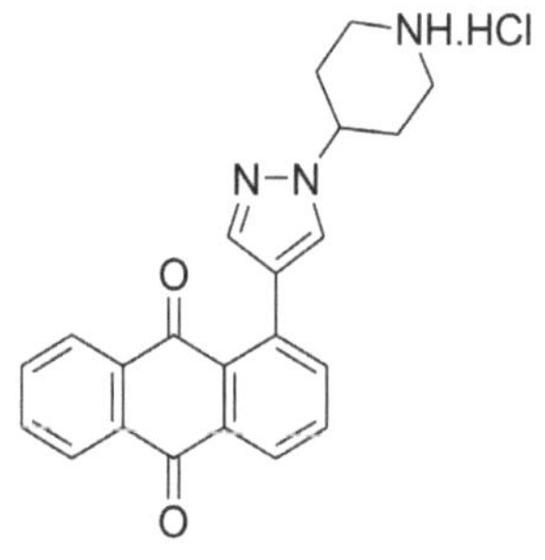

61

IC_{50} = 84 nM.

Figure 66. Structure of compound **61**, a PDK4 inhibitor.

The docking study indicated that compound **61** binds to the allosteric lipoamide site, not the active site. The pyrazole and piperidine rings entered the pocket, while the anthraquinone motif remained at the gate, intercalated between Phe43 and Phe56 on the surface and formed hydrophobic interactions with them. Furthermore, the pyrazole nitrogen atoms formed hydrogen bonds with the Ser53 hydroxyl group and the backbone carbonyl oxygen atom of Gln175 (Figure 67) [74].

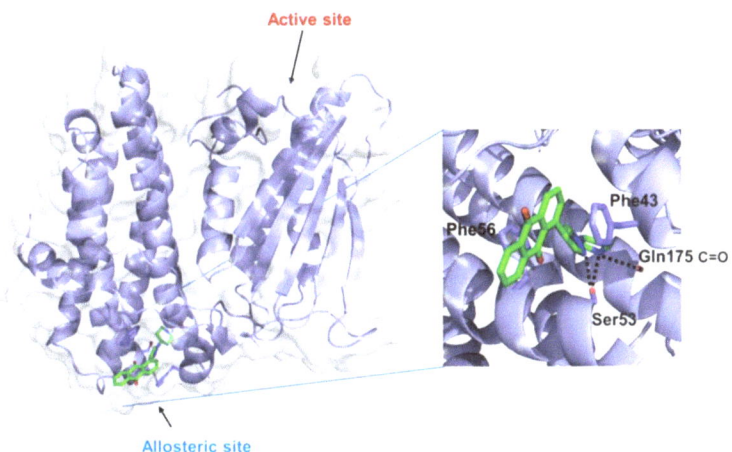

Figure 67. Putative binding mode of compound **61** with the lipoamide allosteric site of PDK4 kinase crystal structure [74].

22. Pyrazole-Based Pim Kinase Inhibitors

22.1. Compound 62

Pim kinases are good targets for management of different disorders including multiple myeloma. Compound **62** (Figure 68) has been reported as a pan-Pim kinase inhibitor. In addition, it demonstrated antiproliferative activity against the MM1.s myeloma cell line (IC_{50} = 0.64 μM). The 6-azaindazole core scaffold is more favorable for activity than indazole. The N-ethylpyrazole is more optimal than other substituted pyrazole rings, and piperazine is better than other alicyclic rings. However, compound **62** suffers from low oral bioavailability (1%) and high plasma protein binding (97.8%). The poor oral bioavailability could be attributed to low permeability. Further structural optimization should be carried out in order to improve the PK profile [75].

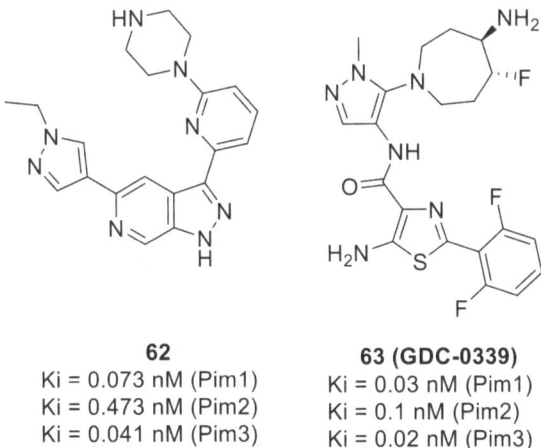

62
Ki = 0.073 nM (Pim1)
Ki = 0.473 nM (Pim2)
Ki = 0.041 nM (Pim3)

63 (GDC-0339)
Ki = 0.03 nM (Pim1)
Ki = 0.1 nM (Pim2)
Ki = 0.02 nM (Pim3)

Figure 68. Structures of pyrazole-based Pim kinase inhibitors and their Ki values.

22.2. Compound 63

Compound **63** (GDC-0339, Figure 68) has been developed as an orally bioavailable pan-Pim kinase inhibitor with antiproliferative activity against multiple myeloma. It was further tested against a panel of 277 kinases at 100 nM concentration, which is 500–5000 times its K_i values against Pim kinases, and showed more than 50% binding to only twelve kinases. In addition, it exerted a high potency against the MM1.s myeloma cell line with an IC_{50} value of 0.07 µM. It was also tested in vivo against MM1.s and RPMI 8226 mice models of multiple myeloma and exhibited promising results. The 2,6-difluorophenyl moiety is more optimal for activity than monofluorophenyl. In addition, the presence of thiazole and pyrazole rings together in the structure is the best combination compared to the 5-membered/6-membered or two 6-membered rings [76].

The docking of compound **63** into the Pim1 crystal structure revealed its fitting into the ATP-binding site. The primary amino group attached to the 7-membered ring forms a salt bridge with Asp128 and Glu171. The other primary amine donates a hydrogen bond to Arg122. Furthermore, the non-methylated pyrazole nitrogen atom accepts a hydrogen bond from Lys67 terminal amine (Figure 69) [76].

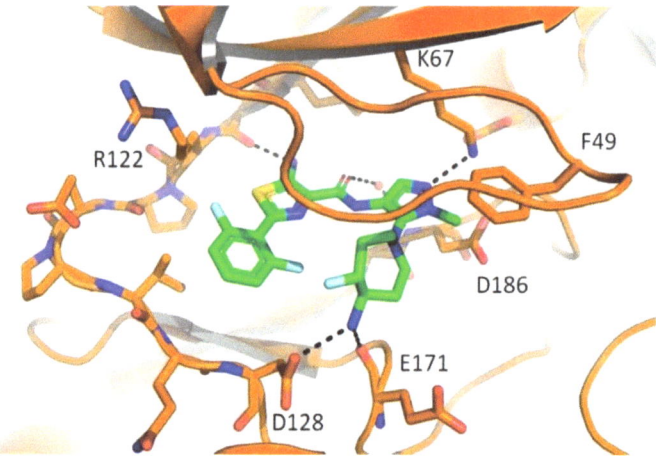

Figure 69. In silico binding interactions of compound **63** with Pim1 crystal structure [76].

23. Pyrazole-Based RAF Kinase Inhibitors

23.1. Compound 64

Compound **64** (Figure 70) is the most potent among a series of 3,4-diarylpyrazole-1-carboxamide derivatives reported as antiproliferative agents against the A375P human melanoma cell line in which mutant V600E-B-RAF kinase is over-expressed. Its IC_{50} value against A375P cell line equals 4.5 µM. The docking of compound **64** into the domain of V600E-B-RAF was carried out to investigate its putative binding mode (Figure 71). The phenolic hydroxyl group forms two hydrogen bonds with Val B590 and Asn B512, pyrazole N2 forms a hydrogen bond as acceptor with the Lys B591 amino acid residue, and the urea carbonyl oxygen accepts a hydrogen bond from Leu B515. The structure-activity relationship (SAR) study showed that terminal dimethylamino is more optimal for activity than bulkier dialkylamino or cyclic amines. In addition, the phenolic group is more favorable than methoxy, and this was supported by the docking study demonstrating the contribution of OH as a hydrogen bond donor. In addition, compound **64** obeys Lipinski's rule of five so it is estimated to be orally bioavailable [77].

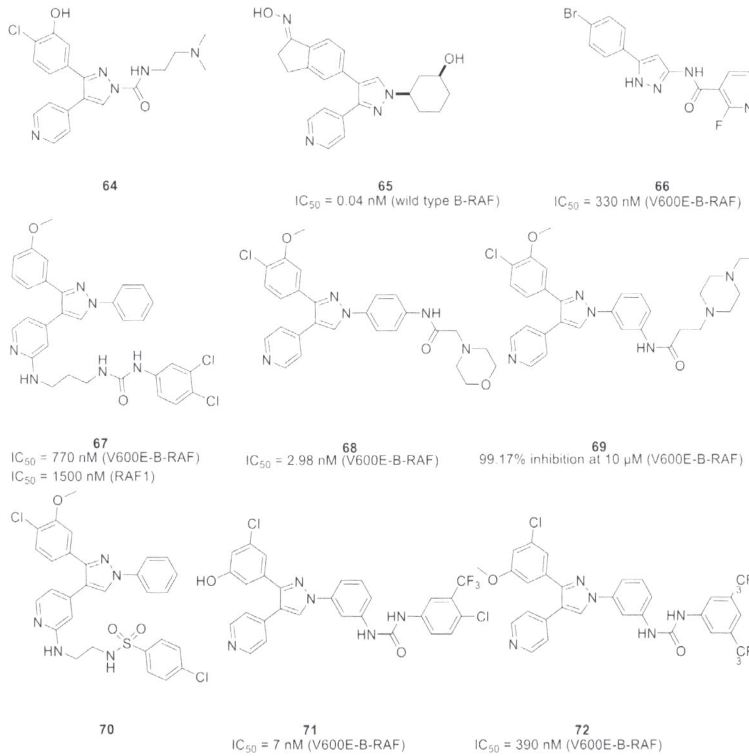

Figure 70. Structures of pyrazole-based RAF kinase inhibitors and their IC_{50}/Ki values or percentage inhibition.

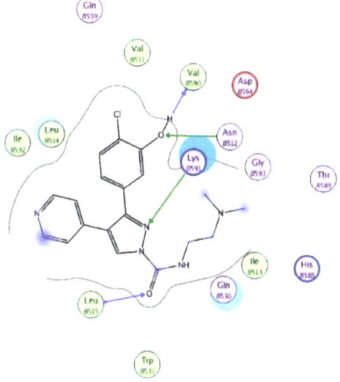

Figure 71. Putative binding interactions of compound **64** with V600E-B-RAF crystal structure [77].

23.2. Compound 65

Compound **65** (Figure 70) is another example of vicinal diarylpyrazole derivatives reported as RAF kinase inhibitors. It showed various B-RAF kinase inhibitory effects when different hydroxylated cycloalkyl groups were placed at the *N1* position of the pyrazole ring. Docking, molecular dynamics (MD) simulations, and hybrid calculation methods (Quantum Mechanics/Molecular Mechanics (QM/MM)) were conducted on the complexes to explain these differences. Compound **65** is the most potent against B-RAF kinase with an IC$_{50}$ value of 0.04 nM. Compound **65** forms hydrogen bonding interactions with Glu501 and Cys532 and is surrounded by Val471, Lys483, Thr529, Leu514, Asp594, Phe583, Ala481, and Trp531. The trans isomer (with the hydroxyl group behind the plane) is less potent against the kinase (IC$_{50}$ = 0.09 nM). Replacement of the cyclohexyl ring with cyclopentyl led to decreased potency [78].

23.3. Compound 66

A series of novel 5-phenyl-1*H*-pyrazole analogues possessing the niacinamide motif have been reported as potential V600E-B-RAF inhibitors. Compound **66** (Figure 70) exhibited the strongest potency against V600E-B-RAF kinase (IC$_{50}$ = 330 nM). Compound **66** also demonstrated the best antiproliferative potency against WM266.4 and A375 melanoma cell lines with IC$_{50}$ values of 2.63 and 3.16 µM, respectively, which are comparable with vemurafenib. Strong electron-withdrawing substituents such as fluoro on the pyridyl ring are beneficial for the activity. The putative binding mode of compound **66** is shown in Figure 72. It neatly binds to V600E-B-RAF via one hydrogen bond with a fluoro substituent and three pi–pi interactions through the pyrazole and phenyl rings [79].

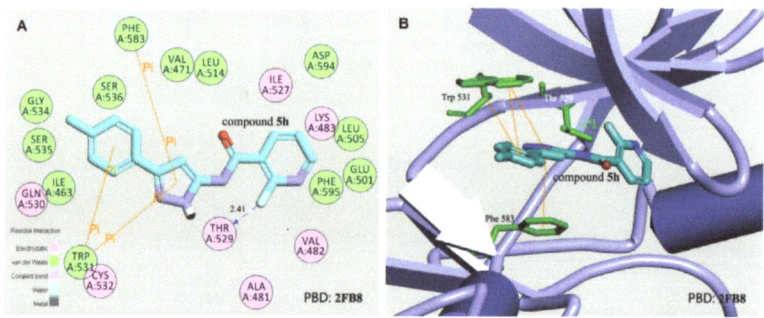

Figure 72. Putative binding interactions of compound **66** with V600E-B-RAF crystal structure [79]. (**A**) 2D interactions; (**B**) 3D interactions.

23.4. Compound 67

A novel series of 1,3,4-triarylpyrazole derivatives containing terminal arylamide or arylurea moieties have been reported as RAF kinase-inhibiting antiproliferative agents. Compound **67** (Figure 70) showed the best mean inhibition percentages values over the National Cancer Institute's (NCI) 58 cell line panel at 10 µM. Compound **67** was tested against seven kinases at 10 µM concentration to profile its kinase inhibitory activities. Compound **67** showed high inhibitory effects (90.44% and 87.71%) against the V600E-B-RAF and RAF1 kinases, respectively. Its IC$_{50}$ values over both kinases are 0.77 and 1.50 µM, respectively. Compound **67** possessing the 3′,4′-dichlorophenylurea terminal moiety showed the most promising results at 5-dose testing. A urea spacer is more favorable for activity in this series than an amide. It exhibited promising potency, efficacy, and broad-spectrum antiproliferative activity against many cancer cell lines of different cancer types (one-digit micromolar IC$_{50}$ values), as well as being superior to sorafenib [80].

23.5. Compound 68

A series of 1,3,4-triarylpyrazoles with an amide spacer were reported as RAF kinase-inhibiting anti-melanoma agents. Among them, compound **68** (Figure 70) is the most potent against A375 melanoma cells (IC$_{50}$ = 1.82 µM), with a selectivity index of 45.83 toward A375 rather than the HS27 normal fibroblasts. Compound **68** showed higher potency against the melanoma cell lines that include B-RAF V600E mutation compared to melanoma cells possessing the NRAS mutation as well as normal epithelial skin cells. Compound **68** is highly potent and selective against the V600E-B-RAF kinase with an IC$_{50}$ value = 2.98 nM. It has one carbon linker between the amide group and the morpholino nitrogen atom in its structure, and it is more active and more potent than the corresponding analogue with no linker. Compound **68** is about two-fold more potent than sorafenib and GW5074 against V600E-B-RAF. The molecular docking study revealed that compound **68** belongs to Type-II kinase inhibitors that bind to the kinase inactive form. Its amide oxygen atom showed an additional hydrogen bond formation with the kinase crystal structures in the docking study that enhances the affinity and potency. In addition, the pyridyl nitrogen forms a hydrogen bonding interaction with the Cys531 amino acid residue (Figure 73) [81].

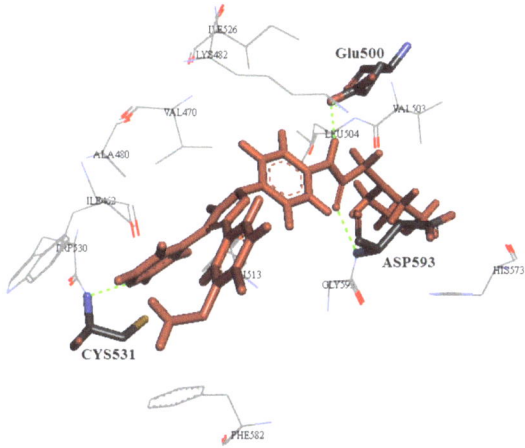

Figure 73. In silico binding interactions of compound **68** with V600E-B-RAF crystal structure [81].

23.6. Compound 69

As an extended study, a series of positional isomers of compound **68** (Figure 70) possessing a *meta*-disubstituted benzene ring at *N1* of the pyrazole ring was reported. These positional isomers are generally more active than the *para*-analogues. Among them, compound **69** (Figure 70) possessing an ethylene spacer between the amide group and the piperazinyl nitrogen is the most promising. It was examined on the NCI-60 cancer cell line panel and showed a 97.72% mean inhibition percentage at 10 µM concentration. Its IC_{50} values are within sub-micromolar range (0.27–0.92 µM) against nine cancer cell lines of nine cancer types. Against the A375 melanoma cell line, its IC_{50} value is 0.82 µM, which is 2.22 times more potent than compound **68**. Furthermore, compound **69** inhibits 99.17% of the V600E-B-RAF kinase activity at 10 µM concentration. The SAR study of this series revealed that N-methylpiperazinyl is more optimal for activity than the higher alkyl-substituted piperazinyl. In both the series of compounds **68** and **69**, the methoxy group is more favorable than hydroxyl [82].

23.7. Compound 70

Compound **70** possessing *p*-chlorobenzenesulfonamido at a terminal position, an ethylene linker, and a 4-chloro-3-methoxyphenyl ring at the C-3 position of the pyrazole core ring is the most promising anticancer agent among its series of compounds (Figure 70). It showed the highest mean percentage inhibition value (66.71%) against the NCI-60 cancer cell line panel at 10 µM concentration. It exerted broad-spectrum activity against various cell lines of different cancer types. Moreover, compound **70** exerted a higher range of selectivity against the HT29 colon cancer cell line than the HL-60 leukemia and MRC-5 lung fibroblasts (normal cells). Upon testing against 12 kinases of different kinase families, compound **70** gave a higher inhibitory effect over three RAF kinases. It produced 78.04%, 74.47%, and 72.46% inhibition at 10 µM concentration against the RAF1, V600E-B-RAF, and V600K-B-RAF kinases, respectively. The SAR study showed that an ethylene linker is more optimum for activity than propylene [83].

23.8. Compounds 71 and 72

Compound **71** (Figure 70) is the most potent RAF kinase-inhibitory derivative among a series of pyrazole-containing diarylureas. Its IC_{50} value against the V600E-B-RAF kinase equals 7 nM. Docking and molecular dynamic simulation studies revealed that compound **71** is a type IIA inhibitor of V600E-B-RAF. The SAR revealed that the phenolic OH on the aryl ring attached to the C-3 of pyrazole is more optimal for activity than OMe. OH forms a bidentate hydrogen bonding with the Cys532 amino acid residue. In addition, a urea linker is more favorable than amide as the two *NH* groups of urea form hydrogen bonds as donors with the αC-helix Glu501amino acid residue (Figure 74). In addition, the pyrazole ring forms a hydrophobic interaction with the Phe595 residue, and the urea oxygen interacts with Asp594 residue (Figure 75) [84]. Moreover, compound **71** was tested for anticancer activity over the NCI-60 cancer cell lines of nine cancer types and showed promising activity. Its mean inhibition percentage over the sixty cell lines is more than 89.54%. In addition, its mean IC_{50} value against the nine subpanels was within the range of 1.98–3.26 µM. Hydrophobic and electron-withdrawing substituents (e.g., Cl & CF_3) on the terminal aryl ring attached to urea spacer are favorable for activity. Furthermore, compound **72** is another promising antiproliferative agent despite its lower potency against the V600E-B-RAF kinase (IC_{50} = 390 nM). It was tested against 58 cancer cell lines of nine different cancer types at the NCI and exerted higher potency than sorafenib against all the 58 tested cell lines. Its IC_{50} values are within the submicromolar range against most of the tested cell lines. It exerted weak potency against the RAW 264.7 non-cancerous cell line, and induced apoptosis in the RPMI-8226 leukemia cell line with an IC_{50} of 1.52 µM [85].

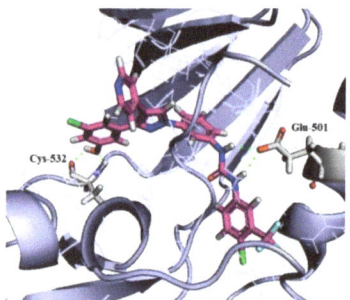

Figure 74. In silico binding interactions of compound **71** with V600E-B-RAF crystal structure [84].

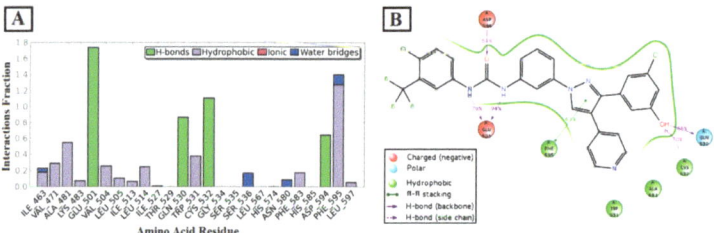

Figure 75. V600E-B-RAF-compound **71** binding interactions throughout the 50 ns simulation period; (**A**) the fractions of interaction happened between compound **71** and V600E-B-RAF kinase. (**B**) 2D interaction diagram of compound **71** within V600E-B-RAF active site [84].

24. Pyrazole-Based ROS Kinase Inhibitors

Compound 73

The ROS1 is a tyrosine kinase whose function is not fully understood, but its role in the development of resistance in some cancers made it a valuable target for management of some cancers. A series of trisubstituted pyrazoles were designed, synthesized and biologically evaluated. The group's previous work on the same scaffold had advanced an understanding of the structure-activity relationship of this scaffold and was summarized in Figure 76 [86].

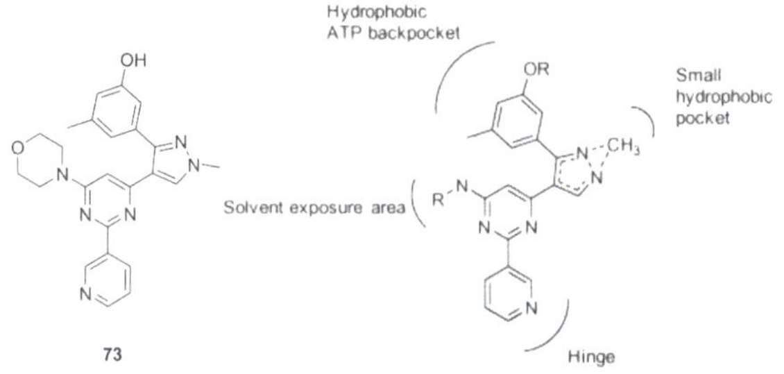

Figure 76. Structure of compound **73** and a simplified top view of a general scheme depicting the binding mode of trisubstituted prazoles in ROS1 and key interactions involved [86].

The key interactions that constitute the SAR of trisubstituted pyrazoles consist of the distal unsubstituted pyridinyl ring, which interacts with the hinge region's Met2029 and loses its activity upon replacing it with a phenyl ring, or there is a deterioration in activity upon the introduction of substituents to the pyridinyl ring due to a steric clash which prevents bonding. The pyrazle's methyl binds to a small hydrophobic pocket, which does not tolerate polar groups, or bigger substituents. Both positional isomers of pyrazole appear to be biologically active with a preference to 1-methylpyrazole over the other isomer. The pyrazole's role is to direct the substituent and the arms into optimal positions to interact with the ROS1 binding site [86].

The series was tested against the ROS1 enzyme. Compound **73** (Figure 76) displayed the highest potency among the series (IC_{50} = 13.6 nM) compared to crizotenib (IC_{50} = 60 nM). Compound **73**'s activity was a strong motivation to investigate the selectivity on a panel of kinases. Using the KINOMEscan™ screening platform, compound **73** was tested on 456 non-mutant and disease related mutant kinases. ROS1, FLT3, JAK2, and TYK2(JH1 domain-catalytic) were shown to be inhibited by **73** at 10 µM, while it did not inhibit the ALK and c-MET enzymes which are the most homologous to the ROS1 kinase. Selectivity was quantitatively measured using the selectivity score parameter, which is obtained by dividing the number of kinases that compounds bind to by the total number of distinct kinases tested, excluding mutant variants. Compound **73** had a selectivity score of 0.076 compared to Imitanib (0.12) and Dasatinib (0.26) [86].

The docking of **73** into the binding site of unphosphorylated ROS1 was performed (Figure 77). The binding mode obtained further strengthened the hypothesis of the proposed SAR generated by the group's work. Pyridinyl bonded with Met2029 of the hinge region via H-bonding, the disubstituted phenyl moiety was directed to a certain hydrophobic pocket under the P-loop, and Morpholine reached out into the solvent [86].

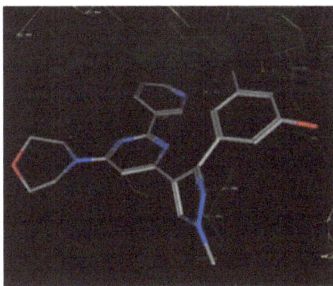

Figure 77. The binding motif of **73** in ROS1 kinase [86].

25. Pyrazole-Based Src Kinase Inhibitor

Compound 74

Compound 74 (Figure 78) was reported as a broad spectrum antiproliferative agent possessing an inhibitory effect against the Src kinase. Upon testing against the NCI-60 cancer cell line panel, it exerted one-digit micromolar IC_{50} values against several cell lines of a variety of cancer types. Its highest potency was against the CCRF-CEM and MOLT-4 leukemia cell lines (IC_{50} = 1.00 µM against both of them). The SAR shows that replacement of the acetyl group with hydrogen diminished the activity. Concerning the pyrazoline ring, expansion or replacement with chalcone decreased the activity while replacement with an isoxazole ring retained it. Compound 74 was further tested against eight kinases and the highest activity was reported against Src (59% inhibition at 10 µM concentration). In silico studies showed that compound 74 obeys Lipinski's rule of five and has an acceptable PK profile. In addition, docking studies demonstrated that compound 74 occupies the ATP-binding pocket of Src. The pyrrole *NH* forms a hydrogen bond with Lys343. Compound 74's pyrazoline nitrogen accepts a hydrogen bond from Ser345. Moreover, the benzofuran benzene ring forms hydrophobic interactions with Leu273 and Gly274 (Figure 79) [87].

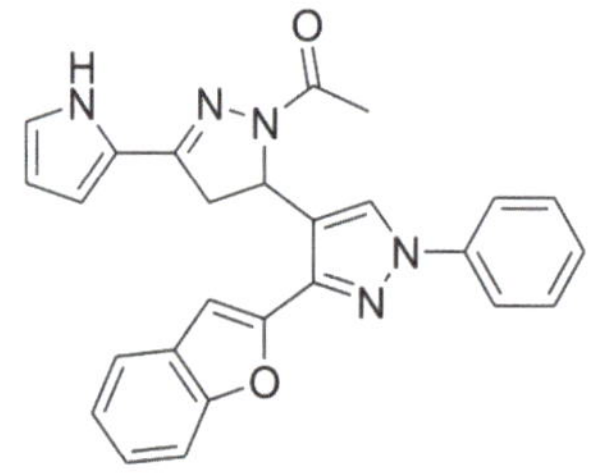

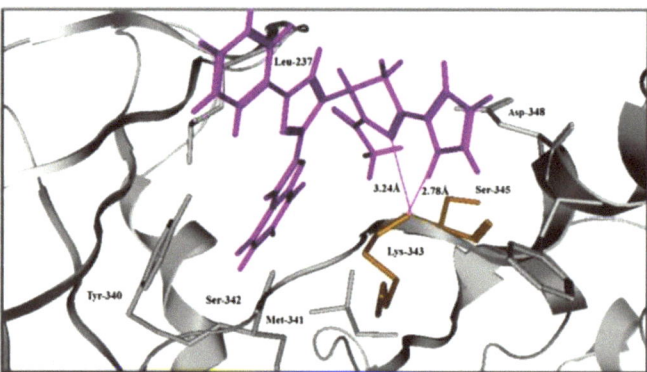

Figure 78. Structure of compound 74, a Src kinase inhibitor.

Figure 79. In silico binding interactions of compound 74 with Src crystal structure [87].

26. Pyrazole-Based TGFβ/ALK Kinase Inhibitors

26.1. Compounds 75 and 76

The motive for the development of compound 76 (Figure 80) was the lack of active compounds with desirable physiochemical properties and oral activity against the R206H mutated ALK2. Through in silico and in vitro investigations, a lead compound 75 (Figure 80) consisting of the vicinal diarylpyrazole compound was identified. The cocrystal structure of the lead with the R206H mutated ALK2 showed the interactions between the aminopyrimidine ring and the hinge region, the hydrogen bond via the water molecule between 3'-pyridyl's nitrogen, and the carboxylate of the Glu248 side chain from the αC helix while the pyrazole ring was embedded inside the sugar pocket and anisidine's methoxy was projected into the solvent region (Figure 81) [88].

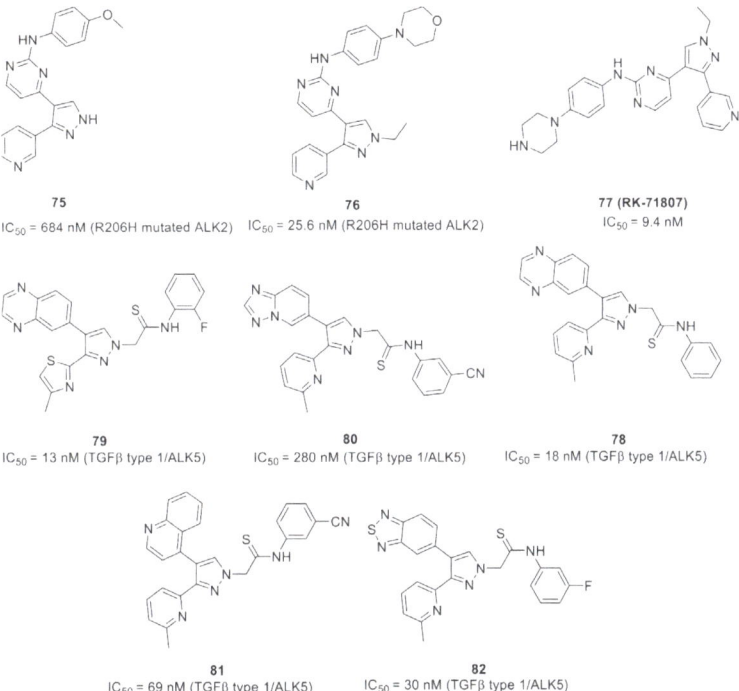

Figure 80. Structures of pyrazole-based TGFβ/ALK inhibitors and their IC$_{50}$ values.

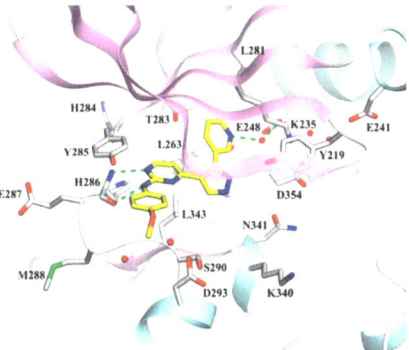

Figure 81. X-ray crystal structure of lead compound **75** in R206H mutant ALK2. White stick model: residues forming ATP binding pockets; Yellow stick model: lead compound; Green dashed lines: the hydrogen bonds between lead compound and active site; Red sphere: water molecules [88].

Using the data from the cocrystal structure, the same research group hypothesized that introduction of polar groups on anisidine and pyrazole moieties would improve activity and physiochemical properties such as aqueous solubility and liver microsomal stability. They started with ring replacement of the 3′-pyridyl ring with different heterocycles, which proved detrimental for activity. Introduction of different chains on the two nitrogens of the pyrazole ring showed that an unsubstituted pyrazole lead compound and an alkyl substituent on *N1* were inferior to an *N2* substituent in terms of inhibitory activity and cell permeability, and *N2*- ethylpyrazole is the best substituent. The group decided to move on to the next step: investigation of the role of substituents on anisidine moiety. It was concluded that compound **76** with *p*-morpholine anisidine had the best activity among the synthesized compounds. Compound **76** had an IC$_{50}$ of 25.6 nM. Permeability was measured using Caco-2 cells which exhibited A to B Papp= 9.12×10^{-6} cm/s. Efflux ratio of compound **76** was 1.0 (calculated by taking the ratio of A to B compared to B to A). Moreover, the multidrug resistance (MDR) was determined using Madin–Darby canine kidney (MDCK) cells which had a ratio of 1.6. Moreover, compound **76** had an aqueous solubility of 200.1 µM and human plasma protein binding of 91.8%. The in vivo study of the pharmacokinetic properties of compound **76** on rate showed good oral bioavailability (F = 56%) [88].

26.2. Compounds 75 and 77

Compounds **75** (RK-59638) and **77** (RK-71807) were reported as ALK2 (R206H) kinase-inhibiting lead compounds for treatment of fibrodysplasia ossificans progressive (Figure 80). The IC$_{50}$ value of compound **75** is 684 nM against the ALK2 (R206H) kinase. The docking study demonstrated hydrogen bonding between the amino pyrimidine moiety and the Ser286 nitrogen in the hinge region. The pyridine ring forms water-mediated hydrogen bonding with Glu248. In addition, its pyrazole ring forms a hydrophobic interaction with Val222 (Figure 82) [89].

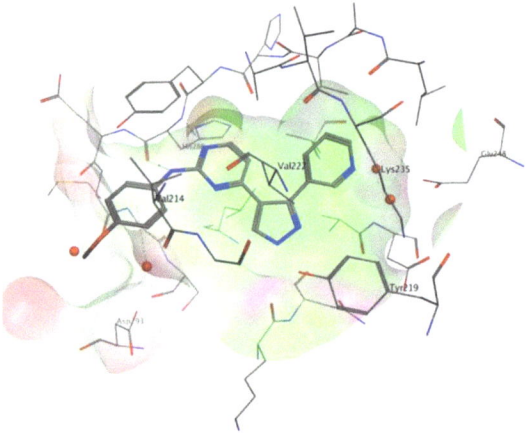

Figure 82. In silico binding interactions of RK-59638 (**75**) with ALK2 (R206H) crystal structure [89].

The *N1* of the pyrazole ring in compound **75** does not contribute to the binding interactions with the kinase. Different substituents on it were investigated, and ethyl was the optimum substituent. The methoxy group was also replaced with a piperazinyl ring to obtain compound **77**. These structural modifications led to improved potency and physicochemical properties. The IC$_{50}$ of compound **77** against the kinase is 9.4 nM, which is about 72.8-fold more potent than compound **75**. The aqueous solubility of compound **77** at pH 7.4 has improved to reach 93.8 µg/mL (vs. 6.4 µg/mL in case of compound **75**). Plasma protein binding decreased from 85% for compound **75** to 65.8% for compound **77**. Compound **77** also showed less inhibitory effects than compound **75** against the cytochrome P450 isozymes. Furthermore, compound **77** exerted only 27% inhibition of hERG upon testing at 10 µM [89].

The putative binding interactions of compound **77** with the kinase crystal structure indicate electrostatic interaction of the protonated piperazine nitrogen with Asp293. The ethyl group exerts a hydrophobic interaction with Tyr219 phenyl ring. Moreover, the pyrazole *N1* forms hydrogen bonding with Lys235 (Figure 83) [89].

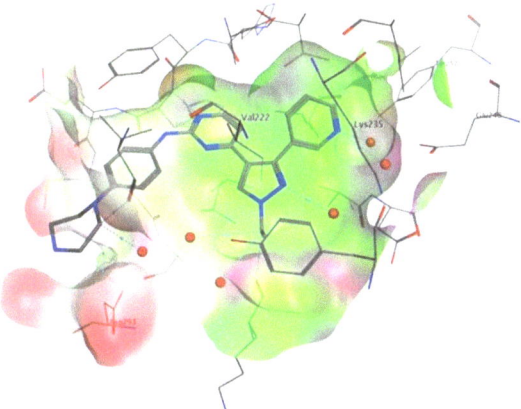

Figure 83. In silico binding interactions of RK-71807 (**77**) with ALK2 (R206H) crystal structure [89].

26.3. Compound 78

The development of TGFβ type 1/ALK5 inhibitors based on their clinical candidate IN-1130 as a lead compound has been reported. That group's previous works had concluded that activity and selectivity were higher in the presence of methyleneamide and methylenethioamide linkers against the ALK5 kinase. They also concluded that although thiazide linkers might be superior in activity in comparison to methylenethioamide, but owing to shelf stability issues during long term storage, the methylenethioamide and methyleneamide are better options for development. To study the tolerability of the ALK5 active domain to the length of the tether between the phenyl ring and central pyrazole ring, the group synthesized few ethyleneamide linkers to be investigated among the synthesized compounds. Another point which was considered during the investigation was the introduction of 2,3-dimethyl substituents on the quinazoline ring, which is thought to improve the H-bonding between the N of the quinazoline ring and the hinge region of ALK5 (Figure 84) [90].

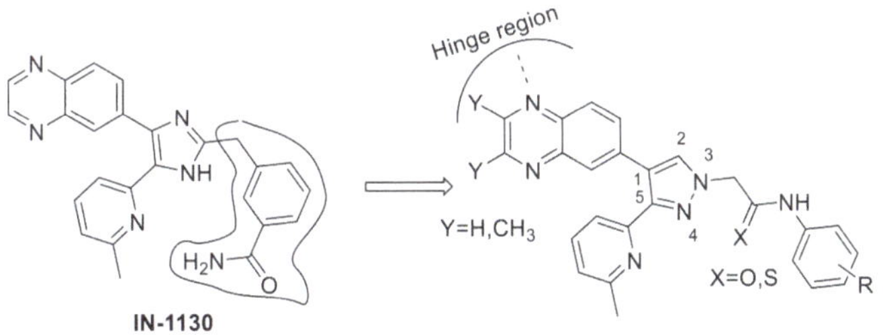

Figure 84. A schematic view of the rationale behind the development, as well as a hypothetical H-bonding between quinazoline's N and hinge region [90].

A total of sixteen compounds were synthesized and biologically evaluated. A kinase assay using purified human ALK5 kinase was produced in Sf9 insect cells to evaluate ALK5 inhibition. All compounds with a 2,3-dimethylquinazoline moiety did not show any activity up to concentration of 1 µM. In addition, the 3-substituted pyrazole ring had superior activity compared to its positional isomer. The ethyleneamide linker experienced a loss of activity compared to methyleneamide, and methylenethioamide derivatives were superior to methyleneamide. The most potent compound against ALK5 was compound **78** (Figure 80). Further investigation through measuring the luciferase activity in a cell-based assay to determine the TGF-β-induced downstream transcriptional activation to

ALK5 signaling was performed. Using HaCaT cells permanently transfected with a p3TP-luciferase reported construct, the results did not differ much from the kinase assay showing a similar trend. Compound **78** inhibited luciferase activity by 80% at 0.1 µM. Compound **78** was further tested and compared to IN-1130 and SB-505154 (a known ALK5 inhibitor) at five different concentrations. Compound **78** inhibited ALK5 in a dose-dependent fashion, it was equipotent with IN-1130, and more potent than SB-505154. The p38α MAP kinase's active site is one of the most homologous to that of the ALK5's, which was chosen to investigate the selectivity of the compounds in this series. The series is devoid of activity towards the p38α MAPK up to a concentration of 1 µM, with compound **78** being the most selective towards ALK5 compared to p38α MAPK (selectivity index > 77) [90].

The docking of compound **78** to study its binding mode and interactions with the active site of ALK5 is shown in (Figure 85). A quinoxalinyl ring mimics the adenine ring of the ATP's pocket and formed H-bonding with the backbone of His283, and the thioamide's NH formed H-bonding with Lys337 in the catalytic domain of ALK5 [90].

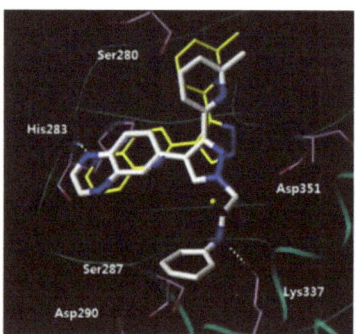

Figure 85. Binding pose of compound **78** in the active site of ALK5, superimposed over the X-ray pose of 1,5-naphthyrine inhibitor (yellow carbon). Yellow dotted lines indicate hydrogen bonding interactions (<2.5 Å) [90].

26.4. Compound 79

Continuing to build on compound **78**, the group went on to modify the *o*-methylpyridinyl motif (Figure 80). The methylpyridinyl motif's importance lies in its ability to form a hydrophobic interaction with Tyr249 of the ALK5's active site, the nitrogen of pyridine forms a water-bridged H-bonding with the side chains of Tyr249 and Glu245 and the backbone of Asp351. Keeping in mind the hypothesis that the inhibitory activity could be improved if the H-bonding of the pyridine motif was stronger, the group sought to replace the methyl group with dimethylamine to study the effect of an electron donating group on improving the H-bonding of the *N* of the pyridine. They also sought bioisosteric replacement of the pyridine ring with the 4-methylthiazol-2-yl and 4-pyrimidinyl groups to study its effect on activity (Figure 86) [91].

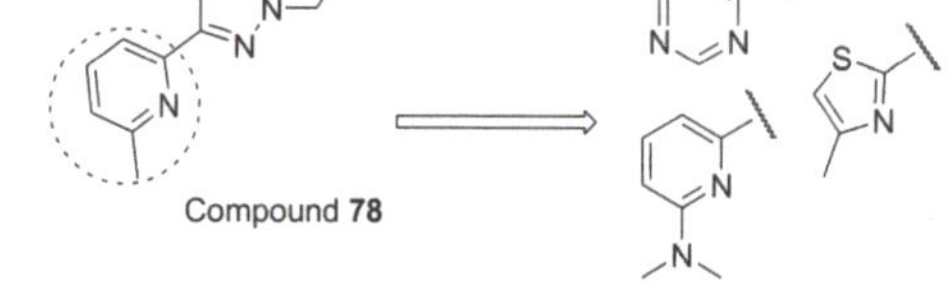

Figure 86. Schematic view showing the design strategy used to modify the *o*-methylpyridinyl motif.

A series compromising of thirty-two compounds was synthesized. The series was tested on a purified human ALK5 kinase domain produced in Sf9 insect cells at 10 µM to evaluate ALK5 activity. The series followed the previously discussed trend in compound **78**, methylenethioamide was superior to methyleneamide, and the 3-substituted pyrazole was superior to its positional isomers. The 6-Methylpyridine was superior to its 6-dimethylaminopyridine counterpart. It is possible that fitting into the enzyme's active site was not achieved due to it being bulkier compared to the methyl group. Nonetheless, the series containing 4-methylthiazol-2-yl showed highly improved activity compared to 6-methylpyridine, with compound **79** (Figure 80) showing the highest inhibition (2% residual activity upon testing at 10 µM concentration) and an IC$_{50}$ of 0.28 µM. Compound **79** was further tested on p38α MAPK at 10 µM since its kinase domain is one of the most homologous to the ALK5's kinase domain, and lacked any inhibitory activity against it. The most potent of all, compound **79** had a selectivity index of >35 against ALK5 compared to p38α MAPK [91].

Compound **79** and its 6-dimethylaminopyridnyl counterpart were docked into ALK5's active site (Figure 87). The docking study explained the higher activity of 4-methylthiazol-2-yl of compound **79** compared to its 6-dimethylaminopyridinyl counterpart with its higher number of bondings, five bonds, in comparison to the two bonds of its dimethylaminopyridinyl counterpart. The phenyl ring of compound **79** bonds with Lys232 via a pi-alkyl bond. The pyrazole ring interacts with the side chains of Leu340 and Val219. Thiazole's contribution to activity was notable as well. The ring's nitrogen bonds with the backbone of Ser287 through a carbon–hydrogen bond. Methyl's involvement with the backbone of Lys337 is through an alkyl bond, as well as with the backbone of Phe289 through a pi-alkyl bond [91].

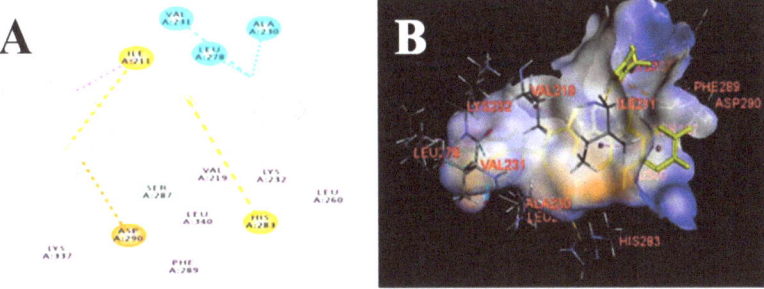

Figure 87. Docking pose of compound **79** in the active site of ALK5. (**A**) 2D binding interactions pro; (**B**) Proposed pose of **79** in the binding pocket of ALK5. The ligands are shown in yellow [91].

26.5. Compound 80

The motivation for carrying out this work stems from the desire to overcome the metabolic oxidation of preclinical candidates IN-1130 (Figure 88). The extensive history of studying and developing a potent and selective ALK5 (Activin receptor-Like Kinase 5) inhibitor by this group had led them to draw a pharmacophore that can effectively and selectively inhibit ALK5. A central five-membered ring with a small tether (e.g., methylene, methylenethioamido and methyleneamide) attached to a substituted phenyl ring (fluorine atom at position 2 or carbonitrile or carboxamido groups at position 3 and 4) and a 2-pyridyl heterocycle attached to the central 5-membered ring can constitute a framework as an ALK5 inhibitor and hinge region binder like the quinazoline ring [92].

It was hypothesized that the bioisosteric replacement of quinazoline to [1,2,4]triazolo[1,5-a]pyridin-6-yl could block oxidation on position 2 and 3 of quinazoline. To investigate the activity of the designed compounds, the group synthesized two series with imidazole or pyrazole central 5-membered rings. Two different tethers (methyleneamido and methylenethioamido) that connect the central 5-membered ring to the terminal phenyl ring were investigated. They were biologically evaluated on a purified human ALK5 kinase domain produced in a Sf9 insect cell kinase assay. The results demonstrated that in both the pyrazole and the imidazole central rings, the activity was improved by methylenethioamide compared to methyleneamide. Additionally, the differences in activity between the pyrazole and the imidazole central rings did not favor one over the other, so they could not conclude which ring is superior. Compound **80** with a pyrazole central ring had the most potent IC$_{50}$ (0.018 µM) in the series (Figure 80). For the evaluation of the activation of ALK5 signaling induced by TGF-β transcriptional activation, HaCaT cells permanently transfected with p3TP-luciferase reporter construct were used for cell-based luciferase activity. Results showed, contrary to the kinase assay, a superior activity exhibited by methyleneamido derivatives compared to the methylenethioamido analogues. Yet, compound **80** had a higher inhibition (95% at 0.03 µM) compared to the other compounds in the series. Further biological evaluation aimed to investigate the selectivity of the compounds over the p38α MAP kinase since its kinase domain is known to be one of the most homologous to that of ALK5. The methyleneamido linkers did not show any activity against the p38α MAP kinase while imidazole containing methylenethioamido linkers did show inhibitory activity against it (IC$_{50}$ of methylenethioamide compounds ranges from 1.05 µM to 5.21 µM). Compound **80** had the best selectivity towards ALK5 over the p38α MAP kinase among the series with a 284 selectivity index. The docking of compound **80** into the X-ray structure of ALK5 and superimposing it on the native ligands (1,5-naphthyrine inhibitor) somehow explained the reason behind the activity of compound **80** (Figure 89). The triazolopyridine ring interacts with the backbone *NH* of His 283 of the hinge region. Moreover, the *N* of the pyrazole ring forms a hydrogen bond with the protonated ammonium group of Lys232. Lastly, the cyano group accepts a hydrogen bond from Ser 287. Compound **80** fits the enzyme's active site and interacts with the key amino acids in it [92].

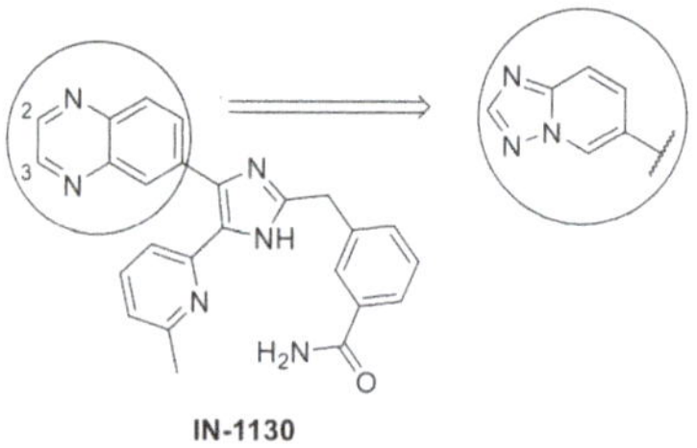

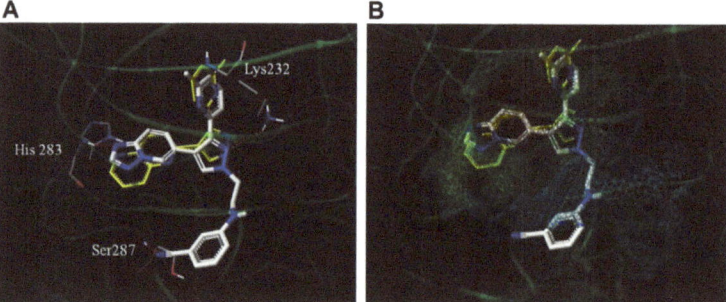

Figure 88. Preclinical candidate IN-1130 and possible oxidation site at position 2 or 3 on the quinazoline's heterocycle.

Figure 89. Putative binding mode of compound **80** with ALK5. (**A**) White, **80**'s binding mode in the active site; Yellow, 1,5-napthyrine; Grey, key amino acid residues represented in line form; Red, hydrogen bond interaction (<2.8 Å); compound **80** is superimposed over 1,5-naphthyrine inhibitor. (**B**) MOLCAD49 lipophilic potential surface map of ALK5's active site in the docking model of **80**. Lipophilicity increases from blue (hydrophilic) to brown (hydrophobic) [92].

26.6. Compound 81

ALK5 inhibitors hold abundant potential for a medicinal chemist to work on. Here, a similar group that worked on the development of compounds **78–80** report yet another study on possible changes and possible modifications that can be performed on the same framework that was used in the previous designs. The group described using a quinolin-4-yl arm which is similar to a previously reported inhibitor of ALK5, and explored the potential biological effect it has. They also planned to replace the quinolin-4-yl with an isostere, the 2-phenylpyridin-4-yl, investigating the depth of design that can be ascertained as a biologically useful agent (Figure 90).

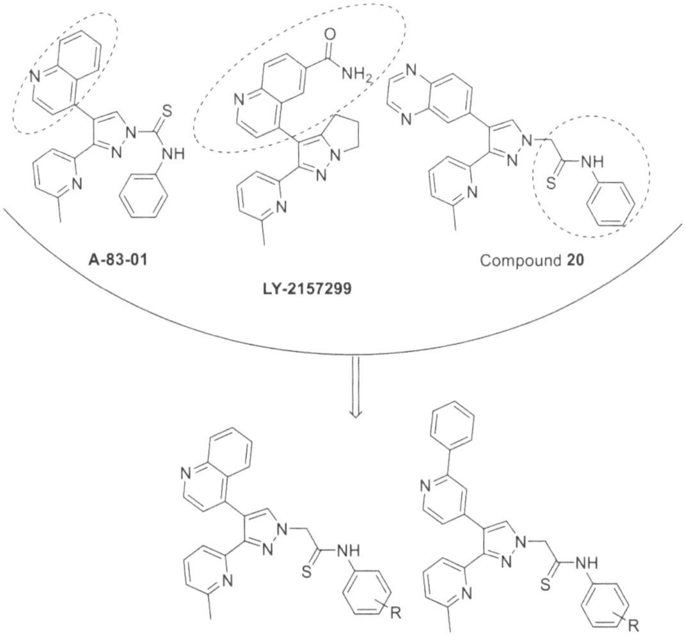

Figure 90. Schematic view of the rationale behind designing the series of compounds as ALK5 inhibitors.

The group synthesized a number of different series and evaluated their ALK5 inhibitory activity using a purified human ALK5 kinase domain produced in the Sf9 insect cell kinase assay at 10 µM, which showed that compound **81** had a promising inhibitory activity (2% residual activity at 10 µM, IC_{50} = 69 nM) (Figure 80). The series containing quinolin-4-yl arm was superior to the one with 2-phenylpyridin-4-yl. Further investigation was carried out on the p38α MAPK since its active site is highly homologous to ALK5's. Most compounds were active against it, following the same trend seen in the ALK5 assay, and had compound **81**'s inhibitory activity at 10 µM as 3% residual activity and an IC_{50} of 104 nM.

26.7. Compound 82

Compound **82** has been reported as a potent and selective inhibitor of ALK5 (Figure 80). Its IC_{50} equals 30 nM. It is 235-fold more selective toward ALK5 than p38α. Moreover, it is 4-fold more potent than the clinical candidate LY-2157299. Compound **82** has also been reported as a potential inhibitor of collagen I and α-SMA protein, and mRNA expressions in TGFβ-induced LX-2 human hepatic stellate cells. Therefore, compound **82** is a potential candidate for treatment of hepatic fibrosis.

The thioamide moiety of compound **82** is more favorable for activity than the corresponding amide. In addition, m-fluorophenyl is more optimal than any other aryl substituent. The docking study demonstrated a formation of hydrogen bonds between the thioamide *NH* and Lys337 and Asn338, in addition to a network of hydrophobic interactions performed by the pyrazole ring and the other rings of the structure (Figure 91) [93].

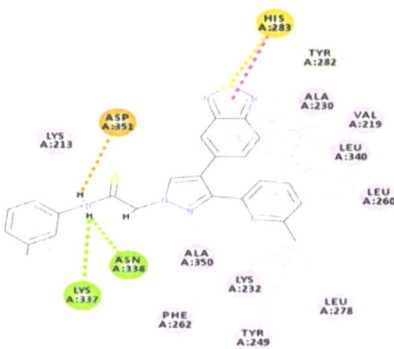

Figure 91. Two-dimensional putative binding interactions of compound **82** with ALK5 crystal structure [93].

27. Pyrazole-Based Trk Inhibitors

27.1. Compounds 83–85

Compound **83** (AZ-23) is a known pyrazole-based ATP-competitive, orally bioavailable Trk kinase inhibitor. Its IC$_{50}$ values against TrkA and TrkB are 2 and 8 nM, respectively (Figure 92). In addition, it inhibits other kinases such as FGFR1, FLT3, Ret, MUSK, and LCK [94].The pyrazole *N* and *NH* of AZ-23 form two hydrogen bonding interactions with Glu590 and Met592. In addition, the *NH* attached to the pyrazole ring donates a hydrogen bond to a backbone amide oxygen. Wang et al., optimized the structure of AZ-23 through ring fusion to get compounds **84** and **85** (Figure 92). Both compounds are potent inhibitors of TrkA with an IC$_{50}$ value of 0.5 nM in a cellular assay. The extended hydroxyl group in both compounds forms an additional hydrogen bond with the backbone amide oxygen of Glu518 in the glycine-rich P loop. The oral bioavailability of both compounds **84** and **85** is 29% and 54%, respectively. In addition, their aqueous solubility values are 250 and 220 μM, respectively. The two compounds were tested against hERG and they were safe enough (IC$_{50}$ values > 25 μM) [95].

27.2. Compound 86

Furuya et al., studied the important interactions of the inhibitor with the juxtamembrane region of the TrkA kinase for selectivity. They studied the interactions of compound **86** with that region (cyan color, Figure 93). The urea oxygen accepts a hydrogen bond from Ile490. In addition, the pyrazole ring with its methyl and methoxy substituents interacts with His489 and Leu486. Moreover, the difluorophenyl moiety interacts with Asn493, Gly488, and Ile490. The presence of moiety that interacts with the juxtamembrane moiety beyond the hinge region is crucial for selectivity. The Trk inhibitors that interact with the ATP-binding (hinge) region are usually non-selective. The selectivity of compound **86** towards TrkA was confirmed by the cell-free biochemical measurements. Its IC$_{50}$ values against TrkA, TrkB, and TrkC are 2.7, 1303.7, and 2483.7 nM, respectively, which confirms its superior selectivity against TrkA [96].

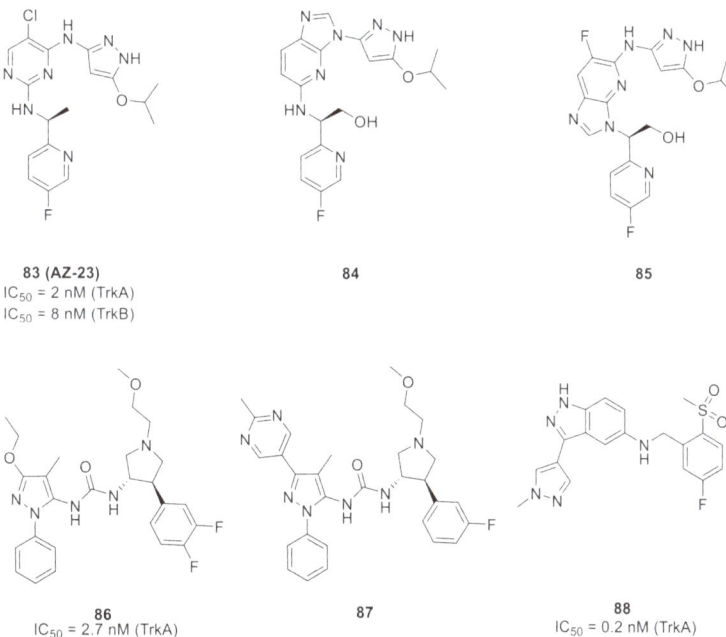

Figure 92. Structures of pyrazole-based TRK inhibitors and their IC$_{50}$ values.

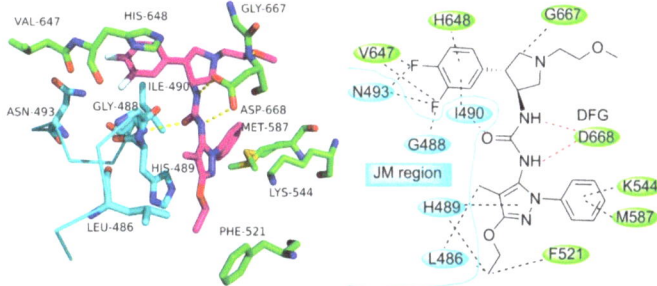

Figure 93. The in silico binding interactions of compound **86** with the juxtamembrane region of TrkA kinase [96].

27.3. Compound **87**

Compound **87** is another pyrazolyl urea derivative that has a structural similarity to compound **86** (Figure 92). Compound **87** was developed with the aim of deciphering the allosteric binding mechanisms of TrkA inhibitors. It possesses the advantage of a rapid association rate with the TrkA crystal structure, thus binding to the inactive conformation of the kinase (i.e., type II TrkA inhibitor). In addition, its off-rate is slow [97].

27.4. Compound **88**

Compound **88** was developed as a potent and peripherally restricted Trk kinase inhibitor for use as an analgesic agent (Figure 92). The main goal of the research group was to have a substrate for the efflux transporter, thus it has a low CNS penetration ability and a higher plasma exposure. The IC$_{50}$ values of compound **88** in cell-free and cell-based Trk kinase assays are 0.2 and 1.7 nM, respectively. It was further tested at 20 nM concentration against a panel of 49 kinases and exerted selectivity against TrkA. Replacement of methylpyrazole with methoxypyridine, the insertion of NHSO$_2$Me instead of the methyl group, and the removal of fluoro led to less potency against TrkA (IC$_{50}$ = 7 and 53 nM in cell-free and cell-based assays, respectively). Furthermore, compound **88** was tested in vivo in Complete Freund's adjuvant (CFA)-induced thermal hypersensitivity model. Compound **88** at a 4 mg/kg oral dose gave anti-pain activity comparable to ibuprofen (100 mg/Kg p.o. dose). The clearance of compound **88** is 127.4 mL/min/kg and its aqueous solubility is 140.7 µM (compared to 15.2–23 µM when there is pyridyl instead of methylpyrazole). After oral administration of a 5 mg/kg of compound **88** in rats, its C$_{max}$ was 161 nM. In addition, its t$_{1/2}$ was 1.46 h following the i.v. administration of 1 mg/kg in rats. The ratio of compound **88** in brain to plasma was found to be only 0.03 after an i.p. injection of 2.5 mg/kg in rats [98].

28. Pyrazole-Based VEGFR Kinase Inhibitors

28.1. Compound 89

The high expenditure of energy, nutrients and oxygen required by tumor cells to survive and grow is met through growing new blood vessels, a process named angiogenesis. Multiple proteins are involved in angiogenesis, but vascular endothelial growth factor receptors (VEGFRs) have been the center of interest as drug targets for their great involvement in tumor neovascularization [99]. Compound **89** was part of a series designed to inhibit the VEGFR-2 kinase (Figure 94). It strongly inhibited the VEGFR-2 kinase (IC$_{50}$ = 0.95 nM) and decreased the proliferation of VEGF-stimulated human umbilical vein endothelial cells (HUVEC) with an IC$_{50}$ of 0.30 nM. The consequences of bioisosteric replacement of amides as well as the tethered phenyl moieties revealed that a smaller aliphatic cyclic system such as cyclopropyl is optimum for activity, heterocyclic pyrazole and generally aromatic systems are better compared to aliphatic cyclic systems, and finally the 2,methylphenyl is optimum for activity compared to other substituents in the tethered phenyl ring. Its kinase selectivity profiling over 250 kinases indicated that compound **89** inhibits VEGFR-1 (IC$_{50}$ = 3.2 nM), VEGFR-3 (IC$_{50}$ = 1.1 nM), PDGFR-α and β (IC$_{50}$ = 4.3 nM and 13 nM, respectively), FMS (IC$_{50}$ = 10 nM) and RET (IC$_{50}$ = 18 nM) kinases while its IC$_{50}$ values against other kinases were above 100 nM. Oral administration of 1 mg/kg twice daily suppressed tumor growth in a mouse xenograft model of human lung adenocarcinoma A549 cells (T/C = 8%) [100].

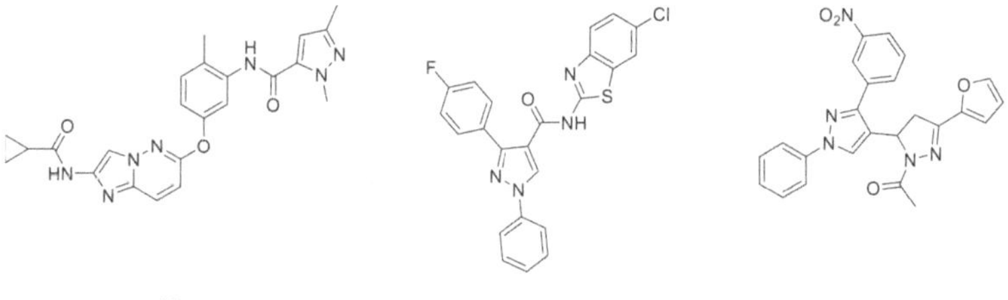

Figure 94. Structures of pyrazole-based VEGFR2 inhibitors and their IC$_{50}$ values.

28.2. Compound 90

Using pyrazole-containing chemotherapeutic agents like crizotinib, axitinib and ibrutinib as a framework, a series of pyrazole-benthothiazole hybrids were designed as antiangiogenic agents. Compound **90** bearing halogens (fluoro and chloro) as substituents, displayed in vitro inhibitory activity against VEGFR-2 (Figure 94). Compound **90** was investigated for cytotoxic activity using the MTT assay against the HT-29 colon cell line (IC$_{50}$ = 3.32 µM), PC-3 prostate cells (IC$_{50}$ = 3.17 µM), A549 lung cells (IC$_{50}$ = 3.87 µM), and U87MG glioblastoma cells (IC$_{50}$ = 6.77 µM). It was also tested against a normal human embryonic kidney cell line (HEK-293T) to investigate selectivity towards tumor cells and revealed 9 to 15-fold more selectivity towards cancer cells compared to axitinib, which is only 2–3 times more selective. The SAR study presented by this series revealed the superiority of electron-withdrawing substituent compared to the electron-donating ones. Further studies such as the colony-forming potential of PC-3 treated with compound **90** showed an inhibition of PC-3 treated with compound **90** at 1, and 5 µM for 7 days, crossed multiple layers of both PC-3 and U87MG spheroids at 1 µM and 5 µM in a 3D multicellular spheroids inhibition assay, inhibited migration in PC-3 cells at 3 µM after 48h as compared to control cells, and almost stopped migration at 5 µM and dose-dependent G_0/G_1 phase cell cycle arrest in PC-3 cells using the flow cytometry analysis. The in vivo antiangiogenic activity was analyzed using Zebrafish embryos treated with compound **90** at 0.1, 0.5 and 1 µM with axitinib used as a positive control 24 h post fertilization (hpf) stage, and it revealed that compound **90** exhibits dose-dependent antiangiogenic activity [101].

28.3. Compound 91

A bi-aryl pyrazole series conjugated with pyrazoline, triazolopyrimidine, and pyrazolone compounds was designed as an antiangiogenic agent, targeting the VEGFR-2 kinase. The best compound of this series in terms of potency was compound **91** (Figure 94) which had in an SRB assay against the MCF-7 cell lines, an IC_{50} of 18.35 µM in comparison to tamoxifen, which has an IC_{50} of 23.31 µM. It also displayed a reduction in the VEGFR-2 levels in the MCF-7 cell lines with 72% inhibition compared to an untreated control. Compared to sorafenib in an ELISA assay, compound **91** had an IC_{50} of 225.13 nM against the VEGFR-2 kinase, while sorafenib's was 186.54 nM. Compound **91** was the most potent in the series [102].

The docking of compound **91** into the VEGFR-2 active pocket was done on the MOE 2008.10 version. The docking results displayed the key interaction of the arms of the pyrazole core, and the contribution made by the N-acetyl pyrazoline and its interactions with different amino acids of the active site. Compounds with the N-acetyl moiety had superior results as compared to the other compounds in this series. The furan centroid interaction with Lys868 could explain the VEGFR-2 inhibitory activity (Figure 95) [102].

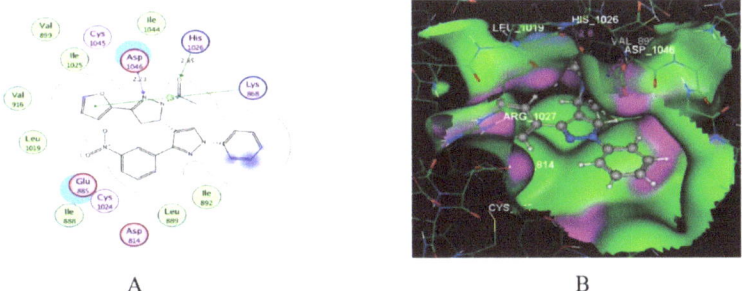

Figure 95. Compound **91** binding mode in the active pocket of VEGFR-2, (**A**) illustrates the 2D interaction and (**B**) the 3D interactions. Green = hydrophobic area, pink = high polar area, blue = mild polar area and dotted lines and arrows = hydrogen bonds [102].

29. Pyrazole-Based Multikinase Inhibitors

29.1. Compound 92

The 1,3,4-triarylpyrazole derivatives with a *p*-fluorophenyl at position 3 of the pyrazole ring and 4-pyridyl at position 4 are potent inhibitors of p38α. Upon a regioisomeric switch from 3-(4-fluorophenyl)-4-(pyridin-4-yl)-1-(aryl)-1*H*-pyrazol-5-amine to 4-(4-fluorophenyl)-3-(pyridin-4-yl)-1-(aryl)-1*H*-pyrazol-5-amine, i.e., an exchange of the locations of the pyridyl and fluorophenyl rings, p38α inhibition was lost, but the new analogues inhibited other kinases over-expressed in tumors. Compound **92** is the most promising kinase inhibitor among this series (Figure 96). It is a multiple inhibitor of VEGFR2, Src, B-RAF (wild-type), V600E-B-RAF, EGFR (wild-type), and L858R-EGFR with IC_{50} values of 34, 399, 270, 592, 113, and 31 nM, respectively. The 2,4,6-trichlorophenyl, 4-fluorophenyl, 4-pyridyl, and the amino group are all together important for the kinase inhibitory effect. Removal of amino, replacement of fluorophenyl with amide or ester, or replacement of the trisubstituted phenyl with a monosubstituted one led to decreased potency against the kinases [103].

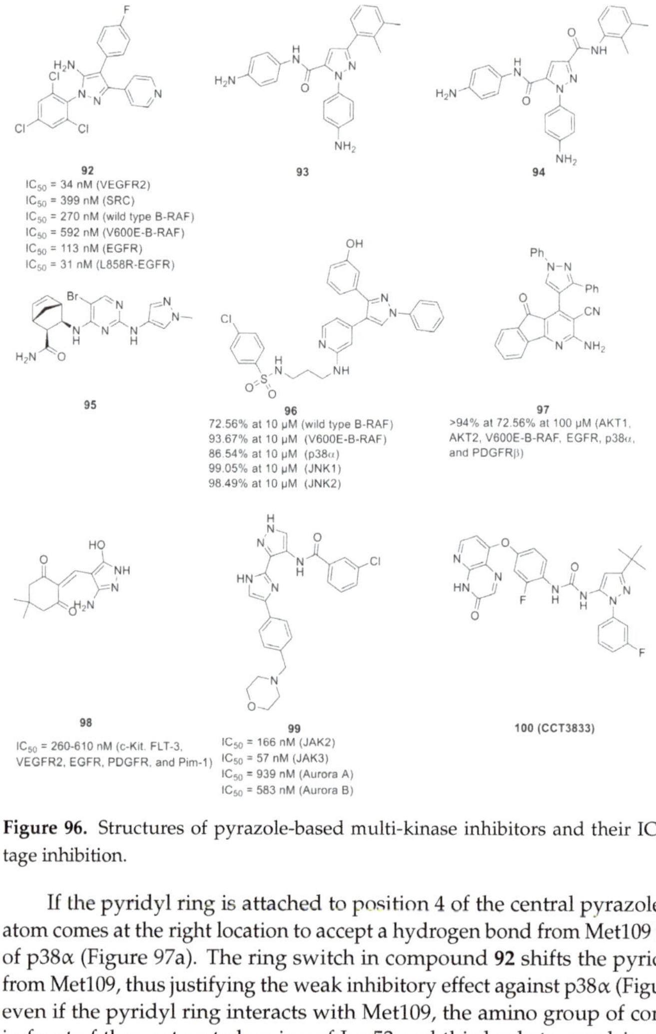

Figure 96. Structures of pyrazole-based multi-kinase inhibitors and their IC$_{50}$ values or percentage inhibition.

If the pyridyl ring is attached to position 4 of the central pyrazole ring, its nitrogen atom comes at the right location to accept a hydrogen bond from Met109 in the hinge region of p38α (Figure 97a). The ring switch in compound **92** shifts the pyridyl nitrogen away from Met109, thus justifying the weak inhibitory effect against p38α (Figure 97b). Moreover, even if the pyridyl ring interacts with Met109, the amino group of compound **92** comes in front of the protonated amino of Lys53 and this leads to repulsion (Figure 97c) [103]. Figure 98 illustrates its binding interactions with B-RAF, Src, and VEGFR2 [103].

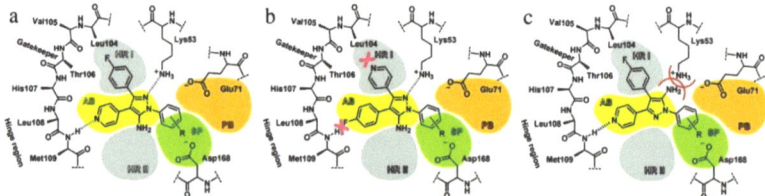

Figure 97. (a) Binding interactions of the regioisomer of compound **92** with p38α. (b,c) Effects of regioisomerism on declined activity against p38α [103].

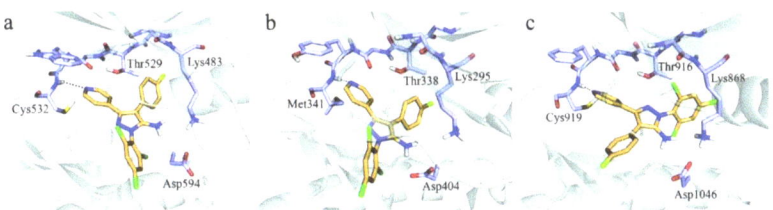

Figure 98. Putative binding interactions of compound **92** with B-RAF (**a**), Src (**b**), and VEGFR2 (**c**) [103].

29.2. Compounds 93 and 94

Both compounds **93** and **94** are antiproliferative agents against the SNU449 hepatocellular carcinoma cell line but with modest potency (IC$_{50}$ 50–100 µM) (Figure 96). In silico studies revealed their potential multikinase inhibitory effects against AKT2, GSK-3β, PI3K, EGFR, IGFR, CDK2, Aurora A, and MAPK. Docking studies demonstrated the formation of 2–3 hydrogen bonds by the terminal amino, the C5-amide O and the *NH* groups. The pyrazole ring and/or the aryl rings interact with the phenyl rings of the Phe or Tyr amino acid residues to form pi-pi interactions [104].

Western blot assays showed that both compounds inhibit the PI3K/AKT/mTOR pathway resulting in a down-regulation of the phosphorylated isoform of both direct and indirect downstream targets such as GSK-3β, ribosomal subunit S6 and MDM2. However, upon testing in real experiments against a 20-kinase panel at 3 µM concentration, no significant inhibition was recorded. The authors recommend kinase testing at high concentrations and we recommend further lead optimization [104].

29.3. Compound 95

A series of novel pyrazole derivatives that are structurally related to kinase inhibitor AS-703569 (cenisertib, Figure 99) were developed in an effort to identify kinase inhibitors with dual KDR/Aurora B activity and enhanced aqueous solubility compared to Abbott's dual inhibitor ABT-348 (ilorasertib) (Figure 99). Compound **95** was found to have a balanced and strong potency against the two kinases (Figures 96 and 99). Compound **95** is also a potent inhibitor of many RTKs and serine/threonine kinases. In fact, this compound has a K$_i$ < 5 nM for thirty-eight kinases, a K$_i$ of 5–10 nM over eleven kinases, and a K$_i$ of 10–20 nM against sixteen kinases. The pan-kinase inhibitory effects of this compound led to a narrow therapeutic index that prohibited its use as an anticancer agent. This is applicable to that series of compounds: the derivatives of compound **95** [105].

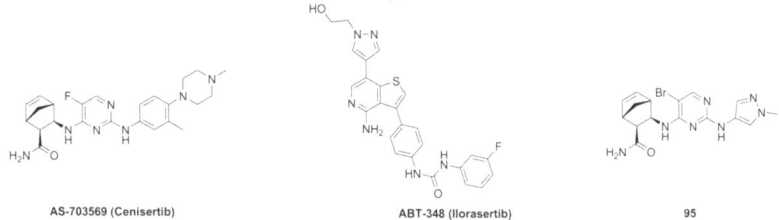

Figure 99. Structures of cenisertib, illorasertib, and compound **95**.

29.4. Compound 96

Compound **96** is the most promising antiproliferative derivative among a series of triarylpyrazoles containing terminal aryl sulfonamide moiety (Figure 96). It was tested against the NCI-60 cancer cell line panel and exerted broad-spectrum activity with a 97.80% mean inhibition percentage. The A498 renal carcinoma cell line is the most sensitive cell line to compound **96** (IC$_{50}$ = 0.33 µM). Upon testing against a 20-kinase panel, it exerted inhibitory effects against B-RAF (wild-type), V600E-B-RAF, p38α, JNK1, and JNK2 kinases (inhibition % values at 10 µM concentration are 72.56%, 93.67%, 86.54%, 99.05%, and 98.49%, respectively). JNK1 and JNK2 are the most sensitive among them (IC_{50} = 350 and 360 nM, respectively). The plasma stability testing of compound **96** showed its high stability profile in both human and rat plasma. However, its oral bioavailability following 10 mg/kg administration in rats is only 9.2%. The SAR study demonstrated that the phenolic *OH*, propylene spacer, and terminal p-chlorobenzene sulfonamide moieties are optimal for the activity of this compound compared to methoxy, ethylene linkers, and other aryl sulfonamide motifs [106].

*29.5. Compound **97***

A series of novel 1,3,4-triarylpyrazole derivatives attached to a tricyclic ring system was reported as multiple kinase-inhibiting antiproliferative agents. Compound **97** is the most promising among them (Figure 96). It was tested against five different cancer cell lines, but its highest potency was exerted against the MCF7 breast cancer cell line (IC_{50} = 6.53 µM). The fused tricyclic ring system with carbonyl was found to be more favorable for antiproliferative activity than a fused bicyclic, monocyclic or even a fused tricyclic ring system lacking a carbonyl group. Compound **97** was further tested against a panel of 12 kinases at 100 µM and was promiscuous. Compound **97** showed more than 94% inhibition against AKT1, AKT2, V600E-B-RAF, EGFR, p38α, and PDGFRβ. The highest activity was against EGFR (99% inhibition) [107].

Docking studies were performed in order to study its binding interactions with AKT1, AKT2, V600E-B-RAF, EGFR, and p38α kinases (Figure 100). The pyrazole ring forms arene–cation interactions with the Lys amino acid residues of the AKT1 and p38α kinases. However, it forms hydrophobic interactions with the Phe163 residue of AKT2. The carbonyl oxygen accepts hydrogen bonds in all kinases except V600E-B-RAF. The cyano and amino groups act as additional hydrogen bond-forming groups, and the fused benzene and pyridine rings form hydrophobic interactions with the EGFR crystal structure. This can rationalize the strong inhibitory effect of compound **97** against the EGFR kinase [107].

*29.6. Compound **98***

Compound **98** is a dimedone-pyrazole hybrid that was reported as multikinase inhibitory antiproliferative agent (Figure 96). It was tested against the A549 (lung), H460 (lung), HT29 (colon), MKN-45 (gastric), U87MG (glioma), and SMMC-77217721 (hepatic) cancer cell lines and showed sub-micromolar IC_{50} values within the range of 0.29–0.42 µM. It was also tested against c-Kit, FLT-3, VEGFR-2, EGFR, PDGFR, and Pim-1 kinases and inhibited all of them with IC_{50} values of 260–610 nM. The highest potency was exerted against Pim-1 (IC_{50} = 260 nM). Phenyl substitution on the *NH* of pyrazole ring or replacement of the amino group with hydroxyl decreased the activity [108].

*29.7. Compound **99***

A series of pyrazole derivatives was reported as multikinase inhibitory antiproliferative agents. These derivatives were designed with a similarity to AT9283, a pyrazolyl urea derivative with JAK/Aurora kinase inhibitory effects (Figure 101). Compound **99**, possessing *m*-chlorobenzamido moiety, exerted more balanced biological results against kinases and cancer cell lines compared to other analogues with substituents except for chloro (Figure 96). The IC_{50} values of compound **99** against JAK2, JAK3, Aurora A, and Aurora B are 166, 57, 939, 583 nM, respectively. Its potency against these kinases is weaker than AT9283 (2.2, 1.2, 26, and 62 nM, respectively). In addition, compound **99** was tested against the K562 leukemia cell line and the HCT116 colon cancer cell line (IC_{50} = 6.726 and 15.054 µM, respectively) but yielded weaker potency than AT9283 (IC_{50} = 0.748 and 0.09 µM, respectively). Against the HCoEpiC and HUVEC normal cells, the IC_{50} values of compound **99** are 31.509 and 28.978 µM, respectively while those of AT9283 are 2.367

and 1.793, respectively. Upon testing the effects of compound **99** on K562 and HCT116 cell cycles, it arrested the G2 phase in a dose-dependent manner [109].

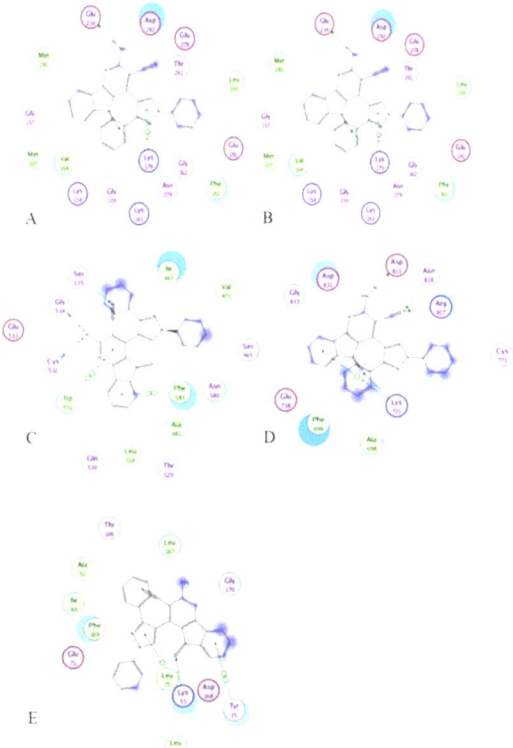

Figure 100. Putative binding interactions of compound **97** with AKT1 (**A**), AKT2 (**B**), V600E-B-RAF (**C**), EGFR (**D**), and p38α kinases (**E**) [107].

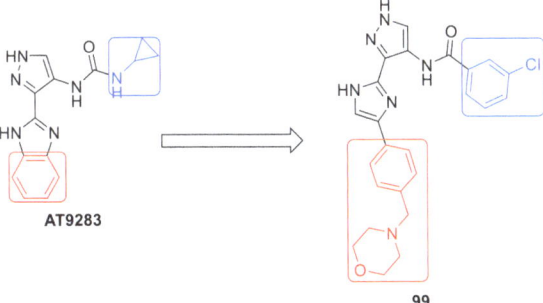

Figure 101. Structures of **AT9283** and compound **99**.

The docking study of compound **99** and AT9283 against the four kinases was carried out (Figure 102). The pyrazole and imidazole rings of compound **99** formed a network of hydrogen bonds with the hinge regions of the four kinases. These interactions are similar to AT9283 but weaker. This explains the weaker potency of compound **99** against the kinase when compared to AT9283. It is noteworthy that the morpholino ring of compound **99** did not contribute to interactions with the kinase crystal structures, and the structure of AT9283 does not possess a similar moiety [109].

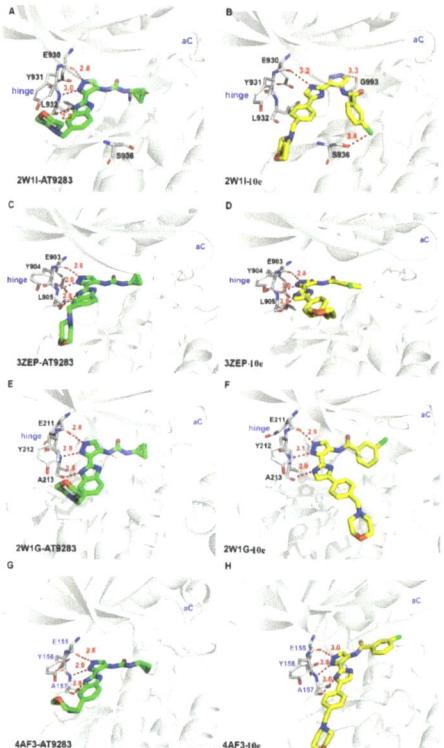

Figure 102. Putative binding interactions of AT9283 and compound **99**. (**A**) AT9283 with JAK2; (**B**) Compound **99** with JAK2; (**C**) AT9283 with JAK3; (**D**) Compound **99** with JAK3; (**E**) AT9283 with Aurora A; (**F**) Compound **99** with Aurora A; (**G**) AT9283 with Aurora B; (**H**) Compound **99** with Aurora B [109].

29.8. Compound **100**

Compound **100** (CCT3833) is a pyrazolyl urea-based pan-RAF kinase inhibitor that possesses inhibitory effects against the Src kinase as well (Figure 96). It inhibited B-RAF, C-RAF, and Src kinases both in vitro and in vivo. In addition, it decreased tumor regression in mouse models. CCT3833 is a clinical candidate that was evaluated in phase I clinical trials for tolerability and safety in volunteer patients with solid tumors [110]. In addition, CCT3833 was reported to increase the progression-free survival in a patient suffering from KRAS (G12V) spindle cell sarcoma [111,112].

30. Conclusions

Pyrazole represents a privileged scaffold with a variety of therapeutic activities. In this article, we reviewed different pyrazole-based kinase inhibitors that were described in the literature in the last decade (2011–2020). During the last decade, pyrazole derivatives were reported to exert a wide spectrum of biological activities including antimicrobial and anticancer activities among others. In the anticancer and anti-inflammatory fields in particular, pyrazoles have been shown to interact at the intracellular level on many pathways, especially against kinases. As reported in the literature from 2011 to 2020, several important results have been obtained, where pyrazole derivatives have been shown to inhibit many kinases such as the Akt, ALK, Aurora, Bcr-Abl, CDK, Chk2, EGFR, ERK/MEK, FGFR, IRAK4, ITK, JAK, JNK, LRRK, Lsrk, MAPK14, PDK4, Pim, RAF, ROS1, Src, VEGFR, and others in the pathways of different diseases. The reviewed compounds were classified according to their kinase targets with some of them being multiple kinase inhibitors. We arranged the compounds chronologically from the oldest to the most recent in each kinase category. Structural modifications of pyrazole derivatives can be optimized to enhance potency, selectivity, and pharmacokinetic properties. The pyrazole ring can replace more hydrophobic (hetero)aromatic rings in the structure to improve aqueous solubility and PK properties. It can also act as a core scaffold for proper orientation of other rings/substituents attached to it inside the kinase crystal structure. The nitrogen atoms of pyrazole can perform hydrogen bonding and its carbons can contribute to hydrophobic interactions. Pyrazole is also an electron-rich ring, so it can contribute to an arene–cation interaction if it comes in front of positively charged amino acid residues in kinase crystal structures. The design and development of pyrazole derivatives as kinase inhibitors have been interesting in research in the field of medicinal chemistry. Azole derivatives including pyrazoles have a potential to inhibit cytochrome P450 enzymes, thus it is recommended for researchers working in this field to test their potential compounds against the CYP450 isozymes. If a significant inhibitory effect is found, the structural design should be reconsidered to decrease affinity to CYP450 with special attention given to decreasing electron density on the pyrazole ring by attaching electron-withdrawing group(s), for example, or replacement of pyrazole with 6-membered ring keeping in mind the possible impact on biological activity. Otherwise, re-adjustment of the doses of co-administered drugs that are metabolized mainly by cytochrome P450 enzymes is recommended to avoid accumulation and toxicity.

Table 1 summarizes the structures of the reviewed pyrazole-based kinase inhibitors, their IC_{50} values against the most sensitive kinases in cell-free assays, and other relevant biological activities.

Table 1. Structures, IC_{50} values, and the most important biological results of the reviewed pyrazole-based kinase inhibitors.

Kinase	Inhibitor	IC_{50} Value in Cell-Free Assay (nM)	Other Biological Activities
AKT1	1	61	Antiproliferative activity against HCT116 and OVCAR-8 cell lines (IC_{50} = 7.76 and 9.76 µM, respectively)
	2	1.3	Antiproliferative activity against HCT116 colon cancer cell line (IC_{50} = 0.95 µM). Reduction of tumor size by 42% in the MM1S model.
ALK	3	2.9	Reduction of phosphorylation of ALK in hippocampus in a dose-dependent manner at 30 mg/kg and higher. Inhibited phosphorylation in prefrontal cortex at 100 mg/kg.
ASK1	4	-	Good CNS penetration. Weak potency against hERG, CYP3A4, and CYP2C9.

Table 1. Cont.

Kinase	Inhibitor	IC$_{50}$ Value in Cell-Free Assay (nM)	Other Biological Activities
Aurora	5 (Barasertib, AZD1152)	0.37 (Aurora B)	Passed phase I clinical trials in Japanese and Western volunteers suffering from advanced acute myeloid leukemia.
	6	160 (Aurora A)	IC$_{50}$ values against HCT116 colon cancer and MCF7 breast cancer cell lines are 0.39 and 0.46 μM, respectively.
	7	28.9 (Aurora A) 2.2 (Aurora B)	IC$_{50}$ values against U937 (leukemia), K562 (leukemia), A549 (lung), LoVo (colon), and HT29 (colon) cancer cell lines are 5.106, 5.003, 0.487, 0.789, and 0.381 μM, respectively.
	8	35 (Aurora A) 75 (Aurora B)	Antiproliferative activity against SW620 and HCT116 colon cancer cell lines (IC$_{50}$ = 0.35 and 0.34 μM, respectively).
	9 (SP-96)	0.316 (Aurora B)	Antiproliferative activity against MDA-MB-468 with IC$_{50}$ value equal to 107 nM.
BCR-ABL	10	14.2	Antiproliferative activity against the K562 leukemia cell line with an IC$_{50}$ value equal to 0.27 μM.
	11	8.5	Antiproliferative activity against the K562 leukemia cell line with an IC$_{50}$ value less than 2 nM.

Table 1. Cont.

Kinase	Inhibitor	IC$_{50}$ Value in Cell-Free Assay (nM)	Other Biological Activities
BCR-ABL	12 (Asciminib, ABL-001)	0.5	IC$_{50}$ = 25 nM against ABL (T315I). Clinical candidate for CML.
Calcium-dependent kinase	13	56	Anti-parasitic activity against *Plasmodium falciparum* with an IC$_{50}$ value of 0.262 µM.
	14 (BKI 1708)	0.7	Anti-parasitic activity against *Cryptosporidium parvum* with an EC$_{50}$ value of 0.41 µM.
	15 (BKI 1770)	2.5	Anti-parasitic activity against *Cryptosporidium parvum* with an EC$_{50}$ value of 0.51 µM.
Checkpoint kinase 2	16	48.4	Antiproliferative activity against HepG2 (hepatocellular carcinoma), HeLa (cervical), and MCF7 (breast) cancer cell lines.
	17	17.9	Antiproliferative activity against HepG2 (hepatocellular carcinoma), HeLa (cervical), and MCF7 (breast) cancer cell lines (IC$_{50}$ = 10.8, 11.8, and 10.4 µM, respectively).
	18	41.64	Modest potency against HepG2, HeLa, and MCF7 cell lines with 2-digit micromolar IC$_{50}$ values.

Table 1. Cont.

Kinase	Inhibitor	IC$_{50}$ Value in Cell-Free Assay (nM)	Other Biological Activities
Cyclin-dependent kinases	19	420 (CDK4)	Modest antiproliferative activity against K562, MCF7, and RPMI-8226 cancer cell lines. Induced apoptosis in RPMI-8226 cells.
	20	-	IC$_{50}$ values against MCF7 cells (IC$_{50}$ = 0.13 µM), MIAPaCa pancreatic cancer cell line (IC$_{50}$ = 0.28 µM), and HeLa cervical cancer cell line (IC$_{50}$ = 0.21 µM).
	21	-	IC$_{50}$ values against MCF7 cells (IC$_{50}$ = 0.15 µM), MIAPaCa pancreatic cancer cell line (IC$_{50}$ = 0.34 µM), and HeLa cervical cancer cell line (IC$_{50}$ = 0 0.73 µM).
	22	24 (CDK2) 23 (CDK5)	Induction of apoptosis in the MiaPaCa2 pancreatic cancer cell line.
	23 (AT7519)	10–210 (multiple CDK inhibitor)	Induction of apoptosis in colon cancer and multiple myeloma cells.
	24	2380 (CDK1)	Antiproliferative activity against hepatocellular carcinoma (HepG2, Huh7, and SNU-475), colon cancer (HCT116), and renal cancer (UO-31) cell lines (IC$_{50}$ = 0.05, 0.065, 1.93, 1.68, and 1.85 µM, respectively).

Table 1. Cont.

Kinase	Inhibitor	IC$_{50}$ Value in Cell-Free Assay (nM)	Other Biological Activities
Cyclin-dependent kinases	25	1520 (CDK1)	Antiproliferative activity against hepatocellular carcinoma (HepG2, Huh7, and SNU-475), colon cancer (HCT116), and renal cancer (UO-31) cell lines (IC$_{50}$ = 0.028, 1.83, 1.70, 0.035, and 2.24 µM, respectively).
	26 (FMF-04-159-2)	88 (CDK14)	Antiproliferative activity against HCT116 colorectal cancer cell line (IC$_{50}$ = 1.14 µM).
	27	8.63 (CDK1) 0.30 (CDK2)	Inhibitory effect against HDAC1, HDAC2, and HDAC3 (IC$_{50}$ = 6.40, 0.25, and 45.0 nM, respectively). Antiproliferative activity against HCT116 colorectal cancer cell line (IC$_{50}$ = 0.71 µM).
	28	9 (CDK12) 5.8 (CDK13)	-
EGFR	29	210	Antiproliferative effect against MCF-7 breast cancer cell line (IC$_{50}$ = 0.30 µM).
FGFR	30 (AZD4547)	0.2 (FGFR1) 2.5 (FGFR2) 1.8 (FGFR3) 165 (FGFR4)	Orally bioavailable, clinical candidate for lymphoma, glioma, lung, breast, gastric, and esophageal types of cancer.
	31 (CH5183284/Debio 1347)	9.3 (FGFR1) 7.6 (FGFR2) 22 (FGFR3) 290 (FGFR4)	Antiproliferative IC$_{50}$ values against gastric SNU-16 and colon HCT116 cancer cell lines are 17 nM and 5.9 µM, respectively.

Table 1. Cont.

Kinase	Inhibitor	IC$_{50}$ Value in Cell-Free Assay (nM)	Other Biological Activities
FGFR	32 (CPL304110)	0.75 (FGFR1) 0.5 (FGFR2) 3.05 (FGFR3) 87.9 (FGFR4)	Antiproliferative activity against FGFR-2-amplified SNU-16 gastric cancer cell line (IC$_{50}$ = 85.64 nM).
IKK	33	-	Antiproliferative activity against HeLa cervical cancer cell line (IC$_{50}$ = 14.2 µg/mL).
IRAK4	34	5	Strong potency (IC$_{50}$ = 83 nM) against lipopolysaccharide-induced THP1-XBlue cells.
	35	0.4	Good permeability (25 × 10^{-6} cm/s) in MDCK cells.
	36	0.51	-
ITK	37	Ki = 0.1 nM	Multi-kinase inhibitor.
	38 (GNE-9822)	Ki = 0.5 nM	Higher kinase selectivity, permeability, and oral bioavailability than compound 37.

Table 1. Cont.

Kinase	Inhibitor	IC$_{50}$ Value in Cell-Free Assay (nM)	Other Biological Activities
ITK	39 (GNE-4997)	Ki = 0.09 nM	Improved potency, selectivity, and less toxicity.
JAK	40	3.4 (JAK1) 2.2 (JAK2) 3.5 (JAK3)	Antiproliferative activity: IC$_{50}$ against PC-3 IC$_{50}$ = 1.08 μM, MCF-7 IC$_{50}$ = 1.33 μM, HEL IC$_{50}$ = 1.08 μM, K562 IC$_{50}$ = 0.77 μM, MOLT4 IC$_{50}$ = 1.61 μM.
	41	-	Antiproliferative activity against HEL (IC$_{50}$ = 0.35 μM) and K562 (IC$_{50}$ = 0.37 μM).
	42	Ki = 2.5 nM (JAK2)	Potent inhibitory activity in a JAK2-driven SET2 cell-based assay (IC$_{50}$ = 131 nM). Low potential for reversible inhibition of five major human CYP450 isozymes, and good in vitro permeability profile.
	43	Ki = 0.21 nM (JAK1) Ki = 0.088 nM (JAK2)	IC$_{50}$ of 4.7 nM in IL-13 stimulated BEAS-2B cells.
	44	Ki = 0.31 nM (JAK1) Ki = 0.14 nM (JAK2)	IC$_{50}$ of 6.4 nM in the IL-13-pSTAT6 cell-based assay.
	45 (BMS-911543)	75 (JAK1) 1.1 (JAK2) 360 (JAK3)	In vivo reduction of reticulocytes and subsequent reductions in red blood cell mass as well as a decrease in platelets.

Table 1. Cont.

Kinase	Inhibitor	IC$_{50}$ Value in Cell-Free Assay (nM)	Other Biological Activities
JNK	46	2800 (JNK1)	In vivo anti-inflammatory activity against carrageenan-induced paw edema model in rats.
	47	227 (JNK3)	-
LRRK	48	9 (LRRK2)	-
	49 (GNE-0877)	0.7 (LRRK2)	Improved human hepatocyte stability, brain exposure, and lower ability to inhibit or induce CYP compared to compound 48.
	50 (GNE-9605)	2 (LRRK2)	Improved human hepatocyte stability, brain exposure, and lower ability to inhibit or induce CYP compared to compound 48.
	51	-	-
	52	K_i = 84 nM (wild-type LRRK2) and 39 nM (G2019S mutant type LRRK2)	98% oral bioavailability.

Table 1. Cont.

Kinase	Inhibitor	IC$_{50}$ Value in Cell-Free Assay (nM)	Other Biological Activities
LsrK	53	119,000	-
MEK/ERK	54	-	Antiproliferative activity against the A375P melanoma cell line (IC$_{50}$ = 6.7 µM).
	55	-	Antiproliferative activity against the MDA-MB-435 melanoma cell line (IC$_{50}$ = 2.7 µM). Kinase inhibition was confirmed by Western blotting. IC$_{50}$ = 0.30 µM against COX-2.
	56	-	IC$_{50}$ = 91 nM against recombinant proteins of the RAF-MEK-ERK cascade. GI$_{50}$ of 1.18, 2.11, and 0.26 µM against HeLa, MCF-7, and A549 cell lines, respectively.
	57	22	Inhibition of TNF-α production in lipopolysaccharide-stimulated THP-1 human cells. In vivo anti-inflammatory activity.
P38α/ MAPK14	58	135	Poor cellular permeability due to its highly charged carboxylate group. Its ethyl ester analogue could inhibit phosphorylation of MK2 in HeLa cells (IC$_{50}$ value = 6 µM) but its IC$_{50}$ value against p38α is 639 nM.
	59 (VPC00628)	7	High selectivity against p38α and p38β.
	60	515	Antiproliferative activity against RPMI-8226 and K-562 leukemia cell lines in addition to the MDA-MB-468 breast cancer cell line (IC$_{50}$ values are 1.71, 3.42, and 6.70 µM, respectively).

Table 1. Cont.

Kinase	Inhibitor	IC$_{50}$ Value in Cell-Free Assay (nM)	Other Biological Activities
PDK4	61	84	Enhanced glucose tolerance in a diet-induced obesity model in mice. Alleviated the allergic reactions in a passive cutaneous anaphylaxis model in mice.
Pim	62	Ki = 0.073 nM (Pim1), 0.473 (Pim2), and 0.041 (Pim3)	Antiproliferative activity against MM1.s myeloma cell line (IC$_{50}$ = 0.64 µM).
	63 (GDC-0339)	Ki = 0.03 nM (Pim1), 0.1 (Pim2), and 0.02 (Pim3)	Promising in vivo activity against MM1.s and RPMI 8226 mice models of multiple myeloma.
RAF	64	-	Antiproliferative activity against the A375P melanoma cell line (IC$_{50}$ = 4.5 µM).
	65	0.04 (wild-type B-RAF)	Its *trans* isomer (with the hydroxyl group behind the plane) is less potent against the kinase (IC$_{50}$ = 0.09 nM).
	66	330 (V600E-B-RAF)	Antiproliferative activity against WM266.4 and A375 melanoma cell lines with IC$_{50}$ values of 2.63 and 3.16 µM, respectively
	67	770 (V600E-B-RAF) and 1500 (RAF1)	One-digit micromolar IC$_{50}$ values against different cancer cell lines.

Table 1. *Cont.*

Kinase	Inhibitor	IC$_{50}$ Value in Cell-Free Assay (nM)	Other Biological Activities
RAF	68	2.98 (V600E-B-RAF)	Antiproliferative activity against the A375 melanoma cells (IC$_{50}$ = 1.82 µM).
	69	99.17% inhibition at 10 µM (V600E-B-RAF)	IC$_{50}$ values within sub-micromolar range (0.27–0.92 µM) against nine cancer cell lines of nine cancer types. Against the A375 melanoma cell line, its IC$_{50}$ value is 0.82 µM.
	70	-	78.04%, 74.47%, and 72.46% inhibition at 10 µM concentration against RAF1, V600E-B-RAF, and V600K-B-RAF kinases, respectively.
	71	7 (V600E-B-RAF)	Mean IC$_{50}$ value against the NCI nine subpanels was within the range of 1.98–3.26 µM.
	72	390 (V600E-B-RAF)	IC$_{50}$ values are within the submicromolar range against most of the tested cell lines (NCI-60 panel). Induced apoptosis in the RPMI-8226 leukemia cell line with an EC$_{50}$ of 1.52 µM.
ROS	73	13.6	-
Src	74	59% inhibition at 10 µM concentration	Antiproliferative activity against CCRF-CEM and MOLT-4 leukemia cell lines (IC$_{50}$ = 1.00 µM against both of them).

227

Table 1. Cont.

Kinase	Inhibitor	IC$_{50}$ Value in Cell-Free Assay (nM)	Other Biological Activities
TGFβ/ALK	75	684 (R206H mutated ALK2)	Promising lead compound for treatment of fibrodysplasia ossificans progressive.
	76	25.6 (R206H mutated ALK2)	Good permeability and in vivo pharmacokinetic properties.
	77 (RK-71807)	9.4	Promising lead compound for treatment of fibrodysplasia ossificans progressive. Improved aqueous solubility compared to compound 75.
	78	13 (TGFβ type 1/ALK5)	Inhibited luciferase activity by 80% at 0.1 μM. In-cell kinase inhibition.
	79	280 (TGFβ type 1/ALK5)	>35-fold more selective against ALK5 compared to p38α MAPK.
	80	18 (TGFβ type 1/ALK5)	In-cell kinase inhibition.
	81	69 (TGFβ type 1/ALK5)	Inhibitory effects against the p38α kinase (IC$_{50}$ = 104 nM).
	82	30 (TGFβ type 1/ALK5)	Potential inhibitor of collagen I and α-SMA protein and mRNA expressions in TGFβ-induced LX-2 human hepatic stellate cells.

Table 1. Cont.

Kinase	Inhibitor	IC$_{50}$ Value in Cell-Free Assay (nM)	Other Biological Activities
Trk	83 (AZ-23)	2 (TrkA) 8 (TrkB)	-
	84	-	Potent inhibitor of TrkA with an IC$_{50}$ value of 0.5 nM in a cellular assay. 29% oral bioavailability. High aqueous solubility and safety against hERG.
	85	-	Potent inhibitor of TrkA with an IC$_{50}$ value of 0.5 nM in a cellular assay. 54% oral bioavailability. High aqueous solubility and safety against hERG.
	86	2.7 (TrkA)	Higher selectivity against TrkA than TrkB and TrkC.
	87	-	Rapid association rate with the TrkA crystal structure, thus binds to the inactive conformation of the kinase (i.e., type II TrkA inhibitor).
	88	0.2 (TrkA)	In vivo activity in CFA-induced thermal hypersensitivity model.

Table 1. Cont.

Kinase	Inhibitor	IC$_{50}$ Value in Cell-Free Assay (nM)	Other Biological Activities
VEGFR	89	0.95 (VEGFR2)	Decreased the proliferation of VEGF stimulated HUVEC with an IC$_{50}$ of 0.30 nM. In vivo anticancer activity in a mouse xenograft model of human lung adenocarcinoma A549 cells.
	90	97 (VEGFR2)	Antiproliferative activity against HT-29 colon cell line (IC$_{50}$ = 3.32 µM), PC-3 prostate cells (IC$_{50}$ = 3.17 µM), A549 lung cells (IC$_{50}$ = 3.87 µM), and U87MG glioblastoma cells (IC$_{50}$ = 6.77 µM).
	91	-	In-cell kinase inhibition. Antiproliferative activity against the MCF-7 cell line (IC$_{50}$ = 18.35 µM).
Multikinase inhibitors	92		Inhibitor of VEGFR2, Src, B-RAF (wild-type), V600E-B-RAF, EGFR (wild-type), and L858R-EGFR with IC$_{50}$ values of 34, 399, 270, 592, 113, and 31 nM, respectively.
	93	Multi-kinase inhibitory effects against AKT2, GSK-3β, PI3K, EGFR, IGFR, CDK2, Aurora A, and MAPK.	Antiproliferative activity against SNU449 hepatocellular carcinoma cell line.
	94	Multikinase inhibitory effects against AKT2, GSK-3β, PI3K, EGFR, IGFR, CDK2, Aurora A, and MAPK.	Antiproliferative activity against SNU449 hepatocellular carcinoma cell line.
	95	Dual KDR/Aurora B activity	Narrow therapeutic index.

Table 1. Cont.

Kinase	Inhibitor	IC$_{50}$ Value in Cell-Free Assay (nM)	Other Biological Activities
Multikinase inhibitors	96	Inhibitory effect against B-RAF (wild-type), V600E-B-RAF, p38α, JNK1, and JNK2 kinases (inhibition % values at 10 μM concentration are 72.56%, 93.67%, 86.54%, 99.05%, and 98.49%, respectively).	Antiproliferative activity against the A498 renal carcinoma cell line (IC$_{50}$ = 0.33 μM). JNK1 and JNK2 are the most sensitive among them (IC$_{50}$ = 350 and 360 nM, respectively).
	97	>94% inhibition of AKT1, AKT2, V600E-B-RAF, EGFR, p38α, and PDGFRβ at 100 μM.	Antiproliferative activity against MCF7 breast cancer cell line (IC$_{50}$ = 6.53 μM).
	98	c-Kit, FLT-3, VEGFR-2, EGFR, PDGFR, and Pim-1 kinases (IC$_{50}$ 260–610 nM).	Antiproliferative activity against A549 (lung), H460 (lung), HT29 (colon), MKN-45 (gastric), U87MG (glioma), and SMMC-77217721 (hepatic) cancer cell lines (IC$_{50}$ values from 0.29–0.42 μM).
	99	JAK2, JAK3, Aurora A, and Aurora B (IC$_{50}$ = 166, 57, 939, 583 nM, respectively).	Antiproliferative activity against K562 leukemia cell line and HCT116 colon cancer cell line (IC$_{50}$ = 6.726 and 15.054 μM, respectively).
	100 (CCT3833)	Inhibited B-RAF, C-RAF, and Src kinases both in vitro and in vivo.	In vivo activity and phase I clinical trials in volunteers with solid tumors. Increased the progression-free survival in a patient suffering from KRAS (G12V) spindle cell sarcoma.

Author Contributions: Conceptualization, M.I.E.-G. and H.S.A.; methodology, M.I.E.-G., S.-O.Z., M.M.M. and H.S.A.; software, S.-O.Z.; validation, M.I.E.-G. and H.S.A.; resources, M.I.E.-G.; writing—original draft preparation, M.I.E.-G., S.-O.Z., M.M.M. and H.S.A.; writing—review and editing, M.I.E.-G., S.-O.Z., M.M.M. and H.S.A.; supervision, M.I.E.-G.; project administration, M.I.E.-G. and H.S.A. All authors have read and agreed to the published version of the manuscript.

Funding: The authors are grateful to University of Sharjah, United Arab Emirates, for financial support.

Institutional Review Board Statement: Not applicable.

Informed Consent Statement: Not applicable.

Data Availability Statement: Not applicable.

Conflicts of Interest: The authors declare no conflict of interest.

Abbreviations

ALK5, Activin receptor-Like Kinase 5; ALS, amyotrophic lateral sclerosis; ASK1, Apoptosis signal-regulating kinase 1; ATP, adenosine triphosphate; CDK, cyclin-dependent kinase; CFA, complete Freund's adjuvant; Chk2, checkpoint kinase 2; CML, chronic myeloid leukemia; COX-1, Cyclooxygenase-1; COX-2, Cyclooxygenase-2; EGFR, Epidermal Growth Factor Receptor; ELISA, enzyme-linked immunosorbent assay; ERK, Extracellular signal-regulated kinase; FDA, Food and Drug Administration; FGFR, fibroblast growth factor receptor; GI_{50}, concentration at which 50% growth inhibition is observed; HDAC, histone deacetylase; HEL, human erythroleukemia; HER-2, human epidermal growth factor receptor 2; hPBMCs, human peripheral blood mononuclear cells; HUVEC, human umbilical vein endothelial cells; IKKβ; inhibitor of nuclear factor kappa-B kinase subunit β; IL, interleukin; IRAK4, interleukin-1 receptor associated kinase 4; ITK, Interleukin-2 inducible T-cell kinase; JAK, Janus kinase; JNK, c-Jun N-terminal kinases; KD, kinase domain; LRRK2, leucine-rich repeat kinase 2; MAPKs, mitogen-activated protein kinases; MDCK, Madin–Darby canine kidney; MDR, multidrug resistance; MM, molecular mechanics; MS, multiple sclerosis; NCI, National Cancer Institute; PDK4, pyruvate dehydrogenase kinase 4; QM, quantum mechanics; QS, quorum sensing; QSAR, quantitative structure-activity relationship; SAR, structure-activity relationship; TDI, time-dependent inhibition; TNF-α, tumor-necrosis factor-α; VEGFR, vascular endothelial growth factor receptors.

References

1. Karrouchi, K.; Radi, S.; Ramli, Y.; Taoufik, J.; Mabkhot, Y.; Al-Aizari, F.; Ansar, M.H. Synthesis and Pharmacological Activities of Pyrazole Derivatives: A Review. *Molecules* **2018**, *23*, 134. [CrossRef]
2. Yerragunta, V.; Suman, D.; Anusha, V.; Patil, P.; Naresh, M. Pyrazole and its biological activity. *PharmaTutor* **2014**, *2*, 40–48.
3. Faria, J.V.; Vegi, P.F.; Miguita, A.G.C.; Dos Santos, M.S.; Boechat, N.; Bernardino, A.M.R. Recently reported biological activities of pyrazole compounds. *Bioorg. Med. Chem.* **2017**, *25*, 5891–5903. [CrossRef]
4. Rauch, J.; Volinsky, N.; Romano, D.; Kolch, W. The secret life of kinases: Functions beyond catalysis. *Cell Commun. Signal.* **2011**, *9*, 23. [CrossRef] [PubMed]
5. Kannaiyan, R.; Mahadevan, D. A comprehensive review of protein kinase inhibitors for cancer therapy. *Expert Rev. Anticancer Ther.* **2018**, *18*, 1249–1270. [CrossRef] [PubMed]
6. Ferguson, F.M.; Gray, N.S. Kinase inhibitors: The road ahead. *Nat. Rev. Drug Discov.* **2018**, *17*, 353–377. [CrossRef]
7. Shaw, A.T.; Yasothan, U.; Kirkpatrick, P. Crizotinib. *Nat. Rev. Drug Discov.* **2011**, *10*, 897–898. [CrossRef] [PubMed]
8. Markham, A. Erdafitinib: First Global Approval. *Drugs* **2019**, *79*, 1017–1021. [CrossRef] [PubMed]
9. Mesa, R.A.; Yasothan, U.; Kirkpatrick, P. Ruxolitinib. *Nat. Rev. Drug Discov.* **2012**, *11*, 103–104. [CrossRef]
10. Zhan, W.; Xu, L.; Dong, X.; Dong, J.; Yi, X.; Ma, X.; Qiu, N.; Li, J.; Yang, B.; Zhou, Y.; et al. Design, synthesis and biological evaluation of pyrazol-furan carboxamide analogues as novel Akt kinase inhibitors. *Eur. J. Med. Chem.* **2016**, *117*, 47–58. [CrossRef]
11. Zhan, W.; Che, J.; Xu, L.; Wu, Y.; Hu, X.; Zhou, Y.; Cheng, G.; Hu, Y.; Dong, X.; Li, J. Discovery of pyrazole-thiophene derivatives as highly Potent, orally active Akt inhibitors. *Eur. J. Med. Chem.* **2019**, *180*, 72–85. [CrossRef]
12. Fushimi, M.; Fujimori, I.; Wakabayashi, T.; Hasui, T.; Kawakita, Y.; Imamura, K.; Kato, T.; Murakami, M.; Ishii, T.; Kikko, Y.; et al. Discovery of Potent, Selective, and Brain-Penetrant 1H-Pyrazol-5-yl-1H-pyrrolo[2,3-b]pyridines as Anaplastic Lymphoma Kinase (ALK) Inhibitors. *J. Med. Chem.* **2019**, *62*, 4915–4935. [CrossRef]
13. Xin, Z.; Himmelbauer, M.K.; Jones, J.H.; Enyedy, I.; Gilfillan, R.; Hesson, T.; King, K.; Marcotte, D.J.; Murugan, P.; Santoro, J.C.; et al. Discovery of CNS-Penetrant Apoptosis Signal-Regulating Kinase 1 (ASK1) Inhibitors. *ACS Med. Chem. Lett.* **2020**, *11*, 485–490. [CrossRef] [PubMed]
14. Tsuboi, K.; Yokozawa, T.; Sakura, T.; Watanabe, T.; Fujisawa, S.; Yamauchi, T.; Uike, N.; Ando, K.; Kihara, R.; Tobinai, K.; et al. A Phase I study to assess the safety, pharmacokinetics and efficacy of barasertib (AZD1152), an Aurora B kinase inhibitor, in Japanese patients with advanced acute myeloid leukemia. *Leuk. Res.* **2011**, *35*, 1384–1389. [CrossRef]
15. Sessa, F.; Villa, F. Structure of Aurora B-INCENP in complex with barasertib reveals a potential transinhibitory mechanism. *Acta Cryst. F Struct. Biol. Commun.* **2014**, *70*, 294–298. [CrossRef]
16. Li, X.; Lu, X.; Xing, M.; Yang, X.-H.; Zhao, T.-T.; Gong, H.-B.; Zhu, H.-L. Synthesis, biological evaluation, and molecular docking studies of N,1,3-triphenyl-1H-pyrazole-4-carboxamide derivatives as anticancer agents. *Bioorg. Med. Chem. Lett.* **2012**, *22*, 3589–3593. [CrossRef]
17. Sharma, M.C.; Sharma, S.; Bhadoriya, K.S. QSAR studies on pyrazole-4-carboxamide derivatives as Aurora A kinase inhibitors. *J. Taibah Univ. Sci.* **2016**, *10*, 107–114. [CrossRef]
18. Zheng, Y.; Zheng, M.; Ling, X.; Liu, Y.; Xue, Y.; An, L.; Gu, N.; Jin, M. Design, synthesis, quantum chemical studies and biological activity evaluation of pyrazole–benzimidazole derivatives as potent Aurora A/B kinase inhibitors. *Bioorg. Med. Chem. Lett.* **2013**, *23*, 3523–3530. [CrossRef]

19. Bavetsias, V.; Pérez-Fuertes, Y.; McIntyre, P.J.; Atrash, B.; Kosmopoulou, M.; O'Fee, L.; Burke, R.; Sun, C.; Faisal, A.; Bush, K.; et al. 7-(Pyrazol-4-yl)-3H-imidazo[4,5-b]pyridine-based derivatives for kinase inhibition: Co-crystallisation studies with Aurora-A reveal distinct differences in the orientation of the pyrazole N1-substituent. *Bioorg. Med. Chem. Lett.* **2015**, *25*, 4203–4209. [CrossRef]
20. Lakkaniga, N.R.; Zhang, L.; Belachew, B.; Gunaganti, N.; Frett, B.; Li, H.-y. Discovery of SP-96, the first non-ATP-competitive Aurora Kinase B inhibitor, for reduced myelosuppression. *Eur. J. Med. Chem.* **2020**, *203*, 112589. [CrossRef]
21. Hu, L.; Zheng, Y.; Li, Z.; Wang, Y.; Lv, Y.; Qin, X.; Zeng, C. Design, synthesis, and biological activity of phenyl-pyrazole derivatives as BCR–ABL kinase inhibitors. *Bioorg. Med. Chem.* **2015**, *23*, 3147–3152. [CrossRef] [PubMed]
22. Hu, L.; Cao, T.; Lv, Y.; Ding, Y.; Yang, L.; Zhang, Q.; Guo, M. Design, synthesis, and biological activity of 4-(imidazo[1,2-b]pyridazin-3-yl)-1H-pyrazol-1-yl-phenylbenzamide derivatives as BCR–ABL kinase inhibitors. *Bioorg. Med. Chem. Lett.* **2016**, *26*, 5830–5835. [CrossRef] [PubMed]
23. Wylie, A.A.; Schoepfer, J.; Jahnke, W.; Cowan-Jacob, S.W.; Loo, A.; Furet, P.; Marzinzik, A.L.; Pelle, X.; Donovan, J.; Zhu, W.; et al. The allosteric inhibitor ABL001 enables dual targeting of BCR–ABL1. *Nature* **2017**, *543*, 733–737. [CrossRef]
24. Schoepfer, J.; Jahnke, W.; Berellini, G.; Buonamici, S.; Cotesta, S.; Cowan-Jacob, S.W.; Dodd, S.; Drueckes, P.; Fabbro, D.; Gabriel, T.; et al. Discovery of Asciminib (ABL001), an Allosteric Inhibitor of the Tyrosine Kinase Activity of BCR-ABL1. *J. Med. Chem.* **2018**, *61*, 8120–8135. [CrossRef] [PubMed]
25. Study of Efficacy and Safety of Asciminib in Combination With Imatinib in Patients with Chronic Myeloid Leukemia in Chronic Phase (CML-CP). Available online: https://clinicaltrials.gov/ct2/show/NCT03578367?id=NCT03578367&draw=2&rank=1&load=cart (accessed on 24 November 2021).
26. Zhan, J.-Y.; Ma, J.; Zheng, Q.-C. Molecular dynamics investigation on the Asciminib resistance mechanism of I502L and V468F mutations in BCR-ABL. *J. Mol. Graph. Model.* **2019**, *89*, 242–249. [CrossRef] [PubMed]
27. Large, J.M.; Osborne, S.A.; Smiljanic-Hurley, E.; Ansell, K.H.; Jones, H.M.; Taylor, D.L.; Clough, B.; Green, J.L.; Holder, A.A. Imidazopyridazines as potent inhibitors of Plasmodium falciparum calcium-dependent protein kinase 1 (PfCDPK1): Preparation and evaluation of pyrazole linked analogues. *Bioorg. Med. Chem. Lett.* **2013**, *23*, 6019–6024. [CrossRef] [PubMed]
28. Huang, W.; Hulverson, M.A.; Choi, R.; Arnold, S.L.M.; Zhang, Z.; McCloskey, M.C.; Whitman, G.R.; Hackman, R.C.; Rivas, K.L.; Barrett, L.K.; et al. Development of 5-Aminopyrazole-4-carboxamide-based Bumped-Kinase Inhibitors for Cryptosporidiosis Therapy. *J. Med. Chem.* **2019**, *62*, 3135–3146. [CrossRef] [PubMed]
29. Galal, S.A.; Abdelsamie, A.S.; Shouman, S.A.; Attia, Y.M.; Ali, H.I.; Tabll, A.; El-Shenawy, R.; El Abd, Y.S.; Ali, M.M.; Mahmoud, A.E.; et al. Part I: Design, synthesis and biological evaluation of novel pyrazole-benzimidazole conjugates as checkpoint kinase 2 (Chk2) inhibitors with studying their activities alone and in combination with genotoxic drugs. *Eur. J. Med. Chem.* **2017**, *134*, 392–405. [CrossRef]
30. Galal, S.A.; Khairat, S.H.M.; Ali, H.I.; Shouman, S.A.; Attia, Y.M.; Ali, M.M.; Mahmoud, A.E.; Abdel-Halim, A.H.; Fyiad, A.A.; Tabll, A.; et al. Part II: New candidates of pyrazole-benzimidazole conjugates as checkpoint kinase 2 (Chk2) inhibitors. *Eur. J. Med. Chem.* **2018**, *144*, 859–873. [CrossRef]
31. Galal, S.A.; Khattab, M.; Shouman, S.A.; Ramadan, R.; Kandil, O.M.; Kandil, O.M.; Tabll, A.; El Abd, Y.S.; El-Shenawy, R.; Attia, Y.M.; et al. Part III: Novel checkpoint kinase 2 (Chk2) inhibitors; design, synthesis and biological evaluation of pyrimidine-benzimidazole conjugates. *Eur. J. Med. Chem.* **2018**, *146*, 687–708. [CrossRef]
32. Jorda, R.; Schütznerová, E.; Cankař, P.; Brychtová, V.; Navrátilová, J.; Kryštof, V. Novel arylazopyrazole inhibitors of cyclin-dependent kinases. *Bioorg. Med. Chem.* **2015**, *23*, 1975–1981. [CrossRef]
33. Ganga Reddy, V.; Srinivasa Reddy, T.; Lakshma Nayak, V.; Prasad, B.; Reddy, A.P.; Ravikumar, A.; Taj, S.; Kamal, A. Design, synthesis and biological evaluation of N-((1-benzyl-1H-1,2,3-triazol-4-yl)methyl)-1,3-diphenyl-1H-pyrazole-4-carboxamides as CDK1/Cdc2 inhibitors. *Eur. J. Med. Chem.* **2016**, *122*, 164–177. [CrossRef] [PubMed]
34. Rana, S.; Sonawane, Y.A.; Taylor, M.A.; Kizhake, S.; Zahid, M.; Natarajan, A. Synthesis of aminopyrazole analogs and their evaluation as CDK inhibitors for cancer therapy. *Bioorg. Med. Chem. Lett.* **2018**, *28*, 3736–3740. [CrossRef] [PubMed]
35. Squires, M.S.; Feltell, R.E.; Wallis, N.G.; Lewis, E.J.; Smith, D.-M.; Cross, D.M.; Lyons, J.F.; Thompson, N.T. Biological characterization of AT7519, a small-molecule inhibitor of cyclin-dependent kinases, in human tumor cell lines. *Mol. Cancer Ther.* **2009**, *8*, 324. [CrossRef]
36. Santo, L.; Vallet, S.; Hideshima, T.; Cirstea, D.; Ikeda, H.; Pozzi, S.; Patel, K.; Okawa, Y.; Gorgun, G.; Perrone, G.; et al. AT7519, A novel small molecule multi-cyclin-dependent kinase inhibitor, induces apoptosis in multiple myeloma via GSK-3beta activation and RNA polymerase II inhibition. *Oncogene* **2010**, *29*, 2325–2336. [CrossRef]
37. Harras, M.F.; Sabour, R. Design, synthesis and biological evaluation of novel 1,3,4-trisubstituted pyrazole derivatives as potential chemotherapeutic agents for hepatocellular carcinoma. *Bioorg. Chem.* **2018**, *78*, 149–157. [CrossRef]
38. Ferguson, F.M.; Doctor, Z.M.; Ficarro, S.B.; Marto, J.A.; Kim, N.D.; Sim, T.; Gray, N.S. Synthesis and structure activity relationships of a series of 4-amino-1H-pyrazoles as covalent inhibitors of CDK14. *Bioorg. Med. Chem. Lett.* **2019**, *29*, 1985–1993. [CrossRef]
39. Cheng, C.; Yun, F.; Ullah, S.; Yuan, Q. Discovery of novel cyclin-dependent kinase (CDK) and histone deacetylase (HDAC) dual inhibitors with potent in vitro and in vivo anticancer activity. *Eur. J. Med. Chem.* **2020**, *189*, 112073. [CrossRef] [PubMed]
40. Poddutoori, R.; Samajdar, S.; Mukherjee, S. Substituted pyrazole derivatives as selective cdk12/13 inhibitors. U.S. Patent No. 10,894,786, 10 October 2019.

41. Zhang, W.-M.; Xing, M.; Zhao, T.-T.; Ren, Y.-J.; Yang, X.-H.; Yang, Y.-S.; Lv, P.-C.; Zhu, H.-L. Synthesis, molecular modeling and biological evaluation of cinnamic acid derivatives with pyrazole moieties as novel anticancer agents. *RSC Adv.* **2014**, *4*, 37197–37207. [CrossRef]
42. Gavine, P.R.; Mooney, L.; Kilgour, E.; Thomas, A.P.; Al-Kadhimi, K.; Beck, S.; Rooney, C.; Coleman, T.; Baker, D.; Mellor, M.J.; et al. AZD4547: An Orally Bioavailable, Potent, and Selective Inhibitor of the Fibroblast Growth Factor Receptor Tyrosine Kinase Family. *Cancer Res.* **2012**, *72*, 2045. [CrossRef]
43. Search Results of the Term AZD4547. Available online: https://clinicaltrials.gov/ct2/results?cond=&term=AZD4547&cntry=&state=&city=&dist= (accessed on 24 November 2021).
44. Tucker, J.A.; Klein, T.; Breed, J.; Breeze, A.L.; Overman, R.; Phillips, C.; Norman, R.A. Structural Insights into FGFR Kinase Isoform Selectivity: Diverse Binding Modes of AZD4547 and Ponatinib in Complex with FGFR1 and FGFR4. *Structure* **2014**, *22*, 1764–1774. [CrossRef]
45. Search Results of the Term CH5183284. Available online: https://clinicaltrials.gov/ct2/results?cond=&term=CH5183284&cntry=&state=&city=&dist= (accessed on 24 November 2021).
46. Ebiike, H.; Taka, N.; Matsushita, M.; Ohmori, M.; Takami, K.; Hyohdoh, I.; Kohchi, M.; Hayase, T.; Nishii, H.; Morikami, K.; et al. Discovery of [5-Amino-1-(2-methyl-3H-benzimidazol-5-yl)pyrazol-4-yl]-(1H-indol-2-yl)methanone (CH5183284/Debio 1347), An Orally Available and Selective Fibroblast Growth Factor Receptor (FGFR) Inhibitor. *J. Med. Chem.* **2016**, *59*, 10586–10600. [CrossRef]
47. Yamani, A.; Zdżalik-Bielecka, D.; Lipner, J.; Stańczak, A.; Piórkowska, N.; Stańczak, P.S.; Olejkowska, P.; Hucz-Kalitowska, J.; Magdycz, M.; Dzwonek, K.; et al. Discovery and optimization of novel pyrazole-benzimidazole CPL304110, as a potent and selective inhibitor of fibroblast growth factor receptors FGFR (1–3). *Eur. J. Med. Chem.* **2020**, *210*, 112990. [CrossRef] [PubMed]
48. Chaudhary, M.; Kumar, N.; Baldi, A.; Chandra, R.; Arockia Babu, M.; Madan, J. Chloro and bromo-pyrazole curcumin Knoevenagel condensates augmented anticancer activity against human cervical cancer cells: Design, synthesis, in silico docking and in vitro cytotoxicity analysis. *J. Biomol. Struct. Dyn.* **2020**, *38*, 200–218. [CrossRef] [PubMed]
49. McElroy, W.T.; Tan, Z.; Ho, G.; Paliwal, S.; Li, G.; Seganish, W.M.; Tulshian, D.; Tata, J.; Fischmann, T.O.; Sondey, C.; et al. Potent and Selective Amidopyrazole Inhibitors of IRAK4 That Are Efficacious in a Rodent Model of Inflammation. *ACS Med. Chem. Lett.* **2015**, *6*, 677–682. [CrossRef] [PubMed]
50. Lim, J.; Altman, M.D.; Baker, J.; Brubaker, J.D.; Chen, H.; Chen, Y.; Kleinschek, M.A.; Li, C.; Liu, D.; Maclean, J.K.F.; et al. Identification of N-(1H-pyrazol-4-yl)carboxamide inhibitors of interleukin-1 receptor associated kinase 4: Bicyclic core modifications. *Bioorg. Med. Chem. Lett.* **2015**, *25*, 5384–5388. [CrossRef]
51. Xue, L.; Huang, L.; Li, H.; Li, T.; Huabin, L.; Huabin, L. Pyrazole Compounds, Pharmaceutical Compositions Thereof And Use Thereof. 2020-03-05, 2020. US Patent No. 20210340124, 4 November 2021.
52. Pastor, R.M.; Burch, J.D.; Magnuson, S.; Ortwine, D.F.; Chen, Y.; De La Torre, K.; Ding, X.; Eigenbrot, C.; Johnson, A.; Liimatta, M.; et al. Discovery and optimization of indazoles as potent and selective interleukin-2 inducible T cell kinase (ITK) inhibitors. *Bioorg. Med. Chem. Lett.* **2014**, *24*, 2448–2452. [CrossRef] [PubMed]
53. Burch, J.D.; Lau, K.; Barker, J.J.; Brookfield, F.; Chen, Y.; Chen, Y.; Eigenbrot, C.; Ellebrandt, C.; Ismaili, M.H.A.; Johnson, A.; et al. Property- and Structure-Guided Discovery of a Tetrahydroindazole Series of Interleukin-2 Inducible T-Cell Kinase Inhibitors. *J. Med. Chem.* **2014**, *57*, 5714–5727. [CrossRef]
54. Burch, J.D.; Barrett, K.; Chen, Y.; DeVoss, J.; Eigenbrot, C.; Goldsmith, R.; Ismaili, M.H.A.; Lau, K.; Lin, Z.; Ortwine, D.F.; et al. Tetrahydroindazoles as Interleukin-2 Inducible T-Cell Kinase Inhibitors. Part II. Second-Generation Analogues with Enhanced Potency, Selectivity, and Pharmacodynamic Modulation In Vivo. *J. Med. Chem.* **2015**, *58*, 3806–3816. [CrossRef] [PubMed]
55. Liang, X.; Zang, J.; Zhu, M.; Gao, Q.; Wang, B.; Xu, W.; Zhang, Y. Design, Synthesis, and Antitumor Evaluation of 4-Amino-(1H)-pyrazole Derivatives as JAKs Inhibitors. *ACS Med. Chem. Lett.* **2016**, *7*, 950–955. [CrossRef]
56. Hoffman, R.; Prchal, J.T.; Samuelson, S.; Ciurea, S.O.; Rondelli, D. Philadelphia Chromosome–Negative Myeloproliferative Disorders: Biology and Treatment. *Biol. Blood Marrow Transplant.* **2007**, *13*, 64–72. [CrossRef]
57. Hanan, E.J.; van Abbema, A.; Barrett, K.; Blair, W.S.; Blaney, J.; Chang, C.; Eigenbrot, C.; Flynn, S.; Gibbons, P.; Hurley, C.A.; et al. Discovery of Potent and Selective Pyrazolopyrimidine Janus Kinase 2 Inhibitors. *J. Med. Chem.* **2012**, *55*, 10090–10107. [CrossRef] [PubMed]
58. Zak, M.; Hanan, E.J.; Lupardus, P.; Brown, D.G.; Robinson, C.; Siu, M.; Lyssikatos, J.P.; Romero, F.A.; Zhao, G.; Kellar, T.; et al. Discovery of a class of highly potent Janus Kinase 1/2 (JAK1/2) inhibitors demonstrating effective cell-based blockade of IL-13 signaling. *Bioorg. Med. Chem. Lett.* **2019**, *29*, 1522–1531. [CrossRef] [PubMed]
59. Wan, H.; Schroeder, G.M.; Hart, A.C.; Inghrim, J.; Grebinski, J.; Tokarski, J.S.; Lorenzi, M.V.; You, D.; McDevitt, T.; Penhallow, B.; et al. Discovery of a Highly Selective JAK2 Inhibitor, BMS-911543, for the Treatment of Myeloproliferative Neoplasms. *ACS Med. Chem. Lett.* **2015**, *6*, 850–855. [CrossRef]
60. Doma, A.; Kulkarni, R.; Palakodety, R.; Sastry, G.N.; Sridhara, J.; Garlapati, A. Pyrazole derivatives as potent inhibitors of c-Jun N-terminal kinase: Synthesis and SAR studies. *Bioorg. Med. Chem.* **2014**, *22*, 6209–6219. [CrossRef]
61. Oh, Y.; Jang, M.; Cho, H.; Yang, S.; Im, D.; Moon, H.; Hah, J.-M. Discovery of 3-alkyl-5-aryl-1-pyrimidyl-1H-pyrazole derivatives as a novel selective inhibitor scaffold of JNK3. *J. Enzym. Inhib. Med. Chem.* **2020**, *35*, 372–376. [CrossRef]

62. Estrada, A.A.; Chan, B.K.; Baker-Glenn, C.; Beresford, A.; Burdick, D.J.; Chambers, M.; Chen, H.; Dominguez, S.L.; Dotson, J.; Drummond, J.; et al. Discovery of Highly Potent, Selective, and Brain-Penetrant Aminopyrazole Leucine-Rich Repeat Kinase 2 (LRRK2) Small Molecule Inhibitors. *J. Med. Chem.* **2014**, *57*, 921–936. [CrossRef] [PubMed]
63. Greshock, T.J.; Sanders, J.M.; Drolet, R.E.; Rajapakse, H.A.; Chang, R.K.; Kim, B.; Rada, V.L.; Tiscia, H.E.; Su, H.; Lai, M.-T.; et al. Potent, selective and orally bioavailable leucine-rich repeat kinase 2 (LRRK2) inhibitors. *Bioorg. Med. Chem. Lett.* **2016**, *26*, 2631–2635. [CrossRef]
64. Stotani, S.; Gatta, V.; Medarametla, P.; Padmanaban, M.; Karawajczyk, A.; Giordanetto, F.; Tammela, P.; Laitinen, T.; Poso, A.; Tzalis, D.; et al. DPD-Inspired Discovery of Novel LsrK Kinase Inhibitors: An Opportunity To Fight Antimicrobial Resistance. *J. Med. Chem.* **2019**, *62*, 2720–2737. [CrossRef]
65. Majik, M.S.; Gawas, U.B.; Mandrekar, V.K. Next generation quorum sensing inhibitors: Accounts on structure activity relationship studies and biological activities. *Bioorg. Med. Chem.* **2020**, *28*, 115728. [CrossRef]
66. Choi, W.-K.; El-Gamal, M.I.; Choi, H.S.; Baek, D.; Oh, C.-H. New diarylureas and diarylamides containing 1,3,4-triarylpyrazole scaffold: Synthesis, antiproliferative evaluation against melanoma cell lines, ERK kinase inhibition, and molecular docking studies. *Eur. J. Med. Chem.* **2011**, *46*, 5754–5762. [CrossRef] [PubMed]
67. El-Gamal, M.I.; Choi, H.S.; Yoo, K.H.; Baek, D.; Oh, C.-H. Antiproliferative Diarylpyrazole Derivatives as Dual Inhibitors of the ERK Pathway and COX-2. *Chem. Biol. Drug Des.* **2013**, *82*, 336–347. [CrossRef] [PubMed]
68. Lv, X.-H.; Ren, Z.-L.; Zhou, B.-G.; Li, Q.-S.; Chu, M.-J.; Liu, D.-H.; Mo, K.; Zhang, L.-S.; Yao, X.-K.; Cao, H.-Q. Discovery of N-(benzyloxy)-1,3-diphenyl-1H-pyrazole-4-carboxamide derivatives as potential antiproliferative agents by inhibiting MEK. *Bioorg. Med. Chem.* **2016**, *24*, 4652–4659. [CrossRef]
69. El-Gamal, M.I.; Anbar, H.S.; Tarazi, H.; Oh, C.-H. Discovery of a potent p38α/MAPK14 kinase inhibitor: Synthesis, in vitro/in vivo biological evaluation, and docking studies. *Eur. J. Med. Chem.* **2019**, *183*, 111684. [CrossRef] [PubMed]
70. Getlik, M.; Grütter, C.; Simard, J.R.; Nguyen, H.D.; Robubi, A.; Aust, B.; van Otterlo, W.A.L.; Rauh, D. Structure-based design, synthesis and biological evaluation of N-pyrazole, N'-thiazole urea inhibitors of MAP kinase p38α. *Eur. J. Med. Chem.* **2012**, *48*, 1–15. [CrossRef]
71. Röhm, S.; Schröder, M.; Dwyer, J.E.; Widdowson, C.S.; Chaikuad, A.; Berger, B.-T.; Joerger, A.C.; Krämer, A.; Harbig, J.; Dauch, D.; et al. Selective targeting of the αC and DFG-out pocket in p38 MAPK. *Eur. J. Med. Chem.* **2020**, *208*, 112721. [CrossRef] [PubMed]
72. Petersen, L.K.; Blakskjær, P.; Chaikuad, A.; Christensen, A.B.; Dietvorst, J.; Holmkvist, J.; Knapp, S.; Kořínek, M.; Larsen, L.K.; Pedersen, A.E.; et al. Novel p38α MAP kinase inhibitors identified from yoctoReactor DNA-encoded small molecule library. *MedChemComm* **2016**, *7*, 1332–1339. [CrossRef]
73. Mohammed, I.E.-G.; Mohammed, S.A.-M.; Mahmoud, M.G.E.-D.; Ji-Sun, S.; Kyung-Tae, L.; Kyung Ho, Y.; Chang-Hyun, O. Synthesis, in vitro Antiproliferative and Antiinflammatory Activities, and Kinase Inhibitory effects of New 1,3,4-triarylpyrazole Derivatives. *Anti-Cancer Agents Med. Chem.* **2017**, *17*, 75–84. [CrossRef]
74. Lee, D.; Pagire, H.S.; Pagire, S.H.; Bae, E.J.; Dighe, M.; Kim, M.; Lee, K.M.; Jang, Y.K.; Jaladi, A.K.; Jung, K.-Y.; et al. Discovery of Novel Pyruvate Dehydrogenase Kinase 4 Inhibitors for Potential Oral Treatment of Metabolic Diseases. *J. Med. Chem.* **2019**, *62*, 575–588. [CrossRef]
75. Hu, H.; Wang, X.; Chan, G.K.Y.; Chang, J.H.; Do, S.; Drummond, J.; Ebens, A.; Lee, W.; Ly, J.; Lyssikatos, J.P.; et al. Discovery of 3,5-substituted 6-azaindoles as potent pan-Pim inhibitors. *Bioorg. Med. Chem. Lett.* **2015**, *25*, 5258–5264. [CrossRef]
76. Wang, X.; Blackaby, W.; Allen, V.; Chan, G.K.Y.; Chang, J.H.; Chiang, P.-C.; Diène, C.; Drummond, J.; Do, S.; Fan, E.; et al. Optimization of Pan-Pim Kinase Activity and Oral Bioavailability Leading to Diaminopyrazole (GDC-0339) for the Treatment of Multiple Myeloma. *J. Med. Chem.* **2019**, *62*, 2140–2153. [CrossRef]
77. El-Gamal, M.I.; Choi, H.S.; Cho, H.-G.; Hong, J.H.; Yoo, K.H.; Oh, C.-H. Design, Synthesis, and Antiproliferative Activity of 3,4-Diarylpyrazole-1-carboxamide Derivatives against Melanoma Cell Line. *Arch. Der Pharm.* **2011**, *344*, 745–754. [CrossRef]
78. Caballero, J.; Alzate-Morales, J.H.; Vergara-Jaque, A. Investigation of the Differences in Activity between Hydroxycycloalkyl N1 Substituted Pyrazole Derivatives as Inhibitors of B-Raf Kinase by Using Docking, Molecular Dynamics, QM/MM, and Fragment-Based De Novo Design: Study of Binding Mode of Diastereomer Compounds. *J. Chem. Inf. Modeling* **2011**, *51*, 2920–2931. [CrossRef]
79. Wang, S.-F.; Zhu, Y.-L.; Zhu, P.-T.; Makawana, J.A.; Zhang, Y.-L.; Zhao, M.-Y.; Lv, P.-C.; Zhu, H.-L. Design, synthesis and biological evaluation of novel 5-phenyl-1H-pyrazole derivatives as potential BRAFV600E inhibitors. *Bioorg. Med. Chem.* **2014**, *22*, 6201–6208. [CrossRef]
80. Gamal El-Din, M.M.; El-Gamal, M.I.; Abdel-Maksoud, M.S.; Yoo, K.H.; Oh, C.-H. Design, synthesis, broad-spectrum antiproliferative activity, and kinase inhibitory effect of triarylpyrazole derivatives possessing arylamides or arylureas moieties. *Eur. J. Med. Chem.* **2016**, *119*, 122–131. [CrossRef] [PubMed]
81. Khan, M.A.; El-Gamal, M.I.; Tarazi, H.; Choi, H.S.; Oh, C.-H. Design and synthesis of a new series of highly potent RAF kinase-inhibiting triarylpyrazole derivatives possessing antiproliferative activity against melanoma cells. *Future Med. Chem.* **2016**, *8*, 2197–2211. [CrossRef] [PubMed]
82. Gamal El-Din, M.M.; El-Gamal, M.I.; Abdel-Maksoud, M.S.; Yoo, K.H.; Oh, C.H. Design, synthesis, in vitro potent antiproliferative activity, and kinase inhibitory effects of new triarylpyrazole derivatives possessing different heterocycle terminal moieties. *J. Enzym. Inhib. Med. Chem.* **2019**, *34*, 1534–1543. [CrossRef] [PubMed]

83. Gamal El-Din, M.M.; El-Gamal, M.I.; Abdel-Maksoud, M.S.; Yoo, K.H.; Baek, D.; Choi, J.; Lee, H.; Oh, C.-H. Design, synthesis, and in vitro antiproliferative and kinase inhibitory effects of pyrimidinylpyrazole derivatives terminating with arylsulfonamido or cyclic sulfamide substituents. *J. Enzym. Inhib. Med. Chem.* **2016**, *31*, 111–122. [CrossRef]
84. Tarazi, H.; El-Gamal, M.I.; Oh, C.-H. Discovery of highly potent V600E-B-RAF kinase inhibitors: Molecular modeling study. *Bioorg. Med. Chem.* **2019**, *27*, 655–663. [CrossRef]
85. El-Gamal, M.I.; Park, B.-J.; Oh, C.-H. Synthesis, in vitro antiproliferative activity, and kinase inhibitory effects of pyrazole-containing diarylureas and diarylamides. *Eur. J. Med. Chem.* **2018**, *156*, 230–239. [CrossRef]
86. Park, B.S.; Al-Sanea, M.M.; Abdelazem, A.Z.; Park, H.M.; Roh, E.J.; Park, H.-M.; Yoo, K.H.; Sim, T.; Tae, J.S.; Lee, S.H. Structure-based optimization and biological evaluation of trisubstituted pyrazole as a core structure of potent ROS1 kinase inhibitors. *Bioorg. Med. Chem.* **2014**, *22*, 3871–3878. [CrossRef] [PubMed]
87. Abd El-Karim, S.S.; Anwar, M.M.; Mohamed, N.A.; Nasr, T.; Elseginy, S.A. Design, synthesis, biological evaluation and molecular docking studies of novel benzofuran–pyrazole derivatives as anticancer agents. *Bioorganic Chem.* **2015**, *63*, 1–12. [CrossRef]
88. Sekimata, K.; Sato, T.; Sakai, N.; Watanabe, H.; Mishima-Tsumagari, C.; Taguri, T.; Matsumoto, T.; Fujii, Y.; Handa, N.; Honma, T.; et al. Bis-Heteroaryl Pyrazoles: Identification of Orally Bioavailable Inhibitors of Activin Receptor-Like Kinase-2 (R206H). *Chem. Pharm. Bull.* **2019**, *67*, 224–235. [CrossRef] [PubMed]
89. Sato, T.; Sekimata, K.; Sakai, N.; Watanabe, H.; Mishima-Tsumagari, C.; Taguri, T.; Matsumoto, T.; Fujii, Y.; Handa, N.; Tanaka, A.; et al. Structural Basis of Activin Receptor-Like Kinase 2 (R206H) Inhibition by Bis-heteroaryl Pyrazole-Based Inhibitors for the Treatment of Fibrodysplasia Ossificans Progressiva Identified by the Integration of Ligand-Based and Structure-Based Drug Design Approaches. *ACS Omega* **2020**, *5*, 11411–11423. [CrossRef] [PubMed]
90. Jin, C.H.; Sreenu, D.; Krishnaiah, M.; Subrahmanyam, V.B.; Rao, K.S.; Nagendra Mohan, A.V.; Park, C.-Y.; Son, J.-Y.; Son, D.-H.; Park, H.-J.; et al. Synthesis and biological evaluation of 1-substituted-3(5)-(6-methylpyridin-2-yl)-4-(quinoxalin-6-yl)pyrazoles as transforming growth factor-β type 1 receptor kinase inhibitors. *Eur. J. Med. Chem.* **2011**, *46*, 3917–3925. [CrossRef]
91. Zhao, L.-M.; Guo, Z.; Xue, Y.-J.; Min, J.Z.; Zhu, W.-J.; Li, X.-Y.; Piao, H.-R.; Jin, C.H. Synthesis and Evaluation of 3-Substituted-4-(quinoxalin-6-yl) Pyrazoles as TGF-β Type I Receptor Kinase Inhibitors. *Molecules* **2018**, *23*, 3369. [CrossRef]
92. Jin, C.H.; Krishnaiah, M.; Sreenu, D.; Subrahmanyam, V.B.; Park, H.-J.; Park, S.-J.; Sheen, Y.Y.; Kim, D.-K. 4-([1,2,4]Triazolo[1,5-a]pyridin-6-yl)-5(3)-(6-methylpyridin-2-yl)imidazole and -pyrazole derivatives as potent and selective inhibitors of transforming growth factor-β type I receptor kinase. *Bioorg. Med. Chem.* **2014**, *22*, 2724–2732. [CrossRef]
93. Zhu, W.-J.; Cui, B.-W.; Wang, H.M.; Nan, J.-X.; Piao, H.-R.; Lian, L.-H.; Jin, C.H. Design, synthesis, and antifibrosis evaluation of 4-(benzo-[c][1,2,5]thiadiazol-5-yl)-3(5)-(6-methyl- pyridin-2-yl)pyrazole and 3(5)-(6-methylpyridin- 2-yl)-4-(thieno-[3,2,-c]pyridin-2-yl)pyrazole derivatives. *Eur. J. Med. Chem.* **2019**, *180*, 15–27. [CrossRef]
94. Thress, K.; MacIntyre, T.; Wang, H.; Whitston, D.; Liu, Z.-Y.; Hoffmann, E.; Wang, T.; Brown, J.L.; Webster, K.; Omer, C.; et al. Identification and preclinical characterization of AZ-23, a novel, selective, and orally bioavailable inhibitor of the Trk kinase pathway. *Mol. Cancer Ther.* **2009**, *8*, 1818. [CrossRef]
95. Wang, T.; Lamb, M.L.; Block, M.H.; Davies, A.M.; Han, Y.; Hoffmann, E.; Ioannidis, S.; Josey, J.A.; Liu, Z.-Y.; Lyne, P.D.; et al. Discovery of Disubstituted Imidazo[4,5-b]pyridines and Purines as Potent TrkA Inhibitors. *ACS Med. Chem. Lett.* **2012**, *3*, 705–709. [CrossRef] [PubMed]
96. Furuya, N.; Momose, T.; Katsuno, K.; Fushimi, N.; Muranaka, H.; Handa, C.; Ozawa, T.; Kinoshita, T. The juxtamembrane region of TrkA kinase is critical for inhibitor selectivity. *Bioorg. Med. Chem. Lett.* **2017**, *27*, 1233–1236. [CrossRef] [PubMed]
97. Subramanian, G.; Johnson, P.D.; Zachary, T.; Roush, N.; Zhu, Y.; Bowen, S.J.; Janssen, A.; Duclos, B.A.; Williams, T.; Javens, C.; et al. Deciphering the Allosteric Binding Mechanism of the Human Tropomyosin Receptor Kinase A (hTrkA) Inhibitors. *ACS Chem. Biol.* **2019**, *14*, 1205–1216. [CrossRef] [PubMed]
98. Shirahashi, H.; Toriihara, E.; Suenaga, Y.; Yoshida, H.; Akaogi, K.; Endou, Y.; Wakabayashi, M.; Takashima, M. The discovery of novel 3-aryl-indazole derivatives as peripherally restricted pan-Trk inhibitors for the treatment of pain. *Bioorg. Med. Chem. Lett.* **2019**, *29*, 2320–2326. [CrossRef] [PubMed]
99. Nishida, N.; Yano, H.; Nishida, T.; Kamura, T.; Kojiro, M. Angiogenesis in cancer. *Vasc. Health Risk Manag.* **2006**, *2*, 213–219. [CrossRef]
100. Miyamoto, N.; Sakai, N.; Hirayama, T.; Miwa, K.; Oguro, Y.; Oki, H.; Okada, K.; Takagi, T.; Iwata, H.; Awazu, Y.; et al. Discovery of N-[5-({2-[(cyclopropylcarbonyl)amino]imidazo[1,2-b]pyridazin-6-yl}oxy)-2-methylph enyl]-1,3-dimethyl-1H-pyrazole-5-carboxamide (TAK-593), a highly potent VEGFR2 kinase inhibitor. *Bioorg. Med. Chem.* **2013**, *21*, 2333–2345. [PubMed]
101. Reddy, V.G.; Reddy, T.S.; Jadala, C.; Reddy, M.S.; Sultana, F.; Akunuri, R.; Bhargava, S.K.; Wlodkowic, D.; Srihari, P.; Kamal, A. Pyrazolo-benzothiazole hybrids: Synthesis, anticancer properties and evaluation of antiangiogenic activity using in vitro VEGFR-2 kinase and in vivo transgenic zebrafish model. *Eur. J. Med. Chem.* **2019**, *182*, 111609. [CrossRef]
102. Dawood, D.H.; Nossier, E.S.; Ali, M.M.; Mahmoud, A.E. Synthesis and molecular docking study of new pyrazole derivatives as potent anti-breast cancer agents targeting VEGFR-2 kinase. *Bioorg. Chem.* **2020**, *101*, 103916. [CrossRef]
103. Thaher, B.A.; Arnsmann, M.; Totzke, F.; Ehlert, J.E.; Kubbutat, M.H.G.; Schächtele, C.; Zimmermann, M.O.; Koch, P.; Boeckler, F.M.; Laufer, S.A. Tri- and Tetrasubstituted Pyrazole Derivates: Regioisomerism Switches Activity from p38MAP Kinase to Important Cancer Kinases. *J. Med. Chem.* **2012**, *55*, 961–965. [CrossRef] [PubMed]

104. Strocchi, E.; Fornari, F.; Minguzzi, M.; Gramantieri, L.; Milazzo, M.; Rebuttini, V.; Breviglieri, S.; Camaggi, C.M.; Locatelli, E.; Bolondi, L.; et al. Design, synthesis and biological evaluation of pyrazole derivatives as potential multi-kinase inhibitors in hepatocellular carcinoma. *Eur. J. Med. Chem.* **2012**, *48*, 391–401. [CrossRef]
105. Curtin, M.L.; Robin Heyman, H.; Frey, R.R.; Marcotte, P.A.; Glaser, K.B.; Jankowski, J.R.; Magoc, T.J.; Albert, D.H.; Olson, A.M.; Reuter, D.R.; et al. Pyrazole diaminopyrimidines as dual inhibitors of KDR and Aurora B kinases. *Bioorg. Med. Chem. Lett.* **2012**, *22*, 4750–4755. [CrossRef]
106. Abdel-Maksoud, M.S.; El-Gamal, M.I.; Gamal El-Din, M.M.; Oh, C.H. Design, synthesis, in vitro anticancer evaluation, kinase inhibitory effects, and pharmacokinetic profile of new 1,3,4-triarylpyrazole derivatives possessing terminal sulfonamide moiety. *J. Enzym. Inhib. Med. Chem.* **2019**, *34*, 97–109. [CrossRef] [PubMed]
107. Nossier, E.S.; Abd El-Karim, S.S.; Khalifa, N.M.; El-Sayed, A.S.; Hassan, E.S.I.; El-Hallouty, S.M. Kinase Inhibitory Activities and Molecular Docking of a Novel Series of Anticancer Pyrazole Derivatives. *Molecules* **2018**, *23*, 3074. [CrossRef] [PubMed]
108. Mohareb, R.M.; Manhi, F.M.; Mahmoud, M.A.A.; Abdelwahab, A. Uses of dimedone to synthesis pyrazole, isoxazole and thiophene derivatives with antiproliferative, tyrosine kinase and Pim-1 kinase inhibitions. *Med. Chem. Res.* **2020**, *29*, 1536–1551. [CrossRef]
109. Zheng, Y.-G.; Wang, J.-A.; Meng, L.; Pei, X.; Zhang, L.; An, L.; Li, C.-L.; Miao, Y.-L. Design, synthesis, biological activity evaluation of 3-(4-phenyl-1H-imidazol-2-yl)-1H-pyrazole derivatives as potent JAK 2/3 and aurora A/B kinases multi-targeted inhibitors. *Eur. J. Med. Chem.* **2021**, *209*, 112934. [CrossRef] [PubMed]
110. A Phase I, First in Man Study to Evaluate the Safety and Tolerability of a panRAF Inhibitor (CCT3833/BAL3833)in Patients with Solid Tumours (PanRAF). Available online: https://clinicaltrials.gov/ct2/show/NCT02437227?id=NCT02437227&draw=2&rank=1&load=cart (accessed on 24 November 2021).
111. Saturno, G.; Lopes, F.; Niculescu-Duvaz, I.; Niculescu-Duvaz, D.; Zambon, A.; Davies, L.; Johnson, L.; Preece, N.; Lee, R.; Viros, A.; et al. The paradox-breaking panRAF plus SRC family kinase inhibitor, CCT3833, is effective in mutant KRAS-driven cancers. *Ann. Oncol.* **2020**, *32*, 269–278. [CrossRef]
112. Dean, E.J.; Banerji, U.; Girotti, R.; Niculescu-Duvaz, I.; Lopes, F.; Davies, L.; Niculescu-Duvaz, D.; Dhomen, N.; Ellis, S.; Ali, Z.; et al. A Phase 1 first-in-human trial to evaluate the safety and tolerability of CCT3833, an oral panRAF inhibitor, in patients with advanced solid tumours, including metastatic melanoma. *J. Clin. Oncol.* **2016**, *34*, TPS9597. [CrossRef]

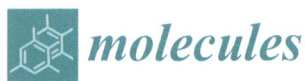

Article

Development of Sustained Release Baricitinib Loaded Lipid-Polymer Hybrid Nanoparticles with Improved Oral Bioavailability

Md. Khalid Anwer [1,*], Essam A. Ali [2], Muzaffar Iqbal [2,3], Mohammed Muqtader Ahmed [1], Mohammed F. Aldawsari [1], Ahmed Al Saqr [1], Mohd Nazam Ansari [4] and M. Ali Aboudzadeh [5,*]

1. Department of Pharmaceutics, College of Pharmacy, Prince Sattam Bin Abdulaziz University, Al-Kharj 11942, Saudi Arabia; mo.ahmed@psau.edu.sa (M.M.A.); moh.aldawsari@psau.edu.sa (M.F.A.); a.alsaqr@psau.edu.sa (A.A.S.)
2. Department of Pharmaceutical Chemistry, College of Pharmacy, King Saud University, Riyadh 11451, Saudi Arabia; esali@ksu.edu.sa (E.A.A.); muziqbal@ksu.edu.sa (M.I.)
3. Bioavailability Laboratory, College of Pharmacy, King Saud University, Riyadh 11451, Saudi Arabia
4. Department of Pharmacology and Toxicology, College of Pharmacy, Prince Sattam Bin Abdulaziz University, Al-Kharj 11942, Saudi Arabia; m.ansari@psau.edu.sa
5. CNRS, Institut des Sciences Analytiques et de Physico-Chimie pour l'Environnement et les Matériaux, University Pau & Pays Adour, E2S UPPA, IPREM, UMR5254, 64000 Pau, France
* Correspondence: m.anwer@psau.edu.sa (M.K.A.); m.aboudzadeh-barihi@univ-pau.fr (M.A.A.)

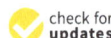

Citation: Anwer, M.K.; Ali, E.A.; Iqbal, M.; Ahmed, M.M.; Aldawsari, M.F.; Saqr, A.A.; Ansari, M.N.; Aboudzadeh, M.A. Development of Sustained Release Baricitinib Loaded Lipid-Polymer Hybrid Nanoparticles with Improved Oral Bioavailability. *Molecules* **2022**, *27*, 168. https://doi.org/10.3390/molecules27010168

Academic Editors: Sumera Zaib and Josef Jampilek

Received: 17 November 2021
Accepted: 24 December 2021
Published: 28 December 2021

Publisher's Note: MDPI stays neutral with regard to jurisdictional claims in published maps and institutional affiliations.

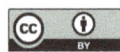

Copyright: © 2021 by the authors. Licensee MDPI, Basel, Switzerland. This article is an open access article distributed under the terms and conditions of the Creative Commons Attribution (CC BY) license (https://creativecommons.org/licenses/by/4.0/).

Abstract: Baricitinib (BTB) is an orally administered Janus kinase inhibitor, therapeutically used for the treatment of rheumatoid arthritis. Recently it has also been approved for the treatment of COVID-19 infection. In this study, four different BTB-loaded lipids (stearin)-polymer (Poly(D,L-lactide-co-glycolide)) hybrid nanoparticles (B-PLN1 to B-PLN4) were prepared by the single-step nanoprecipitation method. Next, they were characterised in terms of physicochemical properties such as particle size, zeta potential (ζP), polydispersity index (PDI), entrapment efficiency (EE) and drug loading (DL). Based on preliminary evaluation, the B-PLN4 was regarded as the optimised formulation with particle size (272 ± 7.6 nm), PDI (0.225), ζP (−36.5 ± 3.1 mV), %EE (71.6 ± 1.5%) and %DL (2.87 ± 0.42%). This formulation (B-PLN4) was further assessed concerning morphology, in vitro release, and in vivo pharmacokinetic studies in rats. The in vitro release profile exhibited a sustained release pattern well-fitted by the Korsmeyer–Peppas kinetic model (R^2 = 0.879). The in vivo pharmacokinetic data showed an enhancement (2.92 times more) in bioavailability in comparison to the normal suspension of pure BTB. These data concluded that the formulated lipid-polymer hybrid nanoparticles could be a promising drug delivery option to enhance the bioavailability of BTB. Overall, this study provides a scientific basis for future studies on the entrapment efficiency of lipid-polymer hybrid systems as promising carriers for overcoming pharmacokinetic limitations.

Keywords: baricitinib; bioavailability; encapsulation; hybrid nanoparticles; poly(D,L-lactide-coglycolide); stearin

1. Introduction

Baricitinib (BTB) is a small molecule that inhibits Janus-associated kinase (JAK) and therapeutically is used for a group of severe inflammatory disorders including resistant rheumatoid arthritis (RA), systemic lupus erythematosus, auto-inflammatory disease, dermatologic disorders, graft versus host disease and uncontrolled infections [1,2]. Recently, it has been reported that BTB interrupts the signalling of multiple cytokines implicated in coronavirus disease-19 (COVID-19) immunopathology. It may also have antiviral efficacies by targeting host factors that viruses rely on for cell entry and by restraining type I interferon driven angiotensin-converting-enzyme-2 up-regulation [3]. Therefore, it has also obtained Emergency Use Authorization (EUA) for the treatment of suspected or laboratory-confirmed critically ill COVID-19 patients solely or together with remdesivir (RDV). BTB is potent and highly effective against JAK 1 and JAK 2 enzymes with half-maximal inhibitory concentration (IC_{50}) values of 5.9 nM and 5.7 nM, respectively, and barely effective counter to JAK 3 (IC_{50} = 400 nM) [4]. Being a small molecule (molecular weight: 371.42 Da), its intra-cellular penetration is appropriate, thus, it can be orally delivered which significantly facilitates regular administration. The oral absorption of BTB is fast with peak plasma concentration achieved within 1 h, but the bioavailability of orally administered BTB varies between different species and were from 48% (dogs), 54% (rats), 47–68% (monkey) to 79% in human (EMEA Assessment report). Its volume of distribution is 76 L with plasma and serum protein binding about 50% and 45 %, respectively and a half-life of nearly 12 h.

As mentioned in the assessment report submitted for regulatory approval, BTB belongs to the biopharmaceutical classification system (BCS) class III substance, which means that it is a highly soluble and poorly permeable drug [5]. In addition, as per the DrugBank identification report, BTB has both solubility (0.357 mg/mL in water) and permeability (Log P = 1.08) issues [6] and drugs with these characteristics may exhibit low (and inconsistent) bioavailability affecting the efficiency of therapeutic benefits [7].

One approach to enhance the bioavailability of bioactive compounds is the encapsulation process in a way that using various coating materials enables target delivery and controlled release [8,9]. Choosing the suitable coating material is vital in the encapsulation process, owing to its impact on target delivery and controlled release, and consequently, on the bioaccessibility of active components. Among different choices, hybrid materials based on polymers are promising therapeutics systems. These hybrid materials have already demonstrated excellent commitment in addressing and offering solutions to the existing challenges in priority areas such as human health, environment and energy [10–12]. However, their design, performance, and practical applications are still ambitious [13,14].

Lipid-polymer hybrid nanoparticles (LP-NPs) are novel hybrid materials that have gained a lot of attention in recent years and they have been developed to achieve an improved therapeutic effect with the least adverse effect [15,16]. Due to their particular core–shell structure, LP-NPs exhibit good storage stability, controlled release profiles due to the polymer core, enhanced therapeutic potency, and biocompatibility because of the lipid–PEG and lipid layers [17]. LP-NPs are effective in encapsulating the hydrophobic molecules with a higher drug payload than biopolymer-based nanoparticles due to their nano-range size and large surface areas [18]. In literature, chitosan polymer-based LP-NPs have been reported to improve drug stability and to improve the oral bioavailability of poorly water-soluble drugs [19–21].

Due to the biodegradable and biocompatible nature of Poly(D,L-lactide-coglycolide) (PLGA), it is considered a smart polymer and is being used extensively for the enhancement of solubility and bioavailability of poorly soluble drugs [22–25]. In addition, PLGA is non-toxic and non-immunogenic and approved by US FDA for pharmaceutical and biomedical applications [26]. However, there are limited reports of PLGA-based LP-NPs for improving the solubility and permeability of bioactive compounds. Recently, PLGA-based LP-NPs has been successfully used for the bioavailability enhancement of poorly water-soluble drugs e.g., paclitaxel (PLGA as polymer and stearyl amine, soya lecithin as lipids) and hydroxy-camptothecin (PLGA as polymer and 1,2-distearoyl-*sn*-glycero-3-phosphoethanolamine-*N*-(methoxy(polyethylene glycol)-2000) ($DSPE-PEG_{2000}$), and lecithin as lipid) [27,28] which resulted for improvement of intracellular uptake of drugs to overcome the multidrug resistance in cancer and enhancement of antitumour activity [29,30]. Previously, PLGA-based BTB nanoparticles have been developed and characterised to show their sustained release performance but without in vivo bioavailability study [31]. To the best of our knowledge, no study has been reported for fabrication of PLGA-based LP-NPs having tristearin and soyalecithin (SL) as lipids aiming at enhancing the bioavailability of poorly soluble and low permeable drugs.

The main goal of this work is to promote the oral bioavailability of BTB through its encapsulation in PLGA-based LP-NPs carriers. Therefore, four different BTB-loaded LP-NPs (B-PLN1 to B-PLN4) were developed by varying the lipid content. Analysing the formulations in terms of physicochemical properties and encapsulation efficiency allowed us to select the optimised nanoparticle carrier which was investigated further in terms of morphology, in vitro release, and in vivo pharmacokinetic studies in rats. The findings in this study may be further sculpted into new encapsulation strategies by employing hybrid materials.

2. Results and Discussion

2.1. Particles Characterisation

BTB-loaded PLGA-based LP-NPs (B-PLNs) were prepared by the single-step nano-precipitation method, consisting of PLGA polymer and tristearin lipid as core and shell parts, respectively. Sonication was employed using a probe sonicator, which produces high-intensity ultrasonic waves that break the big particles into nanoparticles. To optimise B-PLNs, the amount of tristearin (lipid) was varied, utilising a fixed amount of PLGA (polymer) and SL (surfactant). The mean size, PDI and ζP of the B-LPNs at different lipid contents (50–200 mg) are shown in Table 1. The particle size of different formulae (B-PLN1 to B-PLN4) was obtained in the range of 205 ± 5.2 to 272 ± 7.6 nm. The lipids covered the PLGA core, which thickened the shell, thereby increasing the particle size. The purpose of the selection of tristearin as lipid in this formulation as it shows better cellular uptake, low toxicity and greater immune response. [32,33]. The PDI values of PLNs were measured in the range of 0.170–0.299, which indicates a homogenous population of PLNs [34,35]. ζP is the key parameter for the evaluation of the stability of colloidal dispersion. The ζP of the prepared PLNs were measured in the range of -21.1 to -36.5 mV, negative values of ζP are due to negatively charged SL [36]. It is believed that the values of $\zeta P \geq \pm 30$ mV suggest the formation of stable particles, nevertheless, it has to be mentioned that the usual Smoluchowski method to determine ζP is only valid for hard spheres [37]. In this case, due to the soft nature of B-PLNs, ζP calculated by conventional analysis does not reflect the state of agglomeration or stability. Our soft particles were stable despite in some cases (B-PLN1 and B-PLN2) $\zeta P < \pm 30$ mV [38]. As can be seen in Table 1, the particle size, PDI and ζP of formulated B-PLNs increase as the lipid content increases.

Table 1. Physicochemical characterisation of nanoparticles (B-PLNs).

Sample	Size (nm ± SD)	PDI	ζP (±mV)	%EE	%DL
B-PLN1	205 ± 5.2	0.170	−21.1 ± 2.1	57.8 ± 1.1	6.80 ± 0.81
B-PLN2	231 ± 4.3	0.202	−26.5 ± 2.7	45.9 ± 1.9	6.51 ± 1.02
B-PLN3	259 ± 8.6	0.299	−32.4 ± 1.8	68.6 ± 1.9	5.08 ± 0.95
B-PLN4	272 ± 7.6	0.225	−36.5 ± 3.1	71.6 ± 1.5	2.87 ± 0.42

2.2. Percent Drug Entrapment (%EE) and Loading (%DL)

Entrapment efficiency gives an idea about the amount of drug that is successfully entrapped/adsorbed into nanoparticles. Typically, an excellent drug carrier should have high entrapment efficiency (EE). High EE (above 70%) can increase the efficacy of the drug delivery system and decrease the side effects of the drug [39,40]. The %EE and %DL of B-PLNs (B-PLN1 to B-PLN4) were measured in the range of 45.9 ± 1.9 to $71.6 \pm 1.5\%$ and 2.87 ± 0.42 to $6.80 \pm 0.81\%$, respectively (Table 1). The highest drug entrapment ($71.6 \pm 1.5\%$) was found in the case of B-PLN4, a large amount of lipid (200 mg, stearin) formulated in this sample is supposed to prevent the diffusion of the drug from the polymeric core, thereby, enhancing the entrapment of drug [41].

2.3. DSC Studies

DSC thermal studies were performed to investigate the compatibility of drug and excipients (PLGA, tristearin, and SL). The DSC spectra of BTB, PLGA, tristearin, SL and their B-PLNs (B-PLN1-B-PLN4) are presented in Figure 1. The DSC spectra of pure BTB drug exhibited a sharp endothermic peak at 217.97 °C, which confirmed the purity and crystallinity of the drug [31]. PLGA showed a glass transition temperature at 58 °C. The DSC spectrum of tristearin exhibited a distinct endothermic peak at 79 °C, whereas SL showed a merge of multiple peaks between temperatures 180 to 205 °C [42,43]. The endothermic peak of pure BTB were absent in all B-PLNs (B-PLN1-B-PLN4), which clearly indicated successful encapsulation of the drug [44]. The peak associated with tristearin could be seen in all formulations, due to the covering of lipid on the polymeric core.

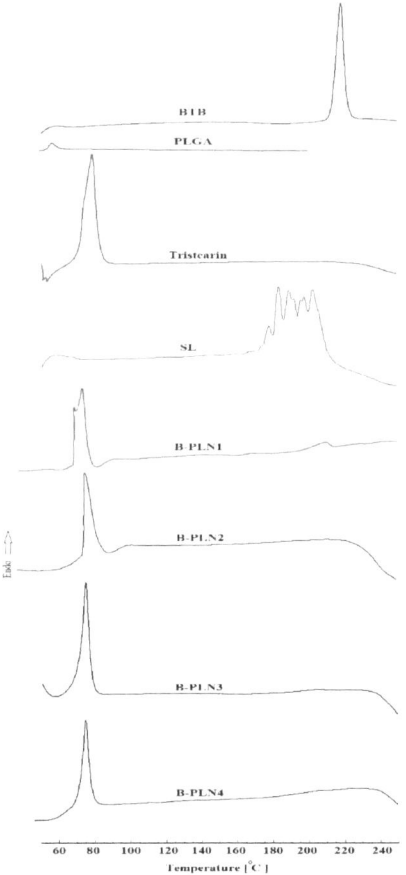

Figure 1. Comparative DSC thermograms of BTB, PLGA, stearin, SL and formulated lipid-polymer nanoparticles (B-PLN1 to B-PLN4).

2.4. FTIR Studies

FTIR spectral studies were performed to investigate the possible chemical interactions between drug and excipients (PLGA, tristearin and SL). The FTIR spectra of BTB, PLGA, tristearin, SL and their corresponding B-PLNs (B-PLN1 to B-PLN4) are presented in Figure 2. The FTIR spectra of pure BTB assigned various characteristics peaks at wave numbers 3207 cm^{-1} (N-H stretching), 3119 cm^{-1} (aromatic =C-H stretching), 2842 cm^{-1} (-C-H stretching), 2263 cm^{-1} (-C=N stretching). FTIR spectra of SL showed a characteristic peak at 2924 cm^{-1} and 2856 cm^{-1} (-C-H stretching), 1738 cm^{-1} (-C=O stretching). FTIR spectra of stearin showed a characteristic peak at 2922 cm^{-1} and 2852 cm^{-1} (-C-H stretching), 1729 cm^{-1} (-C=O stretching) [45]. The FTIR spectra of PLGA indicated a strong peak at

1753 cm^{-1} (C=O stretching). The characteristic peaks of stearin and SL were observed in the spectrum of B-PLNs (B-PLN1 to B-PLN4), suggesting that BTB was successfully loaded inside the lipid shell.

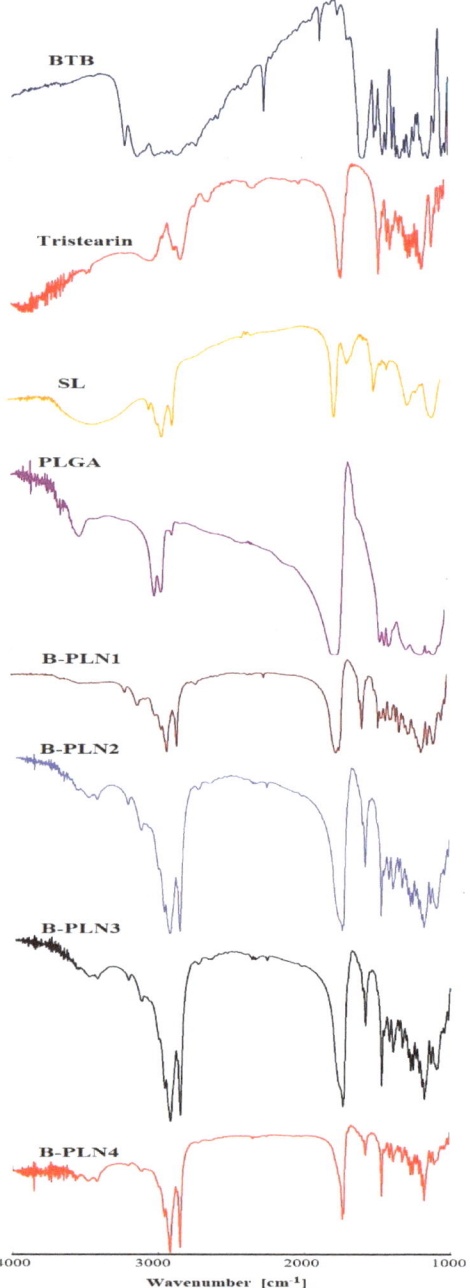

Figure 2. Comparative FTIR spectra of BTB, stearin, PLGA, SL and formulated lipid-polymer nanoparticles (B-PLN1 to B-PLN4).

2.5. XRD Studies

XRD is a frequently used technique for the characterisation that provides the information regarding crystalline and amorphous nature of nanoparticles. Comparative XRD spectra of pure BTB and their polymer-lipid hybrid nanoparticles (B-PLN1 to B-PLN4) are shown in Figure 3. The XRD spectra of pure BTB shows various intense peaks at 12.5° (2θ), 13.6° (2θ), 15.2° (2θ), 17.2° (2θ), 18.9° (2θ) and 26.6° (2θ), which revealed its crystalline nature [31]. The intense XRD peaks of pure BTB were reduced in intensity, broadened or diffused in all B-PLN samples (B-PLN1 to B-PLN4), which clearly indicated amorphisation of the drug, probably due to encapsulation inside polymer and lipid matrix. The polymeric encapsulation layers hinder the drug, which is then not able to crystallise at the solid–air interface. As the result, the coating layer introduces another solid–solid boundary. This process is called amorphous solid dispersion and is certainly the consequence of disrupting intermolecular interactions in the drug's crystal lattice and assembling drug–polymer interactions [46]. Some extra peaks associated with excipients can be seen in all formulations.

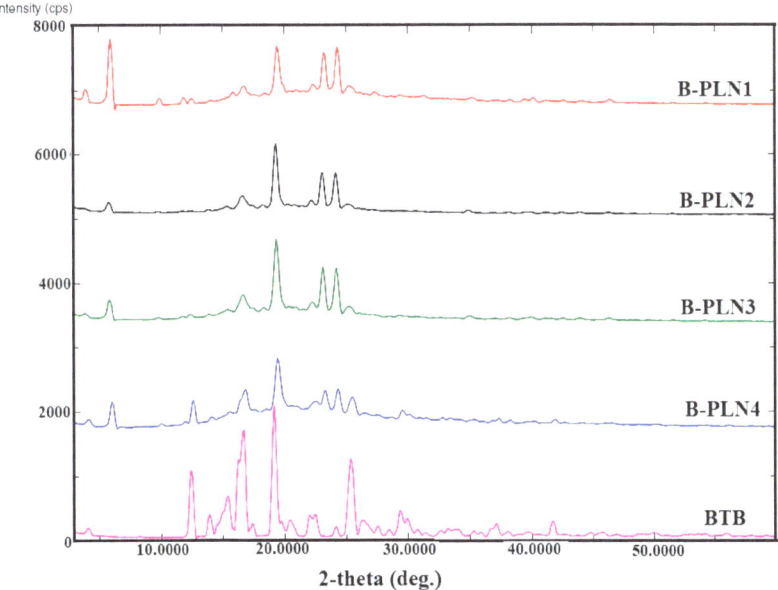

Figure 3. XRD spectra of BTB and formulated lipid-polymer nanoparticles (B-PLN1-B-PLN4).

2.6. In Vitro Release Studies

Comparative in vitro release profiles of pure BTB and B-PLN4 are shown in Figure 4. The first phase burst release of BTB was observed in B-PLN4 formulation in the first 4 h, probably due to surface adsorbed drug on nanoparticles. Thereafter, the second phase has shown sustained release of BTB from lipid-coated polymer hybrid nanoparticles till 48 h. Sustained release of drug was observed due to slow release of drug by diffusion from tristearin and PLGA matrix. However, 100% drug released was observed from pure BTB in the first six hours of the study. The sustained release of BTB may help reduce the frequency of oral administration and in chronic arthritis treatment. The drug release data of optimised formulation (B-PLN4) was treated by employing various kinetic models viz; zero-order (R^2 = 0.4848), first-order (R^2 = 0.6525), Higuchi model (R^2 = 0.7546) and Korsmeyer–Peppas model (R^2 = 0.879). The correlation of coefficient of various models indicated that formulation B-PLN4 was best fitted with the Korsmeyer–Peppas model (R^2 = 0.879) comparison to other kinetic models. Korsmeyer–Peppas model indicated a release simultaneously by diffusion of water into the matrix, swelling of matrix and dissolution of matrix. Additionally, the release data were fitted to the Korsmeyer–Peppas model at a dose of 100% drug release showed the release exponent $n = 0.3619$. The n value less than 0.43 in the spherical encapsulation shape indicates a Fickian diffusion release of the drug [47–50]. The initial burst release followed by sustained release of drug during dissolution also supports the goodness of Korsmeyer–Peppas kinetic models [51].

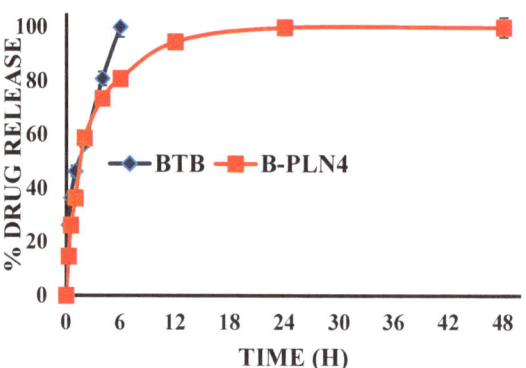

Figure 4. Comparative in vitro release profile of pure drug BTB and optimised B-PLN4 formulation.

2.7. Morphology

SEM images of optimised formulae B-PLN4 represents spherical shapes and with a rough surface. Rough surfaced and agglomerated particles could be seen, probably due to the melting of lipid matrix as stearin melts around 72 °C [52] (Figure 5). The size of the particles was approximately identical as measured by the DLS technique.

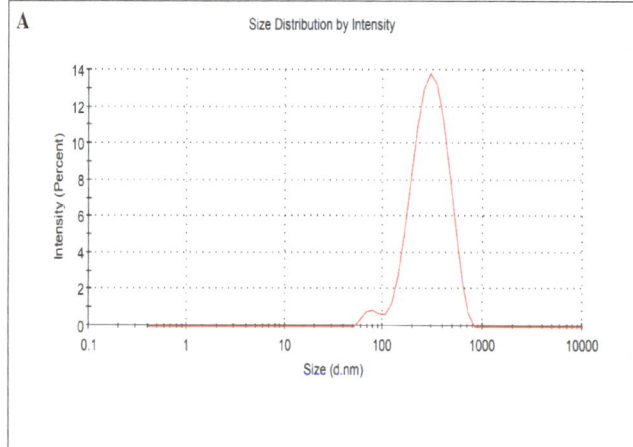
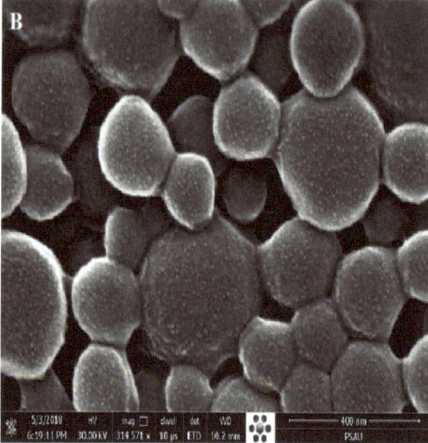

Figure 5. Size distribution plot derived by DLS method (**A**) and SEM images (**B**) of optimised lipid-polymer nanoparticle system (B-PLN4).

2.8. In Vivo Pharmacokinetic Study

The pharmacokinetic parameters calculated after oral administration of pure BTB suspension and B-PLN4 formulation (described by a non-compartmental pharmacokinetic analysis) are presented in Table 2. At the administered dose, both C_{max} ($p < 0.001$) and AUC_{0-24} ($p < 0.005$), $AUC_{0-\infty}$ ($p < 0.05$) values were significantly higher in B-PLN4 formulation compared to pure BTB suspension, without any change in the T_{max} value. This enabled high circulation capability of B-PLN4 formulation and therefore the resulted relative bioavailability was 3-fold higher than pure BTB suspension. Similar results have been also observed in previous PLGA-based polymer-lipid hybrid nanoparticles [27,28]. Moreover, the half-life of B-PLN4 formulation (11.7 h) was higher (although it was not significant) than the plane BTB suspension (8.2 h), indicating that B-PLN4 formulation not only increases the bioavailability of BTB but also facilitates long-term retention i.e., sustain release performance. This was also confirmed by comparing the values of $AUC_{0-\infty}/AUC_{0-24}$ for B-PLN4 (only 75 %) to the one of pure suspension (87 %), implying that a substantial concentration of BTB was still present at the last time point (24 h) and additional timepoint up to 48 h was necessary to be covered for sampling to calculate accurate pharmacokinetic profiles, which is also evident in plasma concentration-time profile (Figure 6). BTB appearance in the circulatory system after administration of B-PLN4 was composed of two steps: the release of the drug from B-PLN4 and the absorption of BTB into the central compartment. The B-PLN4 formulation underwent a slower distribution rate as compared to BTB pure suspension as evidenced from the prolonged half-life. These results confirm that the release of BTB from B-PLN4 formulation was the rate-determining step owing to the protective effects of polymer-lipid hybrid nanoparticles suggesting that BTB loaded lipid polymer nanoparticles were able to enhance BTB in vivo bioavailability. Moreover, the results of the in-vitro release profile of B-PLN4 formulation were also comparable with our pharmacokinetic results. The representative multiple reaction monitoring (MRM) mode chromatograms of BTB and IS (rivaroxaban) after oral administration of BTB (1 mg/Kg) is presented in Figure 7.

Table 2. Pharmacokinetic Parameters after a single oral dose of pure BTB suspension and B-PLN4 administration (1 mg/kg in rats).

Pharmacokinetic Parameters	Pure BTB Suspension	B-PLN4
	Mean ± SD, (n = 6)	Mean ± SD, (n = 6)
C_{max} (ng/mL)	404 ± 58	1020 ± 34 ***
T_{max} (h)	0.5	0.5
AUC_{0-24} (ng·h/mL)	3091 ± 720	9030 ± 1487 **
$AUC_{0-\infty}$ (ng·h/mL)	3536 ± 697	12041 ± 3701 *
K_{el} (h)	0.09 ± 0.02	0.06 ± 0.02
$T_{1/2}$ (h)	8.2 ± 1.7	11.7 ± 4.3
MRT (h)	11.45 ± 2.33	16.29 ± 5.84
Relative Bioavailability (%)	100	292

*** $p < 0.001$, ** $p < 0.005$, * $p < 0.05$.

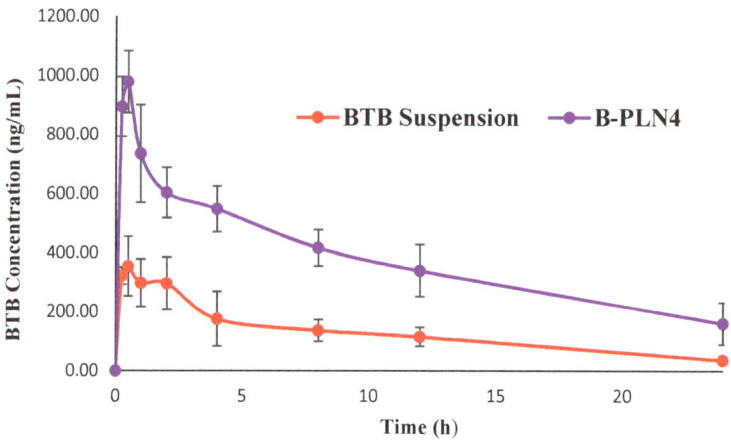

Figure 6. Comparative plasma concentration versus time profile of BTB after oral administration of BTB pure suspension and BPLN4 (1 mg/kg) in rats ($n = 6$).

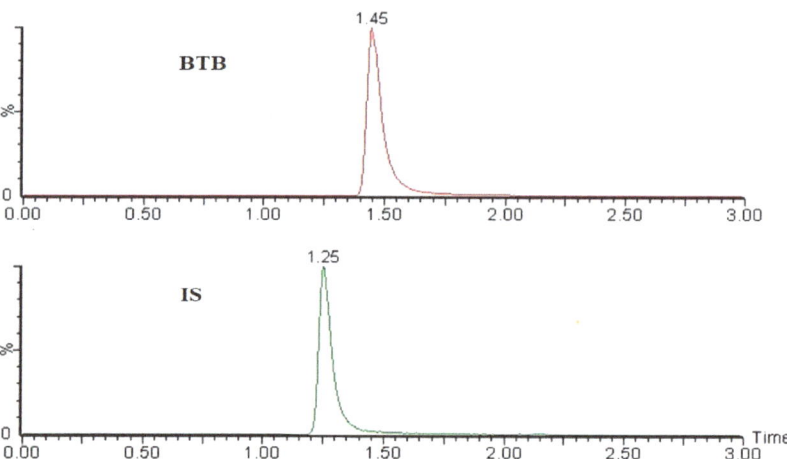

Figure 7. Representative MRM chromatogram of BTB and IS at T_{max} after oral administration of 1 mg/kg of B-PLN4 formulation in rats.

3. Materials and Methods

3.1. Materials

BTB was purchased from "Mesochem Technology" Beijing, China. Tristearin (Dynasan 188), PLGA and Soyalecithin (SL) were purchased from "Sigma Aldrich, St. Louis, MO, USA". All other chemicals and solvents were used as received.

3.2. Preparation of BTB-Loaded PLGA-Lipid Hybrid Nanoparticles

The PLGA-lipid hybrid nanoparticles were prepared using the single-step nano-precipitation method followed by emulsification [22]. Briefly, PLGA (50 mg) and tristearin (lipid) were dissolved in 10 mL of dichloromethane, further drug BTB was added in the above formed organic phase. Separately, the aqueous phase was prepared by adding SL in 20 mL of distilled water. The prepared organic phase was emulsified by adding in aqueous phase dropwise (0.3 mL/min), and sonicated on probe sonicator "(probe # 423, model CL-18, Fisher scientific; Massachusetts, MA, USA)" for 3 min, on/off cycles 10 secs at 60% W power efficiency. The produced emulsion was left under stirring overnight at room temperature to evaporate organic solvent. The resultant suspension was centrifuged "(HermleLabortechnik, Z216MK, Wehingen, Siemensstraße, Germany)" at high speed (12,000 rpm) to separate non-entrapped drugs. The collected sediment was further washed three times with double distilled water and then lyophilised. Four formulations were developed by varying the tristearin content (50–200 mg) (Table 3).

Table 3. Composition of developed lipid-polymer hybrid NPs (B-PLN1 to B-PLN4).

Formulae	PLGA (mg)	Tristearin (mg)	SL (mg)	BTB (mg)
B-PLN1	50	50	50	20
B-PLN2	50	100	50	20
B-PLN3	50	150	50	20
B-PLN4	50	200	50	20

3.3. Particles Characterisation

The particle size, polydispersity index (PDI) and zeta potential (ζP) of synthesised LP-NPs were measured using the DLS method "(Zetasizer Nano ZS instrument, Malvern Instruments, Worcestershire, UK)" at room temperature (25 ± 2 °C). The light scattering angle of measurement was set at $90°$. All the measurements were performed in triplicate and data was presented in mean $\pm$ SD (n = 3).

3.4. Percent Drug Entrapment (%EE) and Loading (%DL)

The freshly prepared dispersion was centrifuged "(HermleLabortechnik, Z216MK, Wehingen, Siemensstraße, Germany)" at 12,000 rpm for 15 min to separate the solid sediment. The obtained supernatant was filtered and diluted appropriately, and analysed for free drug content by UV spectroscopy "(Jasco UV spectrophotometer V-630 Japan)". The %EE and %DL were measured using the following equation:

$$\%EE = \frac{\text{Total BTB loaded} - \text{free BTB in supernatant}}{\text{Total BTB loaded}}$$

$$\%DL = \frac{\text{Intially BTB added} - \text{free BTB in supernatant}}{\text{Total weight of lipid polymer NPs}}$$

3.5. Differential Scanning Calorimetry (DSC) Studies

The thermal properties of pure BTB, PLGA, tristearin, SL and their B-PLNs (B-PLN1-B-PLN4) were examined by DSC "(DSC N-650; Scinco, Seoul, Korea). Accurately weighed (5 mg) of each sample was pressed into a hermetically sealed aluminium pan, placed in a DSC sample holder, and heated for a temperature ranging from 50 °C to 250 °C at a heating rate of 10 °C/min. The instrument was continuously purged with inert nitrogen gas with a flow rate of 20 mL/min during the experiment.

3.6. Fourier Transform Infrared (FTIR) Studies

FTIR spectra of pure BTB, PLGA, tristearin, SL and their B-PLNs (B-PLN1-B-PLN4) were recorded using "FTIR spectrometer (Jasco FTIR Spectrophotometer, Tokyo, Japan)". For the preparation of the sample, each sample was diluted with potassium bromide (KBr) crystal (1:10, w/w) to prepare pellets. FTIR spectra were recorded in the range of 4000 to 1000 cm^{-1}, and peaks were interpreted using "spectral manager" software.

3.7. X-ray Diffraction (XRD) Studies

XRD studies of pure BTB and their polymer-lipid hybrid nanoparticles (B-PLN1-B-PLN4) were recorded using "Ultima IV Diffractometer (Rigaku Inc., Tokyo, Japan at College of Pharmacy, King Saud University, Riyadh, KSA)". The samples equivalent 200 mg of pure BTB were spread on the sample holder and scanned in the range of 0–60° (2θ) at a scan rate of 4°/min.

3.8. In Vitro Release Studies

In vitro release studies of pure BTB drug and synthesised polymer-lipid hybrid nanoparticles (B-PLN1-B-PLN4) were performed using dialysis bag "(cut off of 12 kda)" method over a period of 48 h. Based on preliminary evaluation, B-PLN4 formulae was optimised for release and pharmacokinetic studies. Briefly, pure BTB and B-PLN4 (equivalent to10 mg BTB) was dispersed in a dialysis bag containing 10 mL of phosphate buffer (pH 6.8) and shaken on a biological shaker "(LBS-030S-Lab Tech, Kyonggi, Korea)" at 100 rpm and 37 °C [31]. The supernatant of the samples was collected, centrifuged (12,000 rpm) "(HermleLabortechnik, Z216MK, Wehingen, Germany)" and analysed at 224 nm on different time points (0, 0.25, 0.5, 1, 2, 4, 6, 12, 24 and 48 h). Each analysis was performed in triplicate. To check the kinetic release pattern of BTB from B-PLN4, the obtained release data were fitted with various kinetic models viz. zero order, first order, Higuchi's and Korsemeyer–Peppas kinetic models as follow:

Zero order: ($Q_t = Q_0 + K_0 t$)
First Order: ($\ln Q_t = \ln Q_0 + K_1 t$)
Higuchi: ($Q_t = K_H t^{1/2}$)
Korsmeyer–Peppas: ($Q_t/Q_\infty = K_K t^n$)

3.9. Morphology

The morphology of optimised formulae, B-PLN4 was viewed using Scanning Electron Microscopy (SEM) "(JEOL JSM-5900-LV, Tokyo, Japan)". The sample was homogenously spread and coated with gold-metal in a thin film coater under vacuum "(Quorum Q150R S, East Sussex, UK)". The pre-treated sample was then bombarded with an electron beam and the interaction resulted in the formation of secondary electrons called auger electrons. From this interaction between the electron beam and the specimen's atoms, only the electrons scattered at ≥90° were selected and surface topography was taken at 15 kV acceleration voltage and 314,571× magnification [23].

3.10. Bio-Analytical Methods

BTB was quantified in rat plasma samples by a slight modification of our previous reported UPLC-MS/MS method [50]. The precursor to production ion transition of 372.07 > 251.14 and 440.04 > 4144.9 (quantifier) were used BTB and internal standard (rivaroxaban d-5) quantification in multiple reactions monitoring mode for detection. The capillary voltage was 3.9 kV and the cone voltage and collision energy were set at 50 V and 30 eV for BTB and 46 V and 28 eV for IS, respectively. Before analysis, the method was validated and all parameters were within the acceptable range mentioned in the guideline for bioanalytical method validation.

3.11. Pharmacokinetic Studies

The comparative pharmacokinetic study of newly synthesised B-PLN4 formulation against normal BTB suspension was performed in rats. The experimental protocol involved twelve healthy adult male Wistar albino rats ($n = 6$, weight 200 ± 20 g), randomly divided into two groups: BTB suspension dispersed in 0.5% w/v carboxy methyl cellulose (1 mg/kg, p.o.) and B-PLN4 formulation (1 mg/kg, p.o.). The animals were received from the "Animal Care Centre, College of Pharmacy, Prince Sattam Bin Abdulaziz University, Alkharj" and were kept under the recommended conditions with access to food and water ad libitum. The experimental protocol was reviewed and approved by "Research Ethics Committee, Prince Sattam Bin Abdulaziz University (Approval number: BERC 003-03-21)" and the study was performed following all applicable international guidelines for animal handling and use. The animals were fasted overnight and the blood samples were collected in pre-heparinised tube was at a fixed time span (0, 0.25, 0.5, 1, 2, 4, 8, 12 and 24 h) after administration of respective formations. All blood samples were centrifuged at $4500\times g$ for 5 min to separate the plasma and all the samples were safely stored in a deep freezer ($80 \pm 10\,°C$) until analysis by UPLC-MS/MS.

The non-compartmental pharmacokinetic model was selected to calculate the different pharmacokinetic parameters using "WinNonlin software, Pharsight Co., Mountain View, CA, USA". All the results were presented as mean ± standard deviation (SD). The parameters; peak plasma concentration (C_{max}), time to reach peak concentration (T_{max}), area under cure (AUC) [(AUC_{0-24}) ($AUC_{0-\infty}$)], elimination half-life ($T_{\frac{1}{2}}$) and rate constant (kz), mean residence time (MRT) were calculated. Unpaired t-test was used to compare the results between normal BTB suspension and B-PLN4 formulation ($p < 0.05$) was considered statistically significant.

3.12. Statistical Analysis

"One-way ANOVA using Dunnett's test. However, an unpaired t-test was used for the statistical evaluation of pharmacokinetic parameters. The GraphPad InStat software was used for statistical analysis, and $p < 0.05$ was considered significant".

4. Conclusions

The BTB-loaded lipid-polymer hybrid NPs were prepared using PLGA, lecithin and stearin through a single-step nano-precipitation method to enhance the bioavailability and sustained release profile of BTB. The PLGA precipitated forming hydrophobic core to encapsulate poorly soluble drug (BTB). The SL and stearin assembled around the PLGA polymer core to form a lipid layer shell. The influence of different concentrations of lipid (tristearin) and soya lecithin (surfactant) on particle sizes, zeta potentials and % EE were assessed. Further, all four B-PLN (B-PLN1 to B-PLN4) formulations were characterised by the DSC, FTIR and X-ray diffraction studies. The optimised B-PLN4 formulation was morphologically characterised by SEM study. In vitro release profile of BTB from lipid-coated polymer hybrid nanoparticles showed slow release of drug by diffusion from tristearin and PLGA matrix. In vivo pharmacokinetic study showed that the lipid-coated polymer hybrid nanoparticles prolonged circulation time when compared with pure BTB suspension which results in a 3-fold increase in bioavailability of B-PLN4 formulation. Overall, it can be concluded that the lipid-coated polymer hybrid NPs can open up a new route for drug delivery with improved potential. However, more extended sampling time points need to be added in future pharmacokinetic studies to cover the better pharmacokinetic profile of BTB formulations.

Author Contributions: Conceptualisation, M.K.A., M.I. and M.M.A.; methodology, M.K.A., M.I. and M.N.A.; software, E.A.A. and M.F.A.; validation, A.A.S. and E.A.A.; formal analysis, A.A.S. and M.I.; investigation, M.K.A. and M.M.A.; resources, M.F.A. and A.A.S.; writing—original draft preparation, M.K.A., M.I. and M.A.A.; writing—review and editing, M.A.A., M.I. and M.K.A.; visualisation, M.M.A.; supervision, M.F.A. and M.A.A. All authors have read and agreed to the published version of the manuscript.

Funding: This research was funded by the researchers supporting project at King Saud University via grant number RSP/2021/45.

Institutional Review Board Statement: The study was conducted after approval of the Research Ethics Committee, Prince Sattam Bin Abdulaziz University (Approval number: BERC 003-03-21; dated: March 2021).

Informed Consent Statement: Not applicable.

Data Availability Statement: The data presented in this study are available on request from the corresponding author.

Acknowledgments: The authors wish to thank "Researchers Supporting Project at King Saud University, Riyadh, Saudi Arabia for financial support of this research via grant number RSP/2021/45".

Conflicts of Interest: The authors declare no conflict of interest.

Sample Availability: Not applicable.

References

1. Mogul, A.; Corsi, K.; McAuliffe, L. Baricitinib: The second FDA-approved JAK inhibitor for the treatment of rheumatoid arthritis. *Ann. Pharm.* **2019**, *53*, 947–953. [CrossRef] [PubMed]
2. Assadiasl, S.; Fatahi, Y.; Mosharmovahed, B.; Mohebbi, B.; Nicknam, M.H. Baricitinib: From Rheumatoid Arthritis to COVID-19. *J. Clin. Pharmacol.* **2021**, *61*, 1274–1285. [CrossRef] [PubMed]
3. Jorgensen, S.C.J.; Tse, C.L.Y.; Burry, L.; Dresser, L.D. Baricitinib: A Review of Pharmacology, Safety, and Emerging Clinical Experience in COVID-19. *Pharmacotherapy* **2020**, *40*, 843–856. [CrossRef] [PubMed]
4. Fridman, J.S.; Scherle, P.A.; Collins, R.; Burn, T.C.; Li, Y.; Li, J.; Covington, M.B.; Thomas, B.; Collier, P.; Favata, M.F.; et al. Selective inhibition of JAK1 and JAK2 is efficacious in rodent models of arthritis: Preclinical characterization of INCB028050. *J. Immunol.* **2010**, *184*, 5298–5307. [CrossRef] [PubMed]
5. EMEA Assessment Report: Olumiant. Available online: https://www.ema.europa.eu/en/documents/assessment-report/olumiant-epar-public-assessment-report_en.pdf (accessed on 30 May 2021).
6. Drugbank: Identification of Baricitinib. 2018. Available online: https://www.clearsynth.com/en/CST48553.html; https://go.drugbank.com/drugs/DB11817 (accessed on 30 May 2021).
7. Dahan, A.; Miller, J.M. The solubility–permeability interplay and its implications in formulation design and development for poorly soluble drugs. *AAPS J.* **2012**, *14*, 244–251. [CrossRef] [PubMed]
8. Aboudzadeh, M.A. *Emulsion-Based Encapsulation of Antioxidants*; Springer Nature: Cham, Switzerland, 2021.
9. Aboudzadeh, M.A.; Mehravar, E.; Fernandez, M.; Lezama, L.; Tomovska, R. Low-Energy Encapsulation of α-Tocopherol Using Fully Food Grade Oil-in-Water Microemulsions. *ACS Omega* **2018**, *3*, 10999–11008. [CrossRef] [PubMed]
10. Sabir, F.; Qindeel, M.; Zeeshan, M.; Ul Ain, Q.; Rahdar, A.; Barani, M.; González, E.; Aboudzadeh, M.A. Onco-Receptors Targeting in Lung Cancer via Application of Surface-Modified and Hybrid Nanoparticles: A Cross-Disciplinary Review. *Processes* **2021**, *9*, 621. [CrossRef]
11. Prosheva, M.; Aboudzadeh, M.A.; Leal, G.P.; Gilev, J.B.; Tomovska, R. High-Performance UV Protective Waterborne Polymer Coatings Based on Hybrid Graphene/Carbon Nanotube Radicals Scavenging Filler. *Mater. Sci. Part. Part. Syst. Charact.* **2019**, *36*, 1800555. [CrossRef]
12. Aboudzadeh, M.A.; Iturrospe, A.; Arbe, A.; Grzelczak, M.; Barroso-Bujans, F. Cyclic Polyethylene Glycol as Nanoparticle Surface Ligand. *ACS Macro Lett.* **2020**, *9*, 1604–1610. [CrossRef]
13. Hamzehlou, S.; Aboudzadeh, M.A. Special Issue on "Multifunctional Hybrid Materials Based on Polymers: Design and Performance". *Processes* **2021**, *9*, 1448. [CrossRef]
14. Hamzehlou, S.; Aboudzadeh, M.A. *Multifunctional Hybrid Materials Based on Polymers: Design and Performance*; Book Published in Processes; MDPI: Basel, Switzerland, 2021. [CrossRef]
15. Mukherjee, A.; Waters, A.K.; Kalyan, P.; Achrol, A.S.; Kesari, S.; Yenugonda, V.M. Lipid-polymer hybrid nanoparticles as a next-generation drug delivery platform: State of the art, emerging technologies, and perspectives. *Int. J. Nanomed.* **2019**, *14*, 1937–1952. [CrossRef] [PubMed]
16. Jose, C.; Amra, K.; Bhavsar, C.; Momin, M.; Omri, A. Polymeric Lipid Hybrid Nanoparticles: Properties and Therapeutic Applications. *Crit. Rev. Ther. Drug Carrier Syst.* **2018**, *35*, 555–588. [CrossRef] [PubMed]
17. Chan, J.M.; Zhang, L.; Yuet, K.P.; Liao, G.; Rhee, J.W.; Langer, R.; Farokhzad, O.C. PLGA-lecithin-PEG core-shell nanoparticles for controlled drug delivery. *Biomaterials* **2009**, *30*, 1627–1634. [CrossRef]
18. Zhang, L.; Chan, J.M.; Gu, F.X.; Rhee, J.W.; Wang, A.Z.; Radovic-Moreno, A.F.; Alexis, F.; Langer, R.; Farokhzad, O.C. Self-assembled lipid–polymer hybrid nanoparticles: A robust drug delivery platform. *ACS Nano* **2008**, *2*, 1696–1702. [CrossRef] [PubMed]
19. Anwer, M.K.; Mohammad, M.; Iqbal, M.; Ansari, M.N.; Ezzeldin, E.; Fatima, F.; Alshahrani, S.M.; Aldawsari, M.F.; Alalaiwe, A.; Alzahrani, A.A.; et al. Sustained release and enhanced oral bioavailability of rivaroxaban by PLGA nanoparticles with no food effect. *J. Thromb. Thrombolysis* **2020**, *49*, 404–412. [CrossRef] [PubMed]
20. Dong, W.; Wang, X.; Liu, C.; Zhang, X.; Zhang, X.; Chen, X.; Kou, Y.; Mao, S. Chitosan based polymer-lipid hybrid nanoparticles for oral delivery of enoxaparin. *Int. J. Pharm.* **2018**, *547*, 499–505. [CrossRef]
21. Khan, M.M.; Madni, A.; Torchilin, V.; Filipczak, N.; Pan, J.; Tahir, N.; Shah, H. Lipid-chitosan hybrid nanoparticles for controlled delivery of cisplatin. *Drug Deliv.* **2019**, *26*, 765–772. [CrossRef] [PubMed]
22. Anwer, M.K.; Iqbal, M.; Muharram, M.M.; Mohammad, M.; Ezzeldin, E.; Aldawsari, M.F.; Alalaiwe, A.; Imam, F. Development of Lipomer Nanoparticles for the Enhancement of *Drug* Release, Anti-microbial Activity and Bioavailability of Delafloxacin. *Pharmaceutics* **2020**, *12*, 252. [CrossRef] [PubMed]
23. Anwer, M.K.; Mohammad, M.; Ezzeldin, E.; Fatima, F.; Alalaiwe, A.; Iqbal, M. Preparation of sustained release apremilast-loaded PLGA nanoparticles: In vitro characterization and in vivo pharmacokinetic study in rats. *Int. J. Nanomed.* **2019**, *14*, 1587–1595. [CrossRef] [PubMed]

24. Anwer, M.K.; Al-Shdefat, R.; Ezzeldin, E.; Alshahrani, S.M.; Alshetaili, A.S.; Iqbal, M. Preparation, Evaluation and Bioavailability Studies of Eudragit Coated PLGA Nanoparticles for Sustained Release of Eluxadoline for the Treatment of Irritable Bowel Syndrome. *Front. Pharm.* **2017**, *8*, 844. [CrossRef]
25. Jamil, A.; Aamir Mirza, M.; Anwer, M.K.; Thakur, P.S.; Alshahrani, S.M.; Alshetaili, A.S.; Telegaonkar, S.; Panda, A.K.; Iqbal, Z. Co-delivery of gemcitabine and simvastatin through PLGA polymeric nanoparticles for the treatment of pancreatic cancer: In-vitro characterization, cellular uptake, and pharmacokinetic studies. *Drug Dev. Ind. Pharm.* **2019**, *45*, 745–753. [CrossRef]
26. Makadia, H.K.; Siegel, S.J. Poly Lactic-co-Glycolic Acid (PLGA) as Biodegradable Controlled Drug Delivery Carrier. *Polymers* **2011**, *3*, 1377–1397. [CrossRef]
27. Godara, S.; Lather, V.; Kirthanashri, S.V.; Awasthi, R.; Pandita, D. Lipid-PLGA hybrid nanoparticles of paclitaxel: Preparation, characterization, in vitro and in vivo evaluation. *Mater. Sci. Eng. C Mater. Biol. Appl.* **2020**, *109*, 110576. [CrossRef] [PubMed]
28. Ma, Z.; Liu, J.; Li, X.; Xu, Y.; Liu, D.; He, H.; Wang, Y.; Tang, X. Hydroxycamptothecin (HCPT)-loaded PEGlated lipid-polymer hybrid nanoparticles for effective delivery of HCPT: QbD-based development and evaluation. *Drug Deliv. Transl. Res.* **2021**, *12*, 306–324. [CrossRef] [PubMed]
29. Maghrebi, S.; Joyce, P.; Jambhrunkar, M.; Thomas, N.; Prestidge, C.A. Poly(lactic-*co*-glycolic) Acid-Lipid Hybrid Microparticles Enhance the Intracellular Uptake and Antibacterial Activity of Rifampicin. *ACS Appl. Mat. Interf.* **2020**, *12*, 8030–8039. [CrossRef] [PubMed]
30. Pramual, S.; Lirdprapamongkol, K.; Jouan-Hureaux, V.; Barberi-Heyob, M.; Frochot, C.; Svasti, J.; Niamsiri, N. Overcoming the diverse mechanisms of multidrug resistance in lung cancer cells by photodynamic therapy using pTHPP-loaded PLGA-lipid hybrid nanoparticles. *Eur. J. Pharm. Biopharm.* **2020**, *149*, 218–228. [CrossRef] [PubMed]
31. Ansari, M.J.; Alshahrani, S.M. Nano-encapsulation and characterization of baricitinib using poly-lactic-glycolic acid co-polymer. *Saudi Pharm. J.* **2019**, *27*, 491–501. [CrossRef] [PubMed]
32. Cheow, W.S.; Hadinoto, K. Factors affecting drug encapsulation and stability of lipid-polymer hybrid nanoparticles. *Colloids Surf. B Biointerfaces* **2011**, *85*, 214–220. [CrossRef] [PubMed]
33. Mishra, H.; Mishra, D.; Mishra, P.K.; Nahar, M.; Dubey, V.; Jain, N.K. Evaluation of solid lipid nanoparticles as carriers for delivery of hepatitis B surface antigen for vaccination using subcutaneous route. *J. Pharm. Pharm. Sci.* **2010**, *13*, 495–509. [CrossRef]
34. Badran, M. Formulation and in vitro evaluation of flufenamic acid loaded deformable liposome for improved skin delivery. *Digest J. Nanomater. Biostruct.* **2014**, *9*, 83–91.
35. Chen, M.; Liu, X.; Fahr, A. Skin penetration and deposition of carboxyfluorescein and temoporfin from different lipid vesicular systems: In Vitro study with finite and infinite dosage application. *Int. J. Pharm.* **2011**, *408*, 223–234. [CrossRef]
36. Celia, C.; Cosco, D.; Paolino, D.; Fresta, M. Nanoparticulate devices for brain drug delivery. *Med. Res. Rev.* **2011**, *31*, 716–756. [CrossRef]
37. Pochapski, D.J.; Santos, C.C.D.; Leite, G.W.; Pulcinelli, S.H.; Santilli, C.V. Zeta Potential and Colloidal Stability Predictions for Inorganic Nanoparticle Dispersions: Effects of Experimental Conditions and Electrokinetic Models on the Interpretation of Results. *Langmuir* **2021**, *37*, 13379–13389. [CrossRef] [PubMed]
38. Lerche, D.; Sobisch, T. Evaluation of particle interactions by in situ visualization of separation behavior. *Colloids Surf. A* **2014**, *440*, 122–130. [CrossRef]
39. Rahdar, A.; Sargazi, S.; Barani, M.; Shahraki, S.; Sabir, F.; Aboudzadeh, M.A. Lignin-Stabilized Doxorubicin Microemulsions: Synthesis, Physical Characterization, and In Vitro Assessments. *Polymers* **2021**, *13*, 641. [CrossRef]
40. Rahdar, A.; Taboada, P.; Hajinezhad, M.R.; Barani, M.; Beyzaei, H. Effect of tocopherol on the properties of Pluronic F127 microemulsions: Physico-chemical characterization and in vivo toxicity. *J. Mol. Liq.* **2019**, *277*, 624–630. [CrossRef]
41. Zhang, L.I.; Zhang, L. Lipid–polymer hybrid nanoparticles: Synthesis, Characterization and Applications. *Nano Life* **2010**, *1*, 163–173. [CrossRef]
42. Alsulays, B.B.; Anwer, M.K.; Soliman, G.A.; Alshehri, S.M.; Khafagy, E.S. Impact of Penetratin Stereochemistry On The Oral Bioavailability Of Insulin-Loaded Solid Lipid Nanoparticles. *Int. J. Nanomed.* **2019**, *14*, 9127–9138. [CrossRef]
43. Yassin, A.E.; Anwer, M.K.; Mowafy, H.A.; El-Bagory, I.M.; Bayomi, M.A.; Alsarra, I.A. Optimization of 5-flurouracil solid-lipid nanoparticles: A preliminary study to treat colon cancer. *Int. J. Med. Sci.* **2010**, *7*, 398–408. [CrossRef]
44. Almutairy, B.K.; Alshetaili, A.; Alali, A.S.; Ahmed, M.M.; Anwer, M.K.; Aboudzadeh, M.A. Design of Olmesartan Medoxomil-Loaded Nanosponges for Hypertension and Lung Cancer Treatments. *Polymers* **2021**, *13*, 2272. [CrossRef]
45. Hayeemasae, N.; Sensem, Z.; Surya, I.; Sahakaro, K.; Ismail, H. Synergistic Effect of Maleated Natural Rubber and Modified Palm Stearin as Dual Compatibilizers in Composites based on Natural Rubber and Halloysite Nanotubes. *Polymers* **2020**, *12*, 766. [CrossRef]
46. Pandi, P.; Bulusu, R.; Kommineni, N.; Khan, W.; Singh, M. Amorphous solid dispersions: An update for preparation, characterization, mechanism on bioavailability, stability, regulatory considerations and marketed products. *Int. J. Pharm.* **2020**, *586*, 119560. [CrossRef] [PubMed]
47. Basak, S.C.; Kumar, K.S.; Ramalingam, M. Design and release characteristics of sustained release tablet containing metformin HCl. *Braz. J. Pharm. Sci.* **2008**, *44*, 477–483. [CrossRef]
48. Supramaniam, J.; Adnan, R.; Mohd Kaus, N.H.; Bushra, R. Magnetic nanocellulose alginate hydrogel beads as potential drug delivery system. *Int. J. Biol. Macromol.* **2018**, *118 Pt A*, 640–648. [CrossRef]

49. Bruschi, M.L. 5-Mathematical models of drug release. In *Strategies to Modify the Drug Release from Pharmaceutical Systems*; Woodhead Publishing: Sawston, UK, 2015; pp. 63–86. [CrossRef]
50. Ford Versypt, A.N.; Pack, D.W.; Braatz, R.D. Mathematical modeling of drug delivery from autocatalytically degradable PLGA microspheres—A review. *J. Control. Release* **2013**, *165*, 29–37. [CrossRef] [PubMed]
51. Omwoyo, W.N.; Ogutu, B.; Oloo, F.; Swai, H.; Kalombo, L.; Melariri, P.; Mahanga, G.M.; Gathirwa, J.W. Preparation, characterization, and optimization of primaquine-loaded solid lipid nanoparticles. *Int. J. Nanomed.* **2014**, *9*, 3865–3874. [CrossRef]
52. Ezzeldin, E.; Iqbal, M.; Asiri, Y.A.; Ali, A.A.; Alam, P.; El-Nahhas, T. A Hydrophilic Interaction Liquid Chromatography–Tandem Mass Spectrometry Quantitative Method for Determination of Baricitinib in Plasma, and Its Application in a Pharmacokinetic Study in Rats. *Molecules* **2020**, *25*, 1600. [CrossRef]

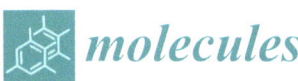

Article

Structural Bases for Hesperetin Derivatives: Inhibition of Protein Tyrosine Phosphatase 1B, Kinetics Mechanism and Molecular Docking Study

Md Yousof Ali [1], Susoma Jannat [2], Hyun-Ah Jung [3],* and Jae-Sue Choi [4],*

1. Department of Physiology and Pharmacology, Hotchkiss Brain Institute and Alberta Children's Hospital Research Institute, Cumming School of Medicine, University of Calgary, Calgary, AB T2N 4N1, Canada; mdyousof.ali@ucalgary.ca
2. Department of Biochemistry and Molecular Biology, University of Calgary, AB T2N 1N4, Canada; jannatacct@gmail.com
3. Department of Food Science and Human Nutrition, Jeonbuk National University, Jeonju 54896, Korea
4. Department of Food and Life Science, Pukyong National University, Busan 48513, Korea
* Correspondence: jungha@jbnu.ac.kr (H.-A.J.); choijs@pknu.ac.kr (J.-S.C.); Tel.: +82-51-629-7547 (J.-S.C.)

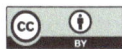

Citation: Ali, M.Y.; Jannat, S.; Jung, H.-A.; Choi, J.-S. Structural Bases for Hesperetin Derivatives: Inhibition of Protein Tyrosine Phosphatase 1B, Kinetics Mechanism and Molecular Docking Study. *Molecules* 2021, 26, 7433. https://doi.org/10.3390/molecules26247433

Academic Editor: Sumera Zaib

Received: 16 November 2021
Accepted: 6 December 2021
Published: 8 December 2021

Publisher's Note: MDPI stays neutral with regard to jurisdictional claims in published maps and institutional affiliations.

Copyright: © 2021 by the authors. Licensee MDPI, Basel, Switzerland. This article is an open access article distributed under the terms and conditions of the Creative Commons Attribution (CC BY) license (https://creativecommons.org/licenses/by/4.0/).

Abstract: In the present study, we investigated the structure-activity relationship of naturally occurring hesperetin derivatives, as well as the effects of their glycosylation on the inhibition of diabetes-related enzyme systems, protein tyrosine phosphatase 1B (PTP1B) and α-glycosidase. Among the tested hesperetin derivatives, hesperetin 5-O-glucoside, a single-glucose-containing flavanone glycoside, significantly inhibited PTP1B with an IC_{50} value of 37.14 ± 0.07 µM. Hesperetin, which lacks a sugar molecule, was the weakest inhibitor compared to the reference compound, ursolic acid (IC_{50} = 9.65 ± 0.01 µM). The most active flavanone hesperetin 5-O-glucoside suggested that the position of a sugar moiety at the C-5-position influences the PTP1B inhibition. It was observed that the ability to inhibit PTP1B is dependent on the nature, position, and number of sugar moieties in the flavonoid structure, as well as conjugation. In the kinetic study of PTP1B enzyme inhibition, hesperetin 5-O-glucoside led to mixed-type inhibition. Molecular docking studies revealed that hesperetin 5-O-glucoside had a higher binding affinity with key amino residues, suggesting that this molecule best fits the PTP1B allosteric site cavity. The data reported here support hesperetin 5-O-glucoside as a hit for the design of more potent and selective inhibitors against PTP1B in the search for a new anti-diabetic treatment.

Keywords: hesperetin derivatives; PTP1B; hesperetin 5-O-glucoside; structure-activity relationship; molecular docking

1. Introduction

Diabetes mellitus (DM) has emerged as a major threat to human health, and the expected number of diabetic patients will exceed 642 million by 2045 globally [1,2]. DM is a chronic metabolic disease, which is characterized by consistently high sugar levels in the bloodstream due to insulin deficiency, insulin resistance, or both [2,3]. Excessive glucose in the blood damages blood vessels and nerves, leading to various diseases, such as hypertension, cardiovascular disease, blindness, stroke, amputations, kidney, and dental diseases [2,4,5]. Despite the fact that there are various treatment options, achieving optimal glycemic control without side effects is difficult.

Recent studies on the pathological mechanism revealed that DM has a close relation to the protein tyrosine phosphatase (PTP) family, which plays a pivotal role in the regulation of insulin function by dephosphorylating the tyrosine residues of proteins [6]. Among the PTP family, PTP1B is a critical member and is in charge of insulin and leptin signaling pathways, and is a negative regulator of the insulin receptor (IR) signal transduction pathway that leads to insulin resistance, which makes this enzyme a promising therapeutic target to manage DM [7,8]. In insulin signaling, PTP1B is known to dephosphorylate the activated insulin receptor and insulin receptor substrates to attenuate the cellular response to insulin binding [7,9]. Mice with PTP1B gene knockouts have enhanced insulin sensitivity and low body weight, even when fed a high-fat diet [10]. For these reasons, PTP1B has become an active therapeutic target for the treatment of type II diabetes. Since PTP1B was discovered more than 25 years ago, it has proven to play a critical role in multiple cellular processes, particularly glucose uptake, body mass regulation, motility, and proliferation [7,11]. Considering the rationale above, PTP1B inhibition may modulate DM, and thus, is an outstanding target for the treatment of this epidemic disease. Thus, PTP1B is an attractive target in the development of new treatments for DM and other related metabolic syndromes.

Flavonoids are phenolic compounds widely distributed in the plant kingdom and are important components of the human diet. Different in vitro and in vivo studies have reported the possible role of citrus fruits and their phenolic components in attenuating metabolic syndrome [12]. Flavonoids are reactive and secondary metabolites abundant in plant-derived foods, particularly fruits, seeds, and vegetables [11,13,14]. The natural flavonoids almost all exist as their O-glycoside or C-glycoside forms in plants. There are several reports that flavonoids can regulate or modulate blood glucose levels after food intake [12,14,15]. Some of these flavonoids can directly induce the secretion of insulin from pancreatic cells in ex vivo assays, but this effect may not translate to in vivo effectiveness because of their low serum bioavailability [12,16]. Flavonoids like hesperidin, neohesperidin, hesperetin, hesperetin 7-O-glucoside, and hesperetin 5-O-glucoside are naturally occurring bioflavonoids found abundantly in citrus fruits [17]. Hesperidin, a flavanone glycoside, possesses antioxidant, anti-inflammatory, antifungal, antiviral, anti-cancer, anti-Alzheimer, anti-hypotensive, neuroprotective, and vasodilator activities [18–22]. Neohesperidin has anti-diabetic, antioxidant, anti-gastritis, anti-cancer, neuroprotective, anti-inflammatory, and anti-Alzheimer activities [23–28]. Moreover, hesperetin and its two glycoside hesperetin 5-O-glucoside, and hesperetin 5-O-glucoside exhibit antioxidant, anti-hyperlipidemic, anti-allergic, anti-bacterial, neuroprotective, anti-cancer, anti-inflammatory activities [29–34].

The primary goal of this study is to examine the effects of the aglycone hesperetin and its various glycosides on the inhibition of diabetes-related enzyme system (PTP1B) and to create an accurate structure-activity link. Molecular docking simulations were also applied to complement the inhibitory activity studies and to predict the binding model of the selected hesperetin derivatives to the three-dimensional structure of PTP1B. We also performed enzyme kinetic analyses of the flavonoids using Lineweaver−Burk plots to confirm the type of enzymatic inhibition.

2. Results

2.1. Inhibition of PTP1B by Hesperetin Derivatives

To evaluate the anti-diabetic activity of hesperetin derivatives, the inhibitory potential of these flavonoids against PTP1B was investigated (Figure 1 and Table 1). Among the tested flavonoids, hesperetin 5-O-glucoside and hesperidin exhibited significant PTP1B inhibitory activity with IC_{50} values of 37.14 ± 0.07 and 58.15 ± 4.18 µM, respectively, compared to the IC_{50} value of ursolic acid (9.65 ± 0.01 µM). In addition, neohesperidin and hesperetin displayed weak PTP1B inhibitory activity with corresponding IC_{50} values of 143.63 ± 3.04 and 288.01 ± 7.98 µM, respectively, while hesperetin 7-O-glucoside was inactive in the PTP1B inhibitory assay.

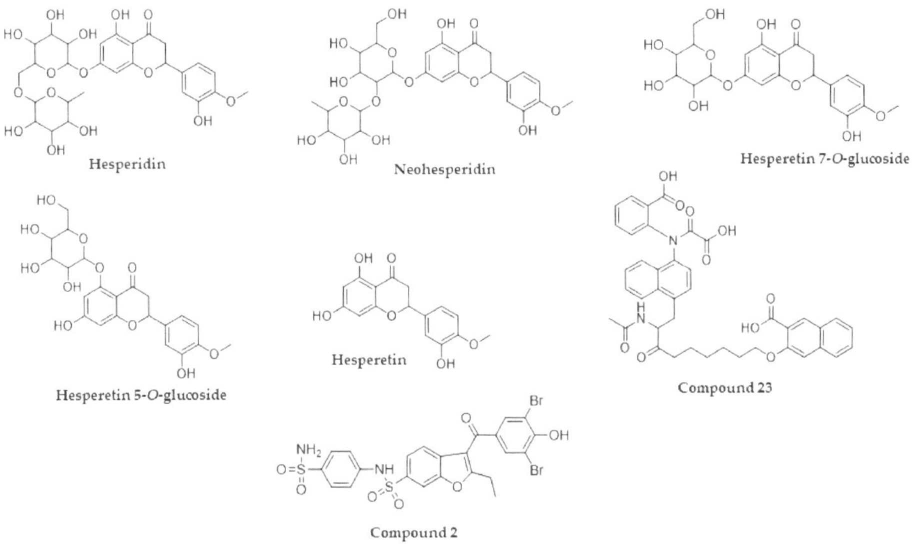

Figure 1. Chemical structures of hesperetin and its glycosylated derivatives.

Table 1. Inhibitory activities of hesperetin derivatives on the tyrosine phosphatase 1B (PTP1B) protein.

Compound	PTP1B		
	IC$_{50}$ (μM) [a]	Type of Inhibition [b]	K$_i$ (μM) [c]
Hesperidin	58.15 ± 4.18	Mixed	50.02
Neohesperidin	143.63 ± 3.04	Uncompetitive	154.28
Hesperetin 7-O-glucoside	>300	-	-
Hesperetin 5-O-glucoside	37.14 ± 0.07	Mixed	81.62
Hesperetin	288.01 ± 7.98	Uncompetitive	295.14
Ursolic acid [d]	9.65 ± 0.01		

[a] The 50% inhibitory concentration (IC$_{50}$) values (μM) were calculated from a log dose inhibition curve and as the mean ± S.E.M of triplicate experiments. [b] Determined by Lineweaver–Burk plots. [c] Determined by Dixon plots. [d] Used as positive control.

2.2. Enzyme Kinetics of PTP1B Inhibition

In an attempt to explain the mode of enzymatic inhibition of active flavonoids, kinetic analysis was performed at different concentrations of the substrate pNPP for PTP1B and the inhibitor. The type of inhibition and inhibition constants (K$_i$) of flavonoids were investigated using Lineweaver–Burk and Dixon plots (Figures 2a–d and 3a–d). Each line of inhibitors intersected at the xy-side, indicating that they are mixed-type inhibitors. Therefore, hesperidin and hesperetin 5-O-glucoside exhibited mixed-type inhibition with K$_i$ values of 50.02 and 81.62 μM, respectively, whereas neohesperidin and hesperetin displayed uncompetitive-type inhibition with K$_i$ values of 154.28 and 295.14 μM, respectively (Table 1).

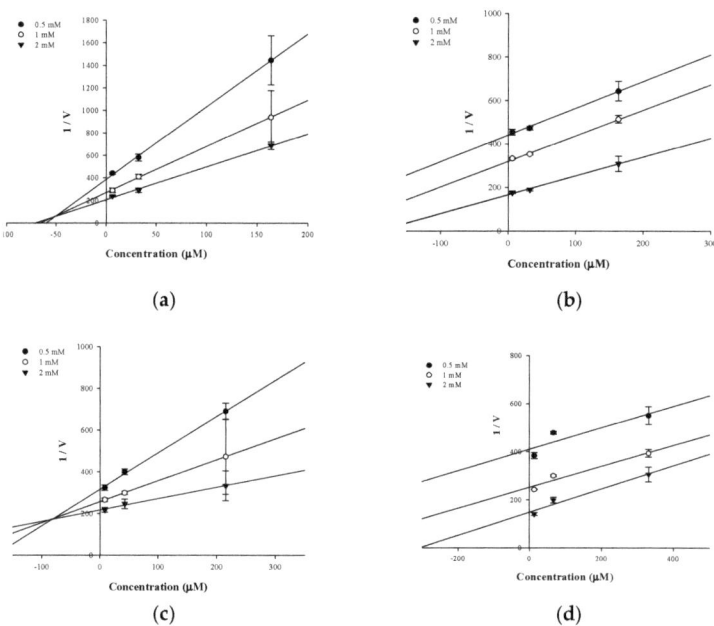

Figure 2. Dixon-plots of the inhibition of PTP1B by the compounds. The results showed the effects of the presence of different concentrations of the substrate (0.5 mM (●), 1 mM (○) and 2 mM (▼) for hesperidin (a), neohesperidin (b), hesperetin 5-O-glucoside (c) and hesperetin (d).

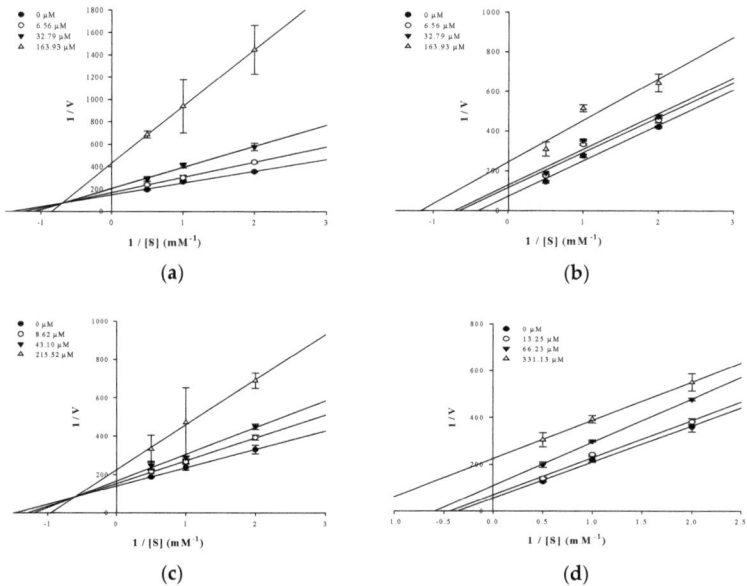

Figure 3. Lineweaver–Burk plots for the inhibition of PTP1B by the flavonoids. The results showed the effects of the presence of different concentrations of the flavonoids (0 μM (●), 6.56 μM (○), 32.79 μM (▼) and 163.93 μM (△) for hesperidin (a) and neohesperidin (b); 0 μM (●), 8.62 μM (○), 43.10 μM (▼) and 215.52 μM (△) hesperetin 5-O-glucoside (c) and 0 μM (●), 13.25 μM (○), 66.23 μM (▼) and 331.13 μM (△) hesperetin (d).

2.3. Molecular-Docking Study of the Inhibition of PTP1B by Flavonoids

Molecular docking is one of the most frequently used approaches in structure-based drug design because of its ability to predict, with a substantial degree of accuracy, the conformation of small-molecule ligands within the appropriate target binding site. To further understand the mechanisms of action of the flavonoids with inhibitory activity against PTP1B, we performed molecular docking simulations. Specifically, we used AutoDock vina to predict and investigate the interactions between five flavonoids (hesperidin, neohesperidin, hesperetin 7-O-glucoside, hesperetin 5-O-glucoside and hesperetin) and PTP1B, whereas 3-({5-[(N-acetyl-3-{4-[(carboxycarbonyl)(2-carboxyphenyl)amino]-1-naphthyl}-L-alanyl)amino]pentyl}oxy)-2-naphthoic acid (compound **23**) and 3-(3,5-dibromo-4-hydroxybenzoyl)-2-ethyl-benzofuran-6-sulfonic acid (4-sulfamoyl-phenyl)-amide (compound **2**), with structures defined in Section 4.4, were considered as the standard ligands for validating the AutoDock vina results (Figure 4).

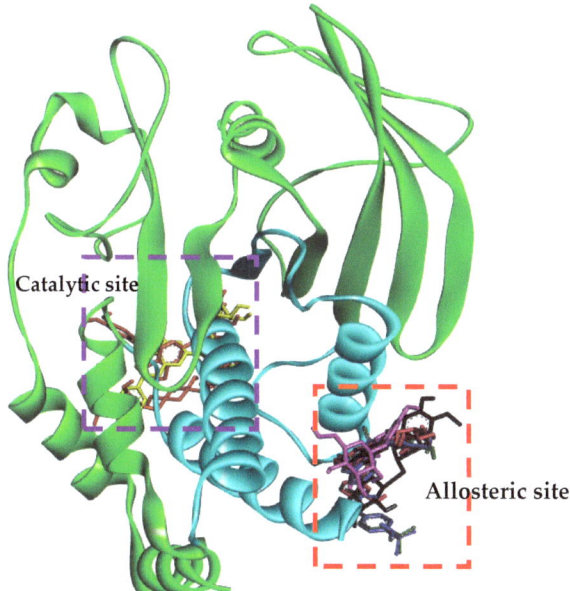

Figure 4. Molecular docking of PTP1B inhibition by compounds (compound **23**, compound **2**, hesperidin, neohesperidin, hesperetin 7-O-glucoside, hesperetin 5-O-glucoside and hesperetin). The tested compounds (compound **23**, compound **2**, hesperidin, neohesperidin, hesperetin 7-O-glucoside, hesperetin 5-O-glucoside and hesperetin) are represented by orange, blue, yellow, red, lavender, purple and green colored structures, respectively.

The ligand-enzyme complexes with flavonoids or compound **23** and compound **2** were stably posed in the catalytic and allosteric pockets of PTP1B by AutoDock vina. As illustrated in Figure 5a, hesperidin exhibited −8.4 kcal/mol binding affinity to the catalytic site of PTP1B. Hesperidin binds to PTP1B via the formation of eight hydrogen bonds, as shown in Figure 5a and Table 2. In particular, the hesperidin sugar moieties were observed to form hydrogen bond interactions with the Glu115, Lys120, Arg221, Phe182, Pro180, Gln266, and Gly183 residues of PTP1B. Moreover, the interacting methoxy group formed single alkyl bond interactions with Ala17. Some other interactions like unfavorable donor-donor with Trp179 and carbon-H bonds with Asp181 were observed. As shown in Figure 5b and Table 2, neohesperidin exhibited a binding affinity of −7.7 kcal/mol for PTP1B. Moreover, the neohesperidin sugar moieties formed three hydrogen bonds interactions with Lys116, Gly183, and Trp179. The neohesperidin sugar moiety was observed to form unfavorable donor-donor bond interaction with the Gln266 residue of PTP1B. Alkyl linkages were noticed with Val49 and Ile219 and π-cation linkage with Arg24. The molecular modeling of cognate ligand, compound **23** of protein tyrosine phosphatase 1B showed a network of π-cation and π-alkyl interactions and hydrogen bonding. As shown in Figure 5c, the amino acid residues six involve in hydrogen bonds were Tyr46, Ser216, Ala217, Gly220, Gln262, and Arg221. While π-cation with Gln266, and π-alkyl with Ala217. Moreover, hesperidin also bound to the allosteric site of PTP1B, showing considerable binding affinity (−7.9 kcal/mol) and illustrating two H-bonds with Glu276 and Asn193, with sugar moieties, whereas the hydroxyl and methoxy groups formed two hydrogen bond interactions with Glu200 and Lys197 (Figure 5d). In addition, π-alkyl interaction by Leu192, and unfavorable acceptor-acceptor interactions with Glu276, and π-π stacked with Phe280, and carbon-H bond with Gly277 were noticed. Furthermore, hesperetin 7-O-glucoside formed five hydrogen bonds with PTP1B and exhibited a binding affinity of −8.0 kcal/mol, as shown in Figure 5e and Table 2, respectively. The Asp236 and Ile281 residues were involved in two hydrogen bonds with the hesperetin 7-O-glucoside sugar moieties, whereas the hydroxyl and methoxy groups formed three hydrogen bond interactions with Ala189, Glu200, and Lys197. While carbon-H bond with Gln276 and π–π stacked with Phe280. Moreover, π-alkyl with Phe280 and Leu192 and alkyl linkages with Leu192 were observed (Figure 5e).

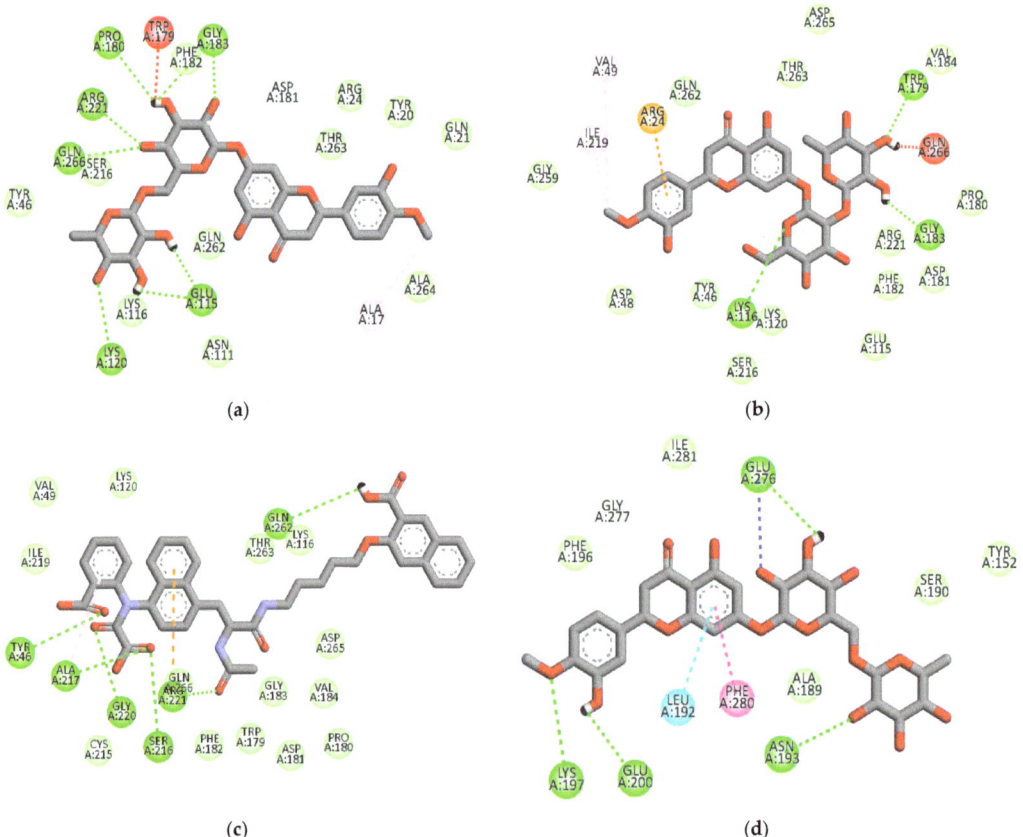

Figure 5. *Cont.*

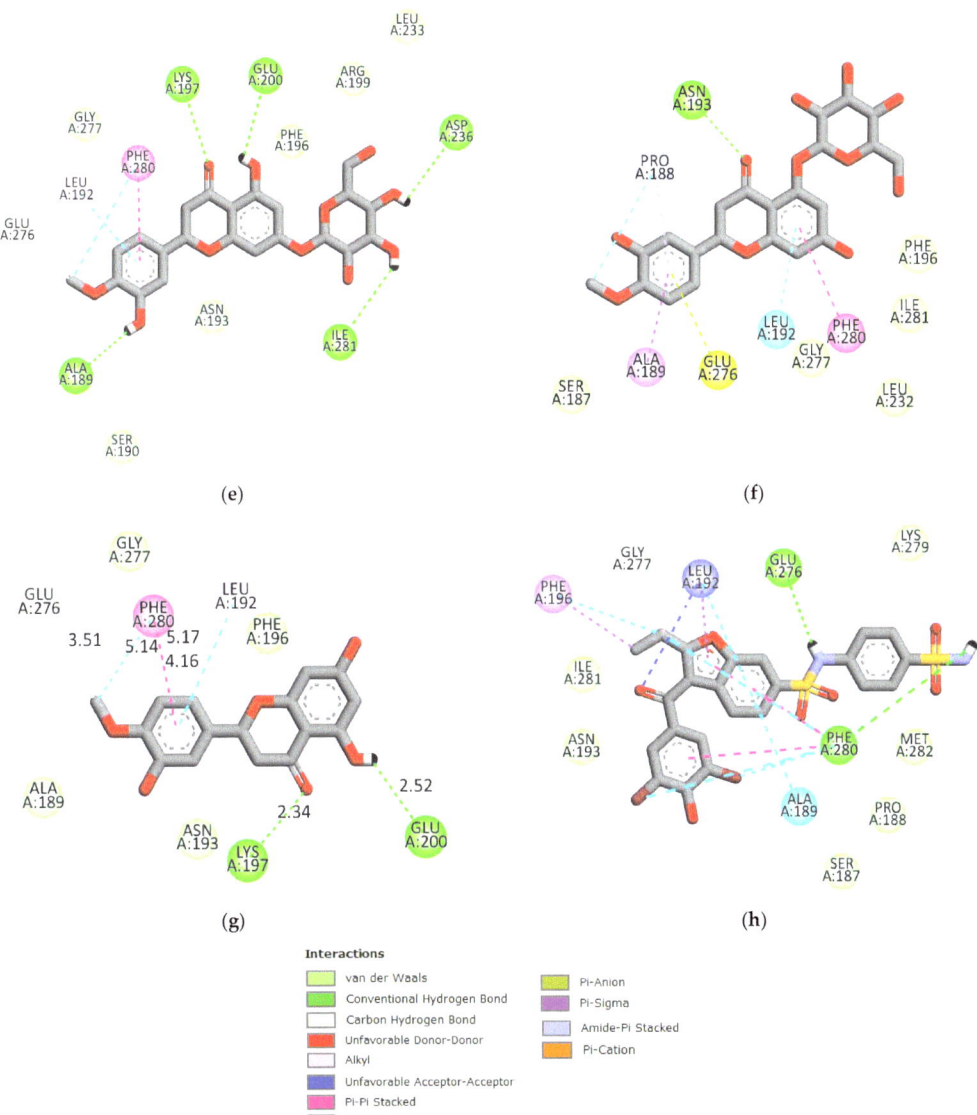

Figure 5. 2D molecular docking models of the catalytic site hesperidin (**a**), neohesperidin (**b**) and compound **23** (**c**), and allosteric site hesperidin (**d**), hesperetin 7-*O*-glucoside (**e**), hesperetin 5-*O*-glucoside (**f**), hesperetin (**g**) and compound **2** (**h**) for PTP1B inhibition.

Table 2. Binding site residues and docking scores of flavonoids in the tyrosine phosphatase 1B protein using the AutoDock vina program.

Compound	Binding Energy [a] (kcal/mol)	H-Bonding Interacting Residues	Other Interactions
Hesperidin [b]	−8.4	Lys120 (2.87 Å), Glu115 (2.04 and 2.12 Å), Arg221 (2.00 Å), Gln266 (2.53 Å), Pro180 (2.79 Å), Gly183 (2.06 and 2.53 Å)	Asp181 (C-H 3.61 Å), Trp179 (Unfavorable donor-donor 2.15 Å) and Ala17 (Alkyl 4.03 Å)
	−7.9	Lys197 (3.01 Å), Glu200 (2.39 Å), Asn193 (2.10 Å), Glu276 (2.70 Å)	Leu192 (π-Alkyl 4.41 Å), Phe280 (π-π stacked 3.81 Å), Glu276 (Unfavorable Aceptor-Aceptor 2.95 Å), Gly277 (C-H 3.10 Å)
Neohesperidin	−7.7	Lys116 (2.59 Å), Trp179 (1.87 Å), Gly183 (1.88 Å)	Ile219 (Alkyl 5.09 Å), Val49 (Alkyl 5.11 Å), Gln266 (Unfavorable donor-donor 1.13 Å), Arg24 (π-cation 3.67 Å)
Hesperetin 7-O-glucoside	−8.0	Ala189 (2.07 Å), Ile281 (2.16 Å), Asp236 (2.78 Å), Glu200 (2.87 Å), Lys197 (2.84 Å)	Glu276 (C-H 3.67 Å), Leu192 (Alkyl 5.05 Å), Leu192 (π-Alkyl 4.53 Å), Phe280 (π-Alkyl 5.18 Å), Phe280 (π-π stacked 4.12 Å)
Hesperetin 5-O-glucoside	−8.3	Asn193 (2.46 Å)	Phe280 (π-π stacked 4.00 Å), Leu192 (π-Alkyl 4.5 Å), Pro188 (π-Alkyl 4.59 Å), Ala189 (π-sigma 3.51 Å), Pro188 (amide π-stacked 4.77 Å), Glu276 (π-anion 4.26 Å)
Hesperetin	−7.6	Lys197 (2.34 Å), Glu200 (2.52 Å)	Leu192 (π-Alkyl 4.53 Å), Phe280 (π-Alkyl 5.14 Å), Phe280 (π-π stacked 4.16 Å), Leu192 (Alkyl 5.17 Å), Glu276 (C-H 3.51 Å)
Compound 2 [c] (Allosteric inhibitor)	−8.8	Glu276 (2.27 Å), Phe280 (2.57 Å)	Phe280 (π-Alkyl 5.48, 5.41 and 5.02 Å), Ala189 (π-Alkyl 4.90 Å), Leu192 (π-Alkyl 4.85 Å), Phe196 (π-Alkyl 3.93 Å), Leu192 (Unfavorable Aceptor-Aceptor 2.69 Å), Leu192 (π-sigma 3.82 Å), Phe196 (π-sigma 3.74 Å), Leu192 (Alkyl 4.40 Å), Phe280 (π-π stacked 4.11 and 4.08 Å), Gly277 (C-H 3.38 Å)
Compound 23 [c] (Catalytic inhibitor)	−8.6	Tyr46 (2.55 Å), Gly220 (2.32 Å), Ala217 (2.72 Å), Ser216 (2.65 Å), Arg221 (2.25 Å), Gln262 (2.41 Å)	Gln266 (π-cation 4.65 Å), Ala217 (Alkyl 3.99 Å)

[a] Estimated the binding free energy of the ligand-receptor complex. [b] Hesperidin showed both types of catalytic (upper) and allosteric (lower) inhibition. [c] Compound 23 (3-((5-[(N-acetyl-3-{4-[(carboxycarbonyl)(2-carboxyphenyl)amino]-1-naphthyl}-L-alanyl]amino]pentyl}oxy)-2-naphthoic acid) and compound 2 (3-(3,5-dibromo-4-hydroxy-benzoyl)-2-ethyl-benzofuran-6-sulfonic acid (4-sulfamoyl-phenyl)-amide) were used as positive ligands.

As illustrated in Figure 5f, hesperetin 5-O-glucoside exhibited a −8.3 kcal/mol binding affinity to PTP1B. The Asn193 residue was involved in a hydrogen bond with the hesperetin 5-O-glucoside ketone group, as shown in Table 2. Some amino acids showed π-alkyl interactions like Pro188 and Leu192. Other exhibited π-π stacked interactions with Phe280 and π-anion with Glu276. Additionally, π-sigma interaction was noticed with Ala189 and amide- π-stacked with Pro188. As shown in Figure 5g and Table 2, hesperetin exhibited a binding affinity of −7.6 kcal/mol for PTP1B. The hesperetin interactions of hydroxyl and ketone groups formed two hydrogen bond interactions with Glu200 and Lys197, respectively. Likewise, amino acids responsible for π-alkyl interactions were Phe280 and Leu192 and alkyl linkage with Leu192. In addition, hesperetin showed π-π stacked interaction with Phe280 and carbon-H with Glu276. On the other hand, the Phe280 and Glu276 enzyme residues participated in hydrogen-bonding interactions with compound 2 (Figure 5h). Some other interactions like unfavorable acceptor-acceptor with Leu192 and π-sigma with Phe196 and Leu192 were observed. Compound 2 made π-π stacked interactions with Phe280 and alkyl with Leu192 and π-alkyl linkage with Phe196, Leu192, Ala189 and Phe280. As shown in Figure 5h and Table 2, the binding energies of compound 2 were negative −8.8 kcal/mol, indicating that the additional hydrogen bonding might stabilize the open form of the enzyme and potentiate tighter binding to the PTP1B active site, resulting in more effective PTP1B inhibition. As shown in Figure 6a–h, the 3D interaction diagrams of flavonoids and we observed various van der Waals interactions between flavonoids and PTP1B residues that further stabilized the protein-ligand interaction.

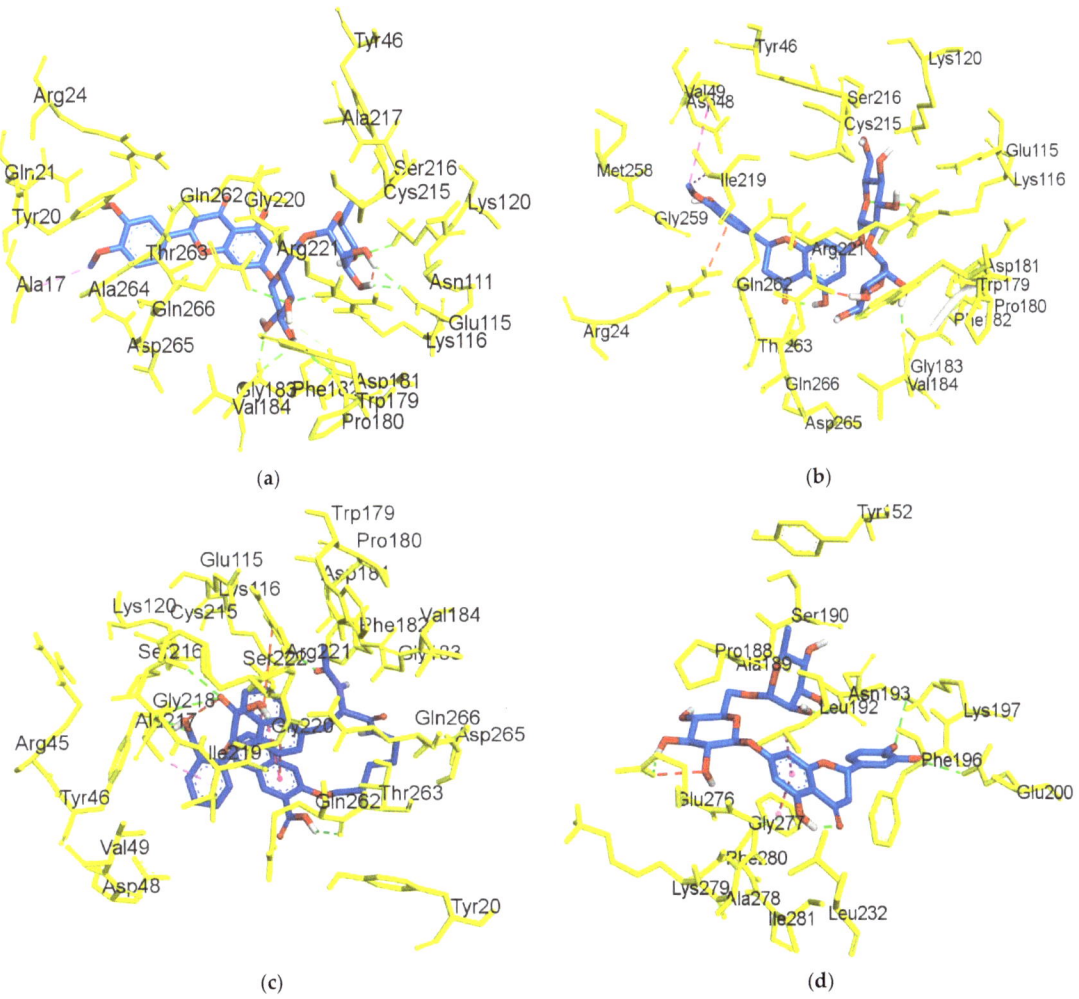

Figure 6. Cont.

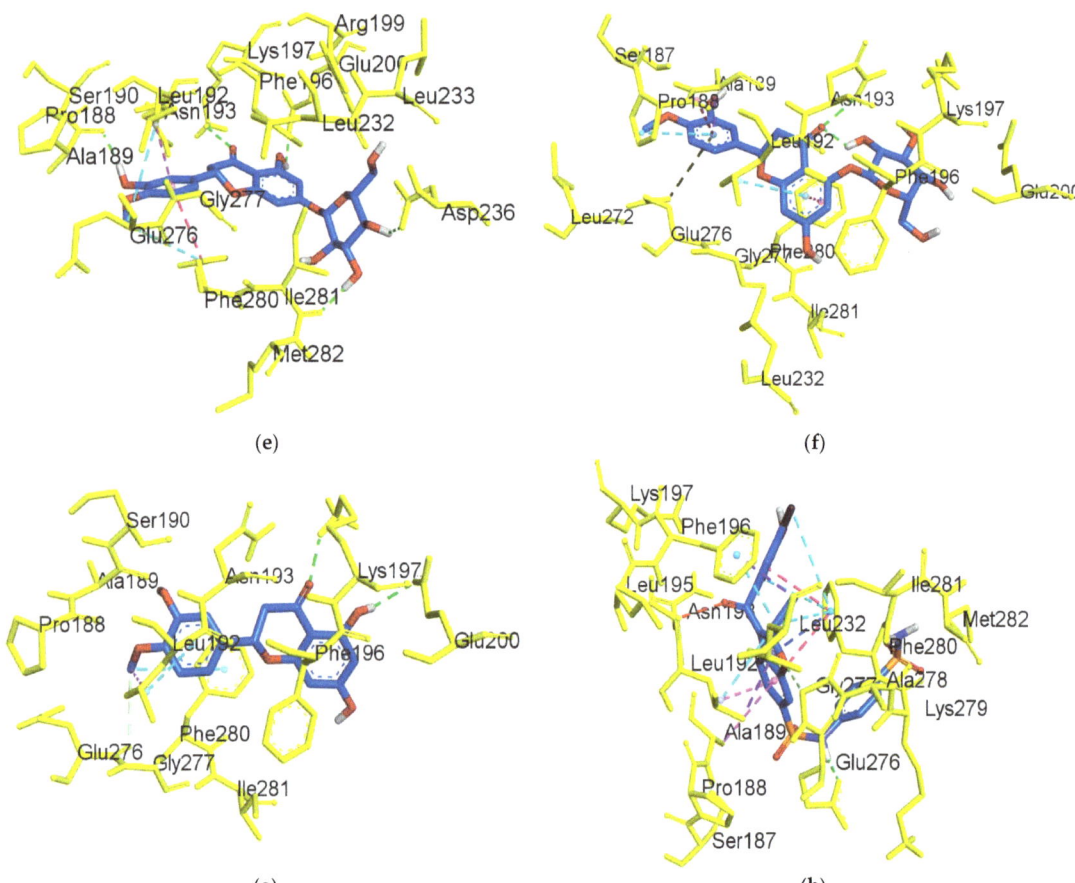

Figure 6. 3D molecular docking models of the catalytic site hesperidin (**a**), neohesperidin (**b**) and compound **23** (**c**), and allosteric site hesperidin (**d**), hesperetin 7-*O*-glucoside (**e**), hesperetin 5-*O*-glucoside (**f**), hesperetin (**g**) and compound **2** (**h**) for PTP1B inhibition.

3. Discussion

Various phytochemicals derived from nature, such as flavonoids, have attracted greater attention due to their numerous health advantages. The dietary flavonoids, especially their glycosides, are the most vital phytochemicals in diets and are of great general interest due to their diverse bioactivity [12,35]. The natural flavonoids almost all exist as their *O*-glycoside or *C*-glycoside forms and the bioavailability, metabolism, and biological activity of flavonoids depend upon the configuration, the total number of sugar moieties, and substitution of functional groups about their nuclear structure [12,35,36]. Recent studies have been demonstrated that the most reactive hydroxyl groups (7-OH or 5-OH in flavones) in flavonoids are generally glycosylated [35]. Glycosylation increases solubility in the aqueous cellular environment and protects the reactive hydroxyl groups from autooxidation [35,37]. It seems as though *O*-glycosylation can enhance certain types of biological benefits, including anti-HIV, anti-tyrosinase, anti-rotavirus, antistress, anti-obesity, anticholinesterase, antiadipogenic, and antiallergic activities [35]. Moreover, several epidemiological and human intervention studies suggest increased consumption of glycosylated flavonoid-rich foods is associated with a reduced risk of type 2 diabetes [12]. Generally, when glycosides are formed, the glycosidic linkage is normally located at position 7 or 5, and the carbohydrate can be L-rhamnose, D-glucose, glucose rhamnose, D-galactose, or L-arabinose [35,38].

In the present study, hesperetin (a flavanone) and its glycosylated derivatives, hesperidin, neohesperidin, hesperetin 7-O-glucoside, and hesperetin 5-O-glucoside, were characterized for their roles in diabetes, and the variation in activity corresponding to their structure was evaluated. PTP1B and α-glucosidase are two key inhibitory assays that were used to assess the anti-diabetic potentials of the hesperetin derivatives. Among hesperetin and its glycosylated derivatives, the most potent inhibitor of PTP1B was found to be hesperetin 5-O-glucoside, a single-glucose-containing flavanone glycosidase with an IC_{50} value of 37.14 ± 0.07 µM (Table 1). On the contrary, hesperetin 7-O-glucoside (7-position glucoside) drastically abolished inhibitory activity against PTP1B. In addition, aglycone hesperetin, which lacks a sugar moiety, showed weak inhibitory activity against PTP1B. Based on these observations, it was clear that the presence of a sugar moiety at the C-5 position is very important for PTP1B inhibitory activity. On the other hand, both hesperidin (hesperetin 7-O-rutinoside) and neohesperidin (hesperetin 7-O-neohesperidoside) contain two disaccharides but exhibited different levels of potency against PTP1B, due to the different positions of the glycosidic linkage. Hesperidin sugars consist of the α-1,6 interglycosidic linkage and showed significant inhibitory activity against PTP1B (IC_{50} = 58.15 ± 4.18 µM), whereas neohesperidin sugar moieties consist of α-1,2 interglycosidic bonds and display weak inhibitory activity against PTP1B (IC_{50} = 143.63 ± 3.04 µM). Thus, based on these results, it was clear that the position of the sugar moiety to be appears important for PTP1B inhibition. Interestingly, all flavonoids were inactive as observed in the α-glucosidase inhibitory assay, hinting that this pathway may be less important for the bioactivity of flavonoids. Thus, the main approach of the present study was to analyze the selective inhibition of PTP1B by naturally occurring flavonoids. Research on PTP1B inhibitors as potential therapeutic options for the treatment of DM and obesity has reached a peak, as approximately 300 PTP1B inhibitors have been developed from a variety of natural sources, with the largest representation from flavonoids [11,39]. Nevertheless, finding a potent and selective molecule, with good oral availability, is still a challenge to be overcome.

Naturally occurring flavonoids co-exist as aglycone and glycoside conjugates, and though certain aglycones have exhibited potent activity against PTP1B, their toxicity at certain concentrations has led researchers to shift their attention to flavonoid glycosides. It was previously suggested that the deglycosylation of flavonoid mono- or di-glucosides, such as prunin, quercetin 4-glucoside, naringin, narirutin, hesperidin, and naringenin greatly facilitated the expression of their bioactivities [12,35,40,41]. Other studies also reported that the influence of the glycosylation of flavonoids affects anti-diabetic activity, such as in the inhibition of advanced glycation end-product formation depending on the conjugation position and the class of sugar moiety [37,42–44]. Moreover, several in vitro and animal studies show that glycosylated flavonoids may have a role in type 2 diabetes therapy by modulating hepatic glucose homeostasis and insulin sensitivity [12]. Moreover, the glycosylation of flavonoids also affected the inhibition against aldose reductase depending on the number and types of sugar moiety and conjugation sites, as well as types of glycosylation [35,42,44–48]. Additionally, the in vivo bioactivity of flavonoids largely depends on their bioavailability, which can vary widely due to the structural diversification of these compounds. According to bioavailability studies, the majority of the flavanones undergo Phase II metabolism and the methylated, sulfated, or glucuronidated metabolites are the primary compounds found in the circulation [12].

The type of inhibition of the active hesperetin derivatives against PTP1B activity was studied using Lineweaver–Burk plots. Analysis of these plots at different substrate and fixed inhibitor concentrations indicated that hesperidin and hesperetin 5-O-glucoside showed a mixed-type and hesperetin and neohesperidin an uncompetitive-type inhibition mechanism. As observed in Figure 3a,c, hesperidin and hesperetin 5-O-glucoside presented mixed-type inhibition, since the K_m value increased while the

V_{max} decreased. This means that both the inhibitor and substrate can be attached to the enzyme, with the inhibitor attached outside of the active site of PTP1B. In this inhibition type, the enzyme binding activity is affected by the binding of the substrate or inhibitor. This indicates that the inhibitor can bind to both the allosteric site of the free enzyme and the substrate–enzyme complex with similar affinity. After kinetic studies, the binding mode and the type of interactions between the flavonoids and the PTP1B were analyzed by molecular docking studies.

The crystal structure of the *human*-PTP1B (PDB ID: 1T49, 1NNY) complex allows the decoding of the active site residues (His214-Cys215-Ser216-Ala217-Gly218-Ile219-Gly220-Arg221) which bind to the phosphorylated tyrosine moiety of the substrate proteins [49]. In addition, a secondary binding site, comprised of amino acid residues (Arg24, Arg254, Gln262 and a few others, such as Tyr46, Asp48, Val49, Met258), has also been reported adjacent to the main active site [50]. The hydrophobic pocket site of PTP1B consists of Tyr46, Asp48, Lys120, Gln262, and Gln266 residues [49]. The molecular docking models of flavonoids, along with compound **23** and compound **2** as the standard ligands, are illustrated in Figure 4 and Table 2. The ligand–enzyme complexes with flavonoids/or compound **23** and compound **2** were stably posed in the same pocket of PTP1B by Autodock vina. The binding energies of flavonoids were −8.4, −7.9, −7.7, −8.0, −8.3, and −7.6 Kcal/mol for hesperidin (catalytic site), hesperdin (allostieric site), neohesperidin, hesperetin 7-O-glucoside, hesperetin 5-O-glucoside, and hesperetin respectively. The PTP1B-hesperidin inhibitor complex had the highest binding energy and the hydroxyl groups of hesperidin showed H-bond interactions with the important residues Arg221, Gln266, and Pro180 of the catalytic and hydrophobic sites of PTP1B, respectively. The sugar moiety −OH groups of neohesperidin formed H-bonds with Gly183, Trp179 and Lys116 at the catalytic active site. Hesperetin 7-O-glucoside showed negative binding energies and high proximity to PTP1B residues, Ile281, Ala189, Asp236, Lys197, and Glu200 in the pocket site. Hesperetin formed two H-bond with two important residues of Lys197 and Glu200. This study also demonstrates that, at the allosteric site of PTP1B, there is a prominent interaction of hesperetin 5-O-glucoside with the key residue Asn193 and confirms the mixed-type allosteric inhibition of PTP1B. The phenyl ring of hesperetin 5-O-glucoside is also stabilized by the π–π interactions, along with the Phe280 and π-sigma with Ala189 residue.

We previously found that prunin is a competitive inhibitor that binds directly to the catalytic active site of PTP1B in the presence of a glucose moiety [51]. Recently, we also reported that naringenin derivatives were tested as PTP1B inhibitors, and that hydrophobic and hydrogen bonding interactions are important for the strength of the protein-ligand interaction, as is the positioning of the inhibitors in the catalytic pocket [41]. Even though hesperidin has a higher number of H-bonds and binding energies that are greater than that of hesperetin 5-O-glucoside, which has fewer H-bonds. However, hesperetin 5-O-glucoside binds to the key residues (Leu192, Asn193, Phe280, Pro188, Ala189, and Glu276) and is the best fit to the PTP1B allosteric site cavity.

Hesperetin 5-O-glucoside, a flavanone glycoside isolated from *Prunus davidiana* that is reported to have biological activities, including antihyperlipidemic and hypocholesterolemic effects [30], and antioxidant activity by inhibition of hydroxyl radicals (OH), reactive oxygen species (ROS), and the scavenging of peroxynitrites [31]. Nevertheless, this is the first work demonstrating the anti-diabetic activity of hesperetin 5-O-glucoside via the inhibition of PTP1B and α-glucosidase. Here we found distinct differences in the IC_{50} values of hesperetin derivatives against PTP1B and identified hesperetin 5-O-glucoside as the best inhibitor. This finding depicts hesperetin 5-O-glucoside as more effective than other hesperetin derivatives, which is our new finding. The novel inhibitory activity of hesperetin 5-O-glucoside, which contains a single glucose molecule at the C-5 position, likely has a favorable conformation and allows it to fit suitably within the allosteric site of the enzyme. These results suggest that hesperetin 5-O-glucoside possesses potential

4. Materials and Methods

4.1. Chemicals and Reagents

Hesperidin, neohesperidin, hesperetin, hesperetin 7-O-glucoside, p-nitrophenyl phosphate (pNPP), and ethylenediaminetetraacetic acid (EDTA) were purchased from Sigma-Aldrich. PTP1B (human recombinant) was purchased from Biomol International LP (Plymouth Meeting, PA, USA), and dithiothreitol (DTT) was purchased from Bio-Rad Laboratories (Hercules, CA, USA). All other chemicals and solvents used were purchased from E. Merck, Fluka, and Sigma-Aldrich, unless otherwise stated.

4.2. PTP1B Inhibitory Assay

The PTP1B inhibitory activity was evaluated using pNPP according to the work of Jung et al. [41]. In each well of a 96-well plate (each with a final volume of 100 µL), 40 µL of PTP1B enzyme [0.5 units diluted with a PTP1B reaction buffer containing 50 mM citrate (pH 6.0), 0.1 M NaCl, 1 mM EDTA, and 1 mM DTT] was added with or without the sample dissolved in 10% DMSO. The plate was preincubated at 37 °C for 10 min and then 50 µL of 2 mM pNPP in the PTP1B reaction buffer was added. Following incubation at 37 °C for 20 min, the reaction was terminated by the addition of 10 M NaOH. The amount of p-nitrophenyl produced after enzymatic dephosphorylation of pNPP was estimated by measuring the absorbance at 405 nm using a microplate spectrophotometer (Molecular Devices). The nonenzymatic hydrolysis of 2 mM of pNPP was corrected by the measured increase in absorbance at 405 nm obtained in the absence of the PTP1B enzyme. The inhibition percentage was obtained using the following equation: % inhibition = (Ac − As)/Ac × 100, where Ac is the absorbance of the control and As is the absorbance of the sample. Ursolic acid was used as a positive control.

4.3. Kinetic Parameters of Hesperetin Derivatives in PTP1B Inhibition

To determine the kinetic mechanism, two kinetic methods using Lineweaver–Burk and Dixon plots were complementarily used. Using Lineweaver–Burk and Dixon plots, the PTP1B inhibition mode was determined at various concentrations of p-NPP substrate (0.5, 1.0 and 2.0 mM) in the absence or presence of different test flavonoid concentrations (0, 6.56, 32.79 and 163.93 µM for hesperidin and neohesperidin; 0, 8.62, 43.10 and 215.52 µM for hesperetin 5-O-glucoside; 0, 13.25, 66.23, 331.13 µM for hesperetin). The enzymatic inhibitions of the test flavonoids were evaluated by monitoring the effects of different concentrations of the substrates in the Dixon plots (single reciprocal plot). The enzymatic procedure consisted of the same, aforementioned, PTP1B assay method. The inhibition constants (K_i) were determined by interpretation of the Dixon plots, where the value of the x-axis implies -K_i.

4.4. Molecular Docking Simulation in PTP1B Inhibition

The X-ray crystallographic structure of PTP1B, with its selective inhibitor 3-(3,5-dibromo-4-hydroxy-benzoyl)-2-ethyl-benzofuran-6-sulfonic acid (4-sulfamoyl-phenyl)-amide (compound **2**) (PDB ID: 1T49) and the 3D structure of catalytic inhibitor 3-({5-[(N-acetyl-3-{4-[(carboxycarbonyl)(2-carboxyphenyl)amino]-1-naphthyl}-L-alanyl)amino]pentyl}oxy)-2-naphthoic acid (compound **23**) were obtained from the RCSB Protein Data Bank (PDB ID: 1NNY) [52,53] website at resolutions of 1.9 Å and the PubChem Compound (NCBI) with compound CID of 447410, respectively. The binding PTP1B inhibitor and water molecules were removed from the structure for the docking simulation using Accelrys Discovery Studio 4.1 (Accelrys, Inc., San Diego, CA, USA). The 3D structures of hesperidin, neohesperidin, hesperetin 7-O-glucoside, hesperetin 5-O-glucoside, and hesperetin were obtained from the PubChem Compound (NCBI), with compound CIDs of 10621, 442439, 147394, 18625123, and 72281, respectively, and were protonated (pH 7.0) using MarvinSketch program (ChemAxon, Budapest, Hungary). The automated docking simulation was performed using AutoDock Tool (ADT) to assess the appropriate binding orientations and conformations of PTP1B with the different compounds. A Lamarckian genetic algorithm method implemented in AutoDock vina was employed. For docking calculations, Gasteiger charges were added by default, the rotatable bonds were set by the ADTs, and all torsions were allowed to rotate. The grid maps were generated by the Autogrid program where the grid box size of 80 × 80 × 80 had a default spacing of 0.375 Å. The respective X, Y, Z coordinates of the center were 56.019, 31.367 and 22.486, respectively. The docking protocol for a rigid and flexible ligand docking consisted of 10 independent genetic algorithms, while the other parameters used were default parameters of the ADT. The binding aspects of the PTP1B residues and their corresponding binding affinity scores were regarded as the best molecular interaction. The results were analyzed using UCSF Chimera [54], while the hydrogen bonds and van der Walls interaction residues were visualized by the Discovery Studio 2016 Client.

4.5. Statistics

All results are expressed as the mean ± SEM of triplicate samples. The statistical significances were analyzed using the one-way ANOVA and Student's t-test (Systat Inc., Evanston, IL, USA), and were noted at $p < 0.05$.

5. Conclusions

In this work, a promising flavonoid scaffold was found as a potential effective PTP1B inhibitor for the treatment of DM. Hesperetin 5-O-glucoside is a potent PTP1B inhibitor with a mixed inhibitory mechanism. Hesperetin 5-O-glucoside, with its single sugar moiety, displayed reasonable binding energy and the highest binding affinity for PTP1B inhibition. The structure-activity relationship studies indicated that the single sugar moiety at the C-5 position was crucial for the activity against PTP1B inhibition. Our results indicated that flavanones containing one sugar moiety at the 5-position, such as hesperetin 5-O-glucoside, best fit the PTP1B allosteric site cavity for PTP1B inhibition. Further in vivo and cellular-based studies are needed to help clarify the detailed mechanism of action of these flavonoids in the brain membrane and other organs.

Author Contributions: M.Y.A. designed and performed the experiments, analyzed the data, and wrote the paper. S.J. provided critical technical input. H.-A.J. and J.-S.C. had primary responsibility for final content. All authors have read and agreed to the published version of the manuscript.

Funding: This research received no external funding.

Institutional Review Board Statement: Not Applicable.

Informed Consent Statement: Not applicable.

Data Availability Statement: This manuscript does not have any data-sharing criteria.

Conflicts of Interest: The authors declare no conflict of interest.

Sample Availability: Samples of the compounds are available from the authors on request.

References

1. Cho, N.H.; Shaw, J.E.; Karuranga, S.; Huang, Y.; da Rocha Fernandes, J.D.; Ohlrogge, A.W.; Malanda, B. IDF Diabetes Atlas: Global estimates of diabetes prevalence for 2017 and projections for 2045. *Diabetes Res. Clin. Pract.* **2018**, *138*, 271–281. [CrossRef]
2. American Diabetes Association. Diabetes Advocacy: Standards of Medical Care in Diabetes-2021. *Diabetes Care.* **2021**, *44*, S221–S222. [CrossRef]
3. Zhang, P.; Gregg, E. Global economic burden of diabetes and its implications. *Lancet Diabetes Endocrinol.* **2017**, *5*, 404–405. [CrossRef]
4. Helgason, C.M. Blood Glucose and Stroke. *Curr. Treat Options Cardiovasc. Med.* **2012**, *14*, 284–287. [CrossRef]

5. Cui, Y.; Zhang, L.; Zhang, M.; Yang, X.; Zhang, L.; Kuang, J.; Zhang, G.; Liu, Q.; Guo, H.; Meng, Q. Prevalence and causes of low vision and blindness in a Chinese population with type 2 diabetes: The Dongguan eye study. *Sci. Rep.* **2017**, *7*, 11195. [CrossRef]
6. Genovese, M.; Nesi, I.; Caselli, A.; Paoli, P. Natural α-glucosidase and protein tyrosine phosphatase 1B inhibitors: A source of scaffold molecules for synthesis of new multitarget antidiabetic drugs. *Molecules* **2021**, *26*, 4818. [CrossRef] [PubMed]
7. Kumar, A.; Rana, D.; Rana, R.; Bhatia, R. Protein Tyrosine Phosphatase (PTP1B): A promising drug target against life-threatening ailments. *Curr. Mol. Pharmacol.* **2020**, *13*, 17–30. [CrossRef]
8. Tamrakar, A.K.; Maurya, C.K.; Rai, A.K. PTP1B inhibitors for type 2 diabetes treatment: A patent review (2011–2014). *Expert Opin. Ther. Pat.* **2014**, *24*, 1101–1115. [CrossRef] [PubMed]
9. Goldstein, B.J.; Bittner-Kowalczyk, A.; White, M.F.; Harbeck, M. Tyrosine dephosphorylation and deactivation of insulin receptor substrate-1 by protein-tyrosine phosphatase 1B. Possible facilitation by the formation of a ternary complex with the Grb2 adaptor protein. *J. Biol. Chem.* **2000**, *275*, 4283–4289. [CrossRef]
10. Elchebly, M.; Payette, P.; Michaliszyn, E.; Cromlish, W.; Collins, S.; Loy, A.L.; Normandin, D.; Cheng, A.; Himms-Hagen, J.; Chan, C.C.; et al. Increased insulin sensitivity and obesity resistance in mice lacking the protein tyrosine phosphatase-1B gene. *Science* **1999**, *283*, 1544–1548. [CrossRef] [PubMed]
11. Zhang, S.; Zhang, Z.Y. PTP1B as a drug target: Recent developments in PTP1B inhibitor discovery. *Drug Discov. Today* **2007**, *12*, 373–381. [CrossRef] [PubMed]
12. Visvanathan, R.; Williamson, G. Citrus polyphenols and risk of type 2 diabetes: Evidence from mechanistic studies. *Crit. Rev. Food Sci. Nutr.* **2021**. [CrossRef] [PubMed]
13. Rasoulia, H.; Hosseini-Ghazvinib, S.M.B.; Adibi, H.; Khodarahmia, R. Differential α-amylase/α-glucosidase inhibitory activities of plant derived phenolic compounds: A virtual screening perspective for the treatment of obesity and diabetes. *Food Funct.* **2017**, *8*, 1942–1954. [CrossRef] [PubMed]
14. Croft, K.D. The chemistry and biological effects of flavonoids and phenolic acids. *Ann. N. Y. Acad. Sci.* **1998**, *854*, 435–442. [CrossRef] [PubMed]
15. Williamson, G.; Nyambe, H. Polyphenol and fiber-rich dried fruits with green tea attenuate starch-derived postprandial blood glucose and insulin; A randomized, controlled, single blind, crossover intervention. *Br. J. Nutr.* **2016**, *116*, 443–450.
16. Khalivulla, S.I.; Mohammed, A.; Mallikarjuna, K. Novel phytochemical constituents and their potential to manage Diabetes. *Curr. Pharm. Des.* **2021**, *27*, 775–788. [CrossRef] [PubMed]
17. Crozier, A.; Jaganath, I.B.; Clifford, M.N. Dietary phenolics: Chemistry, bioavailability and effects on health. *Nat. Prod. Rep.* **2009**, *26*, 1001–1043. [CrossRef]
18. Galati, E.M.; Monforte, M.T.; Kirjavainen, S.; Forestieri, A.M.; Trovato, A.; Tripodo, M.M. Biological effects of hesperidin, a citrus flavonoid. (Note I): Antiinflammatory and analgesic activity. *Farmaco* **1994**, *40*, 709–712. [PubMed]
19. Garg, A.; Garg, S.; Zaneveld, L.J.; Singla, A.K. Chemistry and pharmacology of the citrus bioflavonoid hesperidin. *Phytother. Res.* **2001**, *15*, 655–669. [CrossRef]
20. Li, C.; Zug, C.; Qu, H.; Schluesener, H.; Zhang, Z. Hesperidin ameliorates behavioral impairments and neuropathology of transgenic APP/PS1 mice. *Behav. Brain Res.* **2014**, *281*, 32–42. [CrossRef]
21. Wang, D.; Liu, L.; Zhu, X.; Wu, W.; Wang, Y. Hesperidin alleviates cognitive impairment, mitochondrial dysfunction and oxidative stress in a mouse model of Alzheimer's disease. *Cell Mol. Neurobiol.* **2014**, *34*, 1209–1221. [CrossRef] [PubMed]
22. Pandey, P.; Khan, F. A mechanistic review of the anticancer potential of hesperidin, a natural flavonoid from citrus fruits. *Nutr. Res.* **2021**, *92*, 21–31. [CrossRef] [PubMed]
23. Yang, H.J.; Jeong, S.Y.; Choi, N.S.; Ahn, K.H.; Park, C.S.; Yoon, B.D.; Ryu, Y.W.; Ahn, S.C.; Kim, M.S. Optimization of production yield for neohesperidin by response surface methodology. *J. Life Sci.* **2010**, *20*, 1691–1696. [CrossRef]
24. Xu, F.; Zang, J.; Chen, D.; Zhang, T.; Zhan, H.; Lu, M.; Zhuge, H. Neohesperidin induces cellular apoptosis in human breast adenocarcinoma MDA-MB-231 cells via activating the Bcl-2/Bax-mediated signaling pathway. *Nat. Prod. Commun.* **2012**, *7*, 1475–1478. [CrossRef] [PubMed]
25. Wang, J.J.; Cui, P. Neohesperidin attenuates cerebral ischemia-reperfusion injury via inhibiting the apoptotic pathway and activating the Akt/Nrf2/HO-1 pathway. *J. Asian Nat. Prod. Res.* **2013**, *15*, 1023–1037. [CrossRef]
26. Lee, J.H.; Lee, S.H.; Kim, Y.S.; Jeong, C.S. Protective effects of neohesperidin and poncirin isolated from the fruits of *Poncirus trifoliata* on potential gastric disease. *Phytother. Res.* **2009**, *23*, 1748–1753. [CrossRef] [PubMed]
27. Ho, S.L.; Poon, C.Y.; Lin, C.; Yan, T.; Kwong, D.W.; Yung, K.K.; Wong, M.S.; Bian, Z.; Li, H.W. Inhibition of β-amyloid aggregation by albiflorin, aloeemodin and neohesperidin and their neuroprotective effect on primary hippocampal cells against β-amyloid induced toxicity. *Curr. Alzheimer Res.* **2015**, *12*, 424–433. [CrossRef] [PubMed]
28. Hamdan, D.I.; Mahmoud, M.F.; Wink, M.; El-Shazly, A.M. Effect of hesperidin and neohesperidin from bittersweet orange (*Citrus aurantium* var. bigaradia) peel on indomethacin-induced peptic ulcers in rats. *Environ. Toxicol. Pharmacol.* **2014**, *37*, 907–915. [CrossRef]
29. Jung, H.A.; Jung, M.J.; Kim, J.Y.; Chung, H.Y.; Choi, J.S. Inhibitory activity of flavonoids from *Prunus davidiana* and other flavonoids on total ROS and hydroxyl radical generation. *Arch. Pharm. Res.* **2003**, *26*, 809–815. [CrossRef] [PubMed]
30. Choi, J.S.; Yokozawa, T.; Oura, H. Antihyperlipidemic effect of flavonoids from *Prunus davidiana*. *J. Nat. Prod.* **1991**, *54*, 218–224. [CrossRef]

31. Shimoda, K.; Hamada, H. Production of hesperetin glycosides by *Xanthomonas campestris* and cyclodextrin glucanotransferase and their anti-allergic activities. *Nutrients* **2010**, *2*, 171–180. [CrossRef] [PubMed]
32. Lee, Y.S.; Huh, J.Y.; Nam, S.H.; Moon, S.K.; Lee, S.B. Enzymatic bioconversion of citrus hesperidin by Aspergillus sojae nar inginase: Enhanced solubility of hesperetin-7-O-glucoside with in vitro inhibition of human intestinal maltase, HMG-CoA reductase, and growth of *Helicobacter pylori*. *Food Chem.* **2012**, *135*, 2253–2259. [CrossRef] [PubMed]
33. Cho, J. Antioxidant and neuroprotective effects of hesperidin and its aglycone hesperetin. *Arch. Pharm. Res.* **2006**, *8*, 699–706. [CrossRef] [PubMed]
34. Ding, F.; Peng, W. Biological activity of natural flavonoids as impacted by protein flexibility: An example of flavanones. *Mol. Biosyst.* **2015**, *11*, 1119–1133. [CrossRef] [PubMed]
35. Xiao, J. Dietary flavonoid aglycones and their glycosides: Which show better biological significance. *Crit. Rev. Food Sci. Nutr.* **2017**, *57*, 1874–1905. [CrossRef]
36. Kelly, E.H.; Anthony, R.T.; Dennis, J.B. Flavonoid antioxidants: Chemistry, metabolism and structure-activity relationships. *J. Nutri. Biochem.* **2002**, *13*, 572–584.
37. Kumar, S.; Pandey, A.K. Chemistry and biological activities of flavonoids: An overview. *Sci. World J.* **2013**, *2013*, 162750. [CrossRef] [PubMed]
38. Veitch, N.C.; Grayer, R.J. Flavonoids and their glycosides, including anthocyanins. *Nat. Prod. Rep.* **2011**, *28*, 1626–1695. [CrossRef]
39. Jiang, C.; Liang, L.; Guo, Y. Natural products possessing protein tyrosine phosphatase 1B (PTP1B) inhibitory activity found in the last decades. *Acta Pharmacol. Sin.* **2012**, *33*, 1217–1245. [CrossRef]
40. Chena, L.; Teng, H.; Xie, Z.; Cao, H.; Cheang, W.S.; Skalicka-Woniak, K.; Georgiev, M.I.; Xiao, J. Modifications of dietary flavonoids towards improved bioactivity: An update on structure–activity relationship. *Crit. Rev. Food. Sci. Nutr.* **2016**, *56*, 513–527. [CrossRef]
41. Jung, H.A.; Paudel, P.; Seong, S.H.; Min, B.S.; Choi, J.S. Structure-related protein tyrosine phosphatase 1B inhibition by naringenin derivatives. *Bioorg. Med. Chem. Lett.* **2017**, *27*, 2274–2280. [CrossRef] [PubMed]
42. Jung, S.H.; Lee, J.M.; Lee, H.J.; Kim, C.Y.; Lee, E.H.; Um, L.H. Aldose reductase and advanced glycation endproducts inhibitory effect of *Phyllostachys nigra*. *Biol. Pharm. Bull.* **2007**, *30*, 1569–1572. [CrossRef] [PubMed]
43. Matsuda, H.; Wang, T.; Managi, H.; Yoshikawa, M. Structural requirements of flavonoids for inhibition of protein glycation and radical scavenging activities. *Bioorg. Med. Chem.* **2003**, *11*, 5317–5323. [CrossRef]
44. Choi, J.S.; Islam, M.N.; Ali, M.Y.; Kim, E.J.; Kim, Y.M.; Jung, H.A. Effects of C-glycosylation on anti-diabetic, anti-Alzheimer's disease and anti-inflammatory potential of apigenin. *Food Chem. Toxicol.* **2014**, *64*, 27–33. [CrossRef]
45. Choi, J.S.; Islam, M.N.; Ali, M.Y.; Kim, Y.M.; Park, H.J.; Sohn, H.S.; Jung, H.A. The effects of C-glycosylation of luteolin on its antioxidant, anti-Alzheimer's disease, anti-diabetic, and anti-inflammatory activities. *Arch. Pharm. Res.* **2014**, *37*, 1354–1363. [CrossRef] [PubMed]
46. Jung, S.H.; Kang, S.S.; Shin, K.H.; Kim, Y.S. Inhibitory effects of naturally occurring flavonoids on rat lens aldose reductase. *Nat. Prod. Sci.* **2004**, *10*, 35–39.
47. Lim, S.S.; Jung, Y.J.; Hyun, S.K.; Lee, Y.S.; Choi, J.S. Rat lens aldose reductase inhibitory constituents of *Nelumbo nucifera* stamens. *Phytother. Res.* **2006**, *20*, 825–830. [CrossRef] [PubMed]
48. Matsuda, H.; Morikawa, T.; Toguchida, I.; Yoshikawa, M. Structural requirements of flavonoids and related compounds for aldose reductase inhibitory activity. *Chem. Pharm. Bull.* **2002**, *50*, 788–795. [CrossRef]
49. Johnson, T.O.; Ermolieff, J.; Jirousek, M.R. Protein tyrosine phosphatase 1B inhibitors for diabetes. *Nat. Rev. Drug Discov.* **2002**, *1*, 696–709. [CrossRef] [PubMed]
50. Puius, Y.A.; Zhao, Y.; Sullivan, M.; Lwarence, D.S.; Almo, S.C.; Zhang, Z.Y. Identification of a second aryl phosphate-binding site in protein tyrosine phosphatase 1B: A paradigm for inhibitor design. *Proc. Natl. Acad. Sci. USA* **1997**, *94*, 13420–13425. [CrossRef] [PubMed]
51. Jung, H.A.; Ali, M.Y.; Bhakta, H.K.; Min, B.S.; Choi, J.S. Prunin is a highly potent flavonoid from *Prunus davidiana* stems that inhibits protein tyrosine phosphatase 1B and stimulates glucose uptake in insulin resistant HepG2 cells. *Arch. Pharm. Res.* **2016**, *40*, 37–48. [CrossRef] [PubMed]
52. Berman, H.M.; Battistuz, T.; Bhat, T.N.; Bluhm, W.F.; Bourne, P.E.; Burkhardt, K.; Feng, Z.; Gilliland, G.L.; Iype, L.; Jain, S.; et al. The Protein Data Bank. *Acta Crystallogr. D Biol. Crystallogr.* **2002**, *58*, 899–907. [CrossRef] [PubMed]
53. Bernstein, F.C.; Koetzle, T.F.; Williams, G.J.; Meyer, E.F., Jr.; Brice, M.D.; Rodgers, J.R.; Kennard, O.; Shimanouchi, T.; Tasumi, M. The protein data bank: A computer based archival file for macromolecular structures. *J. Mol. Biol.* **1997**, *112*, 535–542. [CrossRef]
54. Pettersen, E.F.; Goddard, T.D.; Huang, C.C.; Couch, G.S.; Greenblatt, D.M.; Meng, E.C.; Ferrin, T.E. UCSF Chimera-a visualization system for exploratory research and analysis. *J. Comput. Chem.* **2004**, *25*, 1605–1612. [CrossRef] [PubMed]

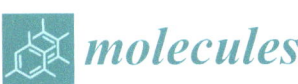

Review

A Review of HER4 (ErbB4) Kinase, Its Impact on Cancer, and Its Inhibitors

Mohammed I. El-Gamal [1,2,3,*], Nada H. Mewafi [1], Nada E. Abdelmotteleb [1], Minnatullah A. Emara [1], Hamadeh Tarazi [1,2], Rawan M. Sbenati [2], Moustafa M. Madkour [2], Seyed-Omar Zaraei [2], Afnan I. Shahin [2] and Hanan S. Anbar [4,*]

1. College of Pharmacy, University of Sharjah, Sharjah 27272, United Arab Emirates; u16103115@sharjah.ac.ae (N.H.M.); u16103110@sharjah.ac.ae (N.E.A.); u16103780@sharjah.ac.ae (M.A.E.); htarazi@sharjah.ac.ae (H.T.)
2. Sharjah Institute for Medical Research, University of Sharjah, Sharjah 27272, United Arab Emirates; u19104619@sharjah.ac.ae (R.M.S.); moustafatrika22@hotmail.com (M.M.M.); holor@live.com (S.-O.Z.); u21102889@sharjah.ac.ae (A.I.S.)
3. Department of Medicinal Chemistry, Faculty of Pharmacy, Mansoura University, Mansoura 35516, Egypt
4. Department of Clinical Pharmacy and Pharmacotherapeutics, Dubai Pharmacy College for Girls, Dubai 19099, United Arab Emirates
* Correspondence: malgamal@sharjah.ac.ae (M.I.E.-G.); dr.hanan@dpc.edu (H.S.A.)

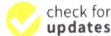

Citation: El-Gamal, M.I.; Mewafi, N.H.; Abdelmotteleb, N.E.; Emara, M.A.; Tarazi, H.; Sbenati, R.M.; Madkour, M.M.; Zaraei, S.-O.; Shahin, A.I.; Anbar, H.S. A Review of HER4 (ErbB4) Kinase, Its Impact on Cancer, and Its Inhibitors. *Molecules* 2021, 26, 7376. https://doi.org/10.3390/molecules26237376

Academic Editors: Imtiaz Khan and Sumera Zaib

Received: 17 November 2021
Accepted: 2 December 2021
Published: 5 December 2021

Publisher's Note: MDPI stays neutral with regard to jurisdictional claims in published maps and institutional affiliations.

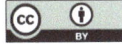

Copyright: © 2021 by the authors. Licensee MDPI, Basel, Switzerland. This article is an open access article distributed under the terms and conditions of the Creative Commons Attribution (CC BY) license (https://creativecommons.org/licenses/by/4.0/).

Abstract: HER4 is a receptor tyrosine kinase that is required for the evolution of normal body systems such as cardiovascular, nervous, and endocrine systems, especially the mammary glands. It is activated through ligand binding and activates MAPKs and PI3K/AKT pathways. HER4 is commonly expressed in many human tissues, both adult and fetal. It is important to understand the role of HER4 in the treatment of many disorders. Many studies were also conducted on the role of HER4 in tumors and its tumor suppressor function. Mostly, overexpression of HER4 kinase results in cancer development. In the present article, we reviewed the structure, location, ligands, physiological functions of HER4, and its relationship to different cancer types. HER4 inhibitors reported mainly from 2016 to the present were reviewed as well.

Keywords: HER4; ErbB4; cancer; kinase inhibitors; structure-activity relationship

1. Introduction

HER4, also known as ErbB4, is a member of epidermal growth factor receptor (EGFR) or ErbB family. HER4 is necessary for normal development of body systems including heart, nervous system, and mammary gland [1]. EGFR/ErbB1/HER1, ErbB2/HER2, ErbB3/HER3, and ErbB4/HER4 are members of this receptor tyrosine kinase family, as shown in Figure 1 [2]. HER4 is the only member of this family of receptors with growth inhibiting properties [2–4]. HER4 can activate related genes in the nucleus when combined with epidermal growth factor (EGF), promoting cell division and proliferation [5].

The binding of ligands to ErbBs causes a change in the receptor shape, which leads to dimerization either with itself to form a homodimer, or with other ErbBs to form a heterodimer [5].

When human epidermal growth factor receptors (HER) are highly expressed and activated; this often results in poor patient prognosis and advances the stages of tumor [3]. However, under normal conditions, this receptor is essential for normal development [2].

Ligand binding activates the HER4 tyrosine kinase like other ErbB receptors, which in turn activates the mitogen-activated protein kinases (MAPKs) and phosphoinositide 3-kinase (PI3K)/AKT pathways [6,7]. As a result, activation of HER4 somatic mutation is significant in a variety of human cancer [6].

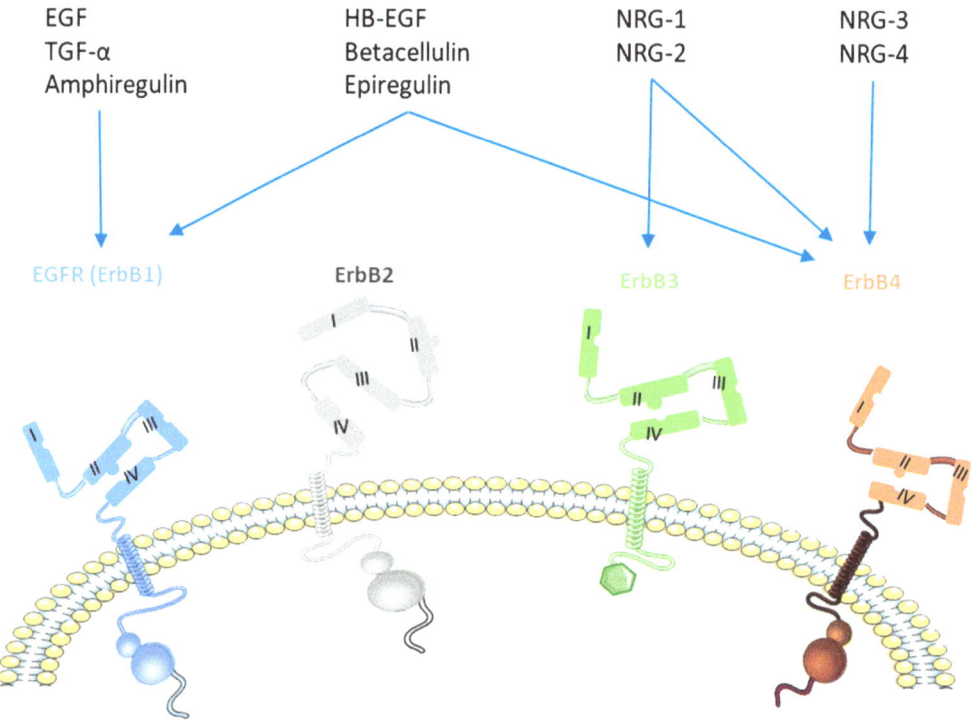

Figure 1. The four members of epidermal growth factor [2]. Reprinted with permission from ref. [2]. Copyright 2020 Springer Nature.

In most cases, overexpression of kinases results in cancer development, therefore, many drugs are being developed by scientists to inhibit these receptors [5]. Most of the drugs that inhibit HER4 usually bind irreversibly to the ATP-binding site.

In the present article, we reviewed the structure, location, ligands, and functions of HER4 kinase, and its relationship to different types of cancer. HER4 inhibitors reported mainly from 2016 to the present were reviewed as well.

2. Structure of HER4 Kinase

The amino acid sequence of receptor protein-tyrosine kinase (EGFR) was first determined by Ullrich et al. using cDNA sequence analysis [8]. The glycosylated extracellular domain of the HER family is divided into four domains: ligand binding takes place in domains I and III, formation of disulfide bond takes place in domains II and IV where multiple cysteine residues are found. Moreover, hetero and homodimer formation takes place in domain II. In total, 19 to 25 amino acid residues in a single transmembrane segment and around 540 amino acid residues in an intracellular section are accompanied by the extracellular domain [9,10]

HER4 has a molar mass of 180 kD where the cytoplasmic domain shows 79% homology with the corresponding domain of EGFR and 77% homology with c-HER2 [11].

Using the homology cloning method, HER4's cDNA sequence was identified after cloning from a human mammary carcinoma cell line [12]. The same-sized ectodomain and cytoplasmic domains are separated by a single transmembrane domain. Ectodomain is made up of a cleaved signal sequence and two cysteine-rich regions; almost all the 50 ectodomain cysteine residues of EGFR are preserved in HER4. Domain III was shown to mediate growth factor binding in comparison with EGFR. HER4 has a comparatively longer stalk region between domain IV and the transmembrane domain, which may make it uniquely susceptible to ectodomain cleavage within this receptor family [13].

All HER receptors have a cytoplasmic ambit that consists of a tyrosine kinase domain, a juxtamembrane region and a carboxy terminal domain. The residues of tyrosine autophosphorylation in EGFR that were found are all preserved in HER4. Although there are mutations in the HER3 kinase domain that considerably lessens its kinase function, these modifications were not found in HER4 kinase domain [14].

All protein kinases, including those of the HER family, are associated with two general forms of conformational movements. The active form of HER4 has the β4νν-lysine– αC-glutamate salt bridge (e.g., 3BCE) and the inactive form has the β4-lysine–DFG-aspartate salt bridge [15].

Crystallographic studies of HER kinase domain reported that the development of asymmetric dimer between a "donor" (activator) monomer's C-lobe and an adjacent "acceptor" (receiver) monomer's N-lobe is a typical structural mechanism necessary to attain maximum kinase activation [16–19].

The local contact density obtained from structure-based network analysis is shown for the Cdk/Src-IF1 and active states of HER4 (Figure 2). The spine residues in the HER4 structures are M747, L758, H816, F837, and D877 [20].

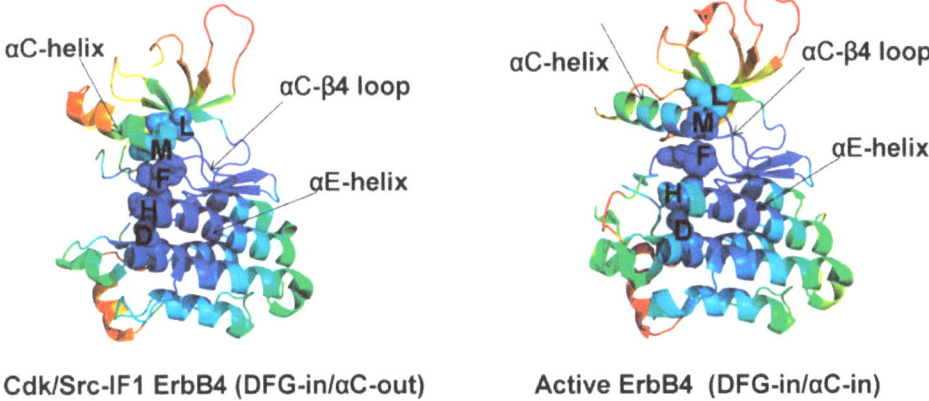

Figure 2. The left panel shows HER4 in Cdk/Src-IF1 form and the right panel shows the active form [20].

The residues of the R spine in EGFR (M766, L777, F856, D896, H835) and HER4 (M747, H816, F837, L758, D877) are closely related, showing the structural integrity of the HRD and DFG motifs, while the residues of the αC-β4/αC-helix interface (M766, L777 in EGFR and M747, L758 in HER4) label the boundary between high and low structural stability regions [20].

Upon mutation of the 19th and 113th amino acid residues at the C-terminal, HER4 protein biological nature was not affected. However, its secondary structure was altered, and protein binding sites were nearby two mutation regions [21].

In addition, additional binding sites were found after mutation introduction. Tertiary modeling of the structure showed that HER4's local structure was modified from an α-helical conformation which is the protein's functional site to a β-chain folding structure. The mutation caused the HER4 receptor to bind to the ligand of neuregulin 1 without forming a dimer, interrupting the signal transduction pathway, and affecting the role of HER4. Expert Protein Analysis System (ExPASy) was used to analyze physiological changes in the properties after the carboxyl end mutation of the intracellular portion of HER4 [21].

3. Location of HER4 Kinase

Localization of HER family members may be the outcome of three basic steps. In the beginning, by targeting receptor-containing vesicles to certain sites, newly synthesized receptors will be delivered to plasma membrane subdomains. To that site, they are anchored by unique intracellular and cell-surface proteins tether receptors. Protein anchoring can also regulate receptor responsiveness to stimulate growth factors or facilitate interactions between the HER family and other signaling pathways. At last, receptors are withdrawn from the cell surface and separated into intracellular compartments responsible for protein recycling or degradation. HER would be provided by cells to the sites responsible for signal transduction and sustain the receptor levels needed for biological activity [22].

Receptor tyrosine kinases are mainly located on the cell surface in limited ranges in order to maintain normal development and maintenance of tissues [22]. The HER4 gene is localized on chromosome 2q33.3–34 [23], but a distinct chromosome is assigned for each one of the HER receptor kinases family. HER4 sites for autophosphorylation are not represented but these sites are localized in the carboxy-terminal domain within other receptors in this family [14]. In mammalian skeletal muscles, HER4 is precisely located on the postsynaptic side of neuromuscular junctions in order to bind to neuregulin growth factors which are secreted by innervating neurons [22]. In addition, HER4 expression was detected in the epidermis, expressed more strongly in the basal layer compared to suprabasal layer. Expression of HER4 was confirmed using four separate antibodies with the same mode of expression in the basal layer of the epidermis [24]. Levels of expression of HER4 extracellular (JM-α and JM-β) were analyzed in invasive breast cancer patients [25]. HER4 was located mainly in the cell membrane of the intact heart [26]. The majority of HER4 cardiac myocytes are present in caveolin-enriched micro domains, most likely caveola [14].

4. Ligands of HER4 Kinase

Seven ligands are known to bind to HER4 proteins provoking conformational changes that result in its activation and signaling. These ligands are divided into two classes: the heregulins, also referred to as neuregulin (NEU) gene, and few ligands of the epidermal growth factor (EGF) family of EGFR/ErbB1. The term heregulins will be used throughout this review for uniformity purposes. Four types of heregulins are found (1, 2, 3, and 4), their recognition of HER4 is variable [26–28]. Several studies have determined the capacity of different heregulins in HER4 activation, particularly heregulins 3 and 4 which demonstrated their high affinity, binding properties, and their role in receptor activation [29,30]. On the other hand, heregulins 1 and 2 fail to recognize HER4 [31,32].

As for the epidermal growth factor (EGF) family of EGFR/ErbB1, few ligands have shown their agonistic potential on HER4, such as epiregulin (EPR), betacellulin (BTC) and heparin binding-EGF (HB-EGF). Epiregulin (EPR) and betacellulin (BTC) are amongst the founding members of the epidermal growth factor (EGF) family of EGFR/ErbB1 [33]. Activation of HER4 by its agonist EPR can be influenced and regulated by EGFR or HER2, due to the proposed mechanism of the receptor trans-modulation and heterodimerization. Low affinity hormone-receptor interactions are controlling the receptor's heterodimerization and heterotypic receptor-receptor contacts, followed by the receptor kinase domains' cross-phosphorylation [34]. There is a chance that EGFR and HER2 are chosen over HER4 proteins for dimerization with HER4 proteins when EPRs are involved. Accordingly, the possibility of forming HER4 dimers is greater in cells expressing the EGFR and HER2 along with them, compared to cells expressing HER4 alone. In other words, the sensitivity of the HER4 protein for EPR increases in the presence of EGFR or HER2. Conversely, betacellulin enhances greater levels of HER4 phosphorylation compared to EPR and does not require the available different proteins to have high-affinity hormone-receptor interactions [35–37].

45K heparin-binding glycoprotein (p45) has similar characteristics to the heregulin proteins that work on HER4 receptor, i.e., proteins' amino terminal sequence induces differentiation of breast cancer cells and has the ability to activate tyrosine phosphorylation in MDA-MB-453 cells [36]. Other EGFR ligands including amphiregulin, EGF and transforming growth factor-α demonstrated their low receptor stimulatory effects. Further studies are currently being performed to explore the role of the newly discovered EGFR agonist, epigen, in inducing receptor activation [31,32].

5. Physiological Roles and Functions of HER4

In many human tissues, both adult and fetal, a survey of HER receptor expression found that HER4 is widely expressed. HER4 plays an important role in different tissues like the heart, nervous system and endocrine system (especially the mammary glands) [2]. HER4 plays an essential role during embryonic development in addition to its involvement in cardiac development [38,39]. HER4's role in cancer is not well understood, with studies supporting anti-proliferative role of HER4 especially in breast cancer, as well as studies supporting proliferative role can be found in the literature. Their differences can be attributed to HER4's complicated biology and variety of ligands that can activate it, different dimerization partners, and different downstream pathways affected by HER4 [2].

6. HER4 Relationship to Different Cancers
6.1. HER4 and Colorectal Cancer (CRC)

According to World Health Organization (WHO), colorectal cancer (CRC) was the third most common type of cancer and the second most common cause of cancer-related death worldwide in 2018 with 1.80 million cases and 862,000 deaths. The peak occurrence occurred in individuals between the ages of 60–79. One of the most critical methods to indicate the early likelihood of CRC is the expansion of the tumor's progression at the time of the diagnosis; depending on the invasion level of the tumor and the spread level to the regional lymph nodes, the prognosis can be worse [40]. Recently, studies aimed to identify possible molecular pathways involved in the progression and development of the pathogenesis of the disease to further enhance diagnostic and therapeutic modalities [41].

Several proteins have been identified and correlated with the development of CRC [42]. Amongst the widely studied proteins are HER proteins. A particular interest has been generated in the effect of HER4 expression in the progression of tumorigenesis in CRC. The effects of several therapeutic entities in the regulation of CRC through their action on these receptors have been investigated [42,43].

It has been found that HER4 proteins protect colon epithelial cells from the tumor necrosis factor (TNF) induced apoptosis by binding to epithelial cells to express anti-apoptotic and cell-protective effects when they are activated [42]. Studies suggested that HER4 overexpression in colorectal cancer is not caused by gene duplication, but due to changes occurring at the transcriptional level or changes related to protein stability [44]. Accordingly, HER4 overexpression is not the first cause of oncogenesis in colorectal cancer.

Additional analysis showed that lower HER4 promoter activity could increase the risk of colorectal cancer [44,45]. Data showed that elevated levels of messenger RNA, including the premalignant adenoma or proteins associated with HER4, are involved in CRC tumorigenesis. Henceforth, low levels of HER4 proteins expressed in a poorly differentiated colorectal cancer cell line caused impairment in its anchorage-independent growth, which is related to different malignant phenotypes [46]. Moreover, evidence suggests that HER4 overexpression may contribute with wingless related integration site (WNT) signaling to boost the human colonocytes growth [45].

HER4 proteins' role has conflicting data on the CRC and its role in proregression and tumor growth. Currently, there are no ideal data explaining and showing its discrepancies. A couple of potential explanations for the discrepancy might be rationalized. HER4 can promote its own expression in a few systems [47]. One of the theories indicates that the role of HER4 in CRC differs among subtypes [48,49].

In summary, studies show that the HER4 receptor is over-expressed at the protein levels and mRNA in colorectal cancer. High HER4 levels are contributing to the activation of phosphatidylinositol 3-kinase (PI3K) and the EGFR pathways along with cyclooxygenase-2

(COX-2) expressions. These results indicate that HER4 can be a valid therapeutic agent and a possible target in CRC and other epithelial-based malignancies [46].

6.2. HER4 and Lung Cancer

According to WHO, lung cancer is the most common cause of cancer-related death worldwide in 2018 with 2.09 million cases and 1.76 million deaths. HER4 mutations in lung cancer have a low rate of clinical significance and are rare [50]. Several somatic HER4 mutations have been explained in non-small cell lung cancer (NSCLC) [51]. Characterization of nine HER4 mutations showed four different mutations, i.e., D931Y, D595V, Y285C, and K935I, along with elevated levels of ligand-induced HER4 phosphorylation levels. These mutations are localized at an important position at the HER4 kinase domain (D931Y and K935I) and in the extracellular ligand binding (Y285C and D595V). Research study has shown that they enhance the HER4 dimerization and phosphorylation whilst stimulating the proteolytic release of the HER4-ICD and enhancing the endurance of 3TE cells when serum is absent [52]. Specific HER4 polymorphisms are linked with a higher risk of lung cancer, i.e., (SNPs rs6747637, rs6740117 and rs6742399), according to that, HER4 variants may be a risk factor to lung cancer development. These data require further studies to identify their activation potential of the HER4 receptor and the possibility of having a therapeutic value of targeting mutated HER4 proteins in regard to this disease [53].

6.3. HER4 and Gastric Cancer

Gastric cancer is among the most widespread types of cancer globally with a significant increase in the morbidity and mortality rate during the last few decades. It is a highly heterogeneous disease. Studies and information on the involvement of HER4 in this type of cancer are still evolving. Out of 294 tested gastric cancer samples, 20 of them showed mutations in the HER4 gene [54]. One of the mutations that has occurred, HER4 p.R50C, has previously been observed in melanoma [55]. In total, 33% of the HER4 mutations in gastric cancer happened in the kinase domain, 20% in the receptor domain, indicating the influence of these mutations on kinase activity or can affect the receptor–ligand interactions [56].

6.4. HER4 and Hepatocellular Carcinoma

Previous reports indicate that HER4 absence in hepatocytes in mice caused an elevation in their likelihood of developing hepatocellular carcinoma (HCC), a response to a toxic stimulus like diethyl nitrosamine (DEN) [57]. Moreover, it has been reported that, compared to control hepatocytes, isolated HER4-null hepatocytes demonstrated a higher proliferation rate in vitro. HER4 activation is down-regulated in tumor samples of patients with HCC, which may be associated with a decreased cellular differentiation and poorer prognosis and quality of life [57]. This could be due to the decreased p53 activity concomitant with the inhibition of the expression of the tumor suppressor tp53inp1 upon loss of the HER4 protein. Further studies showed that loss of HER4 activity has an important role in the progression of hepatic lesions in HCC [58].

6.5. HER4 and Prostate Cancer

The HER family's role in prostate cancer progression is controversial. The HER family plays various roles in prostate cancer [59]. In prostate cancer, the expression of HER4 is upregulated [59–62]. There is a recent study stating that HER4 levels remain the same during the transition from prostate hormone-dependent to hormone-refractory cells [59]. The expression of the HER4 in hormone-sensitive tumors is correlated with a longer time of biochemical relapse. HER4 expression is high in the normal human prostate epithelium and is stated to be related to differentiation, growth arrest and tumor quelling [59,62]. Therefore, the tumor tends to be less aggressive when this receptor is expressed in tumor cells. In contrast, high HER4 expression tends to have a protective function in hormone-sensitive tumors [59].

6.6. HER4 and Bladder Cancer

HER family expression in bladder cancer remains uncertain [63]. However, studies showed that expression of HER4 in bladder cancer is associated with better prognosis. High expression of HER4 protects patients from the effects of high levels of other HER family members including EGFR and HER2. Patients with the highest levels of HER4 had better survival rates compared with patients with lower levels of HER4 expression [64]. Statistically important associations were shown by nuclear HER4 expression, high histologic level and advanced tumor process with non-papillary tumors. Cytoplasmic expression of HER4 was associated with good prognosis [65].

6.7. HER4 and Ovarian Cancer

Limited information and data are present on HER4 impact on ovarian cancer. However, high expression of HER4 was observed at high prevalence of ovarian cancer. HER4 expression was higher in tumor specimens for those with an incomplete response to chemotherapy compared to the complete response. HER4 isoforms enable or suppress downstream molecular pathways that may have similar or opposing roles in developing chemotherapeutic agent resistance. The expression of HER4 was observed mainly in the tumor cell cytoplasm, and in the ovarian cancer cell lines, it is membranous and cytoplasmic. In ovarian cancer cell lines, higher levels of expression than normal cells were reported. Compared with control tissue, HER4 expression was substantially high in the ovarian serous carcinoma specimens [66]. On the other hand, analysis of functionally different isoforms will complicate HER4 cancer biology [66,67].

6.8. HER4 and Breast Cancer

HER receptor family plays a role in mammary epithelial cell growth, and also in malignant transformation and tumor progression [3]. HER4 contributes to the growth and differentiation of a strictly regulated spatiotemporal expression of the mammary gland [3,68]. The significance of HER4 in breast cancer was understood in a series of experimental tests, but the results were contradictory, indicating that HER4 has both oncogenic and tumor suppressive roles [69,70]. Various studies investigating HER4's carcinogenic function have shown that HER4 expression is usually associated with hormone receptor positivity status, including estrogen and progesterone receptors, HER2 negativity, well-differentiated phenotype, and favorable outcome [71–74]. In addition, normal HER4 gene expression and overexpression were claimed to be related to shorter relapse-free survival in comparison to patients with low HER4 gene expression [75] and unfavorable clinical outcome in patients with overexpression of HER4 [76]. Overexpression of HER4 increases the growth of human breast cancer cells by supporting a role in promoting growth [77,78] and changes mice mammary epithelial to form tumors [79].

NRG-1 increases the ratio of cells in the G2/M phase of the cell cycle in HER4-positive but not HER4-negative breast cancer cells and in comparison to HER4/HER2 or HER3/HER2 heterodimers, the G2/M expression checkpoint protein BRCA1 increases, indicating that HER4 homodimers can initiate this mechanism [80]. Activation of HER4 by NRG-1 thus delays mitosis and reduces breast cancer cell proliferation. Interestingly, HER4 mRNA expression has been found to correlate with BRCA1 mRNA expression in human breast cancer samples and requires BRCA1 activity for NRG-1-mediated breast cell growth inhibition, as shown by in vitro and in vivo BRCA1 knockdown studies [80]. These results suggest that by inducing a G2/M checkpoint via a still unknown mechanism involving BRCA1, HER4 impairs the proliferation of breast cancer cells [2]. Other researches have also shown that HER4 activity can induce cell death via mitochondrial accumulation of HER4 in breast cancer-derived cells [81] and the interaction between the BAK pro-apoptotic protein and the BH3- like HER4 domain [2].

In 1993, HER4 was initially cloned from the MDA-MB-4533 line of human breast cancer cells. T-47D, MCF-7, MDA-MB-330, MDA-MB-361, and BT-474 are few other breast cancer cell lines expressed by HER4 [13]. In breast cancer cells, HER4 expression is low compared to EGFR and HER2 expression. Multiple researches have investigated HER4 expression at the protein level in clinical breast cancer through immunohistochemistry with various anti-HER4 antibodies recognizing either the N- or C-terminus of HER4 or the reverse transcription mRNA-PCRRA-level (RT-PCR). Upregulation of HER4 expression has been identified in 7 to 29% of breast cancers, while in 18 to 75% of cases, downregulation of HER4 expression has been observed. The majority of these studies have reported up- and downregulation of HER4 simultaneously. These results suggest that HER4 can be found in breast cancer tissue in vivo in both overexpression and downregulation [82].

In the literature, relatively high HER4 expression has been correlated with estrogen receptor-positive, low-grade, and slowly proliferating breast cancers, while in oestrogen receptor-negative cases, expression of HER4 tends to be downregulated [82].

A study demonstrated that serum HER4 ectodomain concentrations can be measured from ELISA clinical samples, suggesting a different new bioassay for the evaluation of HER signalling [83].

6.9. HER4 and Pancreatic Cancer

HER4 expression in pancreatic cancer is not well understood [84] but it tends to be low in human pancreatic cancers [2]. Moreover, in the early stages of pancreatic cancer, HER4 transcription is diminished, implying that the lack of HER4 expression can be a requirement for tumorigenesis [85]. In pancreatic cancers, higher HER4 expression was also found to correlate with favorable staging [86].

Later studies reported that HER4 is expressed predominantly in the exocrine pancreas duct system and, to less extent, in the cancerous cells of several human pancreatic adenocarcinomas. Moreover, HER4 mRNA expression declines in non-metastatic stages of pancreatic cancer and approaches levels similar to normal control levels in advanced diseases [87].

Tissue obtained after pancreaticoduodenectomy in one study showed that in the normal pancreas, HER4 is highly expressed, but in some cancers the expression is lost [84].

6.10. HER4 and Brain Cancer

Glioblastoma multiforme (GBM) is the most prevalent central nervous system cancer, which is the most common, severe, and difficult to treat [88]. Studies of HER family members show that HER4 is one of the most common proteins in GBM [89]. HER4 mRNA levels were observed to be lower than in normal brain samples, and HER4 protein was found to be widely expressed in GBM, but not related with survival [90].

CCLE data suggests a role of HER4 as a tumor suppressor, by showing copy number loss of HER4 gene through several cell lines of GBM. However, the same variants have been shown to occur at about the same frequencies in the general population [88]. Though GBM has an average low level of HER4 expression, in 11 % of cases, high pHER4 expression was found to be present and associated with reduced survival than no pHER4 expression [90]. Therefore, increased HER4 activity may have prognostic and/or therapeutic effects, considering the low levels of HER4 mRNA in GBM [2].

6.11. HER4 and Melanoma

HER4 is one of the most mutated tyrosine kinase in melanoma. Thus, this receptor plays a crucial role in malignant melanoma. HER4's significance in cancer is debatable due to the receptor's dual oncogenic/tumor-suppressive properties. The findings of the studies indicate that HER4 is oncogenic in malignant melanoma. This is corroborated by the fact that 19% of patients with metastatic melanomas carry a HER4 mutation. As a result of this, HER4 has been proposed as a potential therapeutic target in melanoma [91–94].

6.12. HER4 and Endometrial Cancer

Endometrial cancer is the most prevalent female genital tract cancer, affecting mostly postmenopausal women. Endometrial cancer hits around 2% to 3% of all women throughout their lifetime [95]. In a study examining the expression of the epidermal growth factor system in endometrial cancer, HER4 was found to be overexpressed in endometrial cancer higher than in healthy postmenopausal endometrium. The expression of the HER4 receptor showed no association with tumor grade and stage, nor with the disease's outcome [96].

6.13. HER4 and Osteosarcoma

Osteosarcoma is the most prevalent bone tumor in adolescence. It is characterized by fast progression, metastasis, and poor prognosis [97,98]. In a study investigating the pathway in which HER4 promotes osteosarcoma, HER4 proteins were found to be highly expressed in osteosarcoma cells. It was found that increased HER4 levels highly promoted proliferation, metastasis, and tumor progression in vitro and in vivo. High levels of HER4 were associated with increased expression of other protein kinases that are responsible for osteosarcoma progression, thus, HER4 is considered a potential target for new therapeutic modalities for the treatment of osteosarcoma [99].

7. HER4 Inhibitors

Kinase inhibitors are categorized based on kinase conformation when inhibitors bind (e.g., type1, type $1_{1/2}$, and type 2), and type of inhibition (e.g., reversible or irreversible). Most of the reported drugs that inhibit HER4 are mainly covalent inhibitors, as they bind to the ATP-binding site, covalently/irreversibly making them stronger than reversible drugs. However, the risk of more serious side effects is higher [5].

7.1. Quinazoline Inhibitors

In these derivatives, the quinazoline ring nitrogen atom(s) together with the attached NH are important to mimic the interaction of ATP molecule with the kinases hinge region. Michael acceptor-possessing molecules are designed to act as irreversible inhibitors.

7.1.1. Allitinib (AST-1306)

Allitinib

Allitinib is a novel anilino-quinazoline compound that is orally active and has been synthesized based on the lapatinib chemical structure [100]. It is an irreversible inhibitor of EGFR, HER2 and HER4 with IC_{50} of 0.5, 3, and 0.8 nM, respectively [101]. It is 5 to 15 times more potent compared to dacomitinib and afatinib. In human tumor xenograft models expressing or overexpressing HER family members, allitinib showed antitumor activity, especially in those with HER2 overexpression or EGFR T790M mutant tumors [101]. It binds irreversibly to Cys797 and Cys805 in the catalytic domains of EGFR and HER2, respectively [102]. It has two hydrogen bond donors, six hydrogen bond acceptors, and seven rotatable bonds [103].

It was investigated that allitinib significantly inhibited the proliferation of gastric cancer cells. In vivo, it controls the HER4-PI3K/Akt signaling pathways [4,104].

7.1.2. Poziotinib (HM781-36B)

Poziotinib

Poziotinib is an oral, third-generation, quinazoline-based inhibitor of epidermal growth factor receptors (EGFR, HER2, and HER4) that Hanmi Pharmaceutical has developed, currently being investigated in phase II clinical trials for breast and non-small cell lung cancer treatment [105]. It irreversibly inhibits HERs in vitro with IC_{50} values of 3.2, 5.3, 23.5 nM for EGFR, HER2 and HER4, respectively [106]. At the C6 position, it has a functional α,β-unsaturated carbonyl group like other irreversible EGFR inhibitors that makes covalent modifications to the active site of the EGFR kinase domain [107].

Poziotinib was terminated in 3 clinical studies for NSCLC (patients having EGFR or HER2 exon 20 insertion mutation), breast cancer (In HER2+ breast cancer patients, poziotinib in combination with T-DM1) and adenocarcinoma of lung stage IIIB and IV [108–110]. It is currently active but not recruiting in three clinical studies for solid tumor, breast cancer (HER2+ metastatic BC) and metastatic breast cancer (HER2+ patients with recurrent stage IV cancer who have had at least two previous HER2-directed treatments) [111–113]. Moreover, it is recruiting in five clinical studies and completed seven studies in conditions including metastatic breast cancer, HER2 gene mutation, adenocarcinoma lung stage IV, advanced solid malignancies, HER2+ advanced gastric cancer, increased drug resistance and advanced solid tumor. Unfortunately, there are three studies with unknown status [114].

HER4 is highly expressed in ovarian cancer stem cells. Poziotinib inhibited ovarian CSCs from sphere formation, viability, and proliferation. In addition, it triggered growth 1 (G1) cell cycle arrest and apoptosis. Furthermore, poziotinib decreased the stemming of CSCs and interfered with the pathways of Wnt/β-catenin, Notch, and Hedgehog that lead to CSC self-renewal [115]. Ovarian cancer stem cells have been scientifically shown to survive conventional chemotherapy [116]. Although ovarian CSCs have not been clearly understood in this respect, a small population of chemo-resistant cancer cells may have the properties of cancer stem cells and play an important role in recurrence [117,118]. To interrupt cancer stem cell properties and stem cell signaling pathways, a novel approach is required [115].

It was shown using Chou–Talalay method that combination therapy of poziotinib with manidipine (a dihydropyridine calcium antagonist) showed a synergistic effect in inhibiting ovarian CSCs more than in ovarian cancer cells as shown in Figure 3 [115]. Combination therapy with poziotinib and manidipine inhibited the expression of stem cell markers, especially CD133, NANOG, and KLF4. The two drugs also inhibited the phosphorylation of STAT5, AKT, and ERK, which are involved in CSC self-renewal and β-catenin nuclear translocation [115].

Poziotinib and manidipine combination therapy showed synergistic effect in inhibiting ovarian CSC by inhibiting HER4 and calcium channel mediated STAT5, AKT and ERK signaling [115].

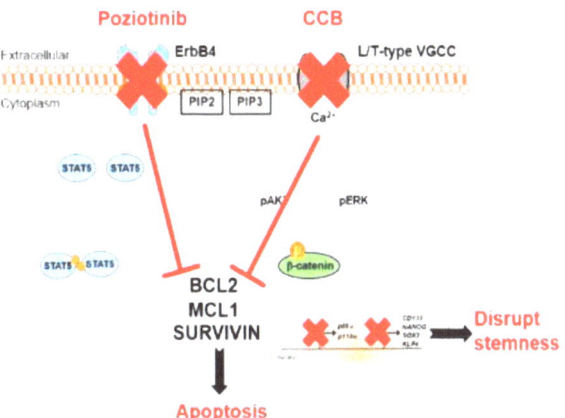

Figure 3. Mechanisms of action of poziotinib and manidipine in ovarian CSCs [115].

7.1.3. Dacomitinib (PF-00299804)

Dacomitinib

Dacomitinib is a second-generation RTK inhibitor used for the treatment of metastatic NSCLC (development phase three), gastric cancer (development phase one/two), head and neck cancer (development phase one/two) and glioblastoma (development phase one/two) [119]. Because of acquired tolerance to first-generation EGFR tyrosine kinase receptor inhibitors, the clinical development of second-generation EGFR tyrosine kinase inhibitors assisted in bypassing many pathways of resistance to first-generation EGFR tyrosine kinase receptor inhibitors. The EGFR kinase domain forms permanent covalent bonds with most second-generation tyrosine kinase receptor inhibitors. Dacomitinib has the ability to inhibit EGFR, HER2, HER3, and HER4 in an irreversible manner [120].

Dacomitinib possesses aminoquinazoline as its adenine pocket moiety. It has a 3-chloro-4-fluoro substituted phenyl that enters a hydrophobic pocket and a Michael acceptor that forms a covalent bond with cysteine [120]. Both HER homodimers and heterodimers are prevented from signaling to the cell. Dacomitinib reduces EGFR signaling in tumors/cells with multiple EGFR mutations but has only a minor effect on tumors with Kirsten rat sarcoma viral mutations, according to preclinical studies. Dacomitinib inhibits the ErbB family of kinases irreversibly and selectively, with IC_{50} values of 6, 45.7, and 73.7 nM against EGFR, HER2, and HER4, respectively.

Second-generation irreversible kinase inhibitors such as afatinib and dacomitinib were initially discovered to be a candidate against diagnosed epidermal growth factor receptor mutated lung cancer. They struggled to resolve T790M-mediated resistance in patients, as they have in monotherapy. The concentrations in which these irreversible inhibitors bypass T790M activation are not preclinically feasible in humans due to the dose-limiting toxicity associated with nonselective inhibition of wild-type EGFR. T790M resistance is induced by these inhibitors, meaning that they are less effective against T790M. As a result, there is a significant unmet need for an inhibitor that can more effectively target T790M tumors while leaving wild-type EGFR alone. As a result, "third-generation" inhibitors have been developed [121,122].

7.1.4. Lapatinib

Lapatinib

Lapatinib is an EGFR double tyrosine kinase inhibitor that is taken orally [123]. It is a type I inhibitor that possesses 4-anilinoquinazoline scaffold. By competing for HER2 and EGFR's ATP binding sites, lapatinib reversibly inhibits their activation. Lapatinib is used to treat advanced or metastatic breast cancer, as well as patients with brain metastases [123]. It interacts with HER4 in a similar way to the EGFR kinase [1]. Lapatinib inhibits EGFR, HER2 and HER4 with IC_{50} values of 10.8, 9.2, and 367 nM, respectively [124].

Lapatinib was terminated in one clinical study as protocol would not be able to approach stated accrual. Tumor cells from around 20% of melanoma patients have a particular mutation of a gene involved in producing HER4, and variations in this gene have been related to cancer. Lapatinib has been shown to substantially delay the growth of melanoma cells with this HER4 gene mutation. Further investigation on whether lapatinib can be beneficial for the treatment of melanoma is needed [5].

For patients with metastatic, EGFR antibody-resistant bowel cancers, a combination of trastuzumab and Lapatinib looks promising, but it is unclear whether the same combination is better than an EGFR antibody for patients who have never been treated for metastatic bowel cancer yet [5].

Binding mode analysis of Lapatinib within the HER4 active site revealed a number of important interactions: the compound was able to form strong hydrogen bond interaction (distance, 1.9 Å) with the corresponding amino acid residue Met-799 (Figure 4 left panel). Other important interactions include the formation of pi–pi stacking between the 3-fluorobenzyloxy terminal arm and the residue Phe-862, formation of pi–sigma interactions between the furan and quinazoline rings and the corresponding residue Leu-724 (Figure 4 right panel).

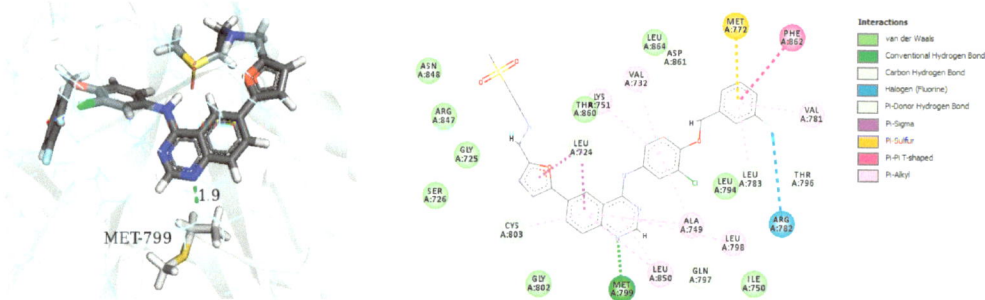

Figure 4. Best-docked pose of Lapatinib within the HER4 (ErbB4) active site, where hydrogen bond interactions are shown as green dashed lines (**left panel**) and its corresponding detailed 2D-interactions map (**right panel**). This docking study was conducted by us, no copyright issues.

7.1.5. Afatinib (BIBW2992)

Afatinib

EGFR, HER2, and HER4 have an effect on tumor cell proliferation and are presumed to be overly expressed in many cancer cells [125]. Five prospective clinical trials had evaluated afatinib's effectiveness in patients with advanced metastatic non-small cell lung cancer. Afatinib is an anilino-quinazoline derivative and works by inhibiting the epidermal growth factor receptor family by utilizing antineoplastic activity. It is used to treat NSCLC. It is an irreversible inhibitor that binds by covalent bonds to the intracellular tyrosine kinase domain of the epidermal growth factor receptors, i.e., EGFR, HER2, HER4, and a few epidermal growth factor receptor mutants such as the ones caused by exon 19 and 21 (L858R) deletion and substitution mutations, respectively [126].

In vitro, Afatinib inhibits HERs irreversibly with IC_{50} values of 0.4, 10, 14, and 1 nM against EGFR (wt), EGFR (L858R), HER2, and HER4, respectively. This is presumed to lead to inhibiting tumor growth and cause angiogenesis in the tumor cells that overexpress RTKs. In addition, trials showed that afatinib improved the overall survival rate and showed inhibition against T790M-mutant EGFR gatekeeper, which is well-known to be resistant to first-generation EGFR inhibitors [127]. Therefore, afatinib along with erlotinib and gefitinib, has been approved as a first-line treatment for patients with metastatic NSCLC [128,129].

Patients are advised to continue the therapy until they experience symptomatic disease progression. However, disease progression does not prevent the physicians from using another agent in its class or possible future reuse of the treatment. Afatinib is known to be correlated with an elevation in serum aminotransferase levels throughout the therapy causing acute liver injury and in rare cases mortality [130].

7.1.6. Canertinib (CI-1033)

Canertinib

Canertinib is an oral pan-HER inhibitor that inhibits all four HER receptors [131]. Canertinib is composed of an aminoquinazoline ring in the adenine pocket, a morpholino ring in the solvent field, and an acrylamide moiety as a Michael acceptor to form a covalent bond with the cysteine residue.

Canertinib irreversibly inhibits the enzymatic activities of EGFR, HER2, and HER4 with IC_{50} values of 0.8, 19, and 7 nM, respectively [132]. Canertinib also has poor clinical results, and the occurrence of side effects including diarrhea and rash in patients with advanced NSCLC has reduced its clinical use [132]. Canertinib has three completed clinical studies including treating patients with metastatic (stage IV) breast cancer (phase II), evaluating the adequate protection and effective dose of canertinib in combination with paclitaxel and carboplatin in patients with advanced NSCLC (phase I) and an open-label review of canertinib as a single agent in patients with severe non-small cell lung cancer [133–135]. Pfizer agreed to stop developing the drug in 2015 because of concerns about its safety and risk/benefit ratio. In the United States, there are currently no canertinib breast cancer studies ongoing [131].

7.2. Quinoline Inhibitors
7.2.1. Neratinib (HKI-272)

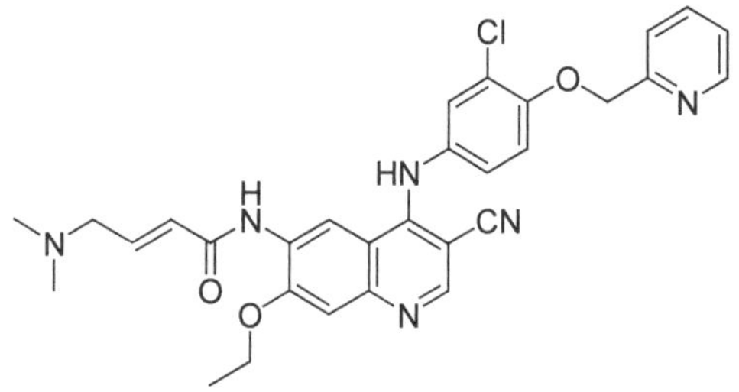

Neratinib

Neratinib is made up of an aminoquinoline ring that binds in the adenine pocket, a pyridine substitution that occupies the solvent regions, and a Michael acceptor, which is needed for covalent inhibitors [136].

Neratinib is an irreversible EGFR inhibitor that has been developed and tested in clinical studies. Neratinib treats some forms of cancer, it inhibits the oncogenic intracellular signaling pathways of EGFR, HER2, and HER4, inhibiting autophosphorylation and activation [137]. Neratinib inhibits the kinase activity of EGFR, HER2, and HER4 (IC_{50} values of 92, 59, and 19 nM, respectively) [138].

Neratinib is currently recruited in one clinical study. This phase I trial focuses on the adverse effects and preferred dose of Neratinib in combination with everolimus, palbociclib, or trametinib in patients who have solid tumors with EGFR mutations/amplification, HER2 mutations/amplification, HER3 and HER4 mutations, or KRAS mutations that affect other body parts and are refractory to treatment (advanced or metastatic). Neratinib, palbociclib, and trametinib can inhibit tumor cell growth by inhibiting certain enzymes required for cell growth. Chemotherapy drugs like everolimus function in a number of ways to stop tumor cells from growing, including destroying them, preventing them from dividing, and preventing them from spreading. In the treatment of solid tumors, Neratinib combined with everolimus, palbociclib, or trametinib may be more effective than neratinib alone [138].

7.2.2. Pyrotinib (SHR1258)

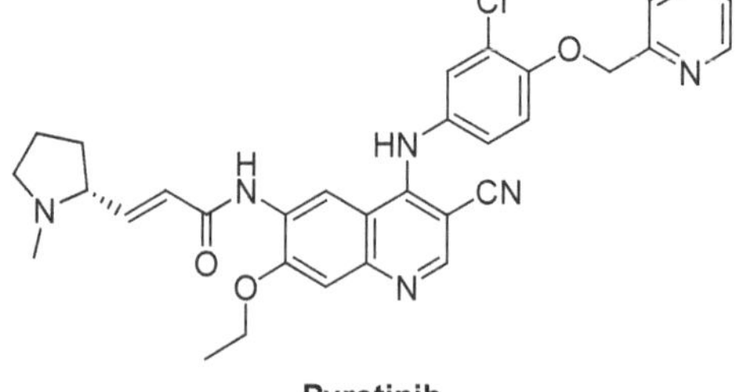

Pyrotinib

Pyrotinib is a second-generation pan-HER receptor tyrosine kinase inhibitor that targets EGFR, HER2, and HER4. It is an irreversible inhibitor and well absorbed [139]. Its

IC$_{50}$ values are 5.6 and 8.1 nM against EGFR and HER2, respectively [140,141]. Clinical trials of pyrotinib/vinorelbine combination therapy of brain metastases from HER2-positive metastatic breast cancer are recruited [142].

Pyrotinib is being examined in another clinical study that is divided into two sections. Investigators will assess the protection and tolerability of pyrotinib plus capecitabine combined with brain radiotherapy in a phase Ib trial. Investigators will study the data after the phase Ib part is completed and determine whether to include this patient before starting the phase II part. Investigators will determine the effectiveness of pyrotinib and capecitabine combined with brain radiotherapy in patients with HER2 positive breast cancer with brain metastases in the phase II portion of the research [139].

Pyrotinib and inetetamab demonstrated high standard anti-tumor efficacy and acceptable protection and optimized ADCC, respectively, in a recruiting study. In order to assess the effectiveness and safety of inetetamab in combination with pyrotinib and chemotherapy for treatment of HER-positive metastatic breast cancer, a phase II single-arm clinical trial is intended to be carried out [143].

7.3. Other Inhibitors
7.3.1. Ibrutinib (PCI-32765)

Ibrutinib

Ibrutinib is an orally delivered, irreversible first-generation Bruton's tyrosine kinase inhibitor (BTK). BTK belongs to the cytoplasmic non-receptor tyrosine kinase class of tyrosine protein kinases (TEC) and is found primarily in hematopoietic cells. Mantle cell lymphoma (MCL), chronic lymphocytic leukemia (CLL), Waldenstrom macroglobulinemia (WM), Marginal zone lymphoma (MZL) and chronic Graft-versus-host disease (GVHD) which are all indications for ibrutinib [144,145].

BTK is a key component of the B-cell receptor signaling pathway and a mediator of pro-inflammatory signals [146]. BTK inhibition can be a treatment tool for B-cell malignancies and autoimmune conditions. BTK is one of 11 tyrosine kinases, including TEC family kinases, EGFR, HER2, HER4, BLK, and JAK3, which all share a conserved cysteine residue adjacent to the ATP-binding site, allowing covalent inhibition by tyrosine kinase inhibitors. Ibrutinib binds covalently to the cysteine-481 at the active site of BTK, inhibiting kinase activity for more than 24 h with an IC$_{50}$ of 0.5 nM [147]. Ibrutinib inhibits HER phosphorylation and the differentiation of HER2 breast cancer cells, implying that it may be used to treat breast cancer [148].

A recent study demonstrated that using the Nucleic Acid Programmable Protein Array (NAPPA) functional protein microarray platform, researchers discovered that HER4 is a promising candidate for ibrutinib. It was discovered that HER4-expressing cells react to ibrutinib via the WNT pathway and that inhibits some WNT activating ligands which help boost ibrutinib reaction. Findings indicate that ibrutinib could be used to treat HER4-expressing cancers in addition to B-cell malignancies, either alone or in conjunction with WNT inhibitors [149–151].

7.3.2. AC-480 (BMS-599626)

AC-480 (BMS-599626)

AC-480 is a small molecule and a pyrrolotriazine analogue that is orally active and has been synthesized by Bristol Myers Squibb Company [152,153]. It reversibly inhibits tyrosine kinase receptors EGFR, HER2, and HER4 with IC_{50} of 22, 32, and 190 nM, respectively, and, to a lesser extent, HER3 [152,154]. AC480 is an ATP competitive inhibitor in EGFR inhibition, according to kinetic studies. AC480, on the other hand, inhibited HER2 via an ATP non-competitive mechanism. Therefore, it acts as a mixed-type inhibitor with Ki values equal 2 and 5 nM, respectively [152].

AC-480 inhibits heterodimerization of EGFR and HER2 receptors, this adds an alternative tumor-inhibiting mechanism in which receptor co-expression and heterodimerization contribute to tumor development. The preclinical studies encourage the development of AC-480 for cancer treatment in humans [152]. AC-480 had completed four clinical studies which are phase I study in patients with HER2-expressing advanced solid malignancies, phase I study in treating patients with metastatic solid tumor, phase I study in patients with advanced solid malignancies, including malignancies that express HER2 at the maximum tolerated dose and/or recommended, phase I dose and pharmacokinetic study of AC480 in patients with recurrent malignant glioma have all been completed [155–158] and safety study for intravenous (IV) AC-480 to treat advanced solid tumors has been withdrawn [159,160].

When comparing the effects of BMS-536924 in addition with AC-480 to the effects of the single agents alone, repeated experiments indicated that the antiproliferative effect of the combination was synergistic [160].

In the five ovarian cancer cell lines that displayed synergistic antiproliferative activity with BMS-536924 and AC480 (BMS-599626), there was a hypothesis that receptor expression and/or phosphorylation modulation occurred. All the five cell lines showed signs of increased HER receptor signaling activity after treatment with BMS-536924. AC480 inhibited the increase in HER receptor signaling in all ovarian cell lines. By Western blotting, there was no observable activation of HER4 in any of the ovarian cell lines [160].

The best docked conformation of compound AC-480 (BMS-599626) within the HER4 (ErbB4) active site revealed strong hydrogen bond (distance, 2.4 Å) formed between the morpholino terminal moiety and the corresponding Arg-847 amino acid residue (Figure 5 left panel). Furthermore, the compound was able to secure large network of weak interactions including van der Waals, pi–sulfur, pi–cation and pi–alkyl interactions as illustrated in (Figure 5 right panel)

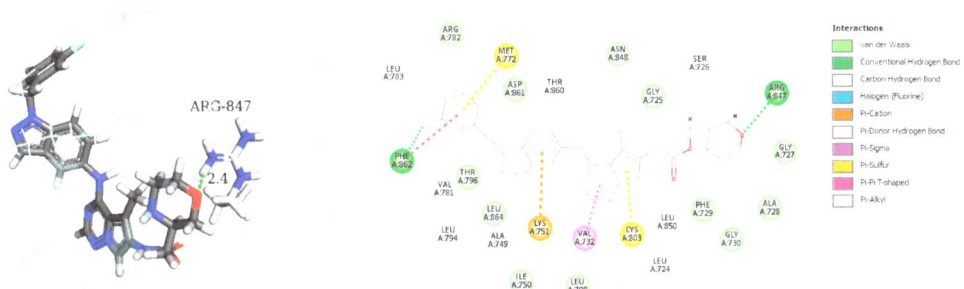

Figure 5. Best-docked pose of compound AC-480 within the HER4 (ErbB4) active site, where hydrogen bond interactions are shown as green dashed lines (**left panel**) and its corresponding detailed 2D-interactions map (**right panel**). This docking study was conducted by us, no copyright issues.

7.3.3. Compounds I and II

These two compounds are first-in-class imidazo[2,1-*b*]thiazole-possessing potent and selective inhibitors of HER4 kinase. This recent study reported selective HER4 inhibitors for the first time, unlike the other previously mentioned inhibitors that are non-selective kinase inhibitors. The IC_{50} values of compounds **I** and **II** against HER4 kinase in cell-free kinase assay are 15.24 and 17.70 nM, respectively. Both exerted relative selectivity against HER4 upon testing against a panel of 63 kinases. Both compounds were tested for antiproliferative activity against NCI-60 cancer cell line panel but compound **I** exerted stronger activity. The mean inhibition percentage values of compounds **I** and **II** against the 60 cell lines upon testing at 10 µM concentration are 36.62% and 21.58%, respectively. Compound **I** was selected for five-dose testing to measure its IC_{50} values against the NCI-60 cell lines, but compound **II** was not selected. Compound **I** exerted high potency against several cell lines of different cancer types. The most sensitive human cancer cell lines to compound **I** are SK-MEL-5 (melanoma), MOLT-4 (leukemia), MDA-MB-468 (breast), UO-31 (renal), DU-145 (prostate), and HCC-2998 (colon) with IC_{50} values of 0.51, 1.02, 1.04, 1.55, 1.67, and 1.78 µM, respectively. It is more potent than sorafenib and ibrutinib, reference standard kinase-inhibiting anticancer agents, against most of these cell lines. Compound **I** was further tested in whole-cell kinase assay against T-47D breast cancer cell line rich in HER4 kinase. The compound showed ability to cross the cell membrane and inhibit HER4 inside the cells. Its IC_{50} value in this assay is 3.30 µM, which is less than its antiproliferative activity against the same cell line (4.08 µM). Moreover, compound **I** exerted other merits such as weak inhibition of hERG, CYP2D6, and CYP3A4 in addition to weak potency against WI-38 normal cells.

Structure–activity relationships of these two compounds and their derivatives against HER4 kinase and the NCI-60 human cancer cell line panel are similar. Pyrimidinyl ring carrying mesyl group is the best option for activity. Pyrimidine ring lacking methylsulfonyl group (e.g., compound **II**) is still favorable for HER4 kinase inhibition. Replacement of this moiety with unsubstituted phenyl or mesyl-substituted phenyl led to a loss of activity.

In addition, imidazo[2,1-*b*]thiazole nucleus is more optimal for activity than the isosteric imidazooxazole. Regarding the benzyloxy substituent, its presence in *meta* position is more favorable for activity than *para* position. Extension of benzyl (e.g., phenethyl, 4-fluorophenethyl, or phenylethanone) led to less activity. Furthermore, *p*-fluoro-substituted benzyl analogue of compound **I** is 47-fold less potent against HER4 in cell-free assay (IC_{50} = 719 nM). Replacement of benzyl substituent with hydrophilic moiety led to complete loss of activity against HER4 kinase and cancer cell lines.

Docking and molecular dynamic simulation of compound **I** bound to HER4 active site revealed the formation of five hydrogen bonds and one hydrophobic interaction (Figure 6). Pyrimidinyl nitrogen, sulfonyl oxygen, imidazo[2,1-*b*]thiazole nitrogen, and benzyloxy oxygen accept the five hydrogen bonds. In addition, the benzyl ring forms hydrophobic interaction with Phe862 [161].

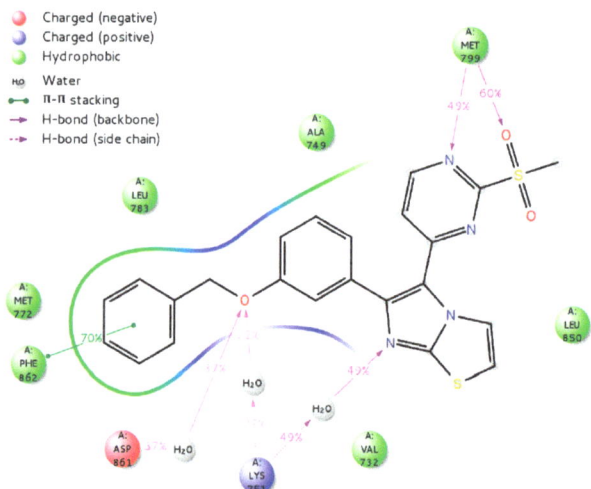

Figure 6. Putative binding interactions of compound **I** with HER4 active site [161]. Reprinted with permission from ref. [161]. Copyright 2021 Elsevier.

Table 1 summarizes the structures, potency, biological activities, and clinical trials (in case of clinical candidate) of the reported HER4 inhibitors.

Table 1. Structures, potency, biological activities, and clinical trials (if any) of the reported HER4 inhibitors.

Name	Structure	Type of Inhibitor	IC$_{50}$ against HER4 Kinase	Other Biological Activity	Status of Clinical Trials	Company
Allitinib	(Allitinib structure)	Irreversible	0.8 nM	**In vitro:** • In HH3T3-EGFR T790M/L858R cells, allitinib effectively suppresses EGFR phosphorylation. • In NCI-H1975 cells with the EGFR T790M/L858R mutation, allitinib inhibits growth in a concentration-dependent manner. **In vivo:** • In SK-OV-3 and Calu-3 xenograft models, allitinib significantly reduced tumor formation. • Blocks phosphorylation of EGFR and downstream pathways. • Tumors in SK-OV-3 models nearly vanish after 1 week of treatment with allitinib. • Slightly inhibits the growth of tumor in HO-8910 and A549 xenograft models.	**Active but not recruiting:** One clinical study to analyze the efficacy and safety of anlotinib in combination with allitinib in the treatment of lung cancer.	Investigational
Poziotinib	(Poziotinib structure)	Irreversible	23.5 nM	**In vitro:** • Inhibits cell growth in HER2-amplification gastric cancer cells as well as phosphorylation of EGFR and key downstream signaling cascade components including STAT3, AKT, and ERK • Causes apoptosis and growth 1 cell cycle arrest in HER2 amplified gastric cancer cells by activating the mitochondrial pathway. • In both HER2 amplified and HER2 non-amplified gastric cancer cells, it has synergistic effects with chemotherapeutic agents. **In vivo:** • Poziotinib (0.5 mg/kg p.o.) inhibits tumor growth in nude mice carrying N87 human gastric cancer xenografts, and coadministration of Poziotinib and 5-FU induces more successful tumor inhibition. Poziotinib has shown to have excellent antitumor activity in a number of EGFR- and HER-2-dependent tumor xenograft models.	**Active but not recruiting:** • Solid tumor • Breast cancer • Metastatic breast cancer. **Recruiting** • Study to allow continued dosing and/or follow-up of patients who have had previous exposure to poziotinib, • EGFR exon 20 mutant advanced nsclc • Study of poziotinib in Japanese patients with NSCLC. • A study of poziotinib in patients with egfr or her2 activating mutations in advanced malignancies • Phase 2 study of poziotinib in patients with nsclc having egfr or her2 exon 20 insertion mutation **Terminated** • 3 clinical trials. **Completed** • 7 clinical trials. **Unknown status** 3 studies	Hanmi Pharmaceutical, South Korea

Table 1. Cont.

Name	Structure	Type of Inhibitor	IC$_{50}$ against HER4 Kinase	Other Biological Activity	Status of Clinical Trials	Company
Dacomitinib	Dacomitinib	Irreversible	73.7 nM	**In vitro:** • At clinically significant concentrations, dacomitinib inhibited the action of DDR1, EPHA6, LCK, DDR2, and MNK1 in vitro. In mice carrying subcutaneously implanted human tumor xenografts driven by HER family targets, including mutated EGFR, dacomitinib inhibited EGFR and HER-2 autophosphorylation and tumor development. **In vivo:** • Dacomitinib showed impressive antitumor efficacy in vivo as a single agent.	**Completed:** • PF-00299804 Monotherapy in Patients With HER-2 positive advanced gastric cancer. **Not yet recruiting:** • An Open Label, Multicentre, Phase II Study of Dacomitinib for EGFR Mutated Non-Small Cell Lung Cancer (NSCLC) With Brain Metastases **Active, not recruiting:** • Study of dacomitinib and osimertinib for patients with advanced EGFR mutant lung cancer. **Recruiting:** • Dacomitinib for treatment of patients in India with metastatic NSCLC with EGFR activating mutations. **Recruiting:** • Phase II study of dacomitinib in NSCLC. • Dacomitinib in lung cancer with uncommon EGFR mutations • A pilot study of dacomitinib with or without osimertinib for patients with metastatic EGFR mutant lung cancers with disease progression on osimertinib. • Dacomitinib treatment followed by 3rd generation EGFR-TKI in patients with EGFR mutation positive advanced NSCLC. **Not yet recruiting:** • Real world utilization and outcomes with dacomitinib first line treatment for EGFR mutation-positive advanced non small cell lung cancer among asian patients-a multi center chart review. **Unknown:** • ARCHER1050: A study of dacomitinib vs. gefitinib in 1st-line treatment of advanced NSCLC. **Completed:** • Safety and efficacy of PF-299804 (Dacomitinib), in patients with recurrent glioblastoma with EGFR amplification or presence of EGFRvIII mutation. a phase II clinical trial.	Pfizer

Table 1. Cont.

Name	Structure	Type of Inhibitor	IC$_{50}$ against HER4 Kinase	Other Biological Activity	Status of Clinical Trials	Company
Lapatinib	Lapatinib	Reversible	3.67 nM	**In vitro:** • Lapatinib weakly inhibits the activity of ErbB4. • Lapatinib inhibits the autophosphorylation of EGFR and ErbB2 receptors in a dose-dependent manner. **In vivo:** The growth of BT474 and HN5 xenografts is significantly inhibited by oral administration of Lapatinib (100 mg/kg) twice daily in a dose-dependent manner.	**Terminated** Study as protocol would not be able to approach stated accrual.	GlaxoSmithKline
Afatinib	Afatinib	Irreversible selective inhibitor	1 nM	**In vitro:** • In cell lines expressing wild-type EGFR as well as chosen EGFR exon 19 deletion mutations, exon 21 L858R mutations, or a less frequent non-resistant mutations, afatinib inhibits autophosphorylation and in some cases along with proliferation. **In vivo:** • Afatinib maintains its inhibitory effects on signal transduction in vivo cancer cell development in tumors prone to reversible EGFR inhibitors, such as those with T790M mutations.	**Completed:** Afatinib Treatment for Patients with EGFR Mutation Positive NSCLC who are age 70 or older. **Terminated:** Afatinib in EGFR+NSCLC (Recurrent or Stage IV)-Patients with Poor performance Status (ECOG 2 or 3). **Completed:** Afatinib Monotherapy in Patients With ERBB-deregulated Metastatic Urothelial Tract Carcinoma After Failure of Platinum Based Chemotherapy.	Boehringer Ingelheim
Canertinib	Canertinib	Irreversible	7 nM	**In vitro:** Canertinib alone suppresses constitutively activated Akt and MAP kinase. **In vivo:** At 5 mg/kg body weight, canertinib displays remarkable activity against A431 xenografts in nude mice.	**Unknown** Canertinib has had poor clinical outcomes, and the presence of side effects such as diarrhea and rash in advanced NSCLC patients has restricted its clinical applications.	Pfizer, development discontinued
Neratinib	Neratinib	Irreversible	19 nM	**In vitro:** • Neratinib weakly inhibits tyrosine kinases and Src. • Neratinib displays no activity against other serine-threonine kinases. **In vivo:** • Oral administration of Neratinib inhibits the development of 3T3/neu xenografts significantly. • Neratinib inhibits the growth of BT474 xenografts • Neratinib is also effective against SK-OV-3 xenografts	**Recruited** Phase I trial that focuses on the side effects and best dose of Neratinib in combination with everolimus, palbociclib, or trametinib in patients who have solid tumors with EGFR mutations/amplification, HER2 mutations/amplification, HER3/4 mutations, or KRAS mutations that have spread to other parts of the body and are refractory to treatment (advanced or metastatic). Neratinib, palbociclib, and trametinib can inhibit tumor cell growth by inhibiting certain enzymes required for cell growth.	Wyeth & Pfizer

Table 1. Cont.

Name	Structure	Type of Inhibitor	IC$_{50}$ against HER4 Kinase	Other Biological Activity	Status of Clinical Trials	Company
Pyrotinib	Pyrotinib	Irreversible	unknown	**In vitro:** Pyrotinib, a dual tyrosine kinase inhibitor for EGFR and HER2, has excellent in vitro potency, selectivity, and PK profiles. **In vivo:** Pyrotinib has shown to have potent anti-tumor effects in HER2-overexpressing xenograft models, as well as adequate safety windows in animals and beneficial pharmacokinetic properties in humans.	**Recruited:** Clinical study of Pyrotinib plus Vinorelbine as the therapy of brain metastases from HER2-positive metastatic breast cancer. **Running:** Pyrotinib, on the other hand, is being examined in another study, which is divided into two sections. Investigators will assess the protection and tolerability of pyrotinib Plus Capecitabine combined with brain radiotherapy in phase Ib trial.	Shanghai Hengrui Pharmaceutical
Ibrutinib	Ibrutinib	Irreversible	Unknown	**In vitro:** • Ibrutinib blocked HER-amplification cell lines as well as main signalling pathways. **In vivo:** • Tumor volumes in ibrutinib-responsive mouse xenograft tumors were reduced with ibrutinib therapy.	**Active, not recruiting:** A phase I/II study of ibrutinib in previously treated EGFR mutant NSCLC.	Janssen
AC-480	AC-480 (BMS-599626)	Reversible	190 nM	**In vitro:** • For HER1, it works as an ATP-competitive inhibitor, and for HER2, it works as an ATP-noncompetitive inhibitor. • By promoting cycle redistribution and inhibiting DNA repair, AC-480 greatly improves the radiosensitivity of HN-5 cells expressing both EGFR and HER2. **In vivo:** • Inhibits Sal2 tumor growth in a dose-dependent manner. • At its maximum tolerated dose of 180 mg/kg, AC-480 has potent antitumor activity in a human breast tumor KPL-4 xenograft.	**Completed:** • Four clinical studies in PK study for recurrent glioma, metastatic solid tumors, advanced solid malignancies and MAD refractory. **Withdrawn:** • One clinical study in safety study to treat advanced solid tumors.	Bristol Myers Squibb

Table 1. *Cont.*

Name	Structure	Type of Inhibitor	IC$_{50}$ against HER4 Kinase	Other Biological Activity	Status of Clinical Trials	Company
Compound I		Reversible	15.24 nM	• Selective HER4 inhibitor. • Potent, broad-spectrum antiproliferative activity against different cell lines of several cancer types. Whole-cell HER4 kinase inhibition effect in T-47D cells. • Weak inhibitor of hERG, CYP2D6, and CYP3A4.	-	Investigational
Compound II		Reversible	17.70 nM	• Selective HER4 inhibitor. • Less active as antiproliferative agent than compound I.	-	Investigational

8. Conclusions

With the ever-growing need for new treatments for the management of cancer, new therapeutic targets have increasingly become an absolute necessity for enhancing the patient's quality of life. HER4 is a tyrosine kinase whose contribution to cancer is still controversial. Several reports highlighted the impact of its overexpression and mutation of several cancer types as reported in this article. However, other articles reported the opposite. Most of the previously reported HER4 inhibitors are non-selective or pan-HER inhibitors. The recent discovery of selective HER4 inhibitors such as the first-in-class imidazo[2,1-*b*]thiazole-based compounds **I** and **II** can be a great addition to this field. Those selective molecules can help molecular biologists and pathologists to better understand whether HER4 is a validated, potential target for cancer therapy or not. The future directions in this domain should involve lead optimization and development of more potent and selective HER4 inhibitors as well as extensive molecular biology research work to conclude whether HER4 inhibition is a potential drug target for cancer treatment or not.

Author Contributions: Conceptualization, M.I.E.-G. and H.S.A.; methodology, N.H.M., N.E.A., M.A.E., R.M.S., M.M.M., S.-O.Z. and A.I.S.; software, H.T.; validation, M.I.E.-G., M.M.M. and H.S.A.; resources, M.I.E.-G.; writing—original draft preparation, all the ten authors; writing—review and editing, all the ten authors; supervision, M.I.E.-G.; project administration, M.I.E.-G. and H.S.A. All authors have read and agreed to the published version of the manuscript.

Funding: The authors are grateful to University of Sharjah, United Arab Emirates, for financial support (grant No. 2101110153).

Institutional Review Board Statement: Not applicable.

Informed Consent Statement: Not applicable.

Data Availability Statement: Not applicable.

Conflicts of Interest: The authors declare no conflict of interest.

Sample Availability: Not available from authors.

Abbreviations

BTC	betacellulin
BTK	Bruton's tyrosine kinase
CLL	chronic lymphocytic leukemia
COX-2	cyclooxygenase-2
CRC	colorectal cancer
DEN	diethyl nitrosamine
EGF	epidermal growth factor
EGFR	epidermal growth factor receptor
EPR	epiregulin
GBM	glioblastoma multiforme
GVHD	Graft-versus-host disease
HCC	hepatocellular carcinoma
HER	human epidermal growth factor receptor
MAPK	mitogen-activated protein kinase
MCL	mantle cell lymphoma
MZL	marginal zone lymphoma
NAPPA	nucleic acid programmable protein assays
NEU	neurogulin
NSCLC	non-small cell lung cancer
PI3K	phosphoinositide 3-kinase
RTK	receptor tyrosine kinase

RT-PCR	reverse transcription mRNA-PCRRA-level	
TNF	tumor necrosis factor	
WHO	World Health Organization	
WM	Waldenstrom macroglobulinemia	
WNT	wingless related integration site	

References

1. Qiu, C.; Tarrant, M.K.; Choi, S.H.; Sathyamurthy, A.; Bose, R.; Banjade, S.; Pal, A.; Bornmann, W.G.; Lemmon, M.A.; Cole, P.A.; et al. Mechanism of Activation and Inhibition of the HER4/ErbB4 Kinase. *Structure* **2008**, *16*, 460–467. [CrossRef] [PubMed]
2. Segers, V.F.M.; Dugaucquier, L.; Feyen, E.; Shakeri, H.; De Keulenaer, G.W. The role of ErbB4 in cancer. *Cell. Oncol.* **2020**, *43*, 335–352. [CrossRef] [PubMed]
3. Muraoka-Cook, R.S.; Feng, S.-M.; Strunk, K.E.; Earp, H.S. ErbB4/HER4: Role in Mammary Gland Development, Differentiation and Growth Inhibition. *J. Mammary Gland. Biol. Neoplasia* **2008**, *13*, 235–246. [CrossRef]
4. Xu, J.; Gong, L.; Qian, Z.; Song, G.; Liu, J. ERBB4 promotes the proliferation of gastric cancer cells via the PI3K/Akt signaling pathway. *Oncol. Rep.* **2018**, *39*, 2892–2898. [CrossRef] [PubMed]
5. Vickers, E. Treatments That Block Proteins Involved in Cell Communication. In *A Beginner's Guide to Targeted Cancer Treatments*; John Wiley & Sons, Ltd.: Cambridge, MA, USA, 2018; pp. 65–109.
6. Haryuni, R.D.; Watabe, S.; Yamaguchi, A.; Fukushi, Y.; Tanaka, T.; Kawasaki, Y.; Zhou, Y.; Yokoyama, S.; Sakurai, H. Negative feedback regulation of ErbB4 tyrosine kinase activity by ERK-mediated non-canonical phosphorylation. *Biochem. Biophys. Res. Commun.* **2019**, *514*, 456–461. [CrossRef] [PubMed]
7. Hynes, N.E.; MacDonald, G. ErbB receptors and signaling pathways in cancer. *Curr. Opin. Cell Biol.* **2009**, *21*, 177–184. [CrossRef]
8. Ullrich, A.; Coussens, L.; Hayflick, J.S.; Dull, T.J.; Gray, A.; Tam, A.W.; Lee, J.; Yarden, Y.; Libermann, T.A.; Schlessinger, J.; et al. Human epidermal growth factor receptor cDNA sequence and aberrant expression of the amplified gene in A431 epidermoid carcinoma cells. *Nature* **1984**, *309*, 418–425. [CrossRef] [PubMed]
9. Roskoski, R. The ErbB/HER family of protein-tyrosine kinases and cancer. *Pharmacol. Res.* **2014**, *79*, 34–74. [CrossRef] [PubMed]
10. Tvorogov, D.; Sundvall, M.; Kurppa, K.; Hollmén, M.; Repo, S.; Johnson, M.S.; Elenius, K. Somatic Mutations of ErbB4: Selective loss-of-function phenotype affecting signal transduction pathways in cancer. *J. Biol. Chem.* **2009**, *284*, 5582–5591. [CrossRef]
11. Walker, R.A. The erbB/HER type 1 tyrosine kinase receptor family. *J. Pathol.* **1998**, *185*, 234–235. [CrossRef]
12. Stamos, J.; Sliwkowski, M.X.; Eigenbrot, C. Structure of the Epidermal Growth Factor Receptor Kinase Domain Alone and in Complex with a 4-Anilinoquinazoline Inhibitor. *J. Biol. Chem.* **2002**, *277*, 46265–46272. [CrossRef] [PubMed]
13. Plowman, G.D.; Culouscou, J.M.; Whitney, G.S.; Green, J.M.; Carlton, G.W.; Foy, L.; Neubauer, M.G.; Shoyab, M. Ligand-specific activation of HER4/p180erbB4, a fourth member of the epidermal growth factor receptor family. *Proc. Natl. Acad. Sci. USA* **1993**, *90*, 1746–1750. [CrossRef]
14. Carpenter, G. ErbB-4: Mechanism of action and biology. *Exp. Cell Res.* **2003**, *284*, 66–77. [CrossRef]
15. Roskoski, R. ErbB/HER protein-tyrosine kinases: Structures and small molecule inhibitors. *Pharmacol. Res.* **2014**, *87*, 42–59. [CrossRef]
16. Bae, J.H.; Boggon, T.J.; Tomé, F.; Mandiyan, V.; Lax, I.; Schlessinger, J. Asymmetric receptor contact is required for tyrosine autophosphorylation of fibroblast growth factor receptor in living cells. *Proc. Natl. Acad. Sci. USA* **2010**, *107*, 2866–2871. [CrossRef] [PubMed]
17. Dawson, J.P.; Bu, Z.; Lemmon, M.A. Ligand-Induced Structural Transitions in ErbB Receptor Extracellular Domains. *Structure* **2007**, *15*, 942–954. [CrossRef] [PubMed]
18. Red Brewer, M.; Choi, S.H.; Alvarado, D.; Moravcevic, K.; Pozzi, A.; Lemmon, M.A.; Carpenter, G. The Juxtamembrane Region of the EGF Receptor Functions as an Activation Domain. *Mol. Cell* **2009**, *34*, 641–651. [CrossRef] [PubMed]
19. Fan, Q.-W.; Cheng, C.K.; Gustafson, W.C.; Charron, E.; Zipper, P.; Wong, R.A.; Chen, J.; Lau, J.; Knobbe-Thomsen, C.; Weller, M.; et al. EGFR Phosphorylates Tumor-Derived EGFRvIII Driving STAT3/5 and Progression in Glioblastoma. *Cancer Cell* **2013**, *24*, 438–449. [CrossRef] [PubMed]
20. James, K.A.; Verkhivker, G.M. Structure-Based Network Analysis of Activation Mechanisms in the ErbB Family of Receptor Tyrosine Kinases: The Regulatory Spine Residues Are Global Mediators of Structural Stability and Allosteric Interactions. *PLoS ONE* **2014**, *9*, e113418. [CrossRef] [PubMed]
21. Chen, C.L.; Zhao, J.W. Analysis of regulatory mechanism after ErbB4 gene mutation based on local modeling methodology. *Genet. Mol. Res.* **2016**, *15*. [CrossRef]
22. Carraway, K.L.; Sweeney, C. Localization and modulation of ErbB receptor tyrosine kinases. *Curr. Opin. Cell Biol.* **2001**, *13*, 125–130. [CrossRef]
23. Karamouzis, M.V.; Badra, F.A.; Papavassiliou, A.G. Breast cancer: The upgraded role of HER-3 and HER-4. *Int. J. Biochem. Cell Biol.* **2007**, *39*, 851–856. [CrossRef] [PubMed]
24. Hoesl, C.; Röhrl, J.M.; Schneider, M.R.; Dahlhoff, M. The receptor tyrosine kinase ERBB4 is expressed in skin keratinocytes and influences epidermal proliferation. *Biochim. Biophys. Acta (BBA)—Gen. Subj.* **2018**, *1862*, 958–966. [CrossRef] [PubMed]

25. Fujiwara, S.; Yamamoto-Ibusuki, M.; Yamamoto, Y.; Yamamoto, S.; Tomiguchi, M.; Takeshita, T.; Hayashi, M.; Sueta, A.; Iwase, H. The localization of HER4 intracellular domain and expression of its alternately-spliced isoforms have prognostic significance in ER+ HER2- breast cancer. *Oncotarget* **2014**, *5*, 3919. [CrossRef] [PubMed]
26. Icli, B.; Bharti, A.; Pentassuglia, L.; Peng, X.; Sawyer, D.B. ErbB4 localization to cardiac myocyte nuclei, and its role in myocyte DNA damage response. *Biochem. Biophys. Res. Commun.* **2012**, *418*, 116–121. [CrossRef]
27. Culouscou, J.M.; Plowman, G.D.; Carlton, G.W.; Green, J.M.; Shoyab, M. Characterization of a breast cancer cell differentiation factor that specifically activates the HER4/p180erbB4 receptor. *J. Biol. Chem.* **1993**, *268*, 18407–18410. [CrossRef]
28. Tzahar, E.; Levkowitz, G.; Karunagaran, D.; Yi, L.; Peles, E.; Lavi, S.; Chang, D.; Liu, N.; Yayon, A.; Wen, D. ErbB-3 and ErbB-4 function as the respective low and high affinity receptors of all Neu differentiation factor/heregulin isoforms. *J. Biol. Chem.* **1994**, *269*, 25226–25233. [CrossRef]
29. Plowman, G.D.; Green, J.M.; Culouscou, J.-M.; Carlton, G.W.; Rothwell, V.M.; Buckley, S. Heregulin induces tyrosine phosphorylation of HER4/p180erbB4. *Nature* **1993**, *366*, 473–475. [CrossRef]
30. Zhang, D.; Sliwkowski, M.X.; Mark, M.; Frantz, G.; Akita, R.; Sun, Y.; Hillan, K.; Crowley, C.; Brush, J.; Godowski, P.J. Neuregulin-3 (NRG3): A novel neural tissue-enriched protein that binds and activates ErbB4. *Proc. Natl. Acad. Sci. USA* **1997**, *94*, 9562–9567. [CrossRef]
31. Ebner, R.; Derynck, R. Epidermal growth factor and transforming growth factor-alpha: Differential intracellular routing and processing of ligand-receptor complexes. *Cell Regul.* **1991**, *2*, 599–612. [CrossRef] [PubMed]
32. Sweeney, C.; Lai, C.; Riese, D.J.; Diamonti, A.J.; Cantley, L.C.; Carraway, K.L. Ligand Discrimination in Signaling through an ErbB4 Receptor Homodimer. *J. Biol. Chem.* **2000**, *275*, 19803–19807. [CrossRef]
33. Riese, D.J.; Kim, E.D.; Elenius, K.; Buckley, S.; Klagsbrun, M.; Plowman, G.D.; Stern, D.F. The Epidermal Growth Factor Receptor Couples Transforming Growth Factor-α, Heparin-binding Epidermal Growth Factor-like Factor, and Amphiregulin to Neu, ErbB-3, and ErbB-4. *J. Biol. Chem.* **1996**, *271*, 20047–20052. [CrossRef] [PubMed]
34. Lemmon, M.A.; Bu, Z.; Ladbury, J.E.; Zhou, M.; Pinchasi, D.; Lax, I.; Engelman, D.M.; Schlessinger, J. Two EGF molecules contribute additively to stabilization of the EGFR dimer. *EMBO J.* **1997**, *16*, 281–294. [CrossRef] [PubMed]
35. Riese, D.J.; van Raaij, T.M.; Plowman, G.D.; Andrews, G.C.; Stern, D.F. The cellular response to neuregulins is governed by complex interactions of the erbB receptor family. *Mol. Cell. Biol.* **1995**, *15*, 5770–5776. [CrossRef] [PubMed]
36. Wen, D.; Peles, E.; Cupples, R.; Suggs, S.V.; Bacus, S.S.; Luo, Y.; Trail, G.; Hu, S.; Silbiger, S.M.; Levy, R.B.; et al. Neu differentiation factor: A transmembrane glycoprotein containing an EGF domain and an immunoglobulin homology unit. *Cell* **1992**, *69*, 559–572. [CrossRef]
37. Tidcombe, H.; Jackson-Fisher, A.; Mathers, K.; Stern, D.F.; Gassmann, M.; Golding, J.P. Neural and mammary gland defects in ErbB4 knockout mice genetically rescued from embryonic lethality. *Proc. Natl. Acad. Sci. USA* **2003**, *100*, 8281–8286. [CrossRef] [PubMed]
38. Chuu, C.-P.; Chen, R.-Y.; Barkinge, J.L.; Ciaccio, M.F.; Jones, R.B. Systems-Level Analysis of ErbB4 Signaling in Breast Cancer: A Laboratory to Clinical Perspective. *Mol. Cancer Res.* **2008**, *6*, 885. [CrossRef] [PubMed]
39. Hollmén, M.; Määttä, J.A.; Bald, L.; Sliwkowski, M.X.; Elenius, K. Suppression of breast cancer cell growth by a monoclonal antibody targeting cleavable ErbB4 isoforms. *Oncogene* **2009**, *28*, 1309–1319. [CrossRef] [PubMed]
40. Kountourakis, P.; Pavlakis, K.; Psyrri, A.; Rontogianni, D.; Xiros, N.; Patsouris, E.; Pectasides, D.; Economopoulos, T. Prognostic significance of HER3 and HER4 protein expression in colorectal adenocarcinomas. *BMC Cancer* **2006**, *6*, 46. [CrossRef] [PubMed]
41. Kishore, C.; Bhadra, P. Current advancements and future perspectives of immunotherapy in colorectal cancer research. *Eur. J. Pharmacol.* **2021**, *893*, 173819. [CrossRef] [PubMed]
42. de Wit, M.; Fijneman, R.J.A.; Verheul, H.M.W.; Meijer, G.A.; Jimenez, C.R. Proteomics in colorectal cancer translational research: Biomarker discovery for clinical applications. *Clin. Biochem.* **2013**, *46*, 466–479. [CrossRef] [PubMed]
43. Yin, H.; Favreau-Lessard, A.J.; deKay, J.T.; Herrmann, Y.R.; Robich, M.P.; Koza, R.A.; Prudovsky, I.; Sawyer, D.B.; Ryzhov, S. Protective role of ErbB3 signaling in myeloid cells during adaptation to cardiac pressure overload. *J. Mol. Cell. Cardiol.* **2021**, *152*, 1–16. [CrossRef] [PubMed]
44. Frey, M.R.; Edelblum, K.L.; Mullane, M.T.; Liang, D.; Polk, D.B. The ErbB4 Growth Factor Receptor Is Required for Colon Epithelial Cell Survival in the Presence of TNF. *Gastroenterology* **2009**, *136*, 217–226. [CrossRef]
45. Keates, S.; Sougioultzis, S.; Keates, A.C.; Zhao, D.; Peek, R.M.; Shaw, L.M.; Kelly, C.P. cag+ Helicobacter pylori Induce Transactivation of the Epidermal Growth Factor Receptor in AGS Gastric Epithelial Cells. *J. Biol. Chem.* **2001**, *276*, 48127–48134. [CrossRef]
46. Williams, C.S.; Bernard, J.K.; Demory Beckler, M.; Almohazey, D.; Washington, M.K.; Smith, J.J.; Frey, M.R. ERBB4 is overexpressed in human colon cancer and enhances cellular transformation. *Carcinogenesis* **2015**, *36*, 710–718. [CrossRef] [PubMed]
47. Zhu, Y.; Sullivan, L.L.; Nair, S.S.; Williams, C.C.; Pandey, A.K.; Marrero, L.; Vadlamudi, R.K.; Jones, F.E. Coregulation of Estrogen Receptor by ERBB4/HER4 Establishes a Growth-Promoting Autocrine Signal in Breast Tumor Cells. *Cancer Res.* **2006**, *66*, 7991–7998. [CrossRef]
48. Thien, C.B.F.; Langdon, W.Y. Tyrosine kinase activity of the EGF receptor is enhanced by the expression of oncogenic 70Z-Cbl. *Oncogene* **1997**, *15*, 2909–2919. [CrossRef] [PubMed]
49. Pawar, A.B.; Sengupta, D. Resolving the conformational dynamics of ErbB growth factor receptor dimers. *J. Struct. Biol.* **2019**, *207*, 225–233. [CrossRef] [PubMed]

50. Tomizawa, K.; Suda, K.; Onozato, R.; Kuwano, H.; Yatabe, Y.; Mitsudomi, T. Analysis of ERBB4 Mutations and Expression in Japanese Patients with Lung Cancer. *J. Thorac. Oncol.* **2010**, *5*, 1859–1861. [CrossRef]
51. Ding, L.; Getz, G.; Wheeler, D.A.; Mardis, E.R.; McLellan, M.D.; Cibulskis, K.; Sougnez, C.; Greulich, H.; Muzny, D.M.; Morgan, M.B.; et al. Somatic mutations affect key pathways in lung adenocarcinoma. *Nature* **2008**, *455*, 1069–1075. [CrossRef]
52. Kurppa, K.J.; Denessiouk, K.; Johnson, M.S.; Elenius, K. Activating ERBB4 mutations in non-small cell lung cancer. *Oncogene* **2016**, *35*, 1283–1291. [CrossRef] [PubMed]
53. Zhang, Y.; Zhang, L.; Li, R.; Chang, D.W.; Ye, Y.; Minna, J.D.; Roth, J.A.; Han, B.; Wu, X. Genetic variations in cancer-related significantly mutated genes and lung cancer susceptibility. *Ann. Oncol.* **2017**, *28*, 1625–1630. [CrossRef] [PubMed]
54. Uchida, T.; Wada, K.; Akamatsu, T.; Yonezawa, M.; Noguchi, H.; Mizoguchi, A.; Kasuga, M.; Sakamoto, C. A Novel Epidermal Growth Factor-like Molecule Containing Two Follistatin Modules Stimulates Tyrosine Phosphorylation of erbB-4 in MKN28 Gastric Cancer Cells. *Biochem. Biophys. Res. Commun.* **1999**, *266*, 593–602. [CrossRef]
55. Song, G.; Zhang, H.; Chen, C.; Gong, L.; Chen, B.; Zhao, S.; Shi, J.; Xu, J.; Ye, Z. miR-551b regulates epithelial-mesenchymal transition and metastasis of gastric cancer by inhibiting ERBB4 expression. *Oncotarget* **2017**, *8*, 45725. [CrossRef]
56. Chen, K.; Yang, D.; Li, X.; Sun, B.; Song, F.; Cao, W.; Brat, D.J.; Gao, Z.; Li, H.; Liang, H.; et al. Mutational landscape of gastric adenocarcinoma in Chinese: Implications for prognosis and therapy. *Proc. Natl. Acad. Sci. USA* **2015**, *112*, 1107–1112. [CrossRef] [PubMed]
57. Liu, Y.; Song, L.; Ni, H.; Sun, L.; Jiao, W.; Chen, L.; Zhou, Q.; Shen, T.; Cui, H.; Gao, T.; et al. ERBB4 acts as a suppressor in the development of hepatocellular carcinoma. *Carcinogenesis* **2017**, *38*, 465–473. [CrossRef] [PubMed]
58. Park, S.T.; Jang, J.W.; Kim, G.D.; Park, J.A.; Hur, W.; Woo, H.Y.; Kim, J.D.; Kwon, J.H.; Yoo, C.R.; Bae, S.H.; et al. Beneficial effect of metronomic chemotherapy on tumor suppression and survival in a rat model of hepatocellular carcinoma with liver cirrhosis. *Cancer Chemother. Pharmacol.* **2010**, *65*, 1029–1037. [CrossRef]
59. Edwards, J.; Traynor, P.; Munro, A.F.; Pirret, C.F.; Dunne, B.; Bartlett, J.M.S. The Role of HER1-HER4 and EGFRvIII in Hormone-Refractory Prostate Cancer. *Clin. Cancer Res.* **2006**, *12*, 123–130. [CrossRef]
60. Hernes, E.; Fosså, S.D.; Berner, A.; Otnes, B.; Nesland, J.M. Expression of the epidermal growth factor receptor family in prostate carcinoma before and during androgen-independence. *Br. J. Cancer* **2004**, *90*, 449–454. [CrossRef]
61. Ping, P.; Zhang, J.; Zheng, Y.-T.; Li, R.C.X.; Dawn, B.; Tang, X.-L.; Takano, H.; Balafanova, Z.; Bolli, R. Demonstration of Selective Protein Kinase C–Dependent Activation of Src and Lck Tyrosine Kinases During Ischemic Preconditioning in Conscious Rabbits. *Circ. Res.* **1999**, *85*, 542–550. [CrossRef] [PubMed]
62. Gallo, R.M.; Bryant, I.; Fry, R.; Williams, E.E.; Riese, D.J. Phosphorylation of ErbB4 on Tyr1056 is critical for inhibition of colony formation by prostate tumor cell lines. *Biochem. Biophys. Res. Commun.* **2006**, *349*, 372–382. [CrossRef]
63. Tsai, Y.-S.; Cheng, H.-L.; Tzai, T.-S.; Chow, N.-H. Clinical Significance of ErbB Receptor Family in Urothelial Carcinoma of the Bladder: A Systematic Review and Meta-Analysis. *Adv. Urol.* **2012**, *2012*, 181964. [CrossRef]
64. Memon, A.A.; Sorensen, B.S.; Meldgaard, P.; Fokdal, L.; Thykjaer, T.; Nexo, E. The relation between survival and expression of HER1 and HER2 depends on the expression of HER3 and HER4: A study in bladder cancer patients. *Br. J. Cancer* **2006**, *94*, 1703–1709. [CrossRef]
65. El Badadawy, N.; Youssef, N.; Ismail, A.; Ragheb, F.; Hakim, S. Evaluation of the role of immunohistochemical expression of EGFR (ERB B1) and HER4 (ERB B4) in urinary bladder urothelial carcinoma. *Pathology* **2016**, *48*, S123. [CrossRef]
66. Saglam, O.; Xiong, Y.; Marchion, D.C.; Strosberg, C.; Wenham, R.M.; Johnson, J.J.; Saeed-Vafa, D.; Cubitt, C.; Hakam, A.; Magliocco, A.M. ERBB4 Expression in Ovarian Serous Carcinoma Resistant to Platinum-Based Therapy. *Cancer Control.* **2017**, *24*, 89–95. [CrossRef] [PubMed]
67. Sundvall, M.; Veikkolainen, V.; Kurppa, K.; Salah, Z.; Tvorogov, D.; Zoelen, E.J.V.; Aqeilan, R.; Elenius, K. Cell Death or Survival Promoted by Alternative Isoforms of ErbB4. *Mol. Biol. Cell* **2010**, *21*, 4275–4286. [CrossRef]
68. Muraoka-Cook, R.S.; Sandahl, M.; Husted, C.; Hunter, D.; Miraglia, L.; Feng, S.-M.; Elenius, K.; Earp, S.I.H. The Intracellular Domain of ErbB4 Induces Differentiation of Mammary Epithelial Cells. *Mol. Biol. Cell* **2006**, *17*, 4118–4129. [CrossRef] [PubMed]
69. Junttila, T.T.; Sundvall, M.; Määttä, J.A.; Elenius, K. ErbB4 and Its Isoforms: Selective Regulation of Growth Factor Responses by Naturally Occurring Receptor Variants. *Trends Cardiovasc. Med.* **2000**, *10*, 304–310. [CrossRef]
70. Gullick, W.J. c-erbB-4/HER4: Friend or foe? *J. Pathol.* **2003**, *200*, 279–281. [CrossRef] [PubMed]
71. Koutras, A.K.; Kalogeras, K.T.; Dimopoulos, M.A.; Wirtz, R.M.; Dafni, U.; Briasoulis, E.; Pectasides, D.; Gogas, H.; Christodoulou, C.; Aravantinos, G.; et al. Evaluation of the prognostic and predictive value of HER family mRNA expression in high-risk early breast cancer: A Hellenic Cooperative Oncology Group (HeCOG) study. *Br. J. Cancer* **2008**, *99*, 1775–1785. [CrossRef] [PubMed]
72. Sassen, A.; Rochon, J.; Wild, P.; Hartmann, A.; Hofstaedter, F.; Schwarz, S.; Brockhoff, G. Cytogenetic analysis of HER1/EGFR, HER2, HER3 and HER4 in 278 breast cancer patients. *Breast Cancer Res.* **2008**, *10*, R2. [CrossRef] [PubMed]
73. Bacus, S.S.; Chin, D.; Yarden, Y.; Zelnick, C.R.; Stern, D.F. Type 1 receptor tyrosine kinases are differentially phosphorylated in mammary carcinoma and differentially associated with steroid receptors. *Am. J. Pathol.* **1996**, *148*, 549–558.
74. Kew, T.Y.; Bell, J.A.; Pinder, S.E.; Denley, H.; Srinivasan, R.; Gullick, W.J.; Nicholson, R.I.; Blamey, R.W.; Ellis, I.O. c-erbB-4 protein expression in human breast cancer. *Br. J. Cancer* **2000**, *82*, 1163–1170. [CrossRef]
75. Bièche, I.; Onody, P.; Tozlu, S.; Driouch, K.; Vidaud, M.; Lidereau, R. Prognostic value of ERBB family mRNA expression in breast carcinomas. *Int. J. Cancer* **2003**, *106*, 758–765. [CrossRef]

76. Lodge, A.J.; Anderson, J.J.; Gullick, W.J.; Haugk, B.; Leonard, R.C.F.; Angus, B. Type 1 growth factor receptor expression in node positive breast cancer: Adverse prognostic significance of c-erbB-4. *J. Clin. Pathol.* **2003**, *56*, 300–304. [CrossRef] [PubMed]
77. Määttä, J.A.; Sundvall, M.; Junttila, T.T.; Peri, L.; Laine, V.J.O.; Isola, J.; Egeblad, M.; Elenius, K. Proteolytic Cleavage and Phosphorylation of a Tumor-associated ErbB4 Isoform Promote Ligand-independent Survival and Cancer Cell Growth. *Mol. Biol. Cell* **2006**, *17*, 67–79. [CrossRef] [PubMed]
78. Junttila, T.T.; Sundvall, M.; Lundin, M.; Lundin, J.; Tanner, M.; Härkönen, P.; Joensuu, H.; Isola, J.; Elenius, K. Cleavable ErbB4 Isoform in Estrogen Receptor–Regulated Growth of Breast Cancer Cells. *Cancer Res.* **2005**, *65*, 1384–1393. [CrossRef]
79. Lynch, C.C.; Vargo-Gogola, T.; Martin, M.D.; Fingleton, B.; Crawford, H.C.; Matrisian, L.M. Matrix Metalloproteinase 7 Mediates Mammary Epithelial Cell Tumorigenesis through the ErbB4 Receptor. *Cancer Res.* **2007**, *67*, 6760–6767. [CrossRef]
80. Muraoka-Cook, R.S.; Caskey, L.S.; Sandahl, M.A.; Hunter, D.M.; Husted, C.; Strunk, K.E.; Sartor, C.I.; Rearick, W.A.; McCall, W.; Sgagias, M.K.; et al. Heregulin-Dependent Delay in Mitotic Progression Requires HER4 and BRCA1. *Mol. Cell. Biol.* **2006**, *26*, 6412–6424. [CrossRef] [PubMed]
81. Naresh, A.; Long, W.; Vidal, G.A.; Wimley, W.C.; Marrero, L.; Sartor, C.I.; Tovey, S.; Cooke, T.G.; Bartlett, J.M.S.; Jones, F.E. The ERBB4/HER4 Intracellular Domain 4ICD Is a BH3-Only Protein Promoting Apoptosis of Breast Cancer Cells. *Cancer Res.* **2006**, *66*, 6412–6420. [CrossRef] [PubMed]
82. Sundvall, M.; Iljin, K.; Kilpinen, S.; Sara, H.; Kallioniemi, O.-P.; Elenius, K. Role of ErbB4 in Breast Cancer. *J. Mammary Gland. Biol. Neoplasia* **2008**, *13*, 259–268. [CrossRef]
83. Hollmén, M.; Liu, P.; Kurppa, K.; Wildiers, H.; Reinvall, I.; Vandorpe, T.; Smeets, A.; Deraedt, K.; Vahlberg, T.; Joensuu, H.; et al. Proteolytic Processing of ErbB4 in Breast Cancer. *PLoS ONE* **2012**, *7*, e39413. [CrossRef] [PubMed]
84. te Velde, E.A.; Franke, A.C.; van Hillegersberg, R.; Elshof, S.M.; de Weger, R.W.; Borel Rinkes, I.H.M.; van Diest, P.J. HER-family gene amplification and expression in resected pancreatic cancer. *Eur. J. Surg. Oncol.* **2009**, *35*, 1098–1104. [CrossRef]
85. Mill, C.P.; Gettinger, K.L.; Riese, D.J. Ligand stimulation of ErbB4 and a constitutively-active ErbB4 mutant result in different biological responses in human pancreatic tumor cell lines. *Exp. Cell Res.* **2011**, *317*, 392–404. [CrossRef] [PubMed]
86. Thybusch-Bernhardt, A.; Beckmann, S.; Juhl, H. Comparative analysis of the EGF-receptor family in pancreatic cancer: Expression of HER-4 correlates with a favourable tumor stage. *Int. J. Surg. Investig.* **2001**, *2*, 393–400. [PubMed]
87. Graber, H.U.; Friess, H.; Kaufmann, B.; Willi, D.; Zimmermann, A.; Korc, M.; Büchler, M.W. ErbB-4 mRNA expression is decreased in non-metastatic pancreatic cancer. *Int. J. Cancer* **1999**, *84*, 24–27. [CrossRef]
88. Jones, D.C.; Scanteianu, A.; DiStefano, M.; Bouhaddou, M.; Birtwistle, M.R. Analysis of copy number loss of the ErbB4 receptor tyrosine kinase in glioblastoma. *PLoS ONE* **2018**, *13*, e0190664. [CrossRef]
89. Andersson, U.; Guo, D.; Malmer, B.; Bergenheim, A.T.; Brännström, T.; Hedman, H.; Henriksson, R. Epidermal growth factor receptor family (EGFR, ErbB2–4) in gliomas and meningiomas. *Acta Neuropathol.* **2004**, *108*, 135–142. [CrossRef]
90. Donoghue, J.F.; Kerr, L.T.; Alexander, N.W.; Greenall, S.A.; Longano, A.B.; Gottardo, N.G.; Wang, R.; Tabar, V.; Adams, T.E.; Mischel, P.S.; et al. Activation of ERBB4 in Glioblastoma Can Contribute to Increased Tumorigenicity and Influence Therapeutic Response. *Cancers* **2018**, *10*, 243. [CrossRef]
91. Prickett, T.D.; Agrawal, N.S.; Wei, X.; Yates, K.E.; Lin, J.C.; Wunderlich, J.R.; Cronin, J.C.; Cruz, P.; Rosenberg, S.A.; Samuels, Y.; et al. Analysis of the tyrosine kinome in melanoma reveals recurrent mutations in ERBB4. *Nat. Genet.* **2009**, *41*, 1127–1132. [CrossRef]
92. Nielsen, T.O.; Poulsen, S.S.; Journe, F.; Ghanem, G.; Sorensen, B.S. HER4 and its cytoplasmic isoforms are associated with progression-free survival of malignant melanoma. *Melanoma Res.* **2014**, *24*, 88–91. [CrossRef]
93. Kurppa, K.; Elenius, K. Mutated ERBB4: A novel drug target in metastatic melanoma? *Pigment. Cell Melanoma Res.* **2009**, *22*, 708–710. [CrossRef] [PubMed]
94. Settleman, J. A Therapeutic Opportunity in Melanoma: ErbB4 Makes a Mark on Skin. *Cancer Cell* **2009**, *16*, 278–279. [CrossRef] [PubMed]
95. Siegel, R.L.; Miller, K.D.; Fuchs, H.E.; Jemal, A. Cancer Statistics, 2021. *CA Cancer J. Clin.* **2021**, *71*, 7–33. [CrossRef]
96. Ejskjær, K.; Sørensen, B.S.; Poulsen, S.S.; Forman, A.; Nexø, E.; Mogensen, O. Expression of the epidermal growth factor system in endometrioid endometrial cancer. *Gynecol. Oncol.* **2007**, *104*, 158–167. [CrossRef]
97. Jaffe, N. Osteosarcoma: Review of the Past, Impact on the Future. The American Experience. In *Pediatric and Adolescent Osteosarcoma*; Jaffe, N., Bruland, O.S., Bielack, S., Eds.; Springer: Boston, MA, USA, 2010; pp. 239–262.
98. Dai, X.; Ma, W.; He, X.; Jha, R.K. Review of therapeutic strategies for osteosarcoma, chondrosarcoma, and Ewing's sarcoma. *Med. Sci. Monit.* **2011**, *17*, RA177–RA190. [CrossRef] [PubMed]
99. Li, X.; Huang, Q.; Wang, S.; Huang, Z.; Yu, F.; Lin, J. HER4 promotes the growth and metastasis of osteosarcoma via the PI3K/AKT pathway. *Acta Biochim. Biophys. Sin.* **2020**, *52*, 345–362. [CrossRef]
100. Xie, H.; Lin, L.; Tong, L.; Jiang, Y.; Zheng, M.; Chen, Z.; Jiang, X.; Zhang, X.; Ren, X.; Qu, W.; et al. AST1306, A Novel Irreversible Inhibitor of the Epidermal Growth Factor Receptor 1 and 2, Exhibits Antitumor Activity Both In Vitro and In Vivo. *PLoS ONE* **2011**, *6*, e21487. [CrossRef] [PubMed]
101. Zhang, J.; Cao, J.; Li, J.; Zhang, Y.; Chen, Z.; Peng, W.; Sun, S.; Zhao, N.; Wang, J.; Zhong, D.; et al. A phase I study of AST1306, a novel irreversible EGFR and HER2 kinase inhibitor, in patients with advanced solid tumors. *J. Hematol. Oncol.* **2014**, *7*, 22. [CrossRef]

102. Sabbah, D.A.; Brattain, M.G.; Zhong, H. Dual Inhibitors of PI3K/mTOR or mTOR-Selective Inhibitors: Which Way Shall We Go? *Curr. Med. Chem.* **2011**, *18*, 5528–5544. [CrossRef]
103. Ahammad, I.; Sarker, M.R.I.; Khan, A.M.; Islam, S.; Hossain, M. Virtual Screening to Identify Novel Inhibitors of Pan ERBB Family of Proteins from Natural Products with Known Anti-tumorigenic Properties. *Int. J. Pept. Res. Ther.* **2020**, *26*, 1923–1938. [CrossRef]
104. To Evaluate the Efficacy and Safety of Anlotinib Combined with Allitinib in Lung Cancer. Available online: https://ClinicalTrials.gov/show/NCT04671303 (accessed on 30 November 2021).
105. Lee, H.; Kim, J.W.; Choi, D.K.; Yu, J.H.; Kim, J.H.; Lee, D.-S.; Min, S.-H. Poziotinib suppresses ovarian cancer stem cell growth via inhibition of HER4-mediated STAT5 pathway. *Biochem. Biophys. Res. Commun.* **2020**, *526*, 158–164. [CrossRef]
106. Subramanian, J.; Katta, A.; Masood, A.; Vudem, D.R.; Kancha, R.K. Emergence of ERBB2 Mutation as a Biomarker and an Actionable Target in Solid Cancers. *Oncologist* **2019**, *24*, e1303–e1314. [CrossRef]
107. Cha, M.Y.; Lee, K.-O.; Kim, M.; Song, J.Y.; Lee, K.H.; Park, J.; Chae, Y.J.; Kim, Y.H.; Suh, K.H.; Lee, G.S.; et al. Antitumor activity of HM781-36B, a highly effective pan-HER inhibitor in erlotinib-resistant NSCLC and other EGFR-dependent cancer models. *Int. J. Cancer* **2012**, *130*, 2445–2454. [CrossRef] [PubMed]
108. A Study of Poziotinib in Combination with T-DM1 in HER2-Positive Breast Cancer. Available online: https://ClinicalTrials.gov/show/NCT03429101 (accessed on 30 November 2021).
109. Poziotinib in Patients with NSCLC Having EGFR or HER2 Exon 20 Insertion Mutation. Available online: https://ClinicalTrials.gov/show/NCT04044170 (accessed on 30 November 2021).
110. NOV120101 (Poziotinib) for 1st Line Monotherapy in Patients with Lung Adenocarcinoma. Available online: https://ClinicalTrials.gov/show/NCT01819428 (accessed on 30 November 2021).
111. Study of Poziotinib in Patients with HER2-Positive Metastatic Breast Cancer. Available online: https://ClinicalTrials.gov/show/NCT02659514 (accessed on 30 November 2021).
112. A Mass Balance and Pharmacokinetics Study of 14C-Labeled Poziotinib in Cancer Patients Suitable for Treatment with Poziotinib. Available online: https://ClinicalTrials.gov/show/NCT03804515 (accessed on 30 November 2021).
113. Poziotinib in Patients with HER2+ Recurrent Stage IV BC Who Have Received at Least 2 Prior HER2-Directed Regimens. Available online: https://ClinicalTrials.gov/show/NCT02418689 (accessed on 30 November 2021).
114. Search Result of Poziotinib in clinicaltrials.gov. Available online: https://clinicaltrials.gov/ct2/results?recrs=&cond=&term=poziotinib&cntry=&state=&city=&dist=%20 (accessed on 30 November 2021).
115. Lee, H.; Kim, J.W.; Lee, D.-S.; Min, S.-H. Combined Poziotinib with Manidipine Treatment Suppresses Ovarian Cancer Stem-Cell Proliferation and Stemness. *Int. J. Mol. Sci.* **2020**, *21*, 7379. [CrossRef] [PubMed]
116. Motohara, T.; Katabuchi, H. Ovarian Cancer Stemness: Biological and Clinical Implications for Metastasis and Chemotherapy Resistance. *Cancers* **2019**, *11*, 907. [CrossRef]
117. Patch, A.-M.; Christie, E.L.; Etemadmoghadam, D.; Garsed, D.W.; George, J.; Fereday, S.; Nones, K.; Cowin, P.; Alsop, K.; Bailey, P.J.; et al. Whole–genome characterization of chemoresistant ovarian cancer. *Nature* **2015**, *521*, 489–494. [CrossRef]
118. Yap, T.A.; Carden, C.P.; Kaye, S.B. Beyond chemotherapy: Targeted therapies in ovarian cancer. *Nat. Rev. Cancer* **2009**, *9*, 167–181. [CrossRef]
119. Rosell, R.; Carcereny, E.; Gervais, R.; Vergnenegre, A.; Massuti, B.; Felip, E.; Palmero, R.; Garcia-Gomez, R.; Pallares, C.; Sanchez, J.M.; et al. Erlotinib versus standard chemotherapy as first-line treatment for European patients with advanced EGFR mutation-positive non-small-cell lung cancer (EURTAC): A multicentre, open-label, randomised phase 3 trial. *Lancet Oncol.* **2012**, *13*, 239–246. [CrossRef]
120. Wu, Y.-L.; Cheng, Y.; Zhou, X.; Lee, K.H.; Nakagawa, K.; Niho, S.; Tsuji, F.; Linke, R.; Rosell, R.; Corral, J.; et al. Dacomitinib versus gefitinib as first-line treatment for patients with EGFR-mutation-positive non-small-cell lung cancer (ARCHER 1050): A randomised, open-label, phase 3 trial. *Lancet Oncol.* **2017**, *18*, 1454–1466. [CrossRef]
121. Girard, N. Optimizing outcomes in EGFR mutation-positive NSCLC: Which tyrosine kinase inhibitor and when? *Future Oncol.* **2018**, *14*, 1117–1132. [CrossRef] [PubMed]
122. Passaro, A.; de Marinis, F. Dacomitinib in EGFR-positive non-small cell lung cancer: An attractive but broken option. *Transl. Lung Cancer Res.* **2018**, *7*, S100–S102. [CrossRef] [PubMed]
123. Bilancia, D.; Rosati, G.; Dinota, A.; Germano, D.; Romano, R.; Manzione, L. Lapatinib in breast cancer. *Ann. Oncol.* **2007**, *18*, vi26–vi30. [CrossRef]
124. Tsang, R.Y.; Sadeghi, S.; Finn, R.S. Lapatinib, a Dual-Targeted Small Molecule Inhibitor of EGFR and HER2, in HER2-Amplified Breast Cancer: From Bench to Bedside. *Clin. Med. Insights Ther.* **2011**, *3*, CMT.S3783. [CrossRef]
125. Wind, S.; Schnell, D.; Ebner, T.; Freiwald, M.; Stopfer, P. Clinical Pharmacokinetics and Pharmacodynamics of Afatinib. *Clin. Pharmacokinet.* **2017**, *56*, 235–250. [CrossRef] [PubMed]
126. Sekhon, N.; Kumbla, R.A.; Mita, M. Chapter 1—Current Trends in Cancer Therapy. In *Cardio-Oncology*; Gottlieb, R.A., Mehta, P.K., Eds.; Academic Press: Boston, MA, USA, 2017; pp. 1–24.
127. Balak, M.N.; Gong, Y.; Riely, G.J.; Somwar, R.; Li, A.R.; Zakowski, M.F.; Chiang, A.; Yang, G.; Ouerfelli, O.; Kris, M.G.; et al. Novel D761Y and Common Secondary T790M Mutations in Epidermal Growth Factor Receptor–Mutant Lung Adenocarcinomas with Acquired Resistance to Kinase Inhibitors. *Clin. Cancer Res.* **2006**, *12*, 6494–6501. [CrossRef] [PubMed]

128. Yang, J.C.-H.; Wu, Y.-L.; Schuler, M.; Sebastian, M.; Popat, S.; Yamamoto, N.; Zhou, C.; Hu, C.-P.; O'Byrne, K.; Feng, J.; et al. Afatinib versus cisplatin-based chemotherapy for EGFR mutation-positive lung adenocarcinoma (LUX-Lung 3 and LUX-Lung 6): Analysis of overall survival data from two randomised, phase 3 trials. *Lancet Oncol.* **2015**, *16*, 141–151. [CrossRef]
129. Manzo, A.; Montanino, A.; Costanzo, R.; Sandomenico, C.; Palumbo, G.; Schettino, C.; Daniele, G.; Morabito, A.; Perrone, F.; Piccirillo, M.C. Chapter 33—EGFR Mutations: Best Results from Second- and Third-Generation Tyrosine Kinase Inhibitors. In *Oncogenomics*; Dammacco, F., Silvestris, F., Eds.; Academic Press: Cambridge, MA, USA, 2019; pp. 477–486.
130. Keating, G.M. Afatinib: A Review of Its Use in the Treatment of Advanced Non-Small Cell Lung Cancer. *Drugs* **2014**, *74*, 207–221. [CrossRef]
131. Sachdev, J.C.; Jahanzeb, M. Blockade of the HER Family of Receptors in the Treatment of HER2-Positive Metastatic Breast Cancer. *Clin. Breast Cancer* **2012**, *12*, 19–29. [CrossRef]
132. Ayati, A.; Moghimi, S.; Salarinejad, S.; Safavi, M.; Pouramiri, B.; Foroumadi, A. A review on progression of epidermal growth factor receptor (EGFR) inhibitors as an efficient approach in cancer targeted therapy. *Bioorg. Chem.* **2020**, *99*, 103811. [CrossRef]
133. A Phase II Study of CI-1033 in Treating Patients with Metastatic (Stage IV) Breast Cancer. Available online: https://ClinicalTrials.gov/show/NCT00051051 (accessed on 30 November 2021).
134. PH 1 Evaluation Of Oral CI-1033 In Combination With Paclitaxel/Carboplatin As 1st Line Chemotherapy In NSCLC Patients. Available online: https://ClinicalTrials.gov/show/NCT00174356 (accessed on 30 November 2021).
135. A Phase 2, Randomized, Open-Label Study Of Single Agent CI-1033 in Patients with Advanced Non-Small Cell Lung Cancer. Available online: https://ClinicalTrials.gov/show/NCT00050830 (accessed on 30 November 2021).
136. Singh, P.K.; Singh, H.; Silakari, O. Kinases inhibitors in lung cancer: From benchside to bedside. *Biochim. Biophys. Acta (BBA)—Rev. Cancer* **2016**, *1866*, 128–140. [CrossRef] [PubMed]
137. Collins, D.M.; Conlon, N.T.; Kannan, S.; Verma, C.S.; Eli, L.D.; Lalani, A.S.; Crown, J. Preclinical Characteristics of the Irreversible Pan-HER Kinase Inhibitor Neratinib Compared with Lapatinib: Implications for the Treatment of HER2-Positive and HER2-Mutated Breast Cancer. *Cancers* **2019**, *11*, 737. [CrossRef] [PubMed]
138. Prové, A.; Dirix, L. Neratinib for the treatment of breast cancer. *Expert Opin. Pharmacother.* **2016**, *17*, 2243–2248. [CrossRef]
139. Xu, B.; Yan, M.; Ma, F.; Hu, X.; Feng, J.; Ouyang, Q.; Tong, Z.; Li, H.; Zhang, Q.; Sun, T.; et al. Pyrotinib plus capecitabine versus lapatinib plus capecitabine for the treatment of HER2-positive metastatic breast cancer (PHOEBE): A multicentre, open-label, randomised, controlled, phase 3 trial. *Lancet Oncol.* **2021**, *22*, 351–360. [CrossRef]
140. Gao, Z.; Song, C.; Li, G.; Lin, H.; Lian, X.; Zhang, N.; Cao, B. Pyrotinib treatment on HER2-positive gastric cancer cells promotes the released exosomes to enhance endothelial cell progression, which can be counteracted by apatinib. *OncoTargets Ther.* **2019**, *12*, 2777–2787. [CrossRef] [PubMed]
141. Blair, H.A. Pyrotinib: First Global Approval. *Drugs* **2018**, *78*, 1751–1755. [CrossRef] [PubMed]
142. A Study of Pyrotinib Plus Vinorelbine in Patients with Brain Metastases from HER2-Positive Metastatic Breast Cancer. Available online: https://ClinicalTrials.gov/show/NCT03933982 (accessed on 30 November 2021).
143. Inetetamab Combined with Pyrotinib and Chemotherapy in the Treatment of HER2 Positive Metastatic Breast Cancer. Available online: https://ClinicalTrials.gov/show/NCT04681911 (accessed on 30 November 2021).
144. Berglöf, A.; Hamasy, A.; Meinke, S.; Palma, M.; Krstic, A.; Månsson, R.; Kimby, E.; Österborg, A.; Smith, C.I.E. Targets for Ibrutinib Beyond B Cell Malignancies. *Scand. J. Immunol.* **2015**, *82*, 208–217. [CrossRef] [PubMed]
145. Blanke, C.D.; Demetri, G.D.; Mehren, M.V.; Heinrich, M.C.; Eisenberg, B.; Fletcher, J.A.; Corless, C.L.; Fletcher, C.D.M.; Roberts, P.J.; Heinz, D.; et al. Long-Term Results From a Randomized Phase II Trial of Standard- Versus Higher-Dose Imatinib Mesylate for Patients With Unresectable or Metastatic Gastrointestinal Stromal Tumors Expressing KIT. *J. Clin. Oncol.* **2008**, *26*, 620–625. [CrossRef] [PubMed]
146. Herman, S.E.M.; Gordon, A.L.; Hertlein, E.; Ramanunni, A.; Zhang, X.; Jaglowski, S.; Flynn, J.; Jones, J.; Blum, K.A.; Buggy, J.J.; et al. Bruton tyrosine kinase represents a promising therapeutic target for treatment of chronic lymphocytic leukemia and is effectively targeted by PCI-32765. *Blood* **2011**, *117*, 6287–6296. [CrossRef] [PubMed]
147. Rushworth, S.A.; Bowles, K.M.; Barrera, L.N.; Murray, M.Y.; Zaitseva, L.; MacEwan, D.J. BTK inhibitor ibrutinib is cytotoxic to myeloma and potently enhances bortezomib and lenalidomide activities through NF-κB. *Cell. Signal.* **2013**, *25*, 106–112. [CrossRef]
148. Wang, X.; Wong, J.; Sevinsky, C.J.; Kokabee, L.; Khan, F.; Sun, Y.; Conklin, D.S. Bruton's Tyrosine Kinase Inhibitors Prevent Therapeutic Escape in Breast Cancer Cells. *Mol. Cancer Ther.* **2016**, *15*, 2198–2208. [CrossRef]
149. Smith, M.R. Ibrutinib in B lymphoid malignancies. *Expert Opin. Pharmacother.* **2015**, *16*, 1879–1887. [CrossRef] [PubMed]
150. Rauf, F.; Festa, F.; Park, J.G.; Magee, M.; Eaton, S.; Rinaldi, C.; Betanzos, C.M.; Gonzalez-Malerva, L.; LaBaer, J. Ibrutinib inhibition of ERBB4 reduces cell growth in a WNT5A-dependent manner. *Oncogene* **2018**, *37*, 2237–2250. [CrossRef] [PubMed]
151. Honigberg, L.A.; Smith, A.M.; Sirisawad, M.; Verner, E.; Loury, D.; Chang, B.; Li, S.; Pan, Z.; Thamm, D.H.; Miller, R.A.; et al. The Bruton tyrosine kinase inhibitor PCI-32765 blocks B-cell activation and is efficacious in models of autoimmune disease and B-cell malignancy. *Proc. Natl. Acad. Sci. USA* **2010**, *107*, 13075–13080. [CrossRef] [PubMed]
152. Wong, T.W.; Lee, F.Y.; Yu, C.; Luo, F.R.; Oppenheimer, S.; Zhang, H.; Smykla, R.A.; Mastalerz, H.; Fink, B.E.; Hunt, J.T.; et al. Preclinical Antitumor Activity of BMS-599626, a pan-HER Kinase Inhibitor That Inhibits HER1/HER2 Homodimer and Heterodimer Signaling. *Clin. Cancer Res.* **2006**, *12*, 6186–6193. [CrossRef] [PubMed]

153. Gill, L.A.; Verdonk, M.; Boyle, G.R.; Taylor, R. A Comparison of Physicochemical Property Profiles of Marketed Oral Drugs and Orally Bioavailable Anti-Cancer Protein Kinase Inhibitors in Clinical Development. *Curr. Top. Med. Chem.* **2007**, *7*, 1408–1422. [PubMed]
154. Ashar, Y.V.; Zhou, J.; Gupta, P.; Teng, Q.-X.; Lei, Z.-N.; Reznik, S.E.; Lusvarghi, S.; Wurpel, J.; Ambudkar, S.V.; Chen, Z.-S. BMS-599626, a Highly Selective Pan-HER Kinase Inhibitor, Antagonizes ABCG2-Mediated Drug Resistance. *Cancers* **2020**, *12*, 2502. [CrossRef] [PubMed]
155. Pharmacokinetics (PK) Study of AC480 for Recurrent Glioma. Available online: https://ClinicalTrials.gov/show/NCT00979173 (accessed on 30 November 2021).
156. BMS-599626 in Treating Patients with Metastatic Solid Tumors. Available online: https://ClinicalTrials.gov/show/NCT00093730 (accessed on 30 November 2021).
157. BMS-599626 in Patients with Advanced Solid Malignancies. Available online: https://ClinicalTrials.gov/show/NCT00095537 (accessed on 30 November 2021).
158. MAD Refractory: Solid Tumor QD w/o Break. Available online: https://ClinicalTrials.gov/show/NCT00207012 (accessed on 30 November 2021).
159. Safety Study for Intravenous (IV) AC480 (AC480IV) to Treat Advanced Solid Tumors. Available online: https://ClinicalTrials.gov/show/NCT01245543 (accessed on 30 November 2021).
160. Haluska, P.; Carboni, J.M.; TenEyck, C.; Attar, R.M.; Hou, X.; Yu, C.; Sagar, M.; Wong, T.W.; Gottardis, M.M.; Erlichman, C. HER receptor signaling confers resistance to the insulin-like growth factor-I receptor inhibitor, BMS-536924. *Mol. Cancer Ther.* **2008**, *7*, 2589–2598. [CrossRef] [PubMed]
161. Zaraei, S.-O.; Sbenati, R.M.; Alach, N.N.; Anbar, H.S.; El-Gamal, R.; Tarazi, H.; Shehata, M.K.; Abdel-Maksoud, M.S.; Oh, C.-H.; El-Gamal, M.I. Discovery of first-in-class imidazothiazole-based potent and selective ErbB4 (HER4) kinase inhibitors. *Eur. J. Med. Chem.* **2021**, *224*, 113674. [CrossRef] [PubMed]

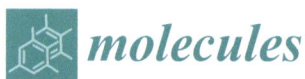

Article

Fabrication and Biological Assessment of Antidiabetic α-Mangostin Loaded Nanosponges: In Vitro, In Vivo, and In Silico Studies

Faisal Usman [1], Hamid Saeed Shah [2,*], Sumera Zaib [3,*], Sirikhwan Manee [4], Jahanzeb Mudassir [1], Ajmal Khan [5], Gaber El-Saber Batiha [6], Khamael M. Abualnaja [7], Dalal Alhashmialameer [7] and Imtiaz Khan [8,*]

[1] Department of Pharmaceutics, Faculty of Pharmacy, Bahauddin Zakariya University, Multan 66000, Pakistan; faisal.usman@bzu.edu.pk (F.U.); jahanzebmudassir@bzu.edu.pk (J.M.)
[2] Institute of Pharmaceutical Sciences, University of Veterinary and Animal Sciences, Lahore 54000, Pakistan
[3] Department of Biochemistry, Faculty of Life Sciences, University of Central Punjab, Lahore 54590, Pakistan
[4] Faculty of Traditional Thai Medicine, Prince of Songkla University, Hat-Yai, Songkhla 90110, Thailand; sirikhwan.m@gmail.com
[5] Natural and Medical Sciences Research Center, University of Nizwa, Nizwa 616, Oman; ajmalkhan@unizwa.edu.om
[6] Department of Pharmacology and Therapeutics, Faculty of Veterinary Medicine, Damanhour University, Damanhour 22511, Albeheira, Egypt; gaberbatiha@gmail.com
[7] Department of Chemistry, College of Science, Taif University, Taif 21944, Saudi Arabia; k.ala@tu.edu.sa (K.M.A.); dsamer@tu.edu.sa (D.A.)
[8] Department of Chemistry and Manchester Institute of Biotechnology, The University of Manchester, 131 Princess Street, Manchester M1 7DN, UK
* Correspondence: hamid.saeed@uvas.edu.pk (H.S.S.); sumera.zaib@ucp.edu.pk (S.Z.); imtiaz.khan@manchester.ac.uk (I.K.)

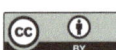

Abstract: Type 2 diabetes mellitus has been a major health issue with increasing morbidity and mortality due to macrovascular and microvascular complications. The urgent need for improved methods to control hyperglycemic complications reiterates the development of innovative preventive and therapeutic treatment strategies. In this perspective, xanthone compounds in the pericarp of the mangosteen fruit, especially α-mangostin (MGN), have been recognized to restore damaged pancreatic β-cells for optimal insulin release. Therefore, taking advantage of the robust use of nanotechnology for targeted drug delivery, we herein report the preparation of MGN loaded nanosponges for anti-diabetic therapeutic applications. The nanosponges were prepared by quasi-emulsion solvent evaporation method. Physico-chemical characterization of formulated nanosponges with satisfactory outcomes was performed with Fourier transform infra-red (FTIR) spectroscopy, differential scanning calorimetry (DSC), and scanning electron microscopy (SEM). Zeta potential, hydrodynamic diameter, entrapment efficiency, drug release properties, and stability studies at stress conditions were also tested. Molecular docking analysis revealed significant interactions of α-glucosidase and MGN in a protein-ligand complex. The maximum inhibition by nanosponges against α-glucosidase was observed to be 0.9352 ± 0.0856 μM, 3.11-fold higher than acarbose. In vivo studies were conducted on diabetic rats and plasma glucose levels were estimated by HPLC. Collectively, our findings suggest that MGN-loaded nanosponges may be beneficial in the treatment of diabetes since they prolong the antidiabetic response in plasma and improve patient compliance by slowly releasing MGN and requiring less frequent doses, respectively.

Keywords: diabetes; drug delivery; α-glucosidase; in vivo studies; α-mangostin; molecular docking; nanosponges; quasi-emulsion method

1. Introduction

Garcinia mangostana Linn., more commonly known as mangosteen (MG), belongs to the family Guttiferae [1,2]. The genus *Garcinia* is native to South-East Asian countries comprising more than 300 distinct species, with each family reported for distinct bioactive compounds such as xanthones, flavonoids, triterpenoids, and benzophenones [3,4]. The mangosteen pericarp possesses a therapeutically active compound named mangostin (MGN) (Figure 1). The two abundant forms (α and γ) are present in the pericarp and xanthone constitutes the core structure of MGN [5,6]. Besides showing antihypertensive and anti-inflammatory potential, xanthone molecule has proved more effective than vitamin C and E in combating reactive oxygen species that are involved in cell damage [7–9]. The xanthone compounds, especially MGN, have been recognized to meliorate damaged pancreatic β-cells for optimal insulin release [10–16].

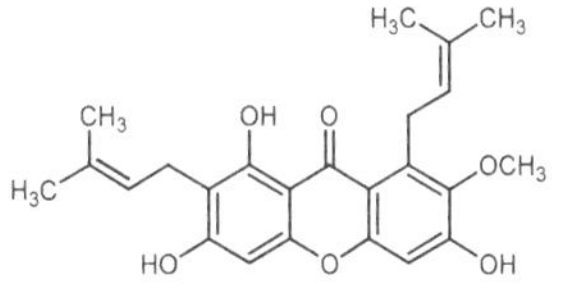

Figure 1. The chemical structure of mangostin.

Type 2 diabetes mellitus (T2DM) with its macrovascular and microvascular complications represent a major wide-reaching health warning with growing morbidity and mortality rate [17]. According to the International Diabetes Federation (IDF), 463 million adults have developed T2DM in 2019 worldwide [18], and this estimate is projected to upsurge to 700 million by 2045 [19]. The largest escalation will come from the countries undergoing monetary evolutions from low-income to middle-income tiers [20]. Over the past few years, natural sources were of high therapeutic interest to avert the impact of free radicals on cells which may be useful in treating various metabolic diseases [21–25].

In recent years, a liaison between phytochemistry and therapeutics has escalated the health-promoting benefits of various plants and their products [26]. The major obstacle of directly utilizing herbal extracts for treating various diseases is their failure to precisely traverse the lipid bilayer that may lead to the impecunious bioavailability of therapeutic agents [27,28]. However, delivering a drug with nanotechnology may improve the bioavailability and therapeutic efficiency of phytochemicals [29–31]. Nanosponges are highly porous nanoparticles composed of hyper-cross-linked polymers and can entrap active molecules. The porous architecture of the nanosponges provides superior drug absorption/complexation properties [32,33]. These tiny structures have the capability of encapsulation of both hydrophilic and hydrophobic drugs and can enhance the solubility of poor water-soluble molecules [34–36]. Their particle size also offers a favorable environment for sustained drug release action for temporal and targeted purposes [37,38].

To the best of our knowledge, no MGN has previously been embedded within a nanosponge system offering a new delivery method for antidiabetic MGN. The goal is to maximize the therapeutic effects of MGN by releasing it in a sustained manner via nanosponges. Because the MGN is not instantly available, the possibility of harmful consequences by over-sensitizing insulin-producing cells could be minimized. The prepared nanosponges were characterized for their hydrodynamic diameter, surface analysis, encapsulation efficiency, and release potential. In vitro enzymatic inhibition, in vivo anti-diabetic effect, and in silico assessment were also carried out to provide an in-depth picture of the targeted therapy.

2. Results and Discussion

2.1. Physical Characterization

2.1.1. Fourier-Transform Infra-Red (FTIR) Spectroscopic Analysis

FTIR spectra of pure MGN and its nanosponges are shown in Figure 2A. In MGN nanosponges (b), a low wide peak at 3915.74 cm^{-1} has been observed, attributable to the presence of trace amounts of water molecules, that may have played a role in hydrogen bonding. Due to O–H stretching, a typically weak and broad peak appeared in the spectra of both pure MGN (3703.81 cm^{-1}) and MGN loaded nanosponges (3709.56 cm^{-1}). Strong and steep peaks were seen as a result of intermolecular O–H stretching at wavenumbers (3458.47 and 3391.52 cm^{-1}) in pure MGN spectrum and wavenumbers (3459.11 and 3390.25 cm^{-1}) in the MGN nanosponges spectrum. The =C–H group stretching vibrations generated small peaks in the MGN spectrum at 2995.63 cm^{-1} whereas the identical peaks were also observed in MGN nanosponges with a minor shift towards lower wavelength (2991.27 cm^{-1}). Additionally, a redshift in the functional group area of the MGN nanosponges (2750.16 cm^{-1}) was observed due to O–H stretching, which was similarly seen in pure MGN (2763.94 cm^{-1}). Due to C=O stretching, a weak and sharp peak emerged in the spectra of pure MGN (1611.45 cm^{-1}), while MGN loaded nanosponges were devoid of this peak due to the possible contact with excipients (EC and PVA). In addition, the presence of C=C aromatic ring (1501.31 and 1496.75 cm^{-1}), C–O–C bond (1223.28 and 1229.37 cm^{-1}), and C–OH bending vibrations (1072.85 and 1076.44 cm^{-1}) was verified in MGN and MGN loaded nanosponges, respectively. The FTIR data for MGN were consistent with earlier reported results [39,40].

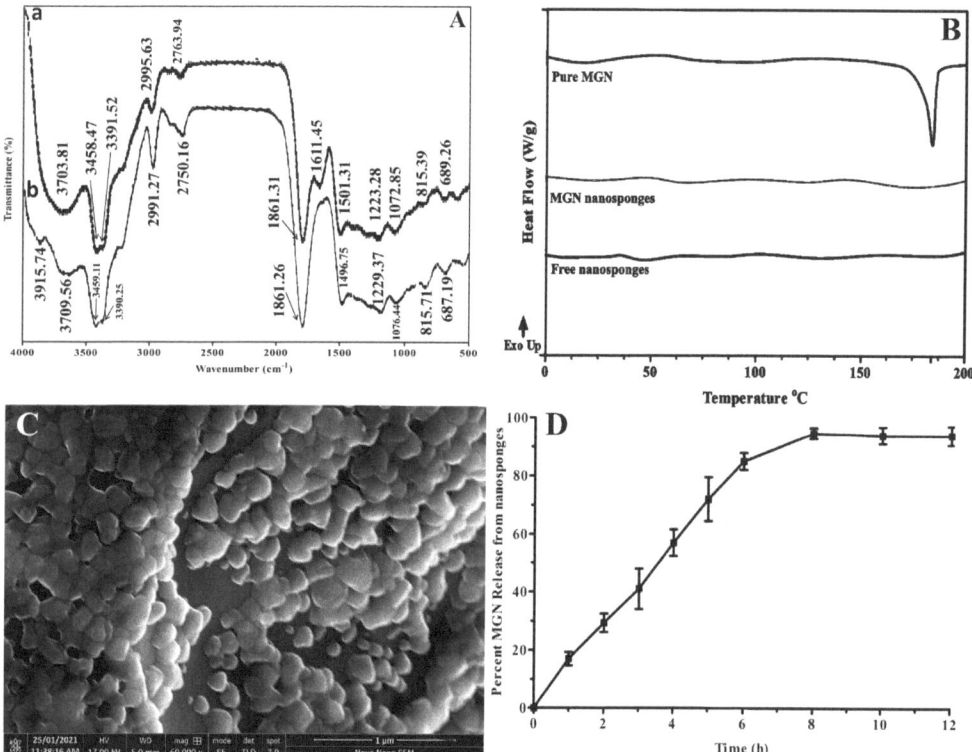

Figure 2. Physico-chemical characterization of prepared MGN nanosponges concerning FTIR (**A**) where spectrum (a) represents pure MGN while (b) shows MGN nanosponges, DSC (**B**), scanning electron microscopy (**C**), and MGN release from nanosponges (**D**).

2.1.2. Differential Scanning Calorimetric (DSC) Analysis

DSC gives important information on the drug's thermal behavior, structural alterations, crystallinity, and interaction with excipients [41]. Thermal imaging of pure MGN and MGN nanosponges was evident for compatibility among drugs and formulation excipients. As demonstrated in Figure 2B, the MGN melting point (T_m) peak was spotted at

183 °C. The characteristic melting point (T_m) peak in the thermogram of MGN nanosponges was disappeared representing the conversion from crystalline to amorphous form inside the nanosponges. The amorphous form of a drug substance improves its solubilization due to increased internal energy and reduction in thermodynamic stability, without affecting its medicinal properties and conformance with its excipients [42,43].

2.1.3. Scanning Electron Microscopic (SEM) Analysis

The physical properties of nanosponges are dependent on the type of excipients used in the formulation [44]. The preparation of nanosponges utilizing the quasi-emulsion solvent evaporation technique mostly gives nanosponges with spherical shapes [45]. The MGN nanosponges portrayed in Figure 2C were characterized by a porous surface that was related to the degree of DCM diffusion from the surface as evident from previous reports [46–48]. It is conspicuous that the lower concentrations of EC and PVA led to better diffusion of the internal phase (dichloromethane) into the exterior phase (aqueous phase), which resulted in a reduction in the time required for the formation of porous structure [49–54].

2.1.4. Nanosponges Size Analysis

The hydrodynamic diameter, zeta potential, and polydispersity index (PDI) of MGN nanosponges were estimated as 113 ± 8 nm, −35.06 ± 4.91 mV, and 0.3890 ± 0.0943, respectively (Table 1). It is evident that increasing the polymer and surfactant (EC and PVA) percentage resulted in a substantial increase in particle size owing to foaming and aggregation [37,44,47]. The zeta potential is influenced by the Brownian motion of suspended particles, and a high scale of zeta potential is associated with better stability of the dispersion [49]. Moreover, viscosity of the system can be improved as the amount of EC in the system is increased, making it more difficult to produce fine dispersion [38,55].

Table 1. Physical characterization and kinetic models of MGN nanosponges.

Properties/Models	Outcomes
Zeta Potential	−35.06 ± 4.91 mV
PDI	0.3890 ± 0.0943
Entrapment Efficiency	89 ± 5 (%)
Production Yield	75 ± 11 (%)
Hydrodynamic Diameter	113 ± 8 nm
Zero-Order	0.7935
First-Order	0.9959
Higuchi Model	0.9121
Korse–Meyer Peppas, n Value	0.9304, 0.4970

In this study, the measurements of zeta potential displayed a reasonable negative charge value −35.06 ± 4.91 mV that revealed an electrostatic stabilization on the surface of nanosponges [50]. A PDI is an exemplification of the size distribution of a given formulation that helps in deciding whether the suspended elements are homogeneous (≤ 0.3) or heterogeneous (>0.3) in nature [51].

The PVA plays a substantial role in deciding the particle size range because an increased amount of PVA improves the viscosity of the medium, thus reducing the shear stress, which is an essential variable in the reduction of particle size [36,48]. Furthermore, PVA adheres to the surface of nanosponges and continues to adhere to them even after repeated washings, resulting in the growth of particle size [46,56].

The generated nanosponges had a PDI value within an acceptable range (0.3890 ± 0.0943); however, if the value exceeds 0.7, the DLS analysis could not be completed due to the high degree of variability in the size distribution [52].

2.1.5. Entrapment Efficiency (%EE)

The EE is usually associated with the modification in the various formulation aspects that affect the ability of the nanosponges to hold a drug molecule [56]. MGN loaded nanosponges exhibited an amicable production yield (75 ± 11%) and entrapment efficiency (89 ± 5%) as shown in Table 1. Higher EE is associated with a slow release of the entrapped drug and quite similar results were exhibited by MGN nanosponges where the ratio of EC and PVA was optimized as 2:1. An optimal quantity of PVA is highly desirable in the nanosponge formation [53].

2.1.6. In Vitro Dissolution Release and Release Kinetics

The release behavior of MGN loaded nanosponges displayed a controlled release of MGN (94% in 12 h) as shown in Figure 2D. Various pharmacokinetic models including zero-order, Higuchi model, first-order, and Korsmeyer Peppas were applied on release profile data using DDSolver to elucidate the MGN release pattern from prepared nanosponges. The values of the regression coefficients for each model are listed in Table 1.

The hydrophobic nature of EC as well as phase transition largely influenced the release kinetics of MGN over an extended time duration (12 h). The cumulative release of nanosponges having MGN (1:1) in 12 h was 94% suggesting that MGN was released in a controlled manner. The results were best suited by the Higuchi model, which had a regression coefficient (R^2) of 0.9121, indicating that drug molecules were distributed equally inside the matrix of nanosponges. The Higuchi model was observed as the best fit depicting the value of 0.9121 for the regression coefficient indicating uniform dispersal of drug metabolism throughout nanosponges. Concentration-dependent release kinetics was shown by regression data from zero-order release (0.793) as well as Korsmeyer Peppas (0.9304; n = 0.497) and first-order (0.9959). The first-order release behavior was supported by aforesaid results whereas the "n" value showed release following non-fickian in which diffusion as well as erosion and swelling both are responsible for drug release [33,44,55,56].

2.2. In Vivo Studies

In vivo studies were conducted on male Wistar rats by strictly adhering to the guidelines as approved by Pharmacy Ethical Committee (12/PEC/2019), Faculty of Pharmacy, Bahauddin Zakariya University, Multan, Pakistan. Diabetes was induced in the rats by intraperitoneal injection of streptozotocin (60 mg/kg body weight) [57]. Plasma glucose, as well as MGN levels, were determined in different animal groups following oral administration of MGN (as free dispersion) and MGN loaded nanosponges using the same dose. A rapid hypoglycemic response was observed upon administration of pure MGN with a maximum response of 28.71% (67.13 ± 4.924 mg/dL blood glucose level p = 0.0032) at T_{max} of 1 h.

A comparatively steady hypoglycemic response was observed with MGN loaded nanosponges with a T_{max} of 8 h and a maximum response of 33.35% with a blood glucose level of 78.42 ± 11.52 mg/dL (p = 0.0028) following oral administration. A significant increase in AUC_{0-12} besides T_{max} and the hypoglycemic response was observed upon oral administration of MGN loaded nanosponges as evident from statistical data (independent samples t-test) in comparison to pure MGN (p < 0.05). The larger hypoglycemic response observed for MGN loaded nanosponges was due to a higher penetrating ability of drug encapsulated via hydrophobic moiety. Our findings (Figure 3 and Table 2) were in accordance with the previous reports [12,16,54,58]. When free nanosponges were given to diabetic rats, the animals expired as a result of acute hyperglycemia, demonstrating that the excipients (EC and PVA) were inert and had no role in lowering plasma glucose levels. Our results were consistent with the outcomes found in enzyme assay where free nanosponges showed no inhibitory potential against α-glucosidase.

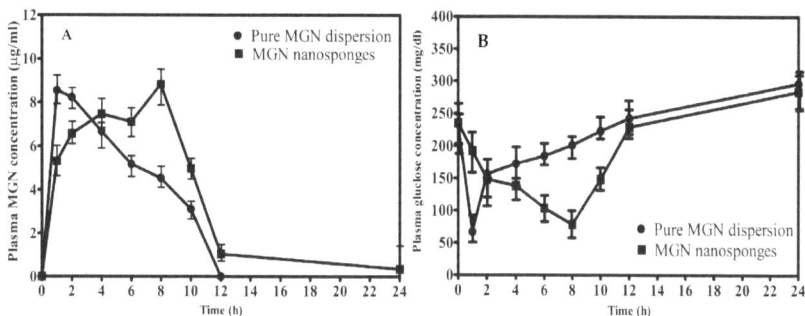

Figure 3. Plasma concentration in experimental rats after administration of pure MGN and MGN nanosponges (**A**), and plasma glucose concentration in experimental rats after administration of pure MGN and MGN nanosponges in different time intervals (**B**).

Table 2. Data of in vivo pharmacokinetic model of pure and MGN loaded nanosponges.

Formulation	Parameters of Activity		
	AUC_{0-12} (mg.h/dL) ± SEM	Max. Hypoglycemic Response (mg/dL) ± SEM	T_{max} (h)
Pure MGN Dispersion	233.8 ± 15.31	67.13 ± 4.925	1
MGN Nanosponges	235.1 ± 17.62	78.42 ± 11.52	8

Sr.No	Groups Description	Glucose Concentration (mg/dL) ± SEM			Plasma MGN Concentration (μg/mL) ± SEM		
		Pure MGN Dispersion	MGN Nanosponges	p-value	Pure MGN Dispersion	MGN Nanosponges	p-value
1	Normal Control	85.64 ± 9.356	87.11 ± 6.579	0.8149	—	—	—
2	Diabetic Control	233.8 ± 15.31	235.1 ± 17.62	0.9736	—	—	—
3	After 1 h	67.13 ± 4.925	192.8 ± 20.71	0.0032	8.551 ± 2.689	5.307 ± 2.851	0.0384
4	After 2 h	156.8 ± 18.61	148.7 ± 24.91	0.4271	8.201 ± 1.662	6.568 ± 1.897	0.1254
5	After 4 h	172.4 ± 15.84	136.6 ± 15.74	0.1845	6.679 ± 3.415	7.462 ± 3.644	0.4918
6	After 6 h	184.7 ± 19.84	103.1 ± 15.32	0.0391	5.162 ± 1.204	7.108 ± 1.927	0.7612
7	After 8 h	201.5 ± 18.69	78.42 ± 11.52	0.0028	4.508 ± 1.691	8.824 ± 2.607	0.0064
8	After 10 h	223.1 ± 17.96	148.5 ± 16.71	0.0414	3.117 ± 1.141	4.971 ± 1.845	0.0217
9	After 11 h	242.6 ± 26.53	229.1 ± 18.24	0.4628	Not detected	1.035 ± 0.360	0.0138
10	After 12 h	296.2 ± 27.38	283.7 ± 31.10	0.4773	Not detected	0.352 ± 0.028	0.0413

The p-value of <0.05 will be considered statistically significant.

2.3. In Vitro Enzyme Inhibition Studies
α-Glucosidase Inhibitory Activity

Enzyme inhibition studies were carried out initially at a single concentration of 10 mM and further, a three-fold serial dilution of each inhibitor was made to estimate IC_{50} (Figure 4C). Both pure MGN and its nanosponges, as well as free nanosponges, were tested against α-glucosidase [53]. The obtained data were compared with the standard inhibitor, acarbose. The maximum inhibition against α-glucosidase was observed by nanosponges (0.9352 ± 0.0856 µM) that was 1.44-fold more potent than pure MGN (1.353 ± 0.3751 µM) and 3.11-fold more potent than acarbose, the standard inhibitor (ANOVA test where $p < 0.05$). Our results corroborated earlier reports of mangostin acting as an α-glucosidase inhibitor [13,59,60]. When tested against α-glucosidase inhibition, the free nanosponges were ineffective, which confirmed their inert nature.

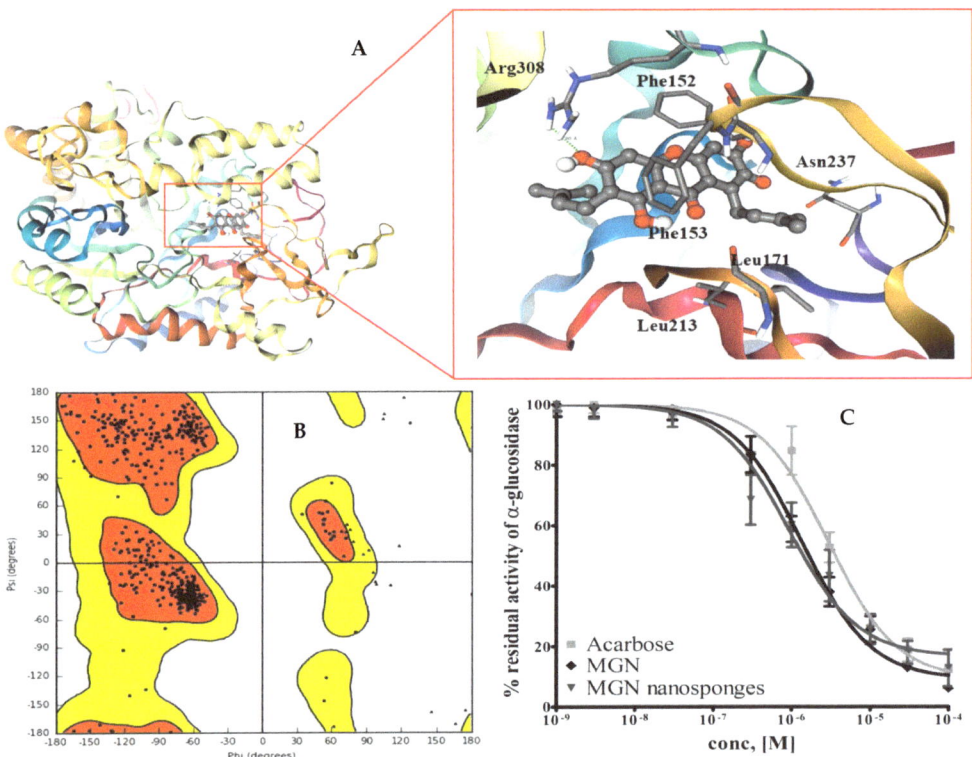

Figure 4. The simulated binding mode of the MGN in the binding site of yeast α-glucosidase. The ligand is presented in a ball and stick model with the hydrogen bond represented with dashed lines. The graphic was rendered using NGL viewer (**A**). The Ramachandran plot of the developed model. The core and outer contours present the allowed and the generously allowed regions (**B**). Inhibition studies of MGN nanosponges against α-glucosidase with IC_{50} values of 1.353 µM (MGN), 0.9352 µM (MGN nanosponges), and 2.909 µM (acarbose) (**C**).

2.4. Molecular Docking Studies

To establish the protein-ligand contact profile of MGN and α-glucosidase complex, molecular docking simulations were carried out. For this purpose, the homology model of the *S. cerevisiae* α-glucosidase was developed using the SWISS-MODEL web-server [61]. The isomaltase from the same species (PDB: 3AJ7) was used as a template. The stereochemical quality of the model was accessed with the help of the Ramachandran plot (Figure 4A) [62]. As evident from the graph, more than 97% of the residues lie in the allowed region which underpins the reliability of the developed model.

To establish the binding mode, the MGN was subjected to molecular docking studies using the homology modeled structure of the yeast α-glucosidase. The pose obtained from docking was refined with the help of MD simulation. Figure 4B presents the post-MD simulation pose of the MGN in the binding site of the *S. cerevisiae* α-glucosidase. As evident from Figure 4, MGN resides comfortably in the binding site of α-glucosidase facilitating contacts with the neighboring residues. The xanthone core structure mediates π-stacking interaction with Phe152 and Phe153 at the binding site. The Phe152 and Phe153 are part of the hydrophobic patch of α-glucosidase that facilitates the catalysis by stacking the face of the saccharide rings. Apart from the stacking interactions, MGN exhibits hydrophobic contacts with the aliphatic chains of the Leu171, Leu213, and Asn237. It has been reported that these hydrophobic interactions are the fundamental interactions responsible for protein-ligand complexation [63]. In addition, our findings revealed that MGN forms a hydrogen connection with the guanidinium cap of the Arg308 molecule.

3. Materials and Methods

3.1. General

The α-mangostin (MGN), ethyl cellulose (EC), dichloromethane (DCM), polyvinyl alcohol (PVA), α-glucosidase, acarbose, streptozotocin, phosphate-buffered saline (PBS) tablets, potassium bromide (KBr), lysozyme, dialysis membrane (10K MWCO), diethyl ether, and ethanol were procured from Merck KGaA (St. Louis, MO, USA) and were utilized without any additional purification.

3.2. Animals

Adult male Sprague Dawley rats (*Rattus norvegicus*) with an average weight of 270–290 g were obtained from the animal house facility at Faculty of Pharmacy, Bahauddin Zakariya University, Multan, Pakistan, and were harbored in appropriate cages and familiarized with the laboratory environment for at least one week before the start of experiments. The test animals were nurtured day and night with standard rodent food and mineralized water. The study design was approved by the committee on animal and research ethics of Bahauddin Zakariya University, Multan, Pakistan.

3.3. Development of MGN Nanosponges

Solvent evaporation technique was utilized to formulate MGN entrapped nanosponges with slight modifications [55]. Briefly, MGN and ethyl cellulose were dissolved in 2:1 molar ratios in dichloromethane (20 mL) while the aqueous phase was comprised of PVA (0.4%). The organic phase was added slowly into the aqueous phase. Subsequently, the mixture was stirred properly at 20000 rpm for 2 h to form nanosponges. The MGN nanosponges were dried into a powder and kept in the refrigerator until further use.

3.4. Physical Characterization of Nanosponges

3.4.1. Fourier Transform Infra-Red (FTIR) Spectroscopic Analysis

KBr disc method was used to obtain the spectra of pure MGN, MGN nanosponges, and free nanosponges recorded on a Shimadzu IR-Prestige FTIR spectrophotometer (Shimadzu IRPrestige-21 Tokyo, Japan) across a range of 4000 to 500 cm^{-1} [64].

3.4.2. Differential Scanning Calorimetric (DSC) Analysis

The physical stability was evaluated with thermal analysis of pure MGN, MGN nanosponges, and blank nanosponges. The heating rate was raised at 10 °C/min together with an uninterrupted nitrogen flow (2 mL/min) to prevent oxidation. The thermogram was produced using DSC 214 Polyma (NETZSCH Instruments, Burlington, USA) by heating to 200 °C using a hollow aluminum pan as a reference [44].

3.4.3. Scanning Electron Microscopic (SEM) Analysis

SEM images of MGN nanosponges were obtained using a Hitachi S-4700 (Houghton, MI, USA) with an acceleration voltage of 10–20 kV. The sample was dispersed in ethanol and instantaneously placed on perfect silicon wafers. For smooth conduction, the sample was sputter-coated with gold [65].

3.4.4. Particle Size Estimation

To determine the hydrodynamic size distribution of MGN nanosponges, the dynamic light scattering (DLS) approach was used. The MGN nanosponges were dispersed in double-distilled water for DLS analysis. A Malvern Zetasizer Nano ZS (Cambridge, UK) equipment was used to determine the zeta potential [66].

3.4.5. Determination of Entrapment Efficiency (%EE)

The entrapment efficiency (%EE) of MGN in nanosponges was calculated as reported previously [67]. Briefly, a dialysis bag containing 5 mL of nano-dispersion was submerged in PBS (100 mL). The setup was placed on a magnetic stirrer (75 rpm) at 37 °C for 1 h. The sample was appropriately diluted before measuring absorbance at 262 nm using a UV-visible spectrophotometer (Shimadzu, Tokyo, Japan). The percent EE was calculated using the following equation [56]:

$$\text{Entrapment Efficiency (\%EE)} = \left[\frac{\text{Total amount of MGN in nanosponges} - \text{Free MGN}}{\text{Total amount of MGN in nanosponges}} \right] \times 100 \quad (1)$$

3.4.6. Determination of Production Yield (%)

The MGN nanosponges obtained after drying were weighed. Percentage yield value was calculated as follows [68]:

$$\text{Production yield (\%)} = \left[\frac{\text{Weight of nanosponges}}{\text{Total amount of solid ingredients}} \right] \times 100 \quad (2)$$

3.4.7. In Vitro Dissolution Studies

The MGN release pattern and kinetic models were studied based on the previously reported method [67]. Briefly, the dialysis membrane (10K MWCO) was filled with nanosponge dispersion (10 mg in 5 mL of PBS) and tied on both ends. The dialysis tube was immersed in 0.1M HCl (250 mL) for 2 h initially and then transferred to PBS (250 mL, pH 6.8) with lysozyme (0.6 g/mL). The experiment was conducted on a magnetic stirrer set at 37 °C with 75 rpm. The samples were collected at predetermined intervals, while MGN release was estimated on a UV-Visible spectrophotometer (Shimadzu, Tokyo, Japan). The acquired data were examined using the DDsolver software for drug release behavior utilizing zero-order, first-order, Higuchi, and Korsmeyer–Peppas models.

3.5. In Vitro Enzyme Inhibition Studies
α-Glucosidase Inhibitory Activity

The α-glucosidase assay was performed using a previously reported method with minor alterations [69]. Briefly, the reaction mixture comprised of 50 µL of enzyme solution (0.4 U/mL) and 50 µL of p-nitrophenyl-α-D-glucopyranoside (pNPG, 1 mM) as substrate was prepared in sodium phosphate buffer (pH 6.8) with the addition of a 10 µL of the test sample. The reaction was terminated by adding 0.1 M NaOH. The control (acarbose) and blank (negative control) wells were also maintained in a 96 well-plate for analysis. The α-glucosidase activity was determined by measuring the extent of hydrolysis of pNPG and estimating the formation of p-nitrophenol measured at 405 nm using ELISA microplate reader ELx808™ (BioTek Instruments, Winooski, VT, USA). The experiment was performed in triplicate and data was presented with the standard error of the mean (SEM). The formulations showed ≥50% enzyme inhibition were further used to calculate IC_{50} value by using GraphPad Prism5 software.

3.6. In Vivo Anti-Diabetic Activity
3.6.1. Induction of Type 2 Diabetes in Rats

T2DM was instigated in overnight starving rats with an intraperitoneal (i.p) injection of streptozotocin (65 mg/kg) dissolved in citrate buffer (pH 4.5). After 72 h of diabetes induction, the rats with persistent high glucose levels (>200 mg/dL) were considered diabetic and included in the study [70].

3.6.2. Experimental Design and Blood Sampling

Healthy male rats were randomly divided into five groups where each group contains five animals and received treatment orally. Among ten, Group I was considered as the control which received the standard anti-diabetic treatment with acarbose while Group II was based on healthy rats that received distilled water orally. Group III was given pure MGN (equivalent to pre-determined IC_{50}) as a test compound while MGN nanosponges (equivalent to IC_{50}) were administered to Group IV. Group V was evaluated to see if the excipients produced the desired hypoglycemic response in diabetic rats by giving free nanosponges.

At specified time intervals (1, 2, 3, 4, 6, 8, 10 and 12 h), the animals were sacrificed after giving anesthesia with diethyl ether and blood was collected into dry clean EDTA containing test tubes. Blood plasma samples were run on HPLC to determine the concentration of free MGN and MGN nanosponges through pharmacokinetic analysis [71,72].

3.6.3. HPLC Assay Method

A 600 µL of blood was removed from rats under investigation and centrifuged at 10,000 rpm for 5 min. The isolated plasma (300 µL) was incubated with methanol (300 µL) to induce protein precipitation. Afterward, the mixture was shaken gently and again centrifuged at 10,000 rpm for 5 min. The supernatant was filtered and diluted with 100 µL of the mobile phase, from which a 20 µL was taken into HPLC to determine the concentration of MGN.

The conditions for the HPLC assay were as follows: The HPLC-LC20A system (Shimadzu, Tokyo, Japan) consisted of an LC-10AT pump, SPD-A20 UV-Vis detector, SIL-20A/C autosampler, and Shimadzu LC-solution software. Chromatographic separation of MGN was achieved by using a Shim-pack MAqC-ODS (150 mm × 4.6 mm × 5 µm) reverse-phase analytical column at ambient temperature. The mobile phase consisted of ammonium acetate (20 mM, pH 6.8) and methanol (5%). An isocratic elution strategy was adopted with a flow rate of 0.5 mL/min. The concentration of eluate (MGN) was calculated and plotted against time using Prism5 software. The pharmacokinetic parameters, area under the concentration-time curve (AUC), maximal response, and period of maximal response were investigated (T_{max}). The in vivo results were reported as SEM (standard error of the mean) [58].

3.7. Molecular Docking Studies

To establish the plausible protein-ligand interaction profile of the MGN and α-glucosidase complex, molecular docking simulations were carried out using a homology model of *S. cerevisiae* α-glucosidase. The SWISS-MODEL web-server was used to develop a homology model using the isomaltase from the same species as a template [73]. The stereochemical quality of the model was assessed by plotting the Ramachandran plot of the Phi and Psi angles. The system was then prepared for docking calculations using the AMBER10: EHT force field implied in the MOE software suite (Chemical computing group, Cambridge, UK).

To benchmark the ability of software to reproduce the crystal pose; the re-docking experiment was carried out using the Protein Data Bank (PDB); 3A4A. After successful re-docking results, MOE was used to establish the binding mode of the MGN. The binding site was identified using the coordinates of the yeast isomaltase complex. The default placement and scoring methods were used in combination with the rigid receptor docking protocol in MOE. The poses generated by the initial placement and scoring methods were subjected to refinement and rescoring. The top-ranked pose was then subjected to post-docking minimization using the MD simulation protocol developed earlier [26]. A short production run of 10 ns was carried out, and the post-MD pose was visually analyzed.

3.8. Statistical Analysis

The results were evaluated using independent samples *t*-test (pharmacokinetics analysis) and one-way analysis of variance (enzyme inhibition assay), with a 95% confidence interval ($p < 0.05$). Certain experimental results, however, were represented as the standard error of the mean (SEM). Microsoft Excel (2010),.(Microsoft Corp, Redmond, WA, USA), SPSS (9.0), (SPSS Inc. Chicago, IL, USA) and Prism (5.0) (GraphPad Software, San Diego, CA, USA) software were used for the statistical analysis.

4. Conclusions

In summary, the present study describes the fabrication of MGN nanosponges for anti-diabetic therapeutic applications. MGN nanosponges were characterized by Fourier-transform infra-red (FTIR) spectroscopy, differential scanning calorimetry (DSC), scanning electron microscopy (SEM), zeta potential, hydrodynamic diameter, entrapment efficiency, controlled drug release, and stability studies at stress conditions. The results demonstrate that the use of MGN loaded nanosponges as a drug delivery system for oral administration would be beneficial since when compared to free drug solution given at the same dosage, a longer and enhanced hypoglycemic impact may be achieved. Thus, the number of dosages that must be administered to patients each day is reduced, and it is anticipated that the number of adverse effects associated with the medication would be reduced as well. This allows for the creation of a convenient dose form. Taken together, the MGN loaded nanosponges described here may function as an archetype for natural materials traditionally used for diabetes treatment. This study may uncover further prospects and exhaust the potential of nutraceuticals.

Author Contributions: Conceptualization, F.U. and H.S.S.; methodology, S.M. and S.Z.; software, S.Z.; validation, H.S.S. and J.M.; formal analysis, I.K. and F.U.; investigation, F.U.; resources, K.M.A. and D.A.; data curation, G.E.-S.B.; K.M.A. and D.A.; writing—original draft preparation, H.S.S. and A.K.; writing—review and editing, I.K.; K.M.A. and D.A.; visualization, S.Z.; supervision, I.K.; project administration, I.K.; funding acquisition, G.E.-S.B.; K.M.A. and D.A. All authors have read and agreed to the published version of the manuscript.

Funding: The authors would like to acknowledge Taif University, Saudi Arabia, for funding this research through Taif University Researchers Supporting Project Number TURSP-2020/267.

Institutional Review Board Statement: The study design entitled "Fabrication and Biological Assessment of Antidiabetic α-Mangostin Loaded Nanosponges: In Vitro, In Vivo, and In Silico Studies" was approved by the committee on animal and research ethics (approval number: 12/PEC/2019), Faculty of Pharmacy, Bahauddin Zakariya University, Multan, Pakistan. The investigators have been directed to ensure the strict adherence to protocols for rats already approved by the ethical committee.

Informed Consent Statement: Not applicable.

Data Availability Statement: The data presented in this study are available from the authors on reasonable request.

Acknowledgments: Taif University, Saudi Arabia, is highly acknowledged for funding this research through Taif University Researchers Supporting Project Number TURSP-2020/267.

Conflicts of Interest: The authors declare no conflict of interest.

Sample Availability: Samples of the compounds (α-mangostin nanosponges) are available from the authors.

References

1. Ibrahim, M.Y.; Hashim, N.M.; Mariod, A.A.; Mohan, S.; Abdulla, M.A.; Abdelwahab, S.I.; Arbab, I.A. α-Mangostin from *Garcinia mangostana* Linn: An updated review of its pharmacological properties. *Arabian J. Chem.* **2016**, *9*, 317–329. [CrossRef]
2. Fatmawati, S.; Ersam, T.; Shimizu, K. The inhibitory activity of aldose reductase in vitro by constituents of *Garcinia mangostana* Linn. *Phytomedicine* **2015**, *22*, 49–51. [CrossRef]

3. Obolskiy, D.; Pischel, I.; Siriwatanametanon, N.; Heinrich, M. *Garcinia mangostana* L.: A phytochemical and pharmacological review. *Phytother. Res.* **2009**, *23*, 1047–1065. [CrossRef] [PubMed]
4. Muhammad, A.A.N.; Amaq, F.; Suhailah, H.; Kuncoroningrat, S.R.J.; Bilqis, I.; Dwi, W.; Akhmad, H.S. A review on medicinal properties of mangosteen (*Garcinia mangostana* L.). *Res. J. Pharm. Technol.* **2020**, *13*, 974–982. [CrossRef]
5. Chin, Y.-W.; Kinghorn, A.D. Structural characterization, biological effects, and synthetic studies on xanthones from mangosteen (*Garcinia mangostana*), a popular botanical dietary supplement. *Mini-Rev. Org. Chem.* **2008**, *5*, 355–364. [CrossRef]
6. Liu, Q.-Y.; Wang, Y.-T.; Lin, L.-G. New insights into the anti-obesity activity of xanthones from *Garcinia mangostana*. *Food Funct.* **2015**, *6*, 383–393. [CrossRef]
7. Panda, S.S.; Chand, M.; Sakhuja, R.; Jain, S. Xanthones as potential antioxidants. *Curr. Med. Chem.* **2013**, *20*, 4481–4507. [CrossRef]
8. Pedraza-Chaverri, J.; Cárdenas-Rodríguez, N.; Orozco-Ibarra, M.; Pérez-Rojas, J.M. Medicinal properties of mangosteen (*Garcinia mangostana*). *Food Chem. Toxicol.* **2008**, *46*, 3227–3239. [CrossRef]
9. Sukatta, U.; Takenaka, M.; Ono, H.; Okadome, H.; Sotome, I.; Nanayama, K.; Thanapase, W.; Isobe, S. Distribution of major xanthones in the pericarp, aril, and yellow gum of mangosteen (*Garcinia mangostana* linn.) fruit and their contribution to antioxidative activity. *Biosci. Biotechnol. Biochem.* **2013**, *77*, 984–987. [CrossRef]
10. Husen, S.A.; Kalqutny, S.H.; Ansori, A.N.M.; Susilo, R.J.K.; Alymandy, A.D.; Winarni, D. Antioxidant and antidiabetic activity of *Garcinia mangostana* L. pericarp extract in streptozotocin-induced diabetic mice. *Biosci. Res.* **2017**, *14*, 1238–1245.
11. Ovalle-Magallanes, B.; Eugenio-Pérez, D.; Pedraza-Chaverri, J. Medicinal properties of mangosteen (*Garcinia mangostana* L.): A comprehensive update. *Food Chem. Toxicol.* **2017**, *109*, 102–122. [CrossRef]
12. Taher, M.; Zakaria, T.M.F.S.T.; Susanti, D.; Zakaria, Z.A. Hypoglycaemic activity of ethanolic extract of *Garcinia mangostana* Linn. in normoglycaemic and streptozotocin-induced diabetic rats. *BMC Complement. Altern. Med.* **2016**, *16*, 1–12. [CrossRef]
13. Ryu, H.W.; Cho, J.K.; Curtis-Long, M.J.; Yuk, H.J.; Kim, Y.S.; Jung, S.; Kim, Y.S.; Lee, B.W.; Park, K.H. α-Glucosidase inhibition and antihyperglycemic activity of prenylated xanthones from *Garcinia mangostana*. *Phytochemistry* **2011**, *72*, 2148–2154. [CrossRef] [PubMed]
14. Jariyapongskul, A.; Areebambud, C.; Suksamrarn, S.; Mekseepralard, C. Alpha-mangostin attenuation of hyperglycemia-induced ocular hypoperfusion and blood retinal barrier leakage in the early stage of type 2 diabetes rats. *BioMed Res. Int.* **2015**, *2015*, 785826. [CrossRef]
15. Bugianesi, E.; McCullough, A.J.; Marchesini, G. Insulin resistance: A metabolic pathway to chronic liver disease. *Hepatology* **2005**, *42*, 987–1000. [CrossRef]
16. Lee, D.; Kim, Y.-M.; Jung, K.; Chin, Y.-W.; Kang, K.S. Alpha-mangostin improves insulin secretion and protects INS-1 cells from streptozotocin-induced damage. *Int. J. Mol. Sci.* **2018**, *19*, 1484. [CrossRef] [PubMed]
17. Zheng, Y.; Ley, S.H.; Hu, F.B. Global aetiology and epidemiology of type 2 diabetes mellitus and its complications. *Nat. Rev. Endocrinol.* **2018**, *14*, 88–98. [CrossRef]
18. International Diabetes Federation. Diabetes in South-East Asia. 2019. Available online: https://idf.org/our-network/regions-members/south-east-asia/diabetes-in-sea.html (accessed on 3 March 2020).
19. Bommer, C.; Sagalova, V.; Heesemann, E.; Manne-Goehler, J.; Atun, R.; Bärnighausen, T.; Davies, J.; Vollmer, S. Global economic burden of diabetes in adults: Projections from 2015 to 2030. *Diabetes Care* **2018**, *41*, 963–970. [CrossRef]
20. Cho, N.; Shaw, J.; Karuranga, S.; Huang, Y.; da Rocha Fernandes, J.; Ohlrogge, A.; Malanda, B. IDF Diabetes Atlas: Global estimates of diabetes prevalence for 2017 and projections for 2045. *Diabetes Res. Clin. Pract.* **2018**, *138*, 271–281. [CrossRef]
21. Ghasemzadeh, A.; Jaafar, H.Z.; Baghdadi, A.; Tayebi-Meigooni, A. Alpha-mangostin-rich extracts from mangosteen pericarp: Optimization of green extraction protocol and evaluation of biological activity. *Molecules* **2018**, *23*, 1852. [CrossRef] [PubMed]
22. Chen, D.-Q.; Feng, Y.-L.; Cao, G.; Zhao, Y.-Y. Natural products as a source for antifibrosis therapy. *Trends Pharmacol. Sci.* **2018**, *39*, 937–952. [CrossRef] [PubMed]
23. Matzinger, M.; Fischhuber, K.; Heiss, E.H. Activation of Nrf2 signaling by natural products-can it alleviate diabetes? *Biotechnol. Adv.* **2018**, *36*, 1738–1767. [CrossRef]
24. Xu, L.; Li, Y.; Dai, Y.; Peng, J. Natural products for the treatment of type 2 diabetes mellitus: Pharmacology and mechanisms. *Pharmacol. Res.* **2018**, *130*, 451–465. [CrossRef]
25. Park, J.; Jang, H.-J. Anti-diabetic effects of natural products an overview of therapeutic strategies. *Mol. Cell. Toxicol.* **2017**, *13*, 1–20. [CrossRef]
26. Faisal, N.A.; Chatha, S.A.S.; Hussain, A.I.; Ikram, M.; Bukhari, S.A. Liaison of phenolic acids and biological activity of escalating cultivars of Daucus carota. *Int. J. Food Prop.* **2017**, *20*, 2782–2792. [CrossRef]
27. Raskin, I.; Ribnicky, D.M.; Komarnytsky, S.; Ilic, N.; Poulev, A.; Borisjuk, N.; Brinker, A.; Moreno, D.A.; Ripoll, C.; Yakoby, N. Plants and human health in the twenty-first century. *Trends Biotechnol.* **2002**, *20*, 522–531. [CrossRef]
28. Saraf, S. Applications of novel drug delivery system for herbal formulations. *Fitoterapia* **2010**, *81*, 680–689. [CrossRef]
29. Daga, M.; de Graaf, I.A.; Argenziano, M.; Barranco, A.S.M.; Loeck, M.; Al-Adwi, Y.; Cucci, M.A.; Caldera, F.; Trotta, F.; Barrera, G. Glutathione-responsive cyclodextrin-nanosponges as drug delivery systems for doxorubicin: Evaluation of toxicity and transport mechanisms in the liver. *Toxicol. In Vitro* **2020**, *65*, 104800. [CrossRef] [PubMed]
30. Ahmad, R.; Srivastava, S.; Ghosh, S.; Khare, S.K. Phytochemical delivery through nanocarriers: A review. *Colloids Surf. B. Biointerfaces* **2020**, *197*, 111389. [CrossRef]

31. Gafur, A.; Sukamdani, G.Y.; Kristi, N.; Maruf, A.; Xu, J.; Chen, X.; Wang, G.; Ye, Z. From bulk to nano-delivery of essential phytochemicals: Recent progress and strategies for antibacterial resistance. *J. Mater. Chem. B* **2020**, *8*, 9825–9835. [CrossRef]
32. Pandey, P.J. Multifunctional nanosponges for the treatment of various diseases: A review. *Asian J. Pharm. Pharmacol.* **2019**, *5*, 235–248. [CrossRef]
33. Almutairy, B.K.; Alshetaili, A.; Alali, A.S.; Ahmed, M.M.; Anwer, M.; Aboudzadeh, M.A. Design of olmesartan medoxomil-loaded nanosponges for hypertension and lung cancer treatments. *Polymers* **2021**, *13*, 2272. [CrossRef]
34. Balwe, M.B. Nanosponge a novel drug delivery system. *Res. J. Pharm. Dosage Forms Technol.* **2020**, *12*, 261–266. [CrossRef]
35. Pawar, S.; Shende, P.; Trotta, F. Diversity of β-cyclodextrin-based nanosponges for transformation of actives. *Int. J. Pharm.* **2019**, *565*, 333–350. [CrossRef]
36. Kumar, M.; Kumar, A.; Kumar, S. Nanosponges: A promising nanocarrier systems for drug delivery. *Curr. Res. Pharm. Sci.* **2020**, 01–05. [CrossRef]
37. Jagtap, S.R.; Bhusnure, O.G.; Mujewar, I.N.; Gholve, S.B.; Panchabai, V. Nanosponges: A novel trend for targeted drug delivery. *J. Drug Delivery Ther.* **2019**, *9*, 931–938. [CrossRef]
38. Silpa, G.; Manohar, R.D.; Mathan, S.; Dharan, S.S. Nanosponges: A potential nanocarrier: A review. *J. Pharm. Sci. Res.* **2020**, *12*, 1341–1344.
39. Asasutjarit, R.; Meesomboon, T.; Adulheem, P.; Kittiwisut, S.; Sookdee, P.; Samosornsuk, W.; Fuongfuchat, A. Physicochemical properties of alpha-mangostin loaded nanomeulsions prepared by ultrasonication technique. *Heliyon* **2019**, *5*, e02465. [CrossRef]
40. Xu, W.-K.; Jiang, H.; Yang, K.; Wang, Y.-Q.; Zhang, Q.; Zuo, J. Development and in vivo evaluation of self-microemulsion as delivery system for α-mangostin. *Kaohsiung J. Med. Sci.* **2017**, *33*, 116–123. [CrossRef] [PubMed]
41. Moin, A.; Roohi, N.F.; Rizvi, S.M.D.; Ashraf, S.A.; Siddiqui, A.J.; Patel, M.; Ahmed, S.; Gowda, D.; Adnan, M. Design and formulation of polymeric nanosponge tablets with enhanced solubility for combination therapy. *RSC Adv.* **2020**, *10*, 34869–34884. [CrossRef]
42. Deb, T.K.; Ramireddy, B.; Moin, A.; Shivakumar, H. In vitro-in vivo evaluation of xanthan gum and eudragit inter polyelectrolyte complex based sustained release tablets. *Intl. J. Pharm. Invest.* **2015**, *5*, 65–72. [CrossRef]
43. Zhang, M.; Li, H.; Lang, B.; O'Donnell, K.; Zhang, H.; Wang, Z.; Dong, Y.; Wu, C.; Williams III, R.O. Formulation and delivery of improved amorphous fenofibrate solid dispersions prepared by thin film freezing. *Eur. J. Pharm. Biopharm.* **2012**, *82*, 534–544. [CrossRef] [PubMed]
44. Ahmed, M.M.; Fatima, F.; Anwer, M.K.; Ansari, M.J.; Das, S.S.; Alshahrani, S.M. Development and characterization of ethyl cellulose nanosponges for sustained release of brigatinib for the treatment of non-small cell lung cancer. *J. Polym. Eng.* **2020**, *40*, 823–832. [CrossRef]
45. Pawar, S.; Shende, P. Design and optimization of cyclodextrin-based nanosponges of antimalarials using central composite design for dry suspension. *J. Incl. Phenom. Macrocycl. Chem.* **2021**, 1–15. [CrossRef]
46. Aldawsari, H.M.; Badr-Eldin, S.M.; Labib, G.S.; El-Kamel, A.H. Design and formulation of a topical hydrogel integrating lemongrass-loaded nanosponges with an enhanced antifungal effect: In vitro/in vivo evaluation. *Int. J. Nanomed.* **2015**, *10*, 893. [CrossRef]
47. Penjuri, S.C.B.; Ravouru, N.; Damineni, S.; Bns, S.; Poreddy, S.R. Formulation and evaluation of lansoprazole loaded Nanosponges. *Turk. J. Pharm. Sci.* **2016**, *13*, 304–310. [CrossRef]
48. Abass, M.M.; Rajab, N.A. Preparation and characterization of etodolac as a topical nanosponges hydrogel. *Iraqi J. Pharm. Sci.* **2019**, *28*, 64–74. [CrossRef]
49. Larsson, M.; Hill, A.; Duffy, J. Suspension stability; why particle size, zeta potential and rheology are important. *Annu. Trans. Nord. Rheol. Soc.* **2012**, *20*, 209–214.
50. Xu, R. Progress in nanoparticles characterization: Sizing and zeta potential measurement. *Particuology* **2008**, *6*, 112–115. [CrossRef]
51. Bachir, Y.N.; Bachir, R.N.; Hadj-Ziane-Zafour, A. Nanodispersions stabilized by β-cyclodextrin nanosponges: Application for simultaneous enhancement of bioactivity and stability of sage essential oil. *Drug Dev. Ind. Pharm.* **2019**, *45*, 333–347. [CrossRef]
52. Shah, H.; Nair, A.B.; Shah, J.; Jacob, S.; Bharadia, P.; Haroun, M. Proniosomal vesicles as an effective strategy to optimize naproxen transdermal delivery. *J. Drug Deliv. Sci. Technol.* **2021**, *63*, 102479. [CrossRef]
53. Danaei, M.; Dehghankhold, M.; Ataei, S.; Davarani, F.H.; Javanmard, R.; Dokhani, A.; Khorasani, S.; Mozafari, M. Impact of particle size and polydispersity index on the clinical applications of lipidic nanocarrier systems. *Pharmaceutics* **2018**, *10*, 57. [CrossRef] [PubMed]
54. Torne, S.J.; Ansari, K.A.; Vavia, P.R.; Trotta, F.; Cavalli, R. Enhanced oral paclitaxel bioavailability after administration of paclitaxel-loaded nanosponges. *Drug Deliv.* **2010**, *17*, 419–425. [CrossRef] [PubMed]
55. Amer, R.I.; El-Osaily, G.H.; Gad, S.S. Design and optimization of topical terbinafine hydrochloride nanosponges: Application of full factorial design, in vitro and in vivo evaluation. *J. Adv. Pharm. Technol. Res.* **2020**, *11*, 13. [CrossRef] [PubMed]
56. Srinivas, P.; Reddy, A.J. Formulation and evaluation of isoniazid loaded nanosponges for topical delivery. *Pharm. Nanotechnol.* **2015**, *3*, 68–76. [CrossRef]
57. Nelli, G.B.; Kilari, E.K. Antidiabetic effect of α-mangostin and its protective role in sexual dysfunction of streptozotocin induced diabetic male rats. *Syst. Biol. Reprod. Med.* **2013**, *59*, 319–328. [CrossRef]
58. Stepensky, D.; Friedman, M.; Raz, I.; Hoffman, A. Pharmacokinetic-pharmacodynamic analysis of the glucose-lowering effect of metformin in diabetic rats reveals first-pass pharmacodynamic effect. *Drug Metab. Dispos.* **2002**, *30*, 861–868. [CrossRef]

59. Lee, S.Y.; Mediani, A.; Nur Ashikin, A.H.; Azliana, A.B.S.; Abas, F. Antioxidant and α-glucosidase inhibitory activities of the leaf and stem of selected traditional medicinal plants. *Intl. Food Res. J.* **2014**, *21*, 379–386.
60. Vongsak, B.; Kongkiatpaiboon, S.; Jaisamut, S.; Machana, S.; Pattarapanich, C. In vitro alpha glucosidase inhibition and free-radical scavenging activity of propolis from Thai stingless bees in mangosteen orchard. *Rev. Bras. Farmacogn.* **2015**, *25*, 445–450. [CrossRef]
61. Shah, S.; Javaid, K.; Zafar, H.; Khan, K.M.; Khalil, R.; Ul-Haq, Z.; Perveen, S.; Choudhary, M.I. Synthesis, and In vitro and in silico α-glucosidase inhibitory studies of 5-chloro-2-aryl benzo[d]thiazoles. *Bioorg. Chem.* **2018**, *78*, 269–279. [CrossRef]
62. Jagannathan, V.; Venkatesan, A.; Viswanathan, P. Kinetics and computational evaluation of eugenol and vanillic acid on inhibition of a potential enzyme of a nosocomial pathogen that promotes struvite formation. *Curr. Enzym. Inhib.* **2020**, *16*, 162–171. [CrossRef]
63. Kerru, N.; Singh-Pillay, A.; Awolade, P.; Singh, P. Current anti-diabetic agents and their molecular targets: A review. *Eur. J. Med. Chem.* **2018**, *152*, 436–488. [CrossRef] [PubMed]
64. Darandale, S.; Vavia, P. Cyclodextrin-based nanosponges of curcumin: Formulation and physicochemical characterization. *J. Incl. Phenom. Macrocycl. Chem.* **2013**, *75*, 315–322. [CrossRef]
65. Omar, S.M.; Ibrahim, F.; Ismail, A. Formulation and evaluation of cyclodextrin-based nanosponges of griseofulvin as pediatric oral liquid dosage form for enhancing bioavailability and masking bitter taste. *Saudi Pharm. J.* **2020**, *28*, 349–361. [CrossRef]
66. Varan, C.; Anceschi, A.; Sevli, S.; Bruni, N.; Giraudo, L.; Bilgiç, E.; Korkusuz, P.; İskit, A.B.; Trotta, F.; Bilensoy, E. Preparation and characterization of cyclodextrin nanosponges for organic toxic molecule removal. *Int. J. Pharm.* **2020**, *585*, 119485. [CrossRef] [PubMed]
67. Shah, H.S.; Usman, F.; Khan, M.A.; Khalil, R.; Ul-Haq, Z.; Mushtaq, A.; Qaiser, R.; Iqbal, J. Preparation and characterization of anticancer niosomal withaferin–A formulation for improved delivery to cancer cells: An in vitro and in vivo evaluation. *J. Drug Deliv. Sci. Technol.* **2020**, 101863. [CrossRef]
68. Swaminathan, S.; Pastero, L.; Serpe, L.; Trotta, F.; Vavia, P.; Aquilano, D.; Trotta, M.; Zara, G.; Cavalli, R. Cyclodextrin-based nanosponges encapsulating camptothecin: Physicochemical characterization, stability and cytotoxicity. *Eur. J. Pharm. Biopharm.* **2010**, *74*, 193–201. [CrossRef]
69. Kim, K.Y.; Nguyen, T.H.; Kurihara, H.; Kim, S.M. α-Glucosidase inhibitory activity of bromophenol purified from the red alga Polyopes lancifolia. *J. Food Sci.* **2010**, *75*, H145–H150. [CrossRef] [PubMed]
70. Sahin, K.; Tuzcu, M.; Orhan, C.; Sahin, N.; Kucuk, O.; Ozercan, I.H.; Juturu, V.; Komorowski, J.R. Anti-diabetic activity of chromium picolinate and biotin in rats with type 2 diabetes induced by high-fat diet and streptozotocin. *Br. J. Nutr.* **2013**, *110*, 197–205. [CrossRef]
71. Furman, B.L. Streptozotocin-induced diabetic models in mice and rats. *Curr. Protoc. Pharmacol.* **2015**, *70*, 5–47. [CrossRef]
72. Asgary, S.; Parkhideh, S.; Solhpour, A.; Madani, H.; Mahzouni, P.; Rahimi, P. Effect of ethanolic extract of Juglans regia L. on blood sugar in diabetes-induced rats. *J. Med. Food* **2008**, *11*, 533–538. [CrossRef] [PubMed]
73. Schwede, T.; Kopp, J.; Guex, N.; Peitsch, M.C. SWISS-MODEL: An automated protein homology-modeling server. *Nucleic Acids Res.* **2003**, *31*, 3381–3385. [CrossRef] [PubMed]

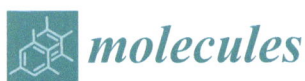

Article

Hybrid Quinoline-Thiosemicarbazone Therapeutics as a New Treatment Opportunity for Alzheimer's Disease-Synthesis, In Vitro Cholinesterase Inhibitory Potential and Computational Modeling Analysis

Sumera Zaib [1,*], Rubina Munir [2,*], Muhammad Tayyab Younas [1], Naghmana Kausar [3], Aliya Ibrar [4], Sehar Aqsa [2], Noorma Shahid [2], Tahira Tasneem Asif [2], Hashem O. Alsaab [5] and Imtiaz Khan [6,*]

[1] Department of Biochemistry, Faculty of Life Sciences, University of Central Punjab, Lahore 54590, Pakistan; muhammadtayyabyounassst@gmail.com
[2] Department of Chemistry, Kinnaird College for Women, Lahore 54000, Pakistan; w14bche002@gmail.com (S.A.); noormashahid@gmail.com (N.S.); tahiratasneem1998@gmail.com (T.T.A.)
[3] Department of Chemistry, University of Gujrat, Gujrat 50700, Pakistan; naghmana.kousar@uog.edu.pk
[4] Department of Chemistry, Faculty of Natural Sciences, The University of Haripur, Haripur 22620, Pakistan; aliya.ibrar@uoh.edu.pk
[5] Department of Pharmaceutics and Pharmaceutical Technology, Taif University, P.O. Box 11099, Taif 21944, Saudi Arabia; h.alsaab@tu.edu.sa
[6] Department of Chemistry, Manchester Institute of Biotechnology, The University of Manchester, 131 Princess Street, Manchester M1 7DN, UK
* Correspondence: sumera.zaib@ucp.edu.pk (S.Z.); rubina.munir@kinnaird.edu.pk (R.M.); imtiaz.khan@manchester.ac.uk (I.K.)

Abstract: Alzheimer's disease (AD) is a progressive neurodegenerative disorder and the leading cause of dementia worldwide. The limited pharmacological approaches based on cholinesterase inhibitors only provide symptomatic relief to AD patients. Moreover, the adverse side effects such as nausea, vomiting, loss of appetite, muscle cramps, and headaches associated with these drugs and numerous clinical trial failures present substantial limitations on the use of medications and call for a detailed insight of disease heterogeneity and development of preventive and multifactorial therapeutic strategies on urgent basis. In this context, we herein report a series of quinoline-thiosemicarbazone hybrid therapeutics as selective and potent inhibitors of cholinesterases. A facile multistep synthetic approach was utilized to generate target structures bearing multiple sites for chemical modifications and establishing drug-receptor interactions. The structures of all the synthesized compounds were fully established using readily available spectroscopic techniques (FTIR, ^{1}H- and ^{13}C-NMR). In vitro inhibitory results revealed compound **5b** as a promising and lead inhibitor with an IC$_{50}$ value of 0.12 ± 0.02 µM, a 5-fold higher potency than standard drug (galantamine; IC$_{50}$ = 0.62 ± 0.01 µM). The synergistic effect of electron-rich (methoxy) group and ethylmorpholine moiety in quinoline-thiosemicarbazone conjugates contributes significantly in improving the inhibition level. Molecular docking analysis revealed various vital interactions of potent compounds with amino acid residues and reinforced the in vitro results. Kinetics experiments revealed the competitive mode of inhibition while ADME properties favored the translation of identified inhibitors into safe and promising drug candidates for pre-clinical testing. Collectively, inhibitory activity data and results from key physicochemical properties merit further research to ensure the design and development of safe and high-quality drug candidates for Alzheimer's disease.

Keywords: quinoline; thiosemicarbazone; molecular design; hybridization; Alzheimer's disease; neurodegeneration; drug therapy; cholinesterases; enzyme inhibition; molecular docking

1. Introduction

Alzheimer's disease (AD), a chronic neurodegenerative disorder, is the leading cause of senile dementia. The typical symptoms include the memory dysfunction, cognitive impairment, psychiatric and behavioral abnormality, and difficulty in performing everyday tasks [1–3]. This multifaceted neurodegenerative disorder is one of the leading causes of death in elderly people and continues to be a social, health and economic burden on society. The exact molecular mechanism for the pathogenesis of AD is not well-understood yet; however, several hypotheses have been proposed explaining the initiation of neurodegeneration in Alzheimer's disease. These include cholinergic hypothesis (pathological changes and the dysfunction of the neuro-cholinergic system), amyloid hypothesis (β-amyloid tangles and aggregations inducing neural apoptosis, tau protein hyperphosphorylation forming senile plaque), oxidative stress hypothesis (neuro-inflammation and increasing level of reactive oxygen radicals), and bio-metal hypothesis (deregulation of transition bio-metals in AD patients). Among these, the design and development of new and potent inhibitors based on central cholinergic hypothesis remains the most common and clinically tested strategy for AD therapy [4–8].

Cholinesterase (ChE), namely acetylcholinesterase (AChE, EC 3.1.1.7) and butyrylcholinesterase (BuChE, EC 3.1.1.8), catalyze the hydrolysis of cholinergic neurotransmitters. Acetylcholine (ACh) is predominantly decomposed by AChE compared to BuChE, thus the inhibition of AChE to increase the level of ACh remains a promising strategy for the treatment of Alzheimer's disease [9,10]. The crystal structure of this enzyme reveals the presence of a catalytic active site (CAS) and a peripheral anionic site (PAS) linked through a 20 Å long gorge. Furthermore, the role of AChE in the induction of AD through the pro-aggregation activity of the Aβ protein, formation of reactive oxygen species (ROS), calcium dysregulation, and neuronal dysfunction has been observed. Therefore, bioactive molecules with a potential to interact specifically with both catalytic site (PAS or CAS) residues can significantly help in the inhibition of AChE while eliminating Aβ aggregation [10].

The current treatment strategy provides only a symptomatic relief to AD patients. The previously approved (marketed) drugs, including tacrine, donepezil, rivastigmine, and galantamine, despite being diverse in structural features and pharmacokinetic profiles, are proving ineffective as medications in stopping or reversing the progression of AD [11]. Although, after 20 years, the approval of Aducanumab, treating the possible cause of the neurodegenerative disorder, rather than just the symptoms, provides a hope against this intractable condition [12], and the design of new and safer therapeutics to address multifactorial disease remains a promising research field. Therefore, employing a well-known pharmacophore hybridization strategy could prove effective in exerting a beneficial role in the treatment of AD [1,13].

Quinoline (1-aza-naphthalene or benzo[b]pyridine) represents a class of nitrogen-containing heterocycles, which are well recognized for a diverse variety of pharmacological applications [14,15]. Various natural products, bioactive drug molecules, pharmaceuticals, and agrochemicals incorporate quinoline pharmacophore [16–18]. Notable medicinal applications associated with the quinoline heterocycle include anticancer, anti-tubercular, anti-proliferative, anti-malarial, antibacterial, anti-inflammatory, anti-protozoal, anti-fungal, anti-tumor, antioxidant, anti-HIV, anti-hypertensive, alkaline phosphatase inhibition and for the treatment of neurodegenerative disorders [19–28]. In parallel, thiosemicarbazones also display a wide plethora of biological properties ranging from anticancer, anti-bacterial, anti-tumor, anti-protozoal, anti-fungal, anti-leishmanial, and antiviral activities [29–34]. Thiosemicarbazone derivatives have also been employed as NDRG1 up-regulators, cathepsin inhibitors, and cholinesterase inhibitors for the treatment of Alzheimer's disease [35–38]. Figure 1 represents illustrative examples of commercial drugs for AD therapy and importance of quinoline as well as thiosemicarbazone in medicinal/pharmaceutical chemistry.

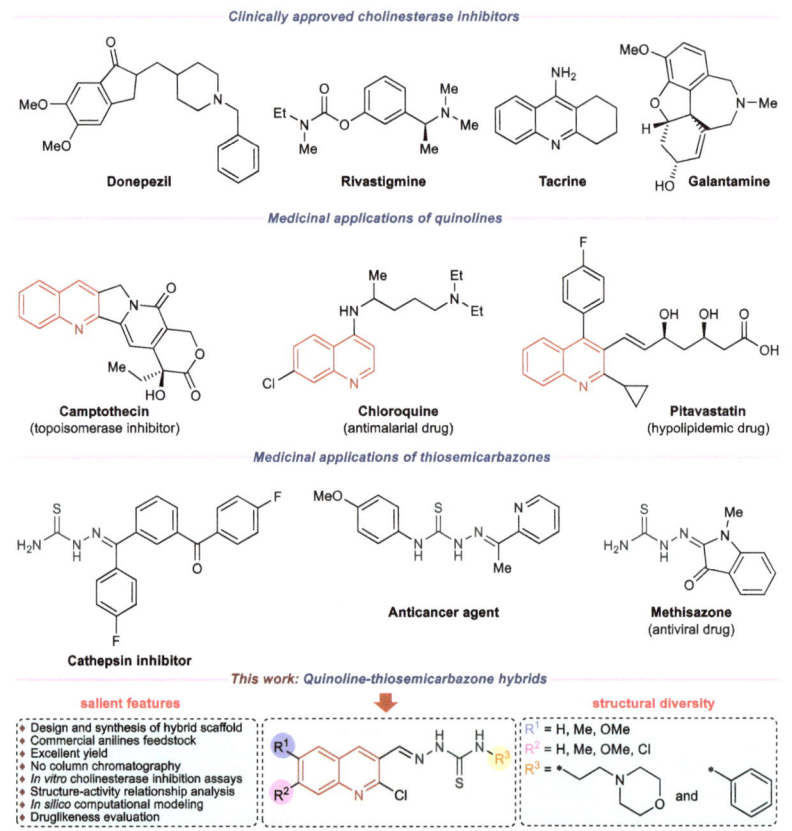

Figure 1. Examples of clinically approved drugs for AD and rationale of current study.

Cognizant of the fact that both quinoline and thiosemicarbazone pharmacophores are promising candidates for the generation of molecular and structural libraries of anti-cholinesterase inhibitors, and taking inspiration from the tacrine scaffold that features a quinoline ring, we herein utilized a pharmacophore hybridization strategy to design and explore the wider chemical space for new and potent cholinesterase inhibitors with less side effects, extending on our previous efforts in the current area of research [39–45]. Furthermore, in view of high demand and omnipresence of nitrogen heterocycles in numerous drugs [46–49], we have introduced an additional morpholine ring of high therapeutic value [50–54] in the target structures to examine the effect on the cholinesterase inhibition (Figure 1). We have also calculated the ADME properties and the results were remarkably good.

2. Results and Discussion

2.1. Synthetic Chemistry

The synthesis of quinoline-thiosemicarbazone hybrids **5a–k** was achieved using a facile and efficient multistep approach, as illustrated in Scheme 1. Several commercially available (un)substituted anilines were acetylated using orthophosphoric acid and acetic acid to afford acetanilides **2a–f** [45]. Subsequent Vilsmeier–Haack formylation using dimethylformamide and phosphoryl chloride provided 2-chloroquinoline-3-carbaldehydes **3a–f** [55]. Acid-catalyzed condensation of formylquinolines with commercially available N-(2-morpholinoethyl)hydrazinecarbothioamide **4a** and N-phenylhydrazinecarbothioamide **4b** gave the desired quinoline-thiosemicarbazone hybrids **5a–e** in excellent yields.

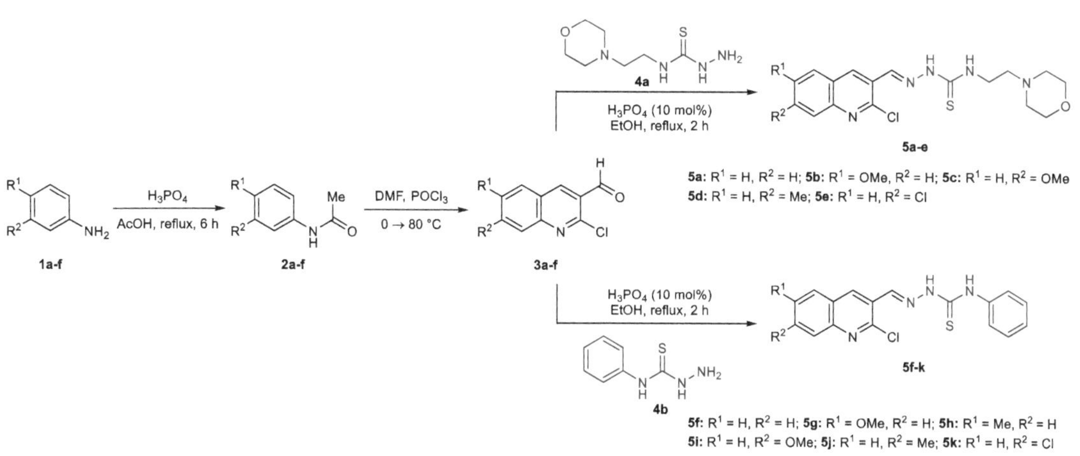

Scheme 1. Synthetic route to quinoline-thiosemicarbazone hybrids **5a–k**.

2.2. Spectroscopic Characterization

The condensation reaction of formylquinolines **3a–f** with thiosemicarbazides **4a** or **4b** affording quinoline-thiosemicarbazones **5a–k** was confirmed through ^{1}H NMR spectroscopy where the target products feature a distinct singlet for azomethine (N=CH) proton (8.26–8.61 ppm). Two additional signals attributable to secondary thioamide protons, out of which =N-NH proton resonated at a relatively more downfield chemical shift as a singlet peak at 11.76–12.23 ppm compared to C-NH proton (10.15–10.29 ppm) also confirmed the structures of thiosemicarbazones **5f–k**. However, in case of compounds **5a–e**, C-NH proton displayed a comparatively upfield triplet signal (8.54–8.70 ppm) due to coupling with the adjacent methylene protons. Moreover, the disappearance of a very distinct aldehyde peak around 10 ppm also confirmed the consumption of **3a–f** during the course of reaction for the formation of target compounds **5a–k**.

The aromatic protons showed chemical shifts between 6.80 and 9.40 ppm according to their chemical environment, with H-4 of quinoline heterocycle appearing as the most deshielded proton. Moreover, in ^{1}H NMR spectra of thiosemicarbazones **5a–e**, the morpholine ring protons gave two sets of signals around 2.45 and 3.60 ppm in addition to linear chain methylene protons that also exhibit a similar pattern.

The structures **5a–e** were further confirmed from ^{13}C NMR data. The C=S carbon resonated at the highest chemical shift near 177 ppm. The signals, referring to aromatic and azomethine carbon atoms, appeared between 106 and 163 ppm. In case of compounds **5a–e**, signals for morpholine ring carbon atoms appeared around 57.0 and 66.0 ppm. The ethyl chain between the morpholine and thioamide group showed peaks near 40.8 and 53.5 ppm, however the former carbon signals were overlapped by NMR solvent signal (DMSO-d_6). Overall, proton integration and appropriate number of carbon signals in ^{1}H and ^{13}C NMR showed complete agreement with the corresponding structures. Furthermore, the elemental analyses of all the quinoline-thiosemicarbazones were in accordance with the proposed structures.

2.3. In Vitro Cholinesterase Inhibition and Structure–Activity Relationship Analyses

The newly prepared quinoline-thiosemicarbazone hybrids **5a–k** were screened in vitro for their ability to inhibit cholinesterase enzymes (AChE and BChE) using Ellman's method [56]. Galantamine was employed as a positive control. The results of inhibitory assays for target compounds are presented in Table 1. The designed molecules consist of two basic components: (i) the quinoline heterocycle with varied degree of structural features (R^1 & R^2), which is mainly involved in π-π stacking and π-alkyl interactions, and

(ii) an acyclic thiosemicarbazone fragment bearing a suitable terminal attachment (R^3) in the form of an aromatic ring (phenyl) and a saturated heterocyclic ring (morpholine) linked through an aliphatic linker (Figure 2). Various nitrogen atoms can act as hydrogen bond donor sites for establishing vital interactions with the amino acid residues in the active site of enzymes. Hence, the hybridization concept not only delivered new and diversified lead structures but also maintained significantly pharmacokinetically relevant parameters, such as molar mass. As such, various dynamic structure-activity relationship analyses could be manifested depicting the effect of functional group/substituent variation on the biological potential.

Table 1. Anti-cholinesterase (AChE and BChE) potential of synthesized compounds 5a–k.

Compound	Substituent			Acetylcholinesterase(AChE)	Butyrylcholinesterse(BChE)
	R^1	R^2	R^3	$IC_{50} \pm$ SEM (µM)/%inhibition	
5a	H	H	ethylmorpholine	2.95 ± 0.24	3.32%
5b	OMe	H	ethylmorpholine	0.12 ± 0.02	8.12%
5c	H	OMe	ethylmorpholine	5.53 ± 0.11	1.33%
5d	H	Me	ethylmorpholine	0.55 ± 0.01	1.52%
5e	H	Cl	ethylmorpholine	10.5 ± 0.16	1.88%
5f	H	H	Ph	23.2 ± 1.28	4.47%
5g	OMe	H	Ph	34.2 ± 1.02	11.3 ± 0.67
5h	Me	H	Ph	49.3 ± 2.49	32.6%
5i	H	OMe	Ph	60.9 ± 6.57	24.0%
5j	H	Me	Ph	46.5 ± 3.12	16.8%
5k	H	Cl	Ph	47.1 ± 1.45	20.3%
Galantamine	—	—	—	0.62 ± 0.01	0.87 ± 0.03

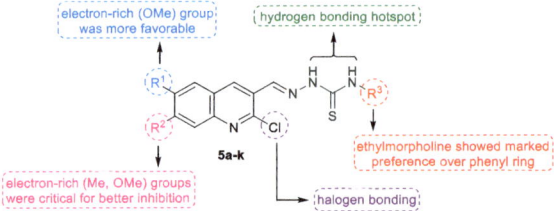

Figure 2. Representation of the diversity points and effect of chemical manipulation on biological activity.

The evaluation of activity results presented in Table 1 revealed that the intricate balance of substituents (R^1, R^2 & R^3) is critical for the strong inhibitory effects. In general, all the tested hybrid derivatives were completely selective towards AChE and showed inhibition in the range of 0.12–60.9 µM. The presence of ethylmorpholine as R^3 on the thioamide unit was significantly preferred over phenyl ring and the derivatives bearing this moiety were identified as the lead candidates. Compound **5b** showed the highest inhibitory efficacy with an IC_{50} value of 0.12 ± 0.02 µM, 5-fold more potent than the standard drug (galantamine; IC_{50} = 0.62 ± 0.01 µM). For further exploration of structure-activity relationships, various alterations were considered taking into account the substituents pattern on different sites of the hybrid structure (Figure 3). For instance, switching the position of methoxy group from 6-position (R^1) to 7-position (R^2) on quinoline ring led to reduced potency (**5c**; IC_{50} = 5.53 ± 0.11 µM), however, the effect of replacing ethylmorpholine with a phenyl ring was completely detrimental (**5i**; IC_{50} = 60.9 ± 6.57 µM). Replacement of methoxy group in **5c** with a methyl substituent reinstated the activity and compound **5d** showed slightly better inhibition profile than galantamine with an IC$_{50}$ value of 0.55 ± 0.01 µM. Similar trend was observed for compound **5j**. Disappointingly, the introduction of a halogen substituent (Cl) as R^2 produced deleterious effect in both cases (**5e** & **5k**); however, the compound bearing an ethylmorpholine (**5e**) was less affected compared to its congener (**5k**), which showed a sharp decrease in potency (IC$_{50}$ = 47.1 ± 1.45 µM). Further modifications to compound **5b**, the lead molecule, were made while removing all the substituents at quinoline ring and the results unveiled the importance of methoxy substituent at 6-position for better in vitro inhibitory properties. The resulting compound **5a** showed significant activity (IC$_{50}$ = 2.95 ± 0.24 µM), but less than lead inhibitor and standard drug (Figure 3). Collectively, the presence of both R^1 and R^2 substituents in combination with ethylmorpholine in an interactive manner is necessary for the quinoline-thiosemicarbazone hybrids to inhibit the acetylcholinesterase with maximum efficiency.

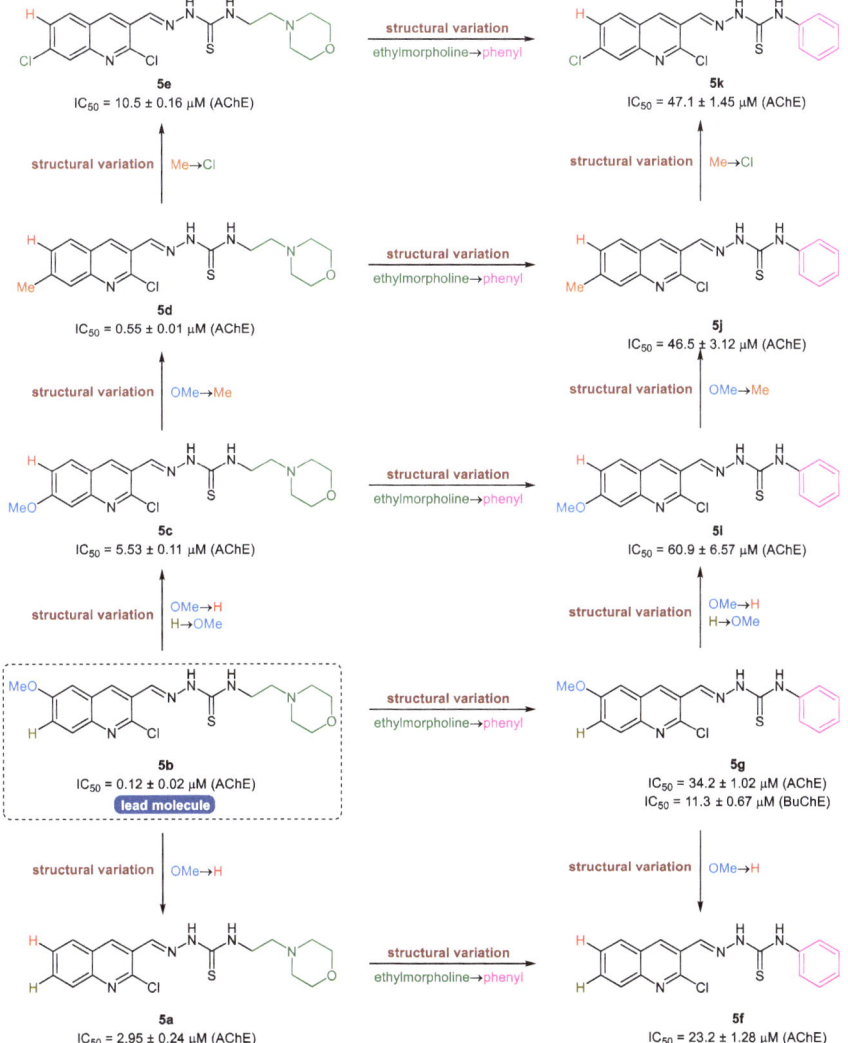

Figure 3. Structure-activity relationship analyses of quinoline-thiosemicarbazones **5a–k**.

The synthesized hybrids **5a–k** have also been investigated for their potential to inhibit butyrylcholinesterase enzyme, however, the compounds showed exclusive selectivity towards acetylcholinesterase. Against butyrylcholinesterase, all the compounds showed <50% inhibition; however, in contrast to AChE results, the modest enhancement in potency preferred the presence of an aromatic (phenyl) ring instead of ethylmorpholine and a methoxy substituent appeared to be crucial for activity. The lead example was compound **5g** with an IC$_{50}$ value of 11.3 ± 0.67 µM while other derivatives **5h–k** showed inhibition of BChE in the range of 16–32%. Hence, the results obtained for BChE confirmed the importance of aromatic moiety on the thioamide core, albeit low activity.

2.4. Mechanism of Inhibition

With the help of kinetics studies, the mode of action of the most potent compounds **5b** and **5d** was determined using acetylthiocholine iodide as a substrate. Enzyme kinetics were used to determine the mechanism of acetylcholinesterase inhibition. Lineweaver-Burk graph (reciprocal of rate of reaction 1/S and reciprocal of substrate concentration 1/V) were used for the determination of the type of inhibition and analysis of effect of inhibitor on V_{max} and K_m. The slope K_m/V_{max} of each line in the Lineweaver-Burk plot was plotted against different concentrations of substrate and chemicals to determine the value of K_i.

Kinetics studies were performed on **5b** and **5d** with different concentrations of compounds and substrate. Four concentrations of 1 mM compound **5b** (0, 0.06, 0.12, 0.18 µM), compound **5d** (0, 0.3, 0.6, 0.9 µM) and four concentrations of substrate (0, 0.5, 1.0, 1.5 and 2.0 mM showing 1/S as 0.0, 2.0, 1.0, 0.667 and 0.5, respectively) were made. Both compounds competes with substrate (acetylthiocholine iodide) for binding in the active site of acetylcholinesterase. V_{max} of enzyme was not affected and K_m of acetylcholinesterase was increased which showed competitive inhibition as shown in Figure 4. In competitive inhibition, lines intersecting at y-axis show no change in V_{max} with an increase in the value of K_m.

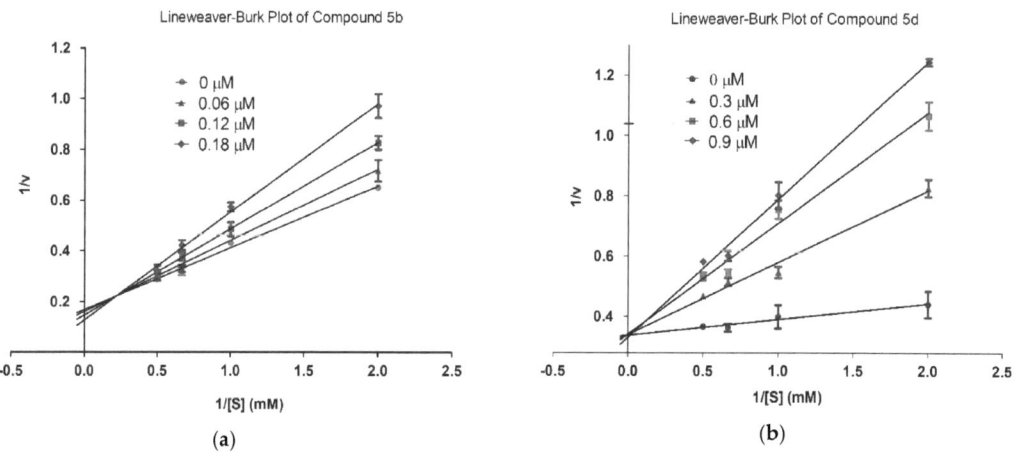

Figure 4. Inhibition of acetylcholinesterase by compounds **5b** (a) and **5d** (b). Lineweaver-Burk graph showing reciprocal rate of reaction 1/V against reciprocal of substrate 1/S.

2.5. Molecular Docking Studies

For docking studies, X-ray structures of human AChE (PDB ID: 4BDT) [57] was selected due to the high crystallographic resolution (3.10 Å) of electric eel AChE. Molecular docking analysis of all the tested compounds was performed against AChE to explore the possible binding modes. An overview of the active site of AChE containing cognate ligand and all the inhibitors was presented in Figure S3. The orientation of the most potent and selective compounds **5b** and **5d** along with the crystallographic inhibitor **huprine W** were presented in the active site of AChE (Figure 5).

The active pocket of AChE was surrounded by amino acid residues Leu76, Tyr124, Phe338, Gly122, Trp286, Tyr337, Val 340, Phe297, Leu289, Tyr72, Ser298, Ser125, Arg 296, Ser203, Tyr341, Ala204 and His447. The hydrogen bonds and π-π interactions were noticed by the most potent inhibitor **5b** as well as by **huprine W** as reported previously [45]. The cognate ligand (**huprine W**) showed two conventional hydrogen bonds with Ser203 (2.33 Å) and Gly122 (2.96 Å) and multiple π-π stacking interactions (4.00, 5.30, 4.41 and 3.69 Å) with Trp86. Additionally, 2-alkyl linkages (4.18 and 4.87 Å) with Trp439 and Tyr449, an alkyl linkage (4.52 Å) with Pro446 were also observed. Moreover, **huprine W** formed a π-π stacked bond (2.54 Å), one π-alkyl bond (4.45 Å) and π-donor hydrogen bond (4.01 Å) with Tyr337. Other interactions like π-alkyl with Met443 (4.89 Å) and a carbon-H bond (3.53 Å) with His447 were also present (Figure 5a).

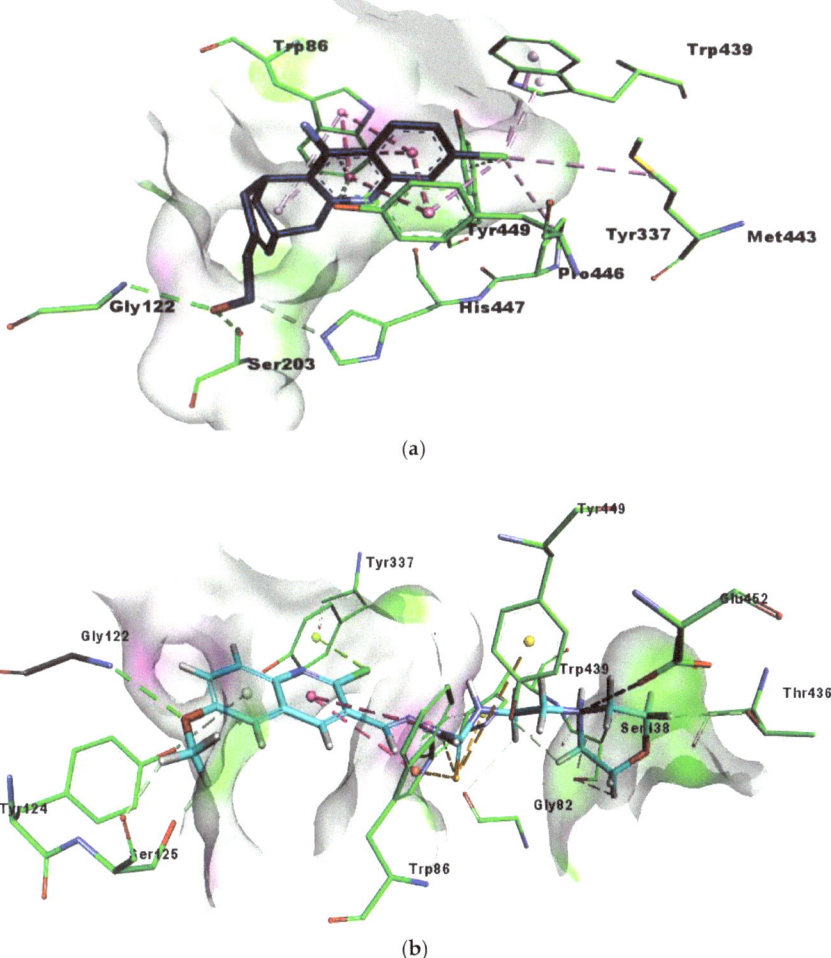

Figure 5. *Cont.*

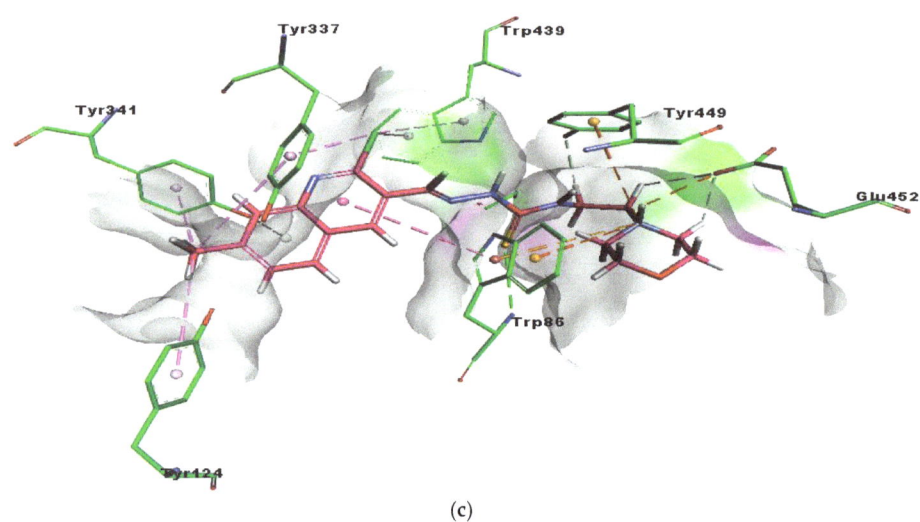

(c)

Figure 5. 3D interactions of **huprine W** (a), compounds **5b** (b) and **5d** (c) with amino acid residues. π-π T-shaped interactions are shown as fuscia, hydrogen bond as green, π-sulfur as yellow and π-alkyl interaction as light green dashed lines.

The most potent compound **5b** presented multiple important interactions with amino acids of active pocket like π-π T-shaped (6.23 Å) by quinoline ring and π-sulfur (4.34 Å) by sulfur atom in the thiosemicarbazone moiety with Trp86, the most important amino acid residue within the active pocket of AChE. Hydrogen bonding was noticed between oxygen atom and Gly122 (2.82 Å). However, Trp439 (4.68 Å) and Tyr449 (5.86 Å) exhibited π-sulfur interactions with sulfur atom in the thiosemicarbazone moiety of **5b**. Methoxy oxygen showed hydrogen bond with Gly122 (2.82 Å), while chloro atom formed π-lone pair (2.80 Å) with Tyr337. Moreover, nitrogen atom of morpholine ring exhibited attractive charge interactions (4.93 Å) with Glu452 (Figure 5b). It was clearly noted that methoxy group did not occupied the deep cleft of catalytic site.

Another potent and selective compound **5d** docked inside the AChE represented several important interactions. These include π-π T-shaped (5.43 Å) by the methyl quinoline ring, hydrogen bond (3.30 Å), by the sulfur atom of thiosemicarbazone moiety and π-cation interactions (5.26 Å), and by the nitrogen atom of morpholine ring with Trp86. Additionally, the nitrogen atom of morpholine ring was involved in the formation of the salt bridge (2.69 Å) and π-cation (4.78 Å), and interactions with Glu452 and Tyr449, respectively. Moreover, multiple π-alkyl (5.14, 5.37 and 3.76 Å) interactions were formed by methyl group with Tyr337, Tyr124 and Tyr341, respectively. The chloro group at the quinoline ring showed π-alkyl interactions (5.43 and 3.32 Å) with Trp439 and Tyr337, respectively, as shown in Figure 5c. Both compounds exhibited mostly similar interactions with the same residues, except for the presence of 6-methoxy and 7-methyl at the quinoline ring. These multiple interactions, especially π-π and strong hydrogen bonds by the potent compounds deep inside the catalytic cleft of acetylcholinesterase, can be the possible reason for their significant inhibitory profile.

The binding poses of all the derivatives were shown in Figure S3, which clearly represents the binding of compound **5b** and **5d** near cognate ligand showing interactions with important residues as **Huprine W** does. However, other residues do not show binding at the same position, instead showed binding with other amino acids and are slightly away from the active pocket

The type of interactions between ligands (**5b** and **5d**) and receptor (4BDT) along with the distance and atoms involved in the interactions are presented in 2D interactions in Figure S4 and Table 2. The docking studies revealed that the most potent compound **5b**, having 6-methoxy at quinoline ring was responsible for the conformational changes and the best binding of compound within the active pocket of enzyme. In vitro results of all the compounds showing variable inhibition against acetylcholinesterase were justified from their binding interactions within the catalytic region of the enzyme. Moreover, the selected compounds presented negative free energy values and were found to bind with significant affinity. Taken together, results presented herein showed that quinoline morpholinoethyl hydrazine carbothioamide derivatives are promising inhibitors of acetylcholinesterase.

Table 2. The types of binding interactions, distance of bonds and atoms involved in interactions.

Compounds	Binding interactions			
	Ligand Atom	Receptor Atom	Interaction Type	Distance (Å)
5b	O26	GLY122	H-bond	2.82
	phenyl ring	TRP86	π-π T-shaped & π-sulfur	6.23 & 4.34
	Cl11	TYR337	π-lone pair	2.80
	S16	TRP439	π-sulfur	4.68
	N20	GLU452	Attractive charges	4.93
	S16	TYR449	π-sulfur	5.86
5d	N20	GLU452	salt bridge	2.69
	N20	TYR449	π-cation	4.78
	S16, phenyl ring & N20	TRP86	H-bond, π-π T-shaped & π-cation	3.30, 5.43 & 5.26
	Cl11	TRP439	π-alkyl	5.43
	Methyl & Cl11	TYR337	π-alkyl	5.14 & 3.32
	Methyl	TYR124	π-alkyl	5.37
	Methyl	TYR341	π-alkyl	3.76
Hup W	O1	GLY122	H-bond	2.96
	O1	SER203	H-bond	2.33
	Quinoline ring	TRP86	π-π Stacked & π-alkyl	4.41, 5.30, 4.00, 3.69 & 4.18, 4.87
	Cl1	PRO446	Alkyl	4.52
	Cl1	TYR337	π-π Stacked & π-alkyl, π-donor	4.47, 2.54 & 4.45, 4.01
	Cl1	MET443	Alkyl	4.89
	Cl1	TRP439	π-alkyl	3.46 & 3.80
	Cl1	TYR449	π-alkyl	5.38

2.6. HYDE Assessment of Potent Inhibitors against Acetylcholinesterase

The top 20 docked conformations were assessed using the HYDE affinity method [58]. The assessment was made for the selected ligands using LeadIT software. The docking scores, binding free energies, and the most favorable poses for all the derivatives were calculated using FlexX (Table 3). The results demonstrated that the potent inhibitors (**5b** and **5d**) have high affinity towards the active site of acetylcholinesterase, as depicted by binding free energies. The potent inhibitors bind to the receptor with a very high binding affinity compared to the cognate ligands of the enzyme. Moreover, moderately and less active compounds exhibited low binding affinity as compared to potent compounds.

Table 3. Docking scores, binding free energies and their corresponding ranks by Hyde affinity assessment.

Compound	Docking Score by FlexX	Pose Rank	Binding Free Energy ΔG (kJ/mol)
5a	−22.12	1	−17
5b	−26.58	2	−25
5c	−21.56	2	−16
5d	−23.01	3	−18
5e	−19.67	2	−16
5f	−14.55	4	−12
5g	−14.62	3	−10
5h	−13.69	1	−8
5i	−12.58	2	−9
5j	−14.24	1	−10
5k	−13.99	2	−9
Huprine W	−16.29	1	−23

2.7. SeeSAR Visual Drug Design

The visual and investigative modes of the docked pose of compounds **5b** and **5d** revealed interpretable, innovative and important conformations using the SeeSAR tool in the LeadIT software [58,59]. Figure 6 represents the iterative and interactive optimization of leads showing the binding and non-binding capacity of compounds. Desolvation and interactions for compounds **5b** and **5d** are also shown in Figure 6. The approach predicts the visual and interpretable feedback for implicit hydrogen bonds and dehydration, and confirms our molecular docking results obtained using FlexX default parameters.

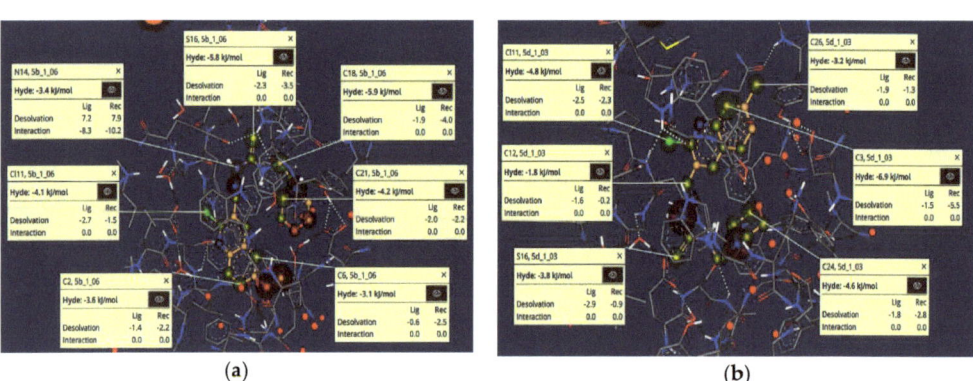

Figure 6. Visual and investigative modes of the docked pose of compounds **5b** (a) and **5d** (b) within the active site of acetylcholinesterase (pdb: 4BDT). The green colour represents the favourable and contributing atoms showing interactions inside the active pocket, while light green are chloride atoms, and yellow are sulfur atoms.

2.8. Molecular Dynamics Simulations

In addition to the molecular docking studies, we have performed molecular simulations for the cognate ligand (**Hup W**) and the most potent compound **5b** showing many fold higher inhibitory activity compared to other inhibitors. The MD simulations of the enzyme in complex with the cognate ligand (**Hup W**) and selected inhibitor **5b** were carried out in an aqueous environment for 30 ns with initial conformations taken from docking pose having the lowest binding free energy. Noncovalent interactions between ligands, **Hup W**, and **5b** and the active site of acetylcholinesterase were monitored in a time dependent manner.

The results of MD simulations are shown in the form of RMSD values, which give information regarding the overall stability of protein and its complex with the inhibitor. As shown in Figure 7, cognate ligand (**Hup W**) exhibited stability from the very start soon after 5 ns and was stable for rest of the time course. The only deviation found was at 2–4.8 ns. The selected ligand (**5b**) showed significant stability and less deviation within the range of 0.3–0.4 nm. The little variations were noticed in the structure of apo protein, whereas the structure of complex was found significantly stable after 4 ns. The structure of **5b**+protein complex showed little deviation between 14–17 ns, while remaining simulations were found stable as compared to protein alone. The consistent slight fluctuations were noted for protein during the whole simulation time (Figure 7).

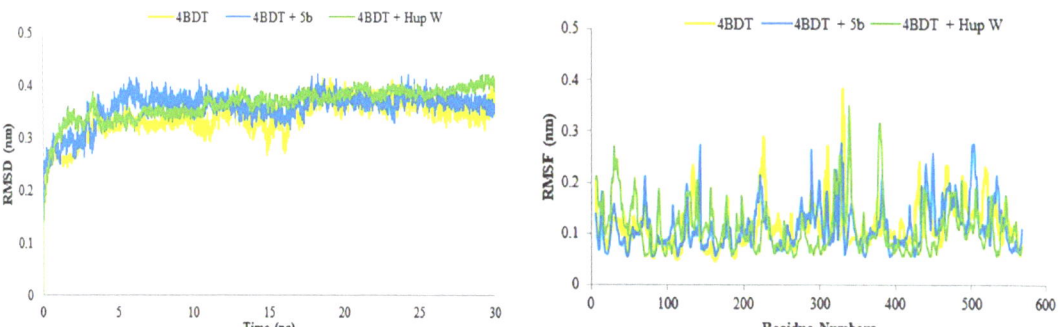

Figure 7. Root mean square deviations (RMSD) and root mean square fluctuations (RMSF) of amino acid residues of protein (4BDT) during 30 ns simulation time in the absence and presence of compound **5b**.

The knowledge of root mean square fluctuation values give the information about the calculations that were carried out to check the flexibility of the structure of receptor in the absence and presence of compound. As shown in Figure 7, the systems having apo and holo proteins presented noteworthy pattern of fluctuations. The apo protein started from 0.2 nm and showed the fluctuation between 0.1 and 0.3 nm during the simulation time with slight increase to 0.4 nm, whereas the holo protein, (protein + **5b**) started from 0.15 nm with fluctuation between 0.1 and 0.28 nm during the simulation time with slight increase. However, the holo protein, (protein + **Hup W**) showed fluctuations within the range of 0.10 to 0.30 during the simulation time course (30 ns). Overall, the system showed stability and less fluctuation. The region having motifs and loops showed less fluctuations, while active site pocket acquired significant stability during the whole time course of simulations. The results recommended the overall stability of complex as compared to protein alone. The results of protein structure depicted the stability of internal motion in protein and complex systems.

The radius of gyration was calculated to determine the compactness of the system during MD simulation time. It also describes the folding and unfolding of protein structure in the absence and presence of cognate ligand (**Hup W**) and compound **5b**. The results provided in Figure 8, demonstrated the compactness of system alone and in the presence of selected cognate ligand and compound. The average scores of Rg for acetylcholinesterase and its complex with **Hup W** and compound **5b** were found to be 2.3 and 2.25 nm, respectively, and showed the compactness of structures throughout the simulations. The results contribute towards the stability and compactness of protein only, with **Hup W** and compound **5b** during the simulation time, therefore playing a significant role in the increased affinity of compound **5b** for acetylcholinesterase enzyme.

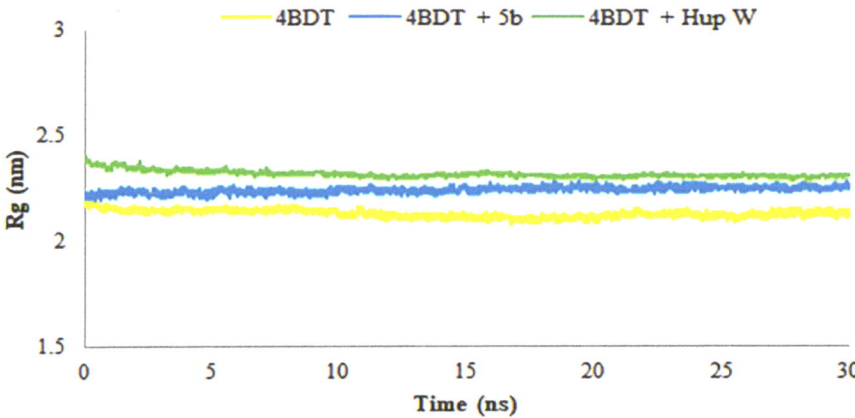

Figure 8. Radius of gyration (Rg) of amino acid residues in the presence and absence of compound **5b** during 30 ns MD simulation run.

2.9. ADME Properties

Pharmacokinetic properties of compounds **5b** and **5d** were predicted to assess the impact of different parameters using previously reported prediction tools [60–63]. These parameters include molecular weight, polar surface area, number of atom types (donor/acceptor), molecular refractivity, and lipophilicity (i.e., the partition coefficient, such as log Po/w, n-octanol, WLOGP, MLOGP and XLOGP3, etc.) representing the free energies of solvation and solvent accessible surface area [64]. Moreover, water solubility predicts solubility of the compounds. These properties predict the drug-likeness and blood-brain barrier permeation of test compounds. The results presented in Table 4 suggested that the tested derivatives are safe to use as drugs. However, in case of BBB permeation, the compounds showed poor pharmacokinetics and may not be able to cross BBB, while all the other properties exhibited by selected compounds are favorable.

Table 4. ADMET prediction scores for the selected compounds.

Properties.	Compounds	
	5b	5d
Physicochemical Properties		
Molecular weight (g/mol)	407.92	391.92
No. of heavy atoms	27	26
No. of aromatic heavy atoms	10	10
Fraction C_{sp3}	0.39	0.39
No. of rotatable bonds	8	7
No. of H-bond acceptors	5	4
No. of H-bond donors	2	2
Molar refractivity	114.72	113.20
TPSA (Å^2)	103.10	93.87
Lipophilicity		
Log $P_{o/w}$ (iLOGP)	3.65	3.21
Log $P_{o/w}$ (XLOGP3)	2.47	2.86
Log $P_{o/w}$ (WLOGP)	1.65	1.95

Table 4. Cont.

Properties.	Compounds	
	5b	5d
Log $P_{o/w}$ (MLOGP)	0.97	1.50
Log $P_{o/w}$ (SILICOS-IT)	3.96	4.41
Consensus Log $P_{o/w}$	2.54	2.79
Water Solubility		
Log S (ESOL)	−3.67	−3.89
Solubility (mg/mL; mol/L)	8.70×10^{-2}; 2.13×10^{-4}	5.00×10^{-2}; 1.28×10^{-4}
Class	Soluble	Soluble
Log S (ALi)	−4.28	−4.49
Solubility(mg/ml; mol/l)	2.14×10^{-2}; 5.26×10^{-5}	1.27×10^{-2}; 3.23×10^{-5}
Class	Moderately soluble	Moderately soluble
Log S (SILICOS-IT)	−5.70	−5.98
Solubility (mg/ml; mol/l)	8.06×10^{-4}; 1.98×10^{-6}	4.13×10^{-4}; 1.05×10^{-6}
Class	Moderately soluble	Moderately soluble
Pharmacokinetics		
GI absorption	High	High
BBB permeant	No	No
P-gp substrate	Yes	Yes
CYP1A2 inhibitor	Yes	Yes
CYP2C19 inhibitor	Yes	Yes
CYP2C9 inhibitor	Yes	Yes
CYP2D6 inhibitor	No	Yes
CYP3A4 inhibitor	Yes	Yes
Log K_p (skin permeation) (cm/s)	−7.03	−6.66
Druglikeness		
Lipinski	Yes; 0 violation	Yes; 0 violation
Ghose	Yes; 0 violation	Yes; 0 violation
Veber	Yes; 0 violation	Yes; 0 violation
Egan	Yes; 0 violation	Yes; 0 violation
Muegge	Yes; 0 violation	Yes; 0 violation
Bioavailability score	0.55	0.55
Medicinal Chemistry		
PAINS	0 alert	0 alert
Brenk	3 alerts: 2-halo_pyridine, imine_1, thiocarbonyl_group	3 alerts: 2-halo_pyridine, imine_1, thiocarbonyl_group
Leadlikeness	No; 2 Violations: MW > 350, Rotors > 7	No; 1 Violation MW > 350
Synthetic accessibility	3.16	3.18

3. Materials and Methods

3.1. General

The chemicals and solvents used were of analytical grade and obtained from commercial suppliers Scharlau (Barcelona, Spain), Merck (Darmstadt, Germany), and Fluka (Buchs, Switzerland), and were used without further purification. Thin layer chromatography was performed using aluminum plates coated with silica gel 60F$_{254}$ (Merck) in an appropriate eluent. The spots were visualized using ultraviolet irradiation. Melting points were recorded on Gallenkamp melting point apparatus (UK) and were uncorrected. ^{1}H NMR spectra were recorded in DMSO-d_6 solvent on a Bruker Avance NMR (300 MHz, Billerica, MA, USA) spectrometer while ^{13}C NMR spectra were recorded at 75 MHz. Chemical shifts are reported as δ values in parts per million (ppm) relative to tetramethylsilane as internal standard. Coupling constant (J) is given in Hertz. FTIR spectra were recorded on an Agilent Technologies Cary 630 FTIR (Santa Clara, CA, USA). Elemental analysis was performed on a LECO 630-200-200 TRUSPEC CHNS micro analyzer (St. Joseph, MI, USA) and the values observed were within ± 0.4% of the calculated results.

Acetylcholinesterase (E.C.3.1.1.7, from electric eel), butyrylcholinesterase (E.C. 3.1.1.8, from horse serum), substrates acetythiocholine chloride, butyrylthiocholine chloride and 5,5-dithio-bis-[2-nitrobenzoic acid] were purchased from Sigma-Aldrich (St. Louis, MO, USA) and Merck (Darmstadt, Germany). Galantamine was used as a standard drug. A 96-well microplate reader (BioTek ELx800, Instruments, Inc. Winooski, VT, USA) was used to determine the biological activities of the compounds.

3.2. Preparation of Acetanilides 2a–f

Orthophosphoric acid (0.2 mol) was added to a stirred solution of substituted anilines **1a–f** (1.0 mol) in glacial acetic acid (2.0 mol, 118 mL) and the resulting mixture was heated to reflux for 6 h. After the completion of the reaction, the mixture was poured into ice cold water with continuous stirring. The precipitated solid was filtered off, washed with excess cold water, and recrystallized from boiling water to produce acetanilides **2a–f** [45].

3.3. Preparation of 2-Chloroquinoline-3-carbaldehydes 3a–f

A Vilsmeier reagent, prepared from dropwise addition of POCl$_3$ (65.3 mL, 0.70 mol) to DMF (19.3 mL, 0.25 mol) at 0 °C with continuous stirring, was added corresponding acetanilide **2a–f** (0.10 mol). The resulting mixture was heated to 80 °C for 6–18 h. After the completion of the reaction (monitored by TLC), the reaction mixture was cautiously poured onto crushed ice (500 g) and stirred for 30 minutes at 0–10 °C. The precipitated solid was filtered off, washed with excess water, dried, and recrystallized from ethyl acetate to produce 2-chloroquinoline-3-carbaldehydes **3a–f** [55].

3.4. General Procedure for the Preparation of Quinoline-Thiosemicarbazones 5a–k

To a stirred solution of N-(2-morpholinoethyl)hydrazinecarbothioamide **4a** or N-phenylhydrazinecarbothioamide **4b** (1 mmol) in absolute ethanol (20 mL) was added 2-chloroquinoline-3-carbaldehyde **3** (1 mmol) followed by orthophosphoric acid (10 mol%). The resulting reaction mixture was heated to reflux for 2 h. The precipitated solid was filtered off and recrystallized from methanol to afford quinoline-thiosemicarbazones **5a–k**.

2-((2-Chloroquinolin-3-yl)methylene)-N-(2-morpholinoethyl)hydrazinecarbothioamide **5a**: Yield 92%. Yellow solid. Mp 250–252 °C. FTIR (cm^{-1}): 3340 (N-H), 3149 (N-H), 2995 (C-H), 1654 (C=N), 1112 (C=S); ^{1}H NMR (DMSO-d_6, 300 MHz) δ$_H$ = 2.46 (t, J = 4.5 Hz, 4H, NCH$_2$ of morpholine ring), 2.55 (t, J = 6.6 Hz, 2H, NH-CH$_2$-CH$_2$-morpholine), 3.61 (t, J = 4.5 Hz, 4H, OCH$_2$ of morpholine ring), 3.70 (q, J = 6.6 Hz, 2H, NH-CH$_2$-CH$_2$-morpholine), 7.23 (td, J = 7.5, 0.9 Hz, 1H, ArH), 7.33 (d, J = 8.1 Hz, 1H, ArH), 7.53 (td, J = 7.5, 1.2 Hz, 1H, ArH), 7.65 (dd, J = 7.8, 0.9 Hz, 1H, ArH), 8.30 (s, 1H, N=CH), 8.54–8.57 (m, 2H, NH, ArH), 11.76 (s, 1H, =N-NH); ^{13}C NMR (DMSO-d_6, 75 MHz) δ$_C$ = 40.8, 53.7, 57.0, 66.8, 115.7, 119.5, 123.0, 125.9, 128.8, 131.5, 134.9, 137.1, 139.4, 161.4, 177.4; Anal. Calcd. for C$_{17}$H$_{20}$ClN$_5$OS: C, 54.03; H, 5.33; N, 18.53; S, 8.49%. Found: C, 53.85; H, 5.01; N, 18.33; S, 8.20%.

2-((2-Chloro-6-methoxyquinolin-3-yl)methylene)-N-(2-morpholinoethyl)hydrazinecarbothioamide
5b: Yield 89%. Off-white solid. Mp 226–228 °C. FTIR (cm^{-1}): 3120 (N-H), 3003 (C-H), 1617 (C=N), 1110 (C=S); ^{1}H NMR (DMSO-d_6, 300 MHz) δ_H = 2.47 (t, J = 4.5 Hz, 4H, NCH$_2$ of morpholine ring), 2.57 (t, J = 6.9 Hz, 2H, NH-CH$_2$-CH$_2$-morpholine), 3.62 (t, J = 4.5 Hz, 4H, OCH$_2$ of morpholine ring), 3.73 (q, J = 6.3 Hz, 2H, NH-CH$_2$-CH$_2$-morpholine), 3.90 (s, 3H, ArOCH$_3$), 7.27 (d, J = 2.7 Hz, 1H, ArH), 7.46 (dd, J = 9.3, 2.7 Hz, 1H, ArH), 7.85 (d, J = 9.3 Hz, 1H, ArH), 8.48 (s, 1H, N=CH), 8.66 (t, J = 5.7 Hz, 1H, NH), 8.93 (s, 1H, ArH), 11.91 (s, 1H, =N-NH); ^{13}C NMR (DMSO-d_6, 75 MHz) δ_C = 40.9, 53.7, 56.1, 56.9, 66.8, 106.1, 124.6, 126.7, 128.4, 129.8, 134.5, 137.2, 143.5, 146.3, 158.5, 177.6; Anal. Calcd. for C$_{18}$H$_{22}$ClN$_5$O$_2$S: C, 53.00; H, 5.44; N, 17.17; S, 7.86%. Found: C, 53.25; H, 5.70; N, 17.34; S, 8.01%.

2-((2-Chloro-7-methoxyquinolin-3-yl)methylene)-N-(2-morpholinoethyl)hydrazinecarbothioamide
5c: Yield 90%. Yellow solid. Mp 242–244 °C. FTIR (cm^{-1}): 3291 (N-H), 3156 (N-H), 3001 (C-H), 1667 (C=N), 1107 (C=S); ^{1}H NMR (DMSO-d_6, 300 MHz) δ_H = 2.46 (t, J = 4.5 Hz, 4H, NCH$_2$ of morpholine ring), 2.56–2.60 (m, 2H, NH-CH$_2$-CH$_2$-morpholine), 3.60–3.72 (m, 6H, OCH$_2$ of morpholine ring, NH-CH$_2$-CH$_2$-morpholine), 3.94 (s, 3H, ArOCH$_3$), 6.82 (d, J = 1.8 Hz, 1H, ArH), 6.87 (dd, J = 8.7, 2.4 Hz, 1H, ArH), 7.55 (d, J = 9.0 Hz, 1H, ArH), 8.26 (s, 1H, N=CH), 8.63 (t, J = 5.4 Hz, 1H, NH), 8.97 (s, 1H, ArH), 11.94 (s, 1H, =N-NH); ^{13}C NMR (DMSO-d_6, 75 MHz) δ_C = 41.0, 53.7, 55.9, 57.0, 66.8, 107.0, 113.8, 122.6, 124.1, 130.4, 134.9, 137.6, 141.4, 149.5, 162.4, 177.2; Anal. Calcd. for C$_{18}$H$_{22}$ClN$_5$O$_2$S: C, 53.00; H, 5.44; N, 17.17; S, 7.86%. Found: C, 52.92; H, 5.30; N, 17.05; S, 7.77%.

2-((2-Chloro-7-methylquinolin-3-yl)methylene)-N-(2-morpholinoethyl)hydrazinecarbothioamide
5d: Yield 87%. Yellow solid. Mp 256–258 °C. FTIR (cm^{-1}): 3332 (N-H), 3197 (N-H), 2851 (C-H), 1655 (C=N), 1106 (C=S); ^{1}H NMR (DMSO-d_6, 300 MHz) δ_H = 2.46–2.53 (m, 9H, NCH$_2$ of morpholine ring, NH-CH$_2$-CH$_2$-morpholine, ArCH$_3$), 3.60 (t, J = 4.2 Hz, 4H, OCH$_2$ of morpholine ring), 3.71 (q, J = 6.6 Hz, 2H, NH-CH$_2$-CH$_2$-morpholine), 7.54 (d, J = 8.4 Hz, 1H, ArH), 7.74 (s, 1H, ArH), 7.89 (d, J = 8.1 Hz, 1H, ArH), 8.49 (s, 1H, N=CH), 8.66 (t, J = 5.4 Hz, 1H, NH), 9.00 (s, 1H, ArH), 11.89 (s, 1H, =N-NH); ^{13}C NMR (DMSO-d_6, 75 MHz) δ_C = 22.0, 41.0, 53.7, 57.0, 66.7, 125.3, 125.8, 127.2, 128.4, 130.7, 135.7, 137.4, 142.6, 147.7, 161.5, 177.5; Anal. Calcd. for C$_{18}$H$_{22}$ClN$_5$OS: C, 55.16; H, 5.66; N, 17.87; S, 8.18%. Found: C, 55.40; H, 5.84; N, 17.98; S, 8.30%.

2-((2,7-Dichloroquinolin-3-yl)methylene)-N-(2-morpholinoethyl)hydrazinecarbothioamide **5e:**
Yield 91%. Pale Yellow solid. Mp 237–239 °C. FTIR (cm^{-1}): 3330 (N-H), 3479 (N-H), 3001 (C-H), 1602 (C=N), 1102 (C=S); ^{1}H NMR (DMSO-d_6, 300 MHz) δ_H = 2.46 (t, J = 3.0 Hz, 4H, NCH$_2$ of morpholine ring), 2.56–2.59 (m, 2H, NH-CH$_2$-CH$_2$-morpholine), 3.58–3.61 (m, 4H, OCH$_2$ of morpholine ring), 3.73 (q, J = 6.4 Hz, 2H, NH-CH$_2$-CH$_2$-morpholine), 7.76 (dd, J = 8.7, 2.1 Hz, 1H, ArH), 8.03–8.09 (m, 2H, ArH), 8.51 (s, 1H, N=CH), 8.70 (t, J = 5.7 Hz, 1H, NH), 9.12 (s, 1H, ArH), 11.95 (s, 1H, =N-NH); ^{13}C NMR (DMSO-d_6, 75 MHz) δ_C = 41.1, 53.7, 57.0, 66.8, 126.0, 127.2, 129.3, 130.7, 132.7, 136.6, 140.1, 147.5, 150.2, 153.7, 177.6; Anal. Calcd. for C$_{17}$H$_{19}$Cl$_2$N$_5$OS: C, 49.52; H, 4.64; N, 16.98; S, 7.78%. Found: C, 49.80; H, 4.88; N, 17.12; S, 7.96%.

2-((2-Chloroquinolin-3-yl)methylene)-N-phenylhydrazinecarbothioamide **5f:** Yield 94%. Yellow solid. Mp 251–253 °C. FTIR (cm^{-1}): 3303 (N-H), 3157 (N-H), 3046 (C-H), 1653 (C=N), 1193 (C=S); ^{1}H NMR (DMSO-d_6, 300 MHz) δ_H = 7.20–7.27 (m, 2H, ArH), 7.32–7.43 (m, 3H, ArH), 7.51–7.60 (m, 3H, ArH), 7.68 (dd, J = 8.1, 0.9 Hz, 1H, ArH), 8.41 (s, 1H, N=CH), 8.85 (s, 1H, ArH), 10.18 (s, 1H, NH), 12.06 (s, 1H, =N-NH); ^{13}C NMR (DMSO-d_6, 75 MHz) δ_C = 115.7, 119.6, 122.9, 125.6, 126.0, 126.6, 128.6, 129.0, 131.6, 135.9, 137.9, 139.5, 161.5, 176.5; Anal. Calcd. for C$_{17}$H$_{13}$ClN$_4$S: C, 59.91; H, 3.84; N, 16.44; S, 9.41%. Found: C, 60.09; H, 4.00; N, 16.72; S, 9.65%.

2-((2-Chloro-6-methoxyquinolin-3-yl)methylene)-N-phenylhydrazinecarbothioamide **5g:** Yield 88%. Light brown solid. Mp 225–227 °C. FTIR (cm^{-1}): 3368 (N-H), 3295 (N-H), 3031 (C-H), 1656 (C=N), 1157 (C=S); ^{1}H NMR (DMSO-d_6, 300 MHz) δ_H = 3.90 (s, 3H, ArOCH$_3$), 7.26 (tt, J = 7.2, 1.2 Hz, 1H, ArH), 7.32 (d, J = 3.0 Hz, 1H, ArH), 7.39–7.50 (m, 3H, ArH), 7.56–7.60 (m, 2H, ArH), 7.87 (d, J = 9.3 Hz, 1H, ArH), 8.61 (s, 1H, N=CH), 9.27 (s, 1H, ArH), 10.28 (s, 1H, NH), 12.21 (s, 1H, =N-NH); ^{13}C NMR (DMSO-d_6, 75 MHz) δ_C = 56.1, 106.3, 124.6, 126.2,

126.5, 126.8, 128.6, 128.7, 129.7, 135.4, 138.1, 139.4, 143.6, 146.5, 158.5, 176.9; Anal. Calcd. for $C_{18}H_{15}ClN_4OS$: C, 58.30; H, 4.08; N, 15.11; S, 8.65%. Found: C, 58.58; H, 4.24; N, 15.33; S, 8.91%.

2-((2-Chloro-6-methylquinolin-3-yl)methylene)-N-phenylhydrazinecarbothioamide **5h**: Yield 92%. Light brown solid. Mp 242–244 °C. FTIR (cm^{-1}): 3303 (N-H), 3151 (N-H), 2995 (C-H), 1651 (C=N), 1123 (C=S); ^{1}H NMR (DMSO-d_6, 300 MHz) δ_H = 2.34 (s, 3H, ArCH$_3$), 7.22–7.28 (m, 3H, ArH), 7.60 (d, J = 8.4 Hz, 2H, ArH), 7.68 (dd, J = 8.4, 1.8 Hz, 1H, ArH), 7.77 (s, 1H, ArH), 7.86 (d, J = 8.7 Hz, 1H, ArH), 8.40 (s, 1H, N=CH), 8.81 (s, 1H, ArH), 10.15 (s, 1H, NH), 12.19 (s, 1H, =N-NH); ^{13}C NMR (DMSO-d_6, 75 MHz) δ_C = 21.6, 126.5, 126.7, 127.4, 128.0, 128.7, 134.3, 136.0, 137.6, 138.0, 139.4, 146.1, 148.2, 161.3, 176.8; Anal. Calcd. for $C_{18}H_{15}ClN_4S$: C, 60.92; H, 4.26; N, 15.79; S, 9.04%. Found: C, 61.14; H, 4.48; N, 15.95; S, 9.18%.

2-((2-Chloro-7-methoxyquinolin-3-yl)methylene)-N-phenylhydrazinecarbothioamide **5i**: Yield 91%. Yellow solid. Mp 224–226 °C. FTIR (cm^{-1}): 3294 (NH), 3149 (NH), 2931 (CH), 1609 (C=O), 1121 (C=S); ^{1}H NMR (DMSO-d_6, 300 MHz) δ_H = 3.94 (s, 3H, ArOCH$_3$), 6.83 (dd, J = 6.0, 2.4 Hz, 1H, ArH), 6.87 (d, J = 2.4 Hz, 1H, ArH), 7.22–7.43 (m, 5H, ArH), 7.91 (d, J = 9.0 Hz, 1H, ArH), 8.61 (s, 1H, N=CH), 9.28 (s, 1H, ArH), 10.25 (s, 1H, NH), 12.14 (s, 1H, =N-NH); ^{13}C NMR (DMSO-d_6, 75 MHz) δ_C = 56.0, 107.1, 113.9, 122.2, 123.9, 125.9, 126.5, 128.6, 130.6, 136.1, 138.4, 139.5, 141.5, 149.6, 162.3, 176.3; Anal. Calcd. for $C_{18}H_{15}ClN_4OS$: C, 58.30; H, 4.08; N, 15.11; S, 8.65%. Found: C, 58.44; H, 4.20; N, 15.30; S, 8.80%.

2-((2-Chloro-7-methylquinolin-3-yl)methylene)-N-phenylhydrazinecarbothioamide **5j**: Yield 90%. Yellow solid. Mp 205–207 °C. FTIR (cm^{-1}): 3301 (N-H), 3143 (N-H), 2936 (C-H), 1653 (C=N), 1197 (C=S); ^{1}H NMR (DMSO-d_6, 300 MHz) δ_H = 2.53 (s, 3H, ArCH$_3$), 7.37–7.44 (m, 3H), 7.53 (dd, J = 8.7, 1.5 Hz, 1H, ArH), 7.59 (d, J = 7.5 Hz, 2H, ArH), 7.75 (s, 1H, ArH), 7.91 (d, J = 8.4 Hz, 1H, ArH), 8.61 (s, 1H, N=CH), 9.31 (s, 1H, ArH), 10.28 (s, 1H, NH), 12.18 (s, 1H, =N-NH); ^{13}C NMR (DMSO-d_6, 75 MHz) δ_C = 22.0, 117.5, 124.5, 125.6, 126.2, 126.8, 127.2, 128.7, 130.6, 136.4, 138.2, 139.4, 142.7, 147.8, 161.6, 176.8; Anal. Calcd. for $C_{18}H_{15}ClN_4S$: C, 60.92; H, 4.26; N, 15.79; S, 9.04%. Found: C, 60.78; H, 4.10; N, 15.57; S, 8.88%.

2-((2,7-Dichloroquinolin-3-yl)methylene)-N-phenylhydrazinecarbothioamide **5k**: Yield 93%. Yellow solid. Mp 237–239 °C. FTIR (cm^{-1}): 3270 (N-H), 3090 (C-H), 1655 (C=N), 1197 (C=S); ^{1}H NMR (DMSO-d_6, 300 MHz) δ_H = 7.36–7.45 (m, 3H, ArH), 7.57–7.59 (m, 3H, ArH), 7.72 (dd, J = 8.7, 2.1 Hz, 1H, ArH), 8.04 (s, 1H, ArH), 8.60 (s, 1H, N=CH), 9.39 (s, 1H, ArH), 10.29 (s, 1H, NH), 12.23 (s, 1H, =N-NH); ^{13}C NMR (DMSO-d_6, 75 MHz) δ_C = 126.0, 126.6, 126.8, 127.1, 128.7, 129.1, 130.8, 135.8, 136.6, 137.6, 139.3, 147.6, 150.3, 161.3, 176.9; Anal. Calcd. for $C_{17}H_{12}Cl_2N_4S$: C, 54.41; H, 3.22; N, 14.93; S, 8.54%. Found: C, 54.63; H, 3.38; N, 15.07; S, 8.70%.

3.5. In Vitro Cholinesterase Inhibition Assay

Inhibition of acetylcholinesterase and butyrylcholinesterase was measured in vitro by spectrophotometric method developed by Ellman [56] with slight modifications [65]. Briefly, the reaction mixture contained 60 µL phosphate buffers (KH$_2$PO$_4$/KOH), pH 7.7, 10 µL of test compound dissolved in DMSO (final DMSO concentration was 2%) and 10 µL of enzyme (0.5 and 3.4 U/mg of AChE or BChE, respectively). Reaction contents were mixed thoroughly and kept for 10 min during pre-incubation at 37 °C. After the pre-incubation, 10 µL of 1 mM acetythiocholine chloride or butyrylthiocholine chloride was added to the respective AChE or BChE enzyme solution to start the enzymatic reactions. DTNB (10 µL, 0.5 mM) was also added as a coloring reagent. The reaction mixture was again incubated for 20 min at 37 °C and the absorbance was measured at 405 nm using 96-well micro-plate reader. All experiments were carried out in triplicate. Galantamine (0.1 mM) was used as a standard inhibitor. In order to measure the activity of enzyme, assay was performed with a blank containing all of the components except inhibitor. The percent inhibition was calculated by the following formula:

$$\text{Inhibition (\%)} = 100 - (A_c/A_f) \times 100 \qquad (1)$$

Where "A_c" and "A_f" are absorbance obtained for the respective enzyme (AChE and BChE) in the presence or absence of inhibitors, after subtracting the respective background (pre-read absorbance). Compounds exhibiting > 50% inhibition against ChEs were further evaluated for the determination of IC_{50} values which were calculated by non-linear curve fitting program PRISM 5.0 (GraphPad, San Diego, CA, USA).

3.6. Kinetics Studies

Michaelis-Menten kinetics experiments were used to determine the type of enzyme inhibition. Detailed kinetics studies of the potent compounds **5b** and **5d** were performed to probe the potential mechanism of action to inhibit the enzyme. For this purpose, the initial rates of the enzyme inhibition at four concentrations of substrate (0, 0.5, 1.0, 1.5, 2.0 mM) in the absence and presence of four different concentrations of compound **5b** (0, 0.06, 0.12, 0.18 µM) and compound **5d** (0, 0.3, 0.6, 0.9 µM) against acetylcholinesterase were measured.

3.7. Molecular Docking Protocols

3.7.1. Structure Selection and Preparation

Molecular docking studies were conducted to investigate the putative interactions of the compounds making complex with the acetylcholinesterase enzyme. In order to perform docking studies, the crystallographic structure of human AChE (PDB ID: 4BDT) was obtained from the RCSB PDB database [57], and prepared for the docking analysis. Prior to the experiments, the structures of the enzyme and compounds were prepared as follows. The enzyme structure was protonated with the Protonate3D [66] algorithm implemented within the molecular modeling tool MOE [67]. The structure was energy minimized using Amber99 force field including all crystallographic solvent molecules. The backbone atoms were restrained with a small force in order to avoid collapse of the binding pockets during energy minimization calculations. Subsequently, the co-crystallized ligands and solvent molecules were removed. The crystallographic water molecules were removed and hypothetical hydrogen atoms were added to the X-ray structure in standard geometries with the MOE.

3.7.2. Compounds Preparation

The 3D structural coordinates of compounds were generated using MOE followed by assignment of protonation and ionization states in physiological pH range by using the "wash" module. Afterwards, the structures of compounds were energy minimized with the MMFF94x force field for docking studies.

3.7.3. Docking Studies

For docking studies, calculations were performed using LeadIT from BioSolveIT, GmbH Germany [68]. Receptor was loaded by Load or Prepare Receptor utility of the LeadIT software. The binding site for the receptor was defined in 9.0 Å spacing of the amino acid residues. By FlexX utility of LeadIT, docking of compounds was performed. For this purpose, compounds were docked inside the active site of receptor and 50 conformations for each ligand-receptor complex were produced based on binding free energies. Default docking parameters were not modified and top 30 highest scoring docked positions were kept for further analysis [58]. Poses with lowest free binding energy values were considered as the most stable ones having the highest affinity to interact with the receptor. Each ligand-protein complex having lowest binding free energy for interactions was examined and 3D putative binding modes were visualized using Discovery Studio Visualizer v4 [69].

3.8. Molecular Dynamics Simulations

The crystallographic structure of human AChE (PDB ID: 4BDT) [57] was obtained from the Protein Data Bank (www.pdb.org, accessed on 14 September 2021). Protein manipulation and protonation were made with the help of GROMOS96 force field having the 43a1 parameter set. The GROMACS (Groningen Machine for Chemical Simulation) simulation packages, 5.1.4 were used for the MD simulations and protocol for molecular dynamics simulations was used according to previously developed methods [70–72] with little modifications. Parameterization of compound 5b and Huprine W were done online using the PRODRG servers [73]. MOE and VMD [74] were used for the visualization and molecular inspection. The crystallographic structure was solvated (addition of water molecule) and counter ions were incorporated to neutralize the receptor. Subsequently, the energy minimization of the system was done, followed by equilibration using two sequential NVT (100 ps) and NPT (100 ps) runs during which protein's heavy atoms were restrained.

After minimization, the resulting ensembles were submitted to 30 ns MD simulations with a time-step of 2 fs for each simulation. Periodic boundary conditions (PBC) were applied during all the simulations. Steepest descent method was used for simple energy minimizations. All NVT and NPT runs used the Berendsen thermostat and the Parrinello-Rahman barostat for temperature (approx. 303 K) and pressure coupling (approx. 1.01 bar), respectively. The cut-off radius of 10 Å and smooth Particle Mesh Ewald (PME) protocol were observed for long-range method. The root mean square deviations, fluctuations and radius of gyration were plotted using XMGRACE v5.1.19 [75].

4. Conclusions

In summary, a series of new quinoline-thiosemicarbazone hybrids was designed and synthesized using a facile multistep protocol. Several commercially available anilines were successfully employed to construct quinoline heterocycle via Vilsmeyer-Haack formylation reaction. Hybridization of quinoline carbaldehydes with thiosemicarbazides afforded target compounds in excellent yields, devoiding the need of column chromatographic purification. Evaluation of cholinesterase inhibitory potential revealed the discovery of numerous potent and highly efficacious inhibitors. In particular, compound **5b** inhibited the acetylcholinesterase selectively showing an IC_{50} value of 0.12 ± 0.02 µM, a 5-fold high potency than galantamine (standard). Structure-activity relationship analysis showed the importance of electron-rich (methoxy) substituent at quinoline ring and ethylmorpholine on the carbothioamide unit, playing a vital role in obtaining high therapeutic efficacy. Docking, physicochemical properties, lipophilicity, water solubility, pharmacokinetics, drug-likeness, and medicinal chemistry properties were also calculated for the potent inhibitors suggesting the safer profile to be investigated as drug molecules and have high probability of blood-brain penetration and absorption. Collectively, our findings established that compound **5b** is a potent, selective and competitive inhibitor of acetylcholinesterase and can serve as a promising candidate for further preclinical development for the therapy of Alzheimer's disease.

Supplementary Materials: ^{1}H and ^{13}C NMR spectra of all the synthesized compounds, dose response curves for enzyme (AChE and BChE) inhibition activity, comparative docking assessment results, 2D interactions of **huprine W**, compounds **5b** and **5d** with amino acid residues and Visual and investigative modes of the docked pose of compounds **5b** and **5d** within the active site of AChE are available online.

Author Contributions: Conceptualization, R.M. and I.K.; methodology, R.M.; software, S.Z.; validation, S.Z.; formal analysis, A.I. and I.K.; investigation, R.M., N.K., S.A. and T.T.A. (synthesis); M.T.Y. (bioactivity); S.Z. (molecular docking, ADME properties); resources, H.O.A., R.M. and S.Z.; data curation, H.O.A.; R.M. and S.Z.; writing—original draft preparation, S.Z. and I.K.; writing—review and editing, A.I.; N.S. and I.K.; visualization, S.Z.; supervision, R.M. and S.Z.; project administration, I.K.; funding acquisition, H.O.A. and S.Z. All authors have read and agreed to the published version of the manuscript.

Funding: Hashem O. Alsaab would like to acknowledge Taif University Researchers Supporting Project number (TURSP-2020/67), Taif University, Taif, Saudi Arabia.

Institutional Review Board Statement: Not applicable.

Informed Consent Statement: Not applicable.

Data Availability Statement: The data presented in this study are available in Supplementary Material.

Acknowledgments: Hashem O. Alsaab would like to acknowledge Taif University Researchers Supporting Project number (TURSP-2020/67), Taif University, Taif, Saudi Arabia. R.M. extends her gratitude to Head of Chemistry Department, Kinnaird College for Women, Lahore, for providing research facilities for synthetic work. S.Z. is grateful to BioSolveIT for the provision of license under Scientific Challenge (16144335733823).

Conflicts of Interest: The authors declare no conflict of interest.

Sample Availability: Samples of the synthetic compounds are available from the authors on reasonable request.

References

1. Sameem, B.; Saeedi, M.; Mahdavi, M.; Shafiee, A. A review on tacrine-based scaffolds as multi-target drugs (MTDLs) for Alzheimer's disease. *Eur. J. Med. Chem.* **2016**, *128*, 332–345. [CrossRef]
2. Ferreira, J.P.; Albuquerque, H.M.; Cardoso, S.M.; Silva, A.M.; Silva, V.L. Dual-target compounds for Alzheimer's disease: Natural and synthetic AChE and BACE-1 dual-inhibitors and their structure-activity relationship (SAR). *Eur. J. Med. Chem.* **2021**, *221*, 113492. [CrossRef] [PubMed]
3. Hroudová, J.; Singh, N.; Fišar, Z.; Ghosh, K.K. Progress in drug development for Alzheimer's disease: An overview in relation to mitochondrial energy metabolism. *Eur. J. Med. Chem.* **2016**, *121*, 774–784. [CrossRef] [PubMed]
4. Singh, M.; Kaur, M.; Kukreja, H.; Chugh, R.; Silakari, O.; Singh, D. Acetylcholinesterase inhibitors as Alzheimer therapy: From nerve toxins to neuroprotection. *Eur. J. Med. Chem.* **2013**, *70*, 165–188. [CrossRef]
5. Li, Q.; He, S.; Chen, Y.; Feng, F.; Qu, W.; Sun, H. Donepezil-based multi-functional cholinesterase inhibitors for treatment of Alzheimer's disease. *Eur. J. Med. Chem.* **2018**, *158*, 463–477. [CrossRef]
6. Wang, L.; Bharti; Kumar, R.; Pavlov, P.F.; Winblad, B. Small molecule therapeutics for tauopathy in Alzheimer's disease: Walking on the path of most resistance. *Eur. J. Med. Chem.* **2021**, *209*, 112915. [CrossRef]
7. Beato, A.; Gori, A.; Boucherle, B.; Peuchmaur, M.; Haudecoeur, R. β-Carboline as a Privileged Scaffold for Multitarget Strategies in Alzheimer's Disease Therapy. *J. Med. Chem.* **2021**, *64*, 1392–1422. [CrossRef]
8. Singh, Y.P.; Rai, H.; Singh, G.; Singh, G.K.; Mishra, S.; Kumar, S.; Srikrishna, S.; Modi, G. A review on ferulic acid and analogs based scaffolds for the management of Alzheimer's disease. *Eur. J. Med. Chem.* **2021**, *215*, 113278. [CrossRef] [PubMed]
9. Li, Q.; Yang, H.; Chen, Y.; Sun, H. Recent progress in the identification of selective butyrylcholinesterase inhibitors for Alzheimer's disease. *Eur. J. Med. Chem.* **2017**, *132*, 294–309. [CrossRef]
10. Bortolami, M.; Pandolfi, F.; de Vita, D.; Carafa, C.; Messore, A.; Di Santo, R.; Feroci, M.; Costi, R.; Chiarotto, I.; Bagetta, D.; et al. New deferiprone derivatives as multi-functional cholinesterase inhibitors: Design, synthesis and in vitro evaluation. *Eur. J. Med. Chem.* **2020**, *198*, 112350. [CrossRef]
11. Grutzendler, J.; Morris, J.C. Cholinesterase inhibitors for Alzheimer's disease. *Drugs* **2001**, *61*, 41–52. [CrossRef]
12. Mullard, A. Landmark Alzheimer's drug approval confounds research community. *Nature* **2021**, *594*, 309–310. [CrossRef]
13. Jalili-Baleh, L.; Babaei, E.; Abdpour, S.; Bukhari, S.N.A.; Foroumadi, A.; Ramazani, A.; Sharifzadeh, M.; Abdollahi, M.; Khoobi, M. A review on flavonoid-based scaffolds as multi-target-directed ligands (MTDLs) for Alzheimer's disease. *Eur. J. Med. Chem.* **2018**, *152*, 570–589. [CrossRef] [PubMed]
14. Bawa, S.; Gupta, H. Biological Activities of Quinoline Derivatives. *Mini-Rev. Med. Chem.* **2009**, *9*, 1648–1654. [CrossRef]
15. Kaur, K.; Jain, M.; Reddy, R.P.; Jain, R. Quinolines and structurally related heterocycles as antimalarials. *Eur. J. Med. Chem.* **2010**, *45*, 3245–3264. [CrossRef] [PubMed]
16. Bawa, S.; Kumar, S.; Drabu, S.; Kumar, R. Structural modifications of quinoline-based antimalarial agents: Recent developments. *J. Pharm. Bioallied Sci.* **2010**, *2*, 64–71. [CrossRef]
17. Boyd, D.R.; Sharma, N.D.; Loke, P.L.; Malone, J.F.; McRoberts, W.C.; Hamilton, J.T.G. Synthesis, structure and stereochemistry of quinoline alkaloids from Choisya ternata. *Org. Biomol. Chem.* **2007**, *5*, 2983–2991. [CrossRef] [PubMed]
18. Cretton, S.; Breant, L.; Pourrez, L.; Ambuehl, C.; Marcourt, L.; Ebrahimi, S.N.; Hamburger, M.; Perozzo, R.; Karimou, S.; Kaiser, M.; et al. Antitrypanosomal Quinoline Alkaloids from the Roots of Waltheria indica. *J. Nat. Prod.* **2014**, *77*, 2304–2311. [CrossRef] [PubMed]
19. Nainwal, L.M.; Tasneem, S.; Akhtar, W.; Verma, G.; Khan, M.F.; Parvez, S.; Shaquiquzzaman, M.; Akhter, M.; Alam, M.M. Green recipes to quinoline: A review. *Eur. J. Med. Chem.* **2018**, *164*, 121–170. [CrossRef]
20. Afzal, O.; Kumar, S.; Haider, R.; Ali, R.; Kumar, R.; Jaggi, M.; Bawa, S. A review on anticancer potential of bioactive heterocycle quinoline. *Eur. J. Med. Chem.* **2014**, *97*, 871–910. [CrossRef]
21. Hu, Y.-Q.; Gao, C.; Zhang, S.; Xu, L.; Xu, Z.; Feng, L.-S.; Wu, X.; Zhao, F. Quinoline hybrids and their antiplasmodial and antimalarial activities. *Eur. J. Med. Chem.* **2017**, *139*, 22–47. [CrossRef]
22. Kaur, R.; Kumar, K. Synthetic and medicinal perspective of quinolines as antiviral agents. *Eur. J. Med. Chem.* **2021**, *215*, 113220. [CrossRef] [PubMed]

23. Lauria, A.; La Monica, G.; Bono, A.; Martorana, A. Quinoline anticancer agents active on DNA and DNA-interacting proteins: From classical to emerging therapeutic targets. *Eur. J. Med. Chem.* **2021**, *220*, 113555. [CrossRef] [PubMed]
24. Khan, I.; Shah, S.J.A.; Ejaz, S.A.; Ibrar, A.; Hameed, S.; Lecka, J.; Millán, J.L.; Sévigny, J.; Iqbal, J. Investigation of quinoline-4-carboxylic acid as a highly potent scaffold for the development of alkaline phosphatase inhibitors: Synthesis, SAR analysis and molecular modelling studies. *RSC Adv.* **2015**, *5*, 64404–64413. [CrossRef]
25. Tomassoli, I.; Ismaili, L.; Pudlo, M.; Ríos, C.D.L.; Soriano, E.; Colmena, I.; Gandía, L.; Rivas, L.; Samadi, A.; Marco-Contelles, J.; et al. Synthesis, biological assessment and molecular modeling of new dihydroquinoline-3-carboxamides and dihydroquinoline-3-carbohydrazide derivatives as cholinesterase inhibitors, and Ca channel antagonists. *Eur. J. Med. Chem.* **2011**, *46*, 1–10. [CrossRef]
26. Pashaei, H.; Rouhani, A.; Nejabat, M.; Hadizadeh, F.; Mirzaei, S.; Nadri, H.; Maleki, M.F.; Ghodsi, R. Synthesis and molecular dynamic simulation studies of novel N-(1-benzylpiperidin-4-yl) quinoline-4-carboxamides as potential acetylcholinesterase inhibitors. *J. Mol. Struct.* **2021**, *1244*, 130919. [CrossRef]
27. Mo, J.; Yang, H.; Chen, T.; Li, Q.; Lin, H.; Feng, F.; Liu, W.; Qu, W.; Guo, Q.; Chi, H.; et al. Design, synthesis, biological evaluation, and molecular modeling studies of quinoline-ferulic acid hybrids as cholinesterase inhibitors. *Bioorganic Chem.* **2019**, *93*, 103310. [CrossRef]
28. Cai, R.; Wang, L.-N.; Fan, J.-J.; Geng, S.-Q.; Liu, Y.-M. New 4-N-phenylaminoquinoline derivatives as antioxidant, metal chelating and cholinesterase inhibitors for Alzheimer's disease. *Bioorganic Chem.* **2019**, *93*, 103328. [CrossRef]
29. Scarim, C.B.; Jornada, D.H.; Machado, M.G.M.; Ferreira, C.M.R.; Santos, J.L.; Chung, M.C. Thiazole, thio and semicarbazone derivatives against tropical infective diseases: Chagas disease, human African trypanosomiasis (HAT), leishmaniasis, and malaria. *Eur. J. Med. Chem.* **2018**, *162*, 378–395. [CrossRef]
30. He, Z.; Qiao, H.; Yang, F.; Zhou, W.; Gong, Y.; Zhang, X.; Wang, H.; Zhao, B.; Ma, L.; Liu, H.-M.; et al. Novel thiosemicarbazone derivatives containing indole fragment as potent and selective anticancer agent. *Eur. J. Med. Chem.* **2019**, *184*, 111764. [CrossRef] [PubMed]
31. Palanimuthu, D.; Poon, R.; Sahni, S.; Anjum, R.; Hibbs, D.; Lin, H.-Y.; Bernhardt, P.; Kalinowski, D.S.; Richardson, D.R. A novel class of thiosemicarbazones show multi-functional activity for the treatment of Alzheimer's disease. *Eur. J. Med. Chem.* **2017**, *139*, 612–632. [CrossRef] [PubMed]
32. Mrozek-Wilczkiewicz, A.; Malarz, K.; Rejmund, M.; Polanski, J.; Musiol, R. Anticancer activity of the thiosemicarbazones that are based on di-2-pyridine ketone and quinoline moiety. *Eur. J. Med. Chem.* **2019**, *171*, 180–194. [CrossRef]
33. Zhang, X.-H.; Wang, B.; Tao, Y.-Y.; Ma, Q.; Wang, H.-J.; He, Z.-X.; Wu, H.-P.; Li, Y.-H.; Zhao, B.; Ma, L.-Y.; et al. Thiosemicarbazone-based lead optimization to discover high-efficiency and low-toxicity anti-gastric cancer agents. *Eur. J. Med. Chem.* **2020**, *199*, 112349. [CrossRef]
34. He, Z.-X.; Huo, J.-L.; Gong, Y.-P.; An, Q.; Zhang, X.; Qiao, H.; Yang, F.-F.; Jiao, L.-M.; Liu, H.-M.; Ma, L.-Y.; et al. Design, synthesis and biological evaluation of novel thiosemicarbazone-indole derivatives targeting prostate cancer cells. *Eur. J. Med. Chem.* **2020**, *210*, 112970. [CrossRef] [PubMed]
35. de Siqueira, L.R.P.; Gomes, P.A.T.D.M.; Ferreira, L.P.D.L.; Rêgo, M.J.B.D.M.; Leite, A.C.L. Multi-target compounds acting in cancer progression: Focus on thiosemicarbazone, thiazole and thiazolidinone analogues. *Eur. J. Med. Chem.* **2019**, *170*, 237–260. [CrossRef]
36. Jawaria, R.; Hussain, M.; Ahmad, H.B.; Ashraf, M.; Hussain, S.; Naseer, M.M.; Khalid, M.; Hussain, M.A.; Al-Rashida, M.; Tahir, M.N.; et al. Probing ferrocene-based thiosemicarbazones and their transition metal complexes as cholinesterase inhibitors. *Inorg. Chim. Acta* **2020**, *508*, 119658. [CrossRef]
37. Ishaq, M.; Taslimi, P.; Shafiq, Z.; Khan, S.; Salmas, R.E.; Zangeneh, M.M.; Saeed, A.; Zangeneh, A.; Sadeghian, N.; Asari, A.; et al. Synthesis, bioactivity and binding energy calculations of novel 3-ethoxysalicylaldehyde based thiosemicarbazone derivatives. *Bioorganic Chem.* **2020**, *100*, 103924. [CrossRef]
38. Hashmi, S.; Khan, S.; Shafiq, Z.; Taslimi, P.; Ishaq, M.; Sadeghian, N.; Karaman, H.S.; Akhtar, N.; Islam, M.; Asari, A.; et al. Probing 4-(diethylamino)-salicylaldehyde-based thiosemicarbazones as multi-target directed ligands against cholinesterases, carbonic anhydrases and α-glycosidase enzymes. *Bioorganic Chem.* **2020**, *107*, 104554. [CrossRef] [PubMed]
39. Khan, I.; Hanif, M.; Hussain, M.T.; Khan, A.A.; Aslam, M.A.S.; Rama, N.H.; Iqbal, J. Synthesis, Acetylcholinesterase and Alkaline Phosphatase Inhibition of Some New 1,2,4-Triazole and 1,3,4-Thiadiazole Derivatives. *Aust. J. Chem.* **2012**, *65*, 1413–1419. [CrossRef]
40. Khan, I.; Ibrar, A.; Zaib, S.; Ahmad, S.; Furtmann, N.; Hameed, S.; Simpson, J.; Bajorath, J.; Iqbal, J. Active compounds from a diverse library of triazolothiadiazole and triazolothiadiazine scaffolds: Synthesis, crystal structure determination, cytotoxicity, cholinesterase inhibitory activity, and binding mode analysis. *Bioorganic Med. Chem.* **2014**, *22*, 6163–6173. [CrossRef]
41. Khan, I.; Zaib, S.; Ibrar, A.; Rama, N.H.; Simpson, J.; Iqbal, J. Synthesis, crystal structure and biological evaluation of some novel 1,2,4-triazolo[3,4-b]-1,3,4-thiadiazoles and 1,2,4-triazolo[3,4-b]-1,3,4-thiadiazines. *Eur. J. Med. Chem.* **2014**, *78*, 167–177. [CrossRef] [PubMed]
42. Khan, I.; Bakht, S.M.; Ibrar, A.; Abbas, S.; Hameed, S.; White, J.M.; Rana, U.A.; Zaib, S.; Shahid, M.; Iqbal, J. Exploration of a library of triazolothiadiazole and triazolothiadiazine compounds as a highly potent and selective family of cholinesterase and monoamine oxidase inhibitors: Design, synthesis, X-ray diffraction analysis and molecular docking studies. *RSC Adv.* **2015**, *5*, 21249–21267. [CrossRef]

43. Ibrar, A.; Khan, A.; Ali, M.; Sarwar, R.; Mehsud, S.; Farooq, U.; Halimi, S.M.A.; Khan, I.; Al-Harrasi, A. Combined in Vitro and in Silico Studies for the Anticholinesterase Activity and Pharmacokinetics of Coumarinyl Thiazoles and Oxadiazoles. *Front. Chem.* **2018**, *6*. [CrossRef]
44. Larik, F.A.; Saeed, A.; Faisal, M.; Hamdani, S.; Jabeen, F.; Channar, P.A.; Mumtaz, A.; Khan, I.; Kazi, M.A.; Abbas, Q.; et al. Synthesis, inhibition studies against AChE and BChE, drug-like profiling, kinetic analysis and molecular docking studies of N-(4-phenyl-3-aroyl-2(3H)-ylidene) substituted acetamides. *J. Mol. Struct.* **2019**, *1203*, 127459. [CrossRef]
45. Munir, R.; Zia-Ur-Rehman, M.; Murtaza, S.; Zaib, S.; Javid, N.; Awan, S.; Iftikhar, K.; Athar, M.; Khan, I. Microwave-Assisted Synthesis of (Piperidin-1-yl)quinolin-3-yl)methylene)hydrazinecarbothioamides as Potent Inhibitors of Cholinesterases: A Biochemical and In Silico Approach. *Molecules* **2021**, *26*, 656. [CrossRef]
46. Vitaku, E.; Smith, D.T.; Njardarson, J.T. Analysis of the Structural Diversity, Substitution Patterns, and Frequency of Nitrogen Heterocycles among U.S. FDA Approved Pharmaceuticals. *J. Med. Chem.* **2014**, *57*, 10257–10274. [CrossRef]
47. Khan, I.; Ibrar, A.; Abbas, N.; Saeed, A. Recent advances in the structural library of functionalized quinazoline and quinazolinone scaffolds: Synthetic approaches and multifarious applications. *Eur. J. Med. Chem.* **2014**, *76*, 193–244. [CrossRef]
48. Khan, I.; Ibrar, A.; Ahmed, W.; Saeed, A. Synthetic approaches, functionalization and therapeutic potential of quinazoline and quinazolinone skeletons: The advances continue. *Eur. J. Med. Chem.* **2014**, *90*, 124–169. [CrossRef]
49. Khan, I.; Zaib, S.; Batool, S.; Abbas, N.; Ashraf, Z.; Iqbal, J.; Saeed, A. Quinazolines and quinazolinones as ubiquitous structural fragments in medicinal chemistry: An update on the development of synthetic methods and pharmacological diversification. *Bioorganic Med. Chem.* **2016**, *24*, 2361–2381. [CrossRef]
50. Arshad, F.; Khan, M.F.; Akhtar, W.; Alam, M.M.; Nainwal, L.M.; Kaushik, S.K.; Akhter, M.; Parvez, S.; Hasan, S.M.; Shaquiquzzaman, M. Revealing quinquennial anticancer journey of morpholine: A SAR based review. *Eur. J. Med. Chem.* **2019**, *167*, 324–356. [CrossRef] [PubMed]
51. Yan, X.-Q.; Wang, Z.-C.; Qi, P.-F.; Li, G.; Zhu, H.-L. Design, synthesis and biological evaluation of 2-H pyrazole derivatives containing morpholine moieties as highly potent small molecule inhibitors of APC–Asef interaction. *Eur. J. Med. Chem.* **2019**, *177*, 425–447. [CrossRef] [PubMed]
52. Doan, P.; Karjalainen, A.; Chandraseelan, J.G.; Sandberg, O.; Yli-Harja, O.; Rosholm, T.; Franzen, R.; Candeias, N.R.; Kandhavelu, M. Synthesis and biological screening for cytotoxic activity of N-substituted indolines and morpholines. *Eur. J. Med. Chem.* **2016**, *120*, 296–303. [CrossRef]
53. Marvadi, S.K.; Krishna, V.S.; Sriram, D.; Kantevari, S. Synthesis of novel morpholine, thiomorpholine and N-substituted piperazine coupled 2-(thiophen-2-yl)dihydroquinolines as potent inhibitors of Mycobacterium tuberculosis. *Eur. J. Med. Chem.* **2018**, *164*, 171–178. [CrossRef]
54. Li, Z.; Wang, Z.-C.; Li, X.; Abbas, M.; Wu, S.-Y.; Ren, S.-Z.; Liu, Q.-X.; Liu, Y.; Chen, P.-W.; Duan, Y.-T.; et al. Design, synthesis and evaluation of novel diaryl-1,5-diazoles derivatives bearing morpholine as potent dual COX-2/5-LOX inhibitors and antitumor agents. *Eur. J. Med. Chem.* **2019**, *169*, 168–184. [CrossRef]
55. Meth-Cohn, O.; Rhouati, S.; Tarnowski, B.; Robinson, A. A versatile new synthesis of quinolines and related fused pyridines, Part 5. The synthesis of 2-chloroquinoline-3-carbaldehydes. *J. Chem. Soc. Perkin Trans. 1* **1981**, 1537–1543. [CrossRef]
56. Ellman, G.L.; Courtney, K.; Andres, V.; Featherstone, R.M. A new and rapid colorimetric determination of acetylcholinesterase activity. *Biochem. Pharmacol.* **1961**, *7*, 88–95. [CrossRef]
57. Nachon, F.; Carletti, E.; Ronco, C.; Trovaslet, M.; Nicolet, Y.; Jean, L.; Renard, P.-Y. Crystal structures of human cholinesterases in complex with huprine W and tacrine: Elements of specificity for anti-Alzheimer's drugs targeting acetyl- and butyrylcholinesterase. *Biochem. J.* **2013**, *453*, 393–399. [CrossRef]
58. Schneider, N.; Lange, G.; Hindle, S.; Klein, R.; Rarey, M. A consistent description of HYdrogen bond and DEhydration energies in protein–ligand complexes: Methods behind the HYDE scoring function. *J. Comput. Mol. Des.* **2012**, *27*, 15–29. [CrossRef]
59. Reulecke, I.; Lange, G.; Albrecht, J.; Klein, R.; Rarey, M. Towards an Integrated Description of Hydrogen Bonding and Dehydration: Decreasing False Positives in Virtual Screening with the HYDE Scoring Function. *ChemMedChem* **2008**, *3*, 885–897. [CrossRef] [PubMed]
60. Daina, A.; Michielin, O.; Zoete, V. SwissADME: A free web tool to evaluate pharmacokinetics, drug-likeness and medicinal chemistry friendliness of small molecules. *Sci. Rep.* **2017**, *7*, 42717. [CrossRef] [PubMed]
61. Daina, A.; Michielin, O.; Zoete, V. iLOGP: A Simple, Robust, and Efficient Description of n-Octanol/Water Partition Coefficient for Drug Design Using the GB/SA Approach. *J. Chem. Inf. Model.* **2014**, *54*, 3284–3301. [CrossRef] [PubMed]
62. Daina, A.; Zoete, V. A BOILED-Egg to Predict Gastrointestinal Absorption and Brain Penetration of Small Molecules. *ChemMedChem* **2016**, *11*, 1117–1121. [CrossRef] [PubMed]
63. Khan, I.; Khan, A.; Halim, S.A.; Khan, M.; Zaib, S.; Al-Yahyaei, B.E.M.; Al-Harrasi, A.; Ibrar, A. Utilization of the common functional groups in bioactive molecules: Exploring dual inhibitory potential and computational analysis of keto esters against α-glucosidase and carbonic anhydrase-II enzymes. *Int. J. Biol. Macromol.* **2020**, *167*, 233–244. [CrossRef]
64. Ertl, P.; Rohde, B.; Selzer, P. Fast Calculation of Molecular Polar Surface Area as a Sum of Fragment-Based Contributions and Its Application to the Prediction of Drug Transport Properties. *J. Med. Chem.* **2000**, *43*, 3714–3717. [CrossRef]
65. Mumtaz, A.; Shoaib, M.; Zaib, S.; Shah, M.S.; Bhatti, H.A.; Saeed, A.; Hussain, I.; Iqbal, J. Synthesis, molecular modelling and biological evaluation of tetrasubstituted thiazoles towards cholinesterase enzymes and cytotoxicity studies. *Bioorganic Chem.* **2018**, *78*, 141–148. [CrossRef] [PubMed]

66. Labute, P. Protonate 3D, Chemical Computing Group. 2007. Available online: http://www.chemcomp.com/journal/proton.htm (accessed on 10 September 2021).
67. Chemical Computing Group's Molecular Operating Environment (MOE). MOE 2019. Available online: http://www.chemcomp.com/MOEMolecular_Operating_Environment.htm (accessed on 10 September 2021).
68. *LeadIT Version 2.3.2*; BioSolveIT GmbH: Sankt Augustin, Germany, 2017; Available online: www.biosolveit.de/LeadIT (accessed on 10 September 2021).
69. BIOVIA. Discovery Studio Client v19.1.0.18287. In *Accelrys Discovery Studio*; Accelrys Software Inc.: San Diego, CA, USA, 2019.
70. Ferreira, R.J.; Ferreira, M.-J.U.; dos Santos, D.J.V.A. Insights on P-Glycoprotein's Efflux Mechanism Obtained by Molecular Dynamics Simulations. *J. Chem. Theory Comput.* **2012**, *8*, 1853–1864. [CrossRef] [PubMed]
71. Ozgeris, B.; Göksu, S.; Köse, L.P.; Gülçin, I.; Salmas, R.E.; Durdagi, S.; Tümer, F.; Supuran, C.T. Acetylcholinesterase and carbonic anhydrase inhibitory properties of novel urea and sulfamide derivatives incorporating dopaminergic 2-aminotetralin scaffolds. *Bioorganic Med. Chem.* **2016**, *24*, 2318–2329. [CrossRef]
72. Mathew, B.; Haridas, A.; Uçar, G.; Baysal, I.; Adeniyi, A.A.; Soliman, M.; Joy, M.; Mathew, G.E.; Lakshmanan, B.; Jayaprakash, V. Exploration of chlorinated thienyl chalcones: A new class of monoamine oxidase-B inhibitors. *Int. J. Biol. Macromol.* **2016**, *91*, 680–695. [CrossRef]
73. Schüttelkopf, A.W.; Van Aalten, D.M.F. PRODRG: A tool for high-throughput crystallography of protein–ligand complexes. *Acta Crystallogr. Sect. D Biol. Crystallogr.* **2004**, *60*, 1355–1363. [CrossRef]
74. Humphrey, W.; Dalke, A.; Schulten, K. VMD: Visual molecular dynamics. *J. Mol. Graph.* **1996**, *14*, 33–38. [CrossRef]
75. Turner, P. *XMGRACE, Version 5.1.19*; Center for Coastal and Land-Margin Research, Oregon Graduate Institute of Science and Technology: Beaverton, OR, USA, 2005.

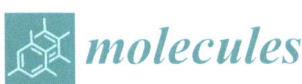

Article

Evaluation of the Inhibitory Effects of Pyridylpyrazole Derivatives on LPS-Induced PGE$_2$ Productions and Nitric Oxide in Murine RAW 264.7 Macrophages

Mahmoud M. Gamal El-Din [1], Mohammed I. El-Gamal [2,3,4], Young-Do Kwon [5,6], Su-Yeon Kim [7,8], Hee-Soo Han [7,8], Sang-Eun Park [7,8], Chang-Hyun Oh [9], Kyung-Tae Lee [7,8,*] and Hee-Kwon Kim [5,6,*]

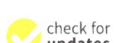

Citation: Gamal El-Din, M.M.; El-Gamal, M.I.; Kwon, Y.-D.; Kim, S.-Y.; Han, H.-S.; Park, S.-E.; Oh, C.-H.; Lee, K.-T.; Kim, H.-K. Evaluation of the Inhibitory Effects of Pyridylpyrazole Derivatives on LPS-Induced PGE$_2$ Productions and Nitric Oxide in Murine RAW 264.7 Macrophages. *Molecules* **2021**, *26*, 6489. https://doi.org/10.3390/molecules26216489

Academic Editors: Imtiaz Khan, Sumera Zaib and William Blalock

Received: 7 September 2021
Accepted: 26 October 2021
Published: 27 October 2021

Publisher's Note: MDPI stays neutral with regard to jurisdictional claims in published maps and institutional affiliations.

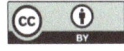

Copyright: © 2021 by the authors. Licensee MDPI, Basel, Switzerland. This article is an open access article distributed under the terms and conditions of the Creative Commons Attribution (CC BY) license (https://creativecommons.org/licenses/by/4.0/).

[1] National Research Centre, Pharmaceutical and Drug Industries Research Division, Dokki-Giza 12622, Egypt; dr.m.g.eldin@hotmail.com
[2] Department of Medicinal Chemistry, College of Pharmacy, University of Sharjah, Sharjah 27272, United Arab Emirates; drmelgamal2002@gmail.com
[3] Sharjah Institute for Medical Research, University of Sharjah, Sharjah 27272, United Arab Emirates
[4] Department of Medicinal Chemistry, Faculty of Pharmacy, Mansoura University, Mansoura 35516, Egypt
[5] Molecular Imaging & Therapeutic Medicine Research Center, Department of Nuclear Medicine, Jeonbuk National University Medical School and Hospital, 20 Geonji-ro, Deokjin-gu, Jeonju 54907, Korea; gskydgo@gmail.com
[6] Research Institute of Clinical Medicine, Jeonbuk National University-Biomedical Research Institute, Jeonbuk National University Hospital, 20 Geonji-ro, Deokjin-gu, Jeonju 54907, Korea
[7] Department of Pharmaceutical Biochemistry, Kyung Hee University, Seoul 02447, Korea; dlstm4@gmail.com (S.-Y.K.); heesu3620@daum.net (H.-S.H.); qkrtkddms0930@naver.com (S.-E.P.)
[8] Department of Life and Nanopharmaceutical Sciences, Graduate School, Kyung Hee University, 26, Kyungheedae-ro, Seoul 02447, Korea
[9] Center for Biomaterials, Korea Institute of Science and Technology, P.O. Box 131, Cheongryang, Seoul 130-650, Korea; choh@kist.re.kr
* Correspondence: ktlee@khu.ac.kr (K.-T.L.); hkkim717@jbnu.ac.kr (H.-K.K.); Tel.: +82-2-961-0860 (K.-T.L.); +82-63-250-2768 (H.-K.K.); Fax: +82-2-961-9580 (K.-T.L.); +82-63-255-1172 (H.-K.K.)

Abstract: A series of thirteen triarylpyrazole analogs were investigated as inhibitors of lipopolysaccharide (LPS)-induced prostaglandin E$_2$ (PGE$_2$) and nitric oxide (NO) production in RAW 264.7 macrophages. The target compounds **1a–m** have first been assessed for cytotoxicity against RAW 264.7 macrophages to determine their non-cytotoxic concentration(s) for anti-inflammatory testing to make sure that the inhibition of PGE$_2$ and NO production would not be caused by cytotoxicity. It was found that compounds **1f** and **1m** were the most potent PGE$_2$ inhibitors with IC$_{50}$ values of 7.1 and 1.1 μM, respectively. In addition, these compounds also showed inhibitory effects of 11.6% and 37.19% on LPS-induced NO production, respectively. The western blots analysis of COX-2 and iNOS showed that the PGE$_2$ and NO inhibitory effect of compound **1m** are attributed to inhibition of COX-2 and iNOS protein expression through inactivation of p38.

Keywords: amide; anti-inflammatory; COX-2; iNOS; NO; PGE$_2$; pyrazole

1. Introduction

Inflammation is considered as a part of our body's defense mechanisms against invasive organisms. It represents an attempt to get rid of such harmful organisms through releasing antibacterial or antiviral from cells close to it to help the body fight against infection [1]. In addition, it enhances injured tissue healing facilitating the return of the cells to their normal conditions. Despite these beneficial effects, it could have harmful effects triggering a list of disorders such as cardiovascular disorders [2], tumors [3], inflammatory bowel syndrome [4], arthritis [5], pulmonary disorders [6], Alzheimer's [7], etc.

In order to treat inflammation, it is crucial to understand the role of inflammatory mediators that directly contribute to inflammatory responses. Inflammatory mediators arise from plasma proteins or some types of cells such as mast cells, platelets, neutrophils, monocytes, and macrophages. They are triggered by bacterial toxins or host cell proteins. The inflammatory mediators bind to particular receptors on the target cells and enhance vascular permeability and neutrophil chemotaxis, induce smooth muscle contraction, directly affect enzymatic activity, produce pain, or induce oxidative damage. The majority of these chemical mediators have short lives but produce harmful effects [1]. The inflammatory chemical mediators are exemplified by vasoactive amines (e.g., histamine and 5-HT), eicosanoids (e.g., prostaglandins and leukotrienes), and cytokines (e.g., tumor necrosis factor (TNF) and interleukin-1 (IL-1)).

Cyclooxygenase-2 (COX-2) converts arachidonic acid into PGE_2, which is the mediator of inflammation [8]. Limiting PGE_2 production *via* inhibition of COX-2 protein expression and/or enzymatic activity is another useful approach for the treatment of inflammation. Moreover, nitric oxide (NO) has another considerable contribution to inflammation development (although it could produce anti-inflammatory effect under other normal physiological conditions) [9–11]. On the other hand, it acts as a proinflammatory mediator to induce localized inflammatory response due to elevated secretion in cases of abnormal conditions. Inducible nitric oxide synthase (iNOS) enzyme forms NO in case of inflammation. NO produces localized vasodilation at the site of inflammation, leading to edema [12]. Therefore, Similar to PGE_2 production inhibition, decreasing NO production *via* iNOS enzymatic activity inhibition, and/or iNOS protein expression inhibition could be a beneficial avenue for the management of inflammation.

Many substituted pyrazole derivatives have been recently reported to possess anti-inflammatory activity [13–16]. In our study, we evaluated a series of substituted pyrazole derivatives with a structural likeness to celecoxib, a pyrazole-based anti-inflammatory agent (Figure 1) as inhibitors of LPS-induced NO and PGE_2 productions. Vicinal diarylheterocycles such as celecoxib have been reported as COX-2-inhibiting anti-inflammatory agents. The presence of vicinal diarylpyrazole scaffold in the structures of our target compounds encouraged us to investigate their anti-inflammatory activity. Our target compounds **1a–m** were previously reported as antiproliferative agents [17]. Moreover, compound **I** (Figure 1) possessing triarylpyrazole nucleus has been reported as inhibitor of PGE_2 and NO release [18].

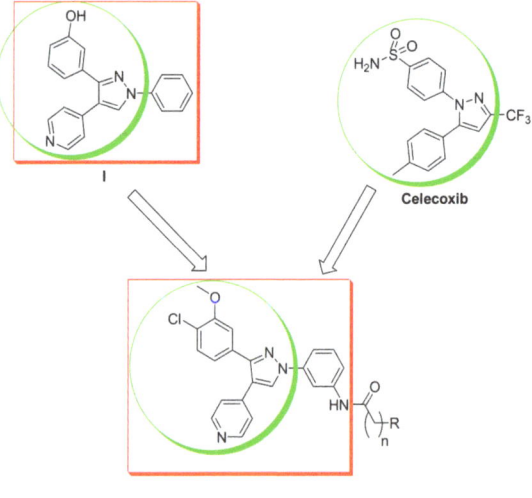

Figure 1. Structures of the lead compound **I** [18], celecoxib, and the target compounds **1a–m**.

2. Results and Discussion

2.1. Chemistry

The final compounds **1a–m** were synthesized *via* the pathway demonstrated in Scheme 1. 2-Chloro-5-methylphenol (**2**) was reacted with dimethyl sulfate/potassium carbonate to obtain methoxy derivative. The methyl group was then oxidized to carboxylic acid by potassium permanganate to 4-chloro-3-methoxy-benzoic acid. Esterification of the resulting acid by methanol and acetyl chloride yielded the corresponding methyl ester **3**. Compound **3** was activated using a strong base; lithium bis(trimethylsilyl)amide (LiH-MDS) followed by slow addition of 4-picoline gave the pyridine ketide intermediate **4**. The reaction of compound **4** with dimethylformamide dimethylacetal (DMF-DMA) produced compound **5**. After that, adding hydrazine monohydrate yielded the pyrazolyl intermediate **6**. Interaction of compound **6** with *meta*-iodonitrobenzene at 90 °C in dimethyl sulfoxide gave the *meta*-nitrophenyl intermediate **7**. Reduction of the NO_2 group of **7** using Pd/C and hydrogen gas produced amino compound **8**. Interaction of the amino intermediate **8** with chloroacetyl chloride or chloropropionyl chloride produced the corresponding amide intermediates **9a,b**, respectively. Interaction of the terminal alkyl halide group of compounds **9a,b** with (substituted) alicyclic amines gave the target compounds **1a–m** [17]. The detailed experimental procedures and the spectral analysis charts are shown in the Supplementary File. Structures of compounds **1a–m** and their cell viability results against RAW 264.7 cells are shown in Table 1.

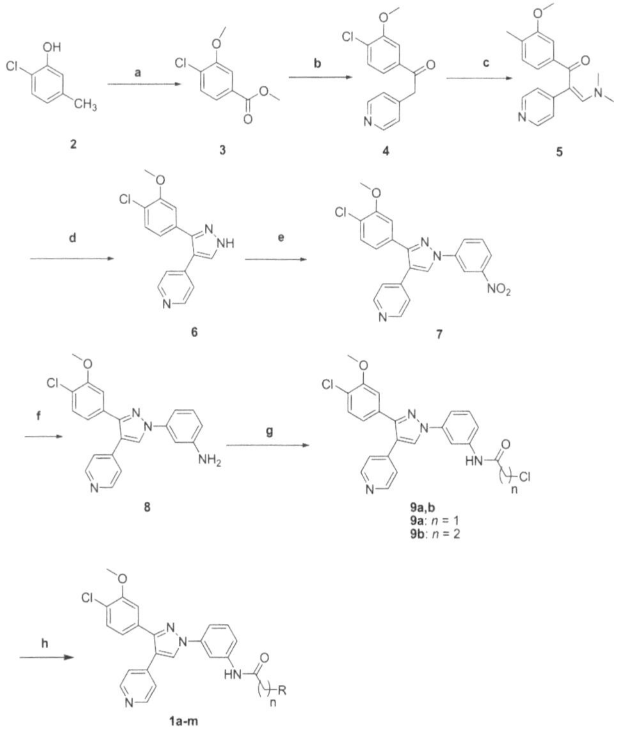

Scheme 1. Reagents and conditions: (**a**) (i) $(CH_3)_2SO_4$, K_2CO_3, acetone, reflux, 1 h, 95%; (ii) $KMnO_4$, C_5H_5N, H_2O, 50 °C, 24 h, then rt, 13 h, 90%; (iii) acetyl chloride, CH_3OH, rt, 15 h, 85%; (**b**) 4-picoline, LiHMDS, THF, rt, overnight, 45%; (**c**) (i) DMF-DMA, rt, 18 h; (**d**) hydrazine monohydrate, C_2H_5OH, rt, overnight, 81%; (**e**) 1-iodo-4-nitrobenzene, K_2CO_3, CuI, L-proline, DMSO, 90 °C, 8 h, 86%; (**f**) H_2, Pd/C, THF, rt, 2 h, 86%; (**g**) chloroacetyl chloride, or chloropropionyl chloride, TEA, CH_2Cl_2, −10 °C, 15 min, 65%; (**h**) appropriate amine derivative, TEA, CH_2Cl_2, rt, 1 h, 46–71%.

Table 1. Structures of compounds **1a–m** and their cell viability results at 1 and 10 μM concentrations against murine RAW 264.7 macrophages.

Compound No.	n	R	Cell Viability (%) 1 μM [a]	Cell Viability (%) 10 μM [a]
1a	1	*–N(piperidine)	99 ± 5.9	10 ± 1.2
1b	1	*–N(morpholine)	92 ± 4.5	65 ± 2.8
1c	1	*–N(piperazine)N–	78 ± 3.3	5 ± 0.8
1d	1	*–N(piperazine)N–CH3	75 ± 2.9	3 ± 0.4
1e	1	*–N(piperazine)N–phenyl	87 ± 4.1	65 ± 4.1
1f	1	*–N(piperazine)N–CH2–phenyl	66 ± 1.8	**107 ± 8.5**
1g	2	*–N(piperidine)	87 ± 3.8	5 ± 1.1
1h	2	*–N(morpholine)	99 ± 2.8	75 ± 1.7
1i	2	*–N(piperazine)N–	99 ± 3.4	5 ± 1.8
1j	2	*–N(piperazine)N–CH3	98 ± 3.1	5 ± 0.8
1k	2	*–N(piperazine)N–phenyl	89 ± 2.8	**112 ± 7.6**
1l	2	*–N(piperazine)N–CH2–phenyl	86 ± 3.7	34 ± 1.1
1m	2	*–N(piperazine)N–CH2–(4-F-phenyl)	90 ± 4.1	**97 ± 3.9**

Data are presented as the means ± SDs of three independent experiments. Bold figures indicate non-cytotoxicity
* Indicates the site of connection to the main structure.

2.2. Biological Evaluation

Before screening the PGE_2 and NO production inhibitory effects of the compounds, the compounds' cytotoxicity was evaluated at 1 and 10 µM concentrations to make sure that the tested concentrations are safe enough and non-cytotoxic to avoid misleading results. All compounds were non-cytotoxic at 1 µM concentration, while by increasing concentration to 10 µM, all the target compounds except **1f**, **1k**, and **1m** started showing cytotoxicity. These three compounds were found to be non-cytotoxic at 10 µM concentration (Figure 2). The three compounds possess N-benzylpiperazinyl, N-phenylpiperazinyl, and N-(4-fluorobenzyl)piperazinyl moieties, respectively. The piperidinyl and the morpholino moieties seem to be unfavorable to avoid cytotoxicity in this series of compounds.

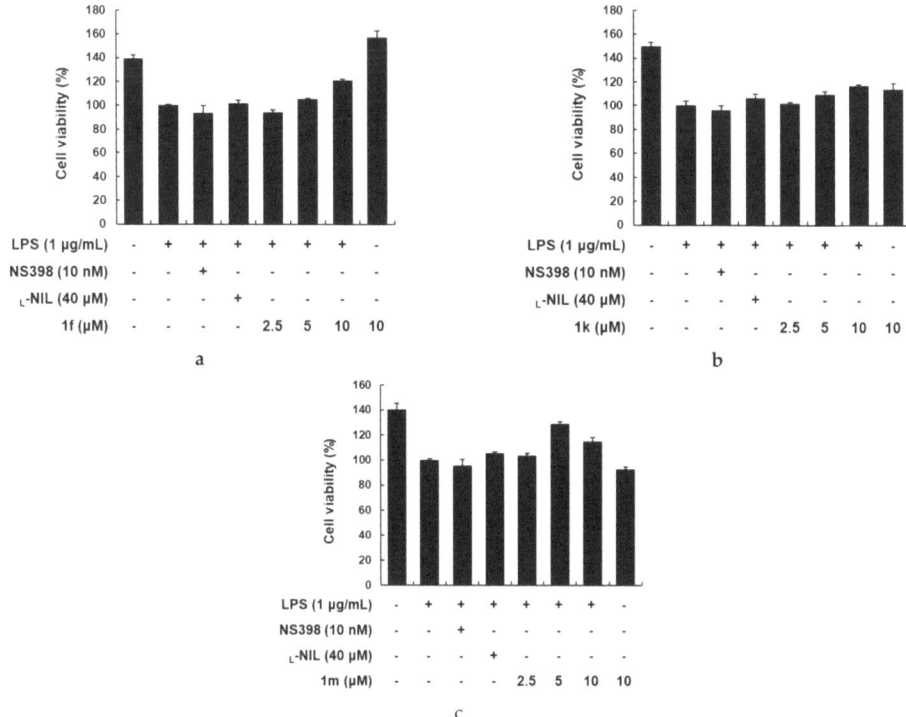

Figure 2. Effects of compounds **1f** (a), **1k** (b), **1m** (c), NS398, and $_L$-NIL on LPS-induced RAW 264.7 cell viability at various concentrations (2.5, 5, or 10 µM).

Upon confirming the non-cytotoxicity of 10 µM concentration of these three derivatives against murine RAW 264.7 macrophages induced by LPS, compounds **1f**, **1k**, and **1m** were tested for inhibitory effect against LPS-induced PGE_2 production together with checking their cell viability. They have shown no cytotoxicity at these levels (2.5, 5, 10 µM) and good inhibition values against PGE_2 production (Figures 2 and 3). Among these selected derivatives, compounds **1f** and **1m** showed dose-dependent inhibition along with increasing its concentration (37.4 at 5 µM to 65.4% at 10 µM) for compound **1f**, and 67% at 2.5 µM and 84.9% at 10 µM for compound **1m**. Furthermore, the IC_{50} values of compounds **1f** and **1m** were 7.6 and 1.1 µM, respectively. This indicates that compound **1m** with ethylene bridge was more active than compound **1f** possessing methylene bridge. The fluorine atom of compound **1m** might confer more lipophilicity that may result in more penetration inside the cell and hence better inhibition of PGE_2 production. The fluorine atom can also add some more merits such as formation of an additional hydrogen bond with a hydrogen bond donor in the target protein and stronger hydrophobic interaction by fluorophenyl compared with unsubstituted phenyl. In addition, *p*-fluoro can prevent aromatic hydroxylation metabolic reaction and hence can elongate the duration of action [19]. Moreover, **1f** and **1m** were evaluated at 1 and 10 µM for inhibitory effects on LPS-induced NO production. It was found that compounds **1f** and **1m** showed inhibition values of 11.06% and 37.19%, respectively on LPS-induced NO production at 10 µM concentration (Table 2). Compound **1m** is slightly more active than L-NIL at 10 µM.

Table 2. Inhibitory effects of compounds **1f** and **1m** against NO production in LPS-induced RAW 264.7 cells.

Compound	Inhibition Rate (%)	
	1 (µM)	10 (µM)
1f	0	11.06 ± 1.5
1m	0	37.19 ± 3.4
L-NIL	3.9 ± 2.1	31.32 ± 2.9

Compounds **1f**, **1k**, and **1m** were also tested for inhibitory effects against LPS-induced PGE_2 production in addition to checking their cell viability. They have shown no cytotoxicity at these levels and good inhibition values against PGE_2 production (Figures 2 and 3). Among these selected derivatives, compounds **1f** and **1m** showed dose-dependent inhibition along with increasing its concentration (37.4% at 5 µM to 65.4% at 10 µM) for compound **1f**, and 67% at 2.5 µM and 84.9% at 10 µM for compound **1m**. Furthermore, the IC_{50} values of compounds **1f** and **1m** were 7.6 and 1.1 µM, respectively. This complies that compound **1m** with ethylene bridge was more active than compound **1f** possessing methylene bridge. The fluorine atom of compound **1m** might confer more lipophilicity that may result in more penetration inside the cell and hence better inhibition of PGE_2 production.

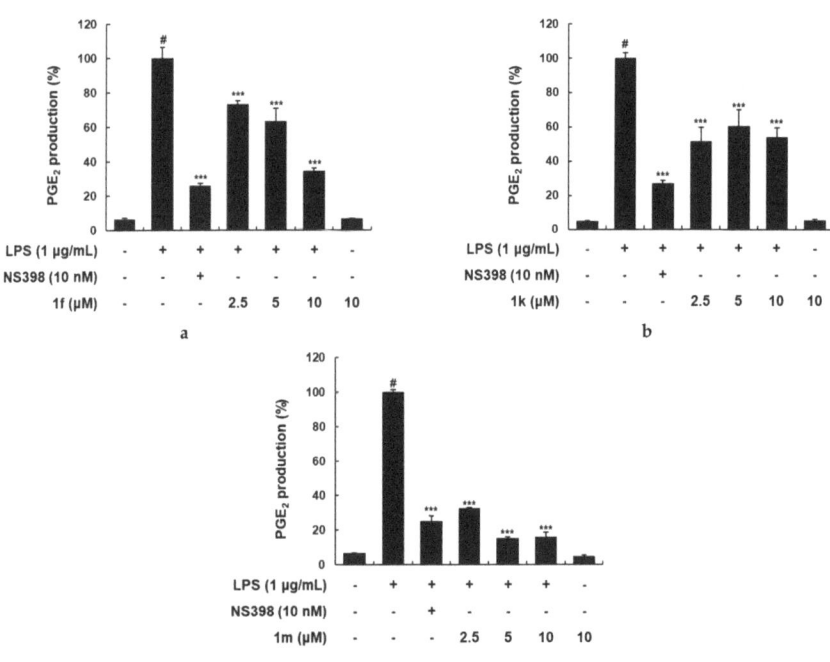

Figure 3. Effects of compounds **1f** (a), **1k** (b), and **1m** (c), and NS398 on LPS-stimulated PGE_2 production in RAW 264.7 macrophages. # means significant difference from the negative control and *** means significant difference from the positive control.

Furthermore, the most promising compound **1m** was chosen for a more extensive investigation of its molecular mechanism(s) of action. It was tested for inhibitory effects on COX-2 and iNOS protein expressions (Figure 4). Compound **1m** showed a concentration-dependent inhibitory effect against COX-2 and iNOS protein expression, especially at 10 µM concentration. Moreover, compound **1m** markedly suppressed the phosphorylation of p38, a key molecule in regulating inflammation [20].

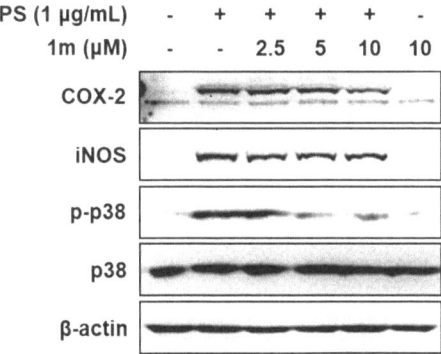

Figure 4. Effect of compound **1m** on COX-2, iNOS, and p-p38 protein expression in LPS-induced RAW 264.7 macrophages.

3. Conclusions

Our target compounds were tested for potential cytotoxicity. We then selected the safest compounds for further investigations as PGE_2 and NO production inhibitors in LPS-induced murine RAW 264.7 macrophages. The two tested compounds (**1f** and **1m**) act more against PGE_2 production than over NO. We identified a couple of potential PGE_2 production inhibitory compounds, namely **1f** and **1m**. The most potent compound, **1m**, exerted a strong inhibitory effect on PGE_2 production with IC_{50} value of 1.1 µM and NO production with 37% at 10 µM. It produces these effects due to inhibition of both COX-2 and iNOS protein expression through inactivation of p38. Further structural optimization is needed in order to optimize activity.

Supplementary Materials: The experimental procedures and the spectral analysis charts are available.

Author Contributions: Conceptualization, C.-H.O., K.-T.L., and H.-K.K.; methodology, M.M.G.E.-D., M.I.E.-G., S.-Y.K., H.-S.H., and S.-E.P.; data curation, Y.-D.K., writing-original draft preparation, M.M.G.E.-D. and M.I.E.-G.; writing-review and editing, M.M.G.E.-D., M.I.E.-G., C.-H.O., K.-T.L., and H.-K.K.; supervision, C.-H.O., K.-T.L., and H.-K.K.; funding acquisition, H.-K.K.; All authors have read and agreed to the published version of the manuscript.

Funding: This research was supported by the National Research Foundation of Korea (NRF) grant funded by the Korea government (MSIT) (NRF-2021R1A2C1011204), and BK21FOUR 21st Century of Medical Science Creative Human Resource Development Center.

Institutional Review Board Statement: Not applicable.

Informed Consent Statement: Not applicable.

Data Availability Statement: Not applicable.

Experimental: The synthetic procedures and the protocols for the biological assay are provided in the Supplementary File.

Conflicts of Interest: The authors declare no conflict of interest.

Sample Availability: Samples of the compounds are available from the authors upon request.

References

1. Abdulkhaleq, L.A.; Assi, M.A.; Abdullah, R.; Zamri-Saad, M. The crucial roles of inflammatory mediators in inflammation: A review. *Vet. World* **2018**, *11*, 627. [CrossRef] [PubMed]
2. Coussens, L.M.; Werb, Z. Inflammation and cancer. *Nature* **2002**, *420*, 860. [CrossRef] [PubMed]
3. Qui, H.; Johansson, A.S.; Sjostrom, M.; Wan, M.; Schroder, O.; Palmbald, J.; Haeggstrom, J.Z. Differential induction of BLT receptor expression on human endothelial cells by lipopolysaccharide, cytokines, and leukotriene B4. *Proc. Natl. Acad. Sci. USA* **2006**, *103*, 6913.
4. Sung, B.; Prasad, S.; Yadav, V.R.; Lavasanifar, A.; Aggarwal, B.B. Cancer and diet: How are they related? *Free Radical Res.* **2011**, *45*, 864. [CrossRef] [PubMed]
5. Lee, I.-A.; Bae, E.-A.; Hyun, Y.-J.; Kim, D.-H. Dextran sulfate sodium and 2,4,6-trinitrobenzene sulfonic acid induce lipid peroxidation by the proliferation of intestinal gram-negative bacteria in mice. *J. Inflamm.* **2010**, *7*, 7. [CrossRef] [PubMed]
6. Hochberg, M.C. Semin. Changes in the incidence and prevalence of rheumatoid arthritis in England and Wales, 1970-1982. *Arthritis Rheum.* **1990**, *19*, 294. [CrossRef]
7. Sastre, M.; Richardson, J.C.; Gentleman, S.M.; Brooks, D.J. Inflammatory risk factors and pathologies associated with Alzheimer's disease. *Curr. Alzheimer Res.* **2011**, *8*, 132. [CrossRef] [PubMed]
8. Hinz, B.; Brune, K.J. Cyclooxygenase-2–10 years later. *Pharmacol. Exp. Ther.* **2002**, *300*, 367. [CrossRef] [PubMed]
9. Bhardwaj, A.; Batchu, S.N.; Kaur, J.; Huang, Z.; Seubert, J.M.; Knaus, E.E. Cardiovascular properties of a nitric oxide releasing rofecoxib analogue: beneficial anti-hypertensive activity and enhanced recovery in an ischemic reperfusion injury model. *ChemMedChem* **2012**, *7*, 1365. [CrossRef] [PubMed]
10. Bhardwaj, A.; Huang, Z.; Kaur, J.; Knaus, E.E. Rofecoxib analogues possessing a nitric oxide donor sulfohydroxamic acid (SO2NHOH) cyclooxygenase-2 pharmacophore: synthesis, molecular modeling, and biological evaluation as anti-inflammatory agents. *ChemMedChem* **2012**, *7*, 62. [CrossRef] [PubMed]
11. Kaur, J.; Bhardwaj, A.; Huang, Z.; Knaus, E.E. Aspirin analogues as dual cyclooxygenase-2/5-lipoxygenase inhibitors: synthesis, nitric oxide release, molecular modeling, and biological evaluation as anti-inflammatory agents. *ChemMedChem* **2011**, *7*, 144. [CrossRef] [PubMed]
12. Yun, H.Y.; Dawson, V.L.; Dawson, T.M. Neurobiology of nitric oxide. *Crit. Rev. Neurobiol.* **1996**, *10*, 291. [CrossRef] [PubMed]
13. Arora, R.K.; Kaur, N.; Bansal, Y.; Bansal, G. Novel coumarin-benzimidazole derivatives as antioxidants and safer anti-inflammatory agents. *Acta Pharm. Sin. B.* **2014**, *4*, 368. [CrossRef] [PubMed]
14. Azelmat, J.; Fiorito, S.; Taddeo, V.A.; Genovese, S.; Epifano, F.; Grenier, D. Synthesis and evaluation of antibacterial and anti-inflammatory properties of naturally occurring coumarins. *Phytochem. Lett.* **2015**, *13*, 399. [CrossRef]
15. Wei, W.; Wu, X.-W.; Deng, G.-G.; Yang, X.-W. Anti-inflammatory coumarins with short- and long-chain hydrophobic groups from roots of Angelica dahurica cv. Hangbaizhi. *Phytochemistry* **2016**, *123*, 58. [CrossRef] [PubMed]
16. Srivastava, P.; Vyas, V.K.; Variya, B.; Patel, P.; Qureshi, G.; Ghate, M. Synthesis, anti-inflammatory, analgesic, 5-lipoxygenase (5-LOX) inhibition activities, and molecular docking study of 7-substituted coumarin derivatives. *Bioorg. Chem.* **2016**, *67*, 130. [CrossRef] [PubMed]
17. Gamal El-Din, M.M.; El-Gamal, M.I.; Abdel-Maksoud, M.S.; Yoo, K.H.; Oh, C.-H. Design, synthesis, in vitro potent antiproliferative activity, and kinase inhibitory effects of new triarylpyrazole derivatives possessing different heterocycle terminal moieties. *J. Enz. Inhibit. Med. Chem.* **2019**, *34*, 1534. [CrossRef] [PubMed]
18. El-Gamal, M.I.; Abdel-Maksoud, M.S.; Gamal El-Din, M.M.; Shin, J.-S.; Lee, K.-T.; Yoo, K.H.; Oh, C.-H. Synthesis, in vitro Antiproliferative and Antiinflammatory Activities, and Kinase Inhibitory effects of New 1,3,4-triarylpyrazole Derivatives. *Anti-Cancer Agents Med. Chem.* **2017**, *17*, 75. [CrossRef]
19. Shah, P.; Westwell, A.D. The role of fluorine in medicinal chemistry. *J. Enz. Inhibit. Med. Chem.* **2007**, *22*, 527. [CrossRef] [PubMed]
20. Madkour, M.M.; Anbar, H.S.; El-Gamal, M.I. Current status and future prospects of p38α/MAPK14 kinase and its inhibitors. *Eur. J. Med. Chem.* **2021**, *213*, 113216. [CrossRef] [PubMed]

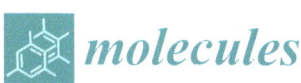

Article

Stereoselective Synthesis of the Di-Spirooxindole Analogs Based Oxindole and Cyclohexanone Moieties as Potential Anticancer Agents

Abdullah Mohammed Al-Majid [1], M. Ali [1], Mohammad Shahidul Islam [1], Saeed Alshahrani [1], Abdullah Saleh Alamary [1], Sammer Yousuf [2], M. Iqbal Choudhary [2] and Assem Barakat [1,3,*]

[1] Department of Chemistry, College of Science, King Saud University, P.O. Box 2455, Riyadh 11451, Saudi Arabia; amajid@ksu.edu.sa (A.M.A.-M.); maly.c@ksu.edu.sa (M.A.); mislam@ksu.edu.sa (M.S.I.); chemistry99y@gmail.com (S.A.); alamary1401@yahoo.com (A.S.A.)
[2] International Center for Chemical and Biological Sciences, H.E.J. Research Institute of Chemistry, University of Karachi, Karachi 75270, Pakistan; dr.sammer.yousuf@gmail.com (S.Y.); iqbal.choudhary@iccs.edu (M.I.C.)
[3] Department of Chemistry, Faculty of Science, Alexandria University, P.O. Box 426, Ibrahimia, Alexandria 21321, Egypt
* Correspondence: ambarakat@ksu.edu.sa; Tel.: +966-11467-5901; Fax: +966-11467-5992

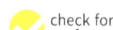

Citation: Al-Majid, A.M.; Ali, M.; Islam, M.S.; Alshahrani, S.; Alamary, A.S.; Yousuf, S.; Choudhary, M.I.; Barakat, A. Stereoselective Synthesis of the Di-Spirooxindole Analogs Based Oxindole and Cyclohexanone Moieties as Potential Anticancer Agents. *Molecules* 2021, 26, 6305. https://doi.org/10.3390/molecules26206305

Academic Editors: Imtiaz Khan and David Barker

Received: 22 June 2021
Accepted: 15 October 2021
Published: 19 October 2021

Publisher's Note: MDPI stays neutral with regard to jurisdictional claims in published maps and institutional affiliations.

Copyright: © 2021 by the authors. Licensee MDPI, Basel, Switzerland. This article is an open access article distributed under the terms and conditions of the Creative Commons Attribution (CC BY) license (https://creativecommons.org/licenses/by/4.0/).

Abstract: A new series of di-spirooxindole analogs, engrafted with oxindole and cyclohexanone moieties, were synthesized. Initially, azomethine ylides were generated via reaction of the substituted isatins **3a–f** (isatin, **3a**, 6-chloroisatin, **3b**, 5-fluoroisatin, **3c**, 5-nitroisatin, **3d**, 5-methoxyisatin, **3e**, and 5-methylisatin, **3f**, and (2S)-octahydro-1H-indole-2-carboxylic acid **2**, in situ azomethine ylides reacted with the cyclohexanone based-chalcone **1a–f** to afford the target di-spirooxindole compounds **4a–n**. This one-pot method provided diverse structurally complex molecules, with biologically relevant spirocycles in a good yields. All synthesized di-spirooxindole analogs, engrafted with oxindole and cyclohexanone moieties, were evaluated for their anticancer activity against four cancer cell lines, including prostate PC3, cervical HeLa, and breast (MCF-7, and MDA-MB231) cancer cell lines. The cytotoxicity of these di-spirooxindole analogs was also examined against human fibroblast BJ cell lines, and they appeared to be non-cytotoxic. Compound **4b** was identified as the most active member of this series against prostate cancer cell line PC3 (IC$_{50}$ = 3.7 ± 1.0 μM). The cyclohexanone engrafted di-spirooxindole analogs **4a** and **4l** (IC$_{50}$ = 7.1 ± 0.2, and 7.2 ± 0.5 μM, respectively) were active against HeLa cancer cells, whereas NO$_2$ substituted isatin ring and *meta*-fluoro-substituted (2E,6E)-2,6-dibenzylidenecyclohexanone containing **4i** (IC$_{50}$ = 7.63 ± 0.08 μM) appeared to be a promising agent against the triple negative breast cancer MDA-MB231 cell line. To explore the plausible mechanism of anticancer activity of di-spirooxindole analogs, molecular docking studies were investigated which suggested that spirooxindole analogs potentially inhibit the activity of MDM2.

Keywords: spirooxindole; azomethine ylides; [3+2] cycloaddition reaction; anti-cancer activity

1. Introduction

According to GLOBOCAN report in 2018, there were 9.6 million mortalities and 18 million new cases of cancer. In addition, the report describes cancer as the second leading cause of death worldwide. Therefore, development of anticancer agents with low toxicity, high efficacy, low drug resistance, and acceptable bioavailability is an urgent need to meet this global health challenge [1]. Drug discovery based on medicinal chemistry of natural and synthetic products have gained much attention [2,3]. In the past century, there has been an enormous success in drug innovation in the area of oral availability and biological compatibility, but drug resistance has emerged as a challenge for the medicinal chemists. Therefore, pharmacologists and chemists are focussing on functional diversity of drug leads [4], nano-formulation, and drug delivery development [5–7], with an aim of overcoming the existing problems. Specifically, the alkaloids spirooxindole scaffold, as a member of the oxindole class of natural products [8] has received much attention. The first member of this series was isolated from Apocynaceae and Rubiaceae plants. The spirooxindole scaffold is a privileged structure consisting of two basic sub-units: the first is oxindole with multiple functionalities, which can interact as acceptors or donors with the biological targets via hydrogen bonding. The second unit is a carbocyclic or heterocyclic moiety fused with oxindole ring at the C-3 position. It provides an opportunity to regulate many physicochemical properties and the liposolubility of spirooxindoles [9]. Accordingly, the significant biological activities (e.g., anti-inflammatory, anticancer, analgesic, antimicrobial, antimalarial, antioxidant, antiviral, antidiabetic, antiatherosclerotic, and insecticidal properties) and unique spatial architecture of spirooxindoles have attracted a remarkable attention of pharmacologists and chemists [10,11]. In the last few decades, several approaches towards new of spirooxindole analogs with structural diversity have been explored [12]. Based on the literature survey, the spirooxindole scaffold has shown to be a promising candidate for anti-cancer drug discovery.

In 2014, Santos's group reported the synthesis of some novel spiropyrazoline based oxindole scaffold, and subsequently examined the cytotoxicity in vitro toward MCF-7 breast cancer cell line (Figure 1). The hit with high efficacy towards the breast cancer line was checked against MDA-MB-231 cell line. The results demonstrated that compound **I** exhibited a high activity with higher selectivity between the two cell lines with $GI_{50} < 7.4$ μM and >10-fold than the MDA-MB-231 cell line. Interestingly, the promising compound **I** behaved safely, and was noncytotoxic to HEK293T normal cell line [13].

Zhou's group synthesized a family of spirooxindoles **II**, grafted with five-membered carbocyclic, with substituted oxindoles via set of chemical transformations, including Knoevenagel condensation/Michael cyclization (Figure 1). The synthesized compounds were evaluated for anticancer activity against three cancer cell lines, lung A549, human leukemia K562, and prostate-cancer cell lines PC-3. From this study, some representative compounds showed a comparable or stronger inhibitory effect against human leukemia cells K562 (IC_{50} = 7.4 to 32.8 μM) as compared to cisplatin (up to 3.4-fold). Moreover, other hits have either shown equivalent inhibition toward A549 cell line or slightly increased inhibitory activity against prostate cancer PC-3 cell line as compared to cisplatin [14].

In 2018, Barakat et al. reported a family of functionalized spirooxindoles. Representative compounds having the substituent on the benzene ring, such as 4-Me, 3-Br, and 4-CF$_3$, exhibited potent cytotoxic activity against HCT-116 cells (IC_{50} = 7 μM, 9 μM, and 9 μM, respectively) and high selectivity index (SI) toward normal cells (SI > 2) [15]. On the other hand, the research group reported that the 2,4-diCl substituted benzene showed high cytotoxic activity and selectivity against PC-3 and HepG2 with IC_{50} = 2 μM for both cancer cells (SI = 4.5 and 4.5, respectively), and was more potent as compared to positive control, such as cisplatin (IC_{50} = 5 μM and 5.5 μM, respectively). In our previous reports, we explored the anticancer activity of the spriooxindole scaffold-based cyclohexanone against two cancer cell lines, MCF-7 breast and K562-leukemia cancer cells. We found that the compound **VII**, with a 4-methoxy group substituted benzene, was the most potent compound (IC_{50} = 13.38 ± 0.14 μM), targeting K562 leukemia cancer cells more selectively than 5-FU (IC_{50} = 38.58 ± 0.02 μM) Additionally, we noted that the hit with the *p*-Br-substituted benzene **VIII** had a higher efficacy for targeting MCF-7 breast cancer cells (IC_{50} = 15.32 ± 0.02 μM) as compared to the standard drug, 5-fluorouracil (5-FU) (IC_{50} = 78.28 ± 0.2 μM) (Figure 1) [16,17].

In 2019, Tumskiy et al. synthesized five spirooxindolepyrrolidines and examined the cytotoxic activity against some cell lines (Vero normal and HeLa cancer cells). The results demonstrated that hit **III** having a pyridine moiety with the chlorine atom in the *ortho* position exhibited a moderate selectivity (3-fold) between HeLa cancer cells and Vero healthy cells [18].

In continuation of research work, Barakat et al. reported the synthesis of spirooxindole–pyrrolothiazoles having a 3-cinnamoyl moiety. The results of cytotoxicity activities assay disclosed that compound **V** was the most active member of the series towards HCT-116, HepG2, and PC-3 cancer cells ($IC_{50} < 4$ μM). The selectivity index for the cancer cells versus the normal cells was superior to 2. Additionally, the research group carried out a set of biological assays which indicated that compound **V** could inhibit cell migration, colony formation, arrest cancer cell growth at the G2/M phase and induce apoptosis through extrinsic and intrinsic pathways [19] (Figure 1).

In 2019, Barakat et al. reported the synthesis and cytotoxicity activities (HeLa) of the hit depicted in Figure 1 (i.e., **VI**). The antiproliferative assay showed that the compound can inhibit the proliferation of HeLa cancer cell line ($IC_{50} = 11.2$ μM), but less than the anticancer drug, doxorubicin ($IC_{50} = 1.2$ μM) [20].

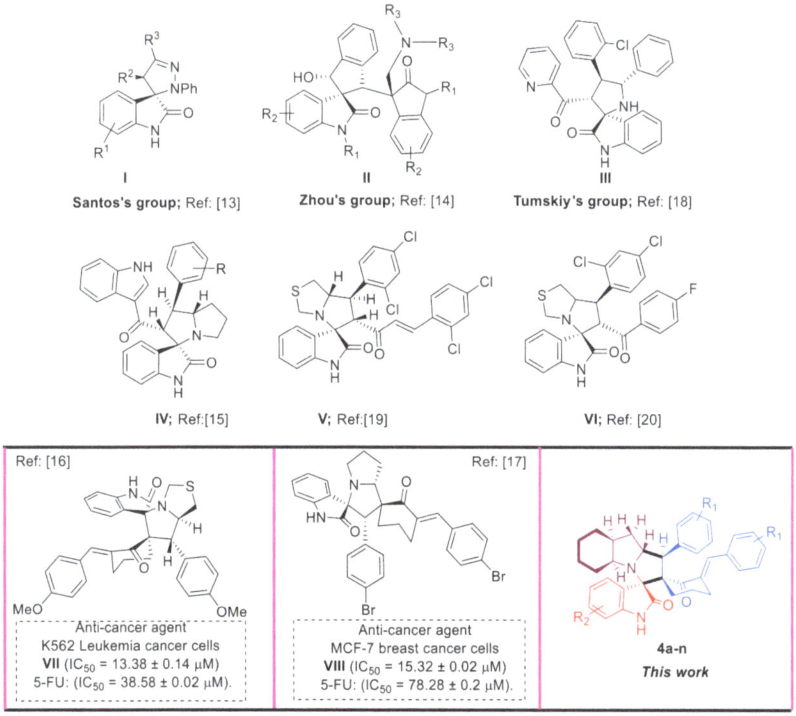

Figure 1. The anticancer activity of some reported spirooxindoles analogs.

The large library of the spirooxindole scaffold was generated with diverse pharmaceutical activities including low toxicity, acceptable bioavailability, and high efficiency [21–29]. In this paper, we describe in detail the synthesis of the spirooxindole analogs with significant bioactivities against the cancer cell in vitro. Molecular docking studies were also carried out to explore the plausible mechanism of anticancer activity of di-spirooxindole analogs.

2. Results and Discussion

2.1. Synthesis of (4a–n)

The main objective of this study was to synthesize a new series of dispirooxindole scaffold and to examine their anticancer activity. For this purpose, desired dispirooxindole derivatives (**4a–n**) were synthesized via one-pot multicomponent reaction approach proceeded through [3+2] cycloaddition reaction (Scheme 1), and the plausible mechanism described in Scheme 2 [17,30–35]. Fourteen members with different electronic effects were prepared according to our previously reported protocol. The reaction proceeded smoothly via mixing the α,β-unsaturated ketones (**1a–f**), with the substituted isatin (**3a–f**) (Isatin (**3a**), 6-chloroisatin (**3b**), 5-fluoroisatin (**3c**), 5-nitroisatin (**3d**), 5-methoxyisatin (**3e**), and 5-methylisatin (**3f**), and (2*S*)-octahydro-1*H*-indole-2-carboxylic acid (**2**) in MeOH under reflux conditions at 60 °C for 1–1.5 h to afford the requisite di-spirooxindoles in high chemical yields (up to 75%) with regio- and diastereoselective manner. This led to the generation of indoline analogs which are isosteric derivatives of previously synthesized compounds [12,13]. The aromatic substituents (R_1 = H, F, Br, and CF_3) in the cyclohexanone based-chalcones were employed in the [3+2]-dipolar cycloaddition reaction approach [31–35]. The chemical structures were deduced on the basis of spectroscopic techniques, including NMR, IR, and MS as well as CHN elemental analysis. Optical rotation of the synthesized compounds were carried out and confirmed the optical purity of the dispirooxindoles (**4a–n**).

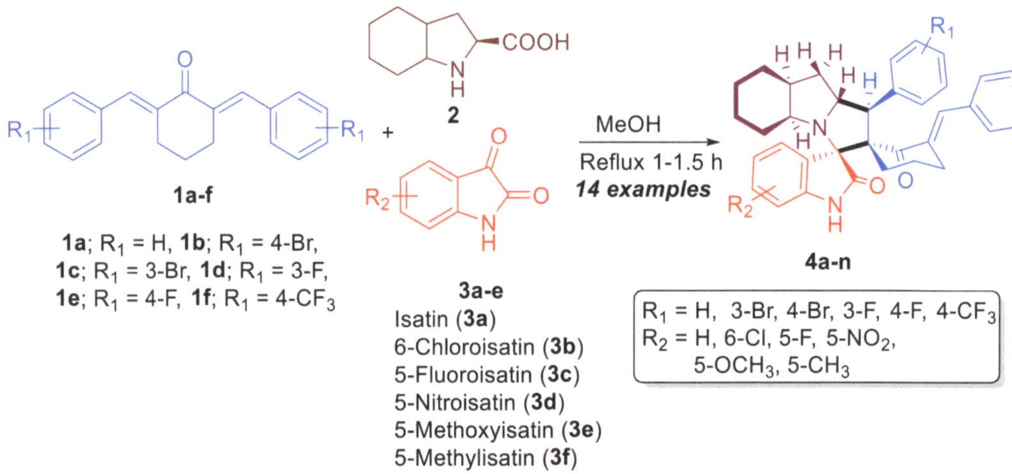

Scheme 1. Enantio-selective synthesis of the di-spirooxindoles **4a–n**-based oxindole and cyclohexanone moieties.

To assign the stereochemistry of the final compounds, several attempts were carried out to obtain a suitable single crystal for X-ray diffraction analysis but unfortunately, it failed as it provided amorphous materials. Then, extensive analysis by 1D- and 2D-NMR spectroscopy were investigated (Supplementary Materials Figures S15–S19). Compound **4f** was chosen as a model example to reach the stereochemistry assignment of the final compounds (Figure 2). As shown in Supplementary Materials Figure S15, ^{1}H- and ^{13}C-NMR confirmed the only desired regioisomer which confirm the proposed [3+2] cycloaddition reaction approach (*ortho/endo*-Pathway) [31–35] (Scheme 2).

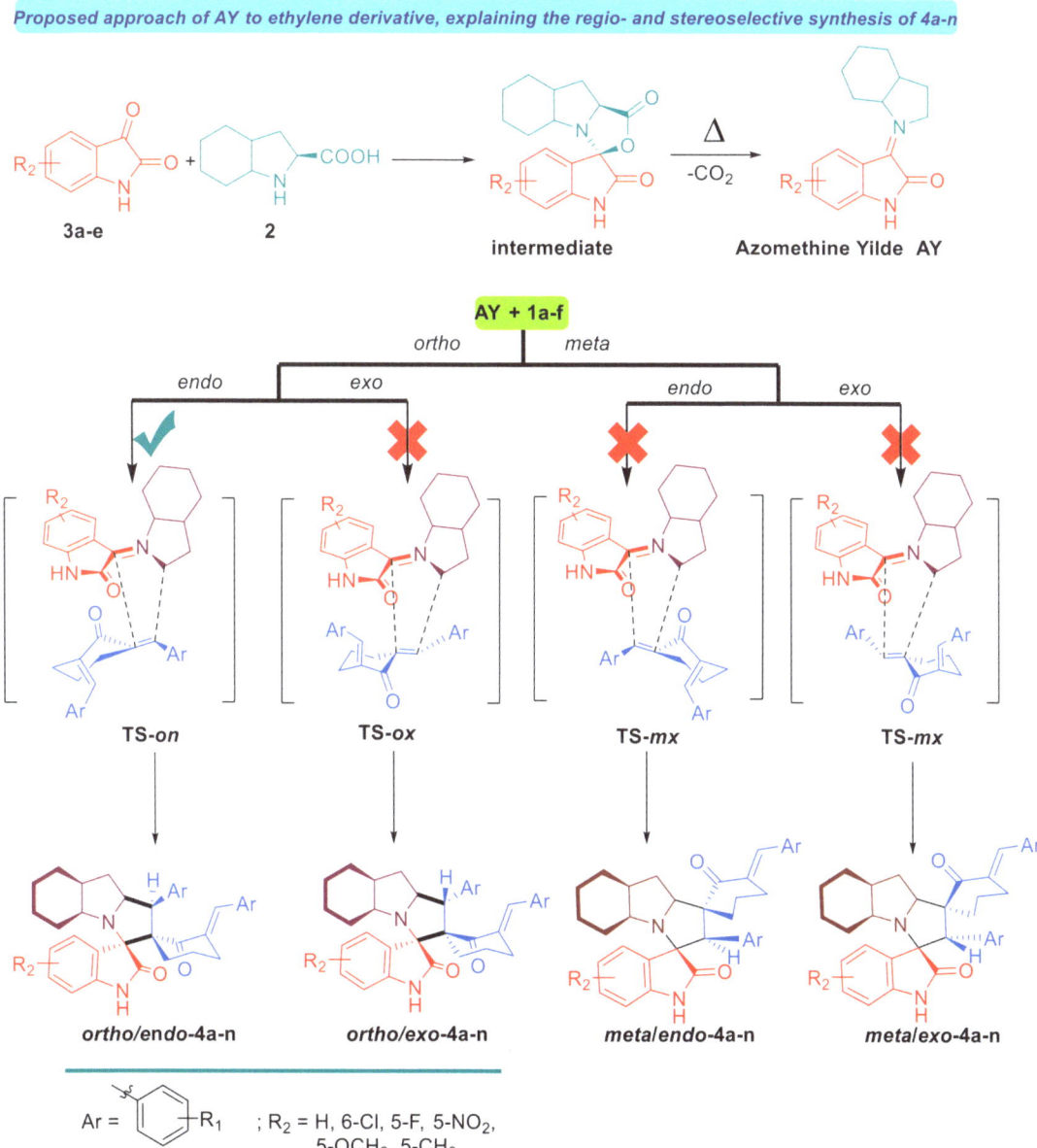

Scheme 2. Plausible approach of **AY** to ethylene derivative, explaining the regio- and stereoselective synthesis of the target compounds **4a–n**.

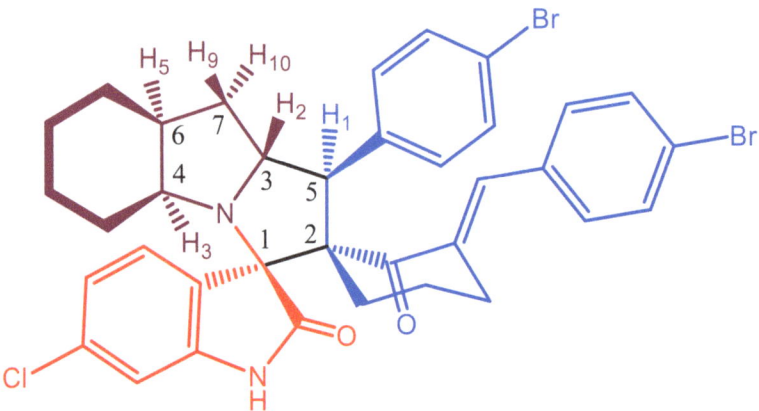

Figure 2. Chemical structure of 4f.

It was clearly evident from the ^{13}C- and DEPT-135 spectra by comparison that the molecule **4f** having 4 CH carbon (C_3, C_4, C_5, and C_6) at δ (ppm) = 64.29, 58.08, 51.44, and 42.51, respectively (+ve peaks) and 8 **CH$_2$** carbon (C_7–C_{14}) at δ (ppm) = 36.17, 28.47, 28.32, 28.02, 26.63, 24.67, 21.59, and 20.31, respectively (-ve peaks) which are clearly observed in DEPT-135 spectra, while two quaternary carbons C_1 and C_2 appear at δ(ppm) = 79.58 and 69.30, respectively in ^{13}C-NMR, while those peaks disappeared from the DEPT-135 spectra (Supplementary Materials Figure S16).

HMQC (Supplementary Materials Figure S17) analysis confirmed that C_1 and C_2 carbon do not have any proton attached to these carbons but C_3, C_4, C_5, and C_6, bear single proton H_2, H_3, H_1, H_5, respectively, while for eight carbons C_7–C_{14}, each of them is attached to two protons (C_7-$H_{9,10}$; C_8-$H_{18,20}$; C_9-$H_{11,13}$; C_{10}-$H_{7,8}$; C_{11}-$H_{4,6}$; C_{12}-$H_{12,17}$; C_{13}-$H_{15,19}$; C_{14}-$H_{14,16}$). By this observation, we excluded the two diastereoisomeres formed via *meta*-approach in the [3+2] cycloaddition reaction (32CA) (Scheme 2) [31–35].

Next, COSY analysis mapping helped us to find the neighboring protons association. H_1 and H_2 coupled with each other while H_2 also coupled with two other protons ($H_{9,10}$). Proton H_3 had three strong coupling signals with H_5 and $H_{18,20}$. Similarly, proton H_5 had five adjacent protons since it had five coupling signals with H_3, $H_{9,10}$, and $H_{11,13}$ (Figure S18, Supplementary Materials). HMQC Spectra explain the 1–3 and 1–4 interaction of H_1 with C_2, C_3, C_7, C_{11}, and CO which further confirm the position of H_1 proton (Supplementary Materials Figure S19).

2.2. Biological Activity

All synthesized di-spirooxindole analogs **4a–n**, attached with substituted cyclohexanone moiety, were initially examined for toxicity against human fibroblast BJ cell line and appeared to be non-toxic except compound **4g** which was slightly toxic (IC$_{50}$ = 21.7 $\pm$ 0.2) at 30 µM concentration. The antiproliferative activity against four cancer cell lines, including prostate PC3, cervical HeLa, and triple-negative breast cancer (MCF-7 and MDA-MB231) was evaluated by MTT assay, while standard drug doxorubicin was used as a reference for comparison (Table 1).

Table 1. Results of anticancer assay against BJ, PC3, HeLa, MCF-7, and MDA-MB231 cells.

#	Chemical Structure 4a-n	Cancer Type/Cell Line (IC$_{50}$, μM) [a,b]				
		Human Fibroblast BJ	Prostate PC3	Cervical HeLa	Breast MCF-7	Breast MDA-MB231
4a		NA	24.1 ± 1.1	7.1 ± 0.2	25.04 ± 0.57	19.50 ± 0.56
4b		NA	3.7 ± 1.0	NA	27.72 ± 0.59	24.08 ± 0.02
4c		NA	17.9 ± 0.2	NA	27.82 ± 1.02	20.62 ± 2.16
4d		NA	29.8 ± 0.1	NA	NA	NA
4e		NA	19.6 ± 1.2	26.5 ± 0.04	NA	NA
4f		NA	NA	NA	NS [c]	NS
4g		21.7 ± 0.2	14.3 ± 1.0	NA	NA	NS

Table 1. Cont.

#	Chemical Structure 4a-n	Cancer Type/Cell Line (IC$_{50}$, µM) [a,b]				
		Human Fibroblast BJ	Prostate PC3	Cervical HeLa	Breast MCF-7	Breast MDA-MB231
4h		NA	NA	NA	NA	14.43 ± 0.09
4i		NA	NA	NA	NA	7.63 ± 0.08
4j		NA	NA	11.9 ± 0.04	NA	10.49 ± 0.71
4k		NA	NA	NA	NA	NA
4l		NA	NA	7.2 ± 0.5	NA	14.45 ± 0.08
4m		NA	NA	24.6 ± 0.4	NA	NA
4n		NA	NA	NA	NA	NA
STD.	Doxorubicin	NA	1.9 ± 0.4	0.9 ± 0.14	0.79 ± 0.05	0.32 ± 0.002

[a] IC$_{50}$ (µM) was evaluated using MTT assay and ± is the standard deviation from three independent experiments. [b] NA means that the tested compound did not show anticancer activity at 30 µM. [c] NS: Not soluble.

Among synthesized di-spirooxindole analogs **4a–n**, compound **4b** (IC$_{50}$ = 3.7 ± 1.0 µM) was found to be the most active candidate against prostate cancer PC3 cell line in comparison to standard drug doxorubicin (IC$_{50}$ = 1.9 ± 0.4 µM) and non-substituted spirooxindole analogue **4a** (IC$_{50}$ = 24.1 ± 1.1 µM). Structurally, in comparison to **4a**, compound **4b** consisted of 6-chloro substituted isatin moiety attached to non-substituted phenyl rings containing (2E,6E)-2,6-dibenzylidenecyclohexanone. The change of 6-chloro phenyl substituents of isatin moiety with 5-flouro, 5-methoxy, and 5 nitro phenyl rings contributed towards a gradual decrease in activity as in compounds **4c** (IC$_{50}$ = 17.9 ± 0.2 µM), **4e** (IC$_{50}$ = 19.6 ± 1.2 µM), and **4d** (IC$_{50}$ = 29.8 ± 0.1 µM), respectively. However, a major increase in activity was observed in compound **4g** (IC$_{50}$ = 14.3 ± 1.0 µM) having a *para*-bromo-substituted benzene rings attached to 5 nitro isatin moiety instead of 5 nitro isatin moiety containing compound **4d** (IC$_{50}$ was 29.8 ± 0.1 µM). All other compounds, i.e., **4f**, and **4h–n** appeared to be inactive against prostate cancer cell line PC3.

The anticancer potential of the spirooxindole analogs **4a–n**, attached with cyclohexanone moiety, was also evaluated against cervical cancer HeLa cell line in comparison to the standard drug doxorubicin (IC$_{50}$ = 0.9 ± 0.14 µM). The most active spirooxindole analog appeared to be compound **4a** (IC$_{50}$ = 7.1 ± 0.2 µM), having un-substituted isatin and aromatic ring of chlacones moieties. No change in activity was observed for compound **4l** incorporated with 6-choloro isatin and *p*-fluoro-substituted aromatic ring of chlacones moieties (IC$_{50}$ = 7.2 ± 0.5 µM). However, substitution of *p*-fluoro atom of aromatic ring of chlacone moieties with *p*-trifluoromethyl groups contributed towards a decrease in activity as observed in compound **4m** (IC$_{50}$ = 24.6 ± 0.4 µM). The incorporation of methoxy group on isatin ring (**4e**; IC$_{50}$ = 26.5 ± 0.04 µM) also contributed towards a decrease in activity in comparison to **4a** (IC$_{50}$ = 7.1 ± 0.2 µM), having un-substituted isatin and aromatic ring of chlacone moieties. However, a significant improvement of anticancer potential was observed for compound **4j** (IC$_{50}$ = 11.9 ± 0.04 µM) having 6-methoxy isatin and *p*-fluoro-substituted aromatic ring. All other compounds **4b–d**, **4f–i**, **4k**, and **4n** appeared to be inactive.

Many of the tested di-spirooxindole analogs **4a–n** attached with cyclohexanone moiety appeared to be inactive against breast cancer MCF-7 cancer cell line, except compounds **4a** (IC$_{50}$ = 25.04 ± 0.57 µM), **4b** (IC$_{50}$ = 27.72 ± 0.59 µM), and **4c** (IC$_{50}$ = 27.82 ± 1.02 µM), which appeared to be weakly active against the MCF-7 cell line in comparison to standard drug, doxorubicin (IC$_{50}$ = 0.79 ± 0.4 µM).

Finally, all synthesized di-spirooxindole analogues **4a–n** were evaluated against MDA-MB231 triple negative breast cancer cell line. 5-Nitro isatin and *m*-fluoro-phenyl ring containing chlacone **4i** (IC$_{50}$ = 7.63 ± 0.08 µM) appeared to be the most active member of the series. A gradual decrease in activity was observed for compounds **4j** (IC$_{50}$ = 10.49 ± 0.71 µM) and **4h** (IC$_{50}$ = 14.43 ± 0.09 µM) having 5-nitro isatin and 6-chloro isatin moieties, instead of 5-nitro isatin as observed in **4i** (IC$_{50}$ = 7.63 ± 0.08 µM). However, change of position of fluoro substituent from *meta* **4h** (IC$_{50}$ = 14.43 ± 0.09 µM) to *para* **4l** (IC$_{50}$ = 14.45 ± 0.08 µM) on phenyl rings of dibenzylidenecyclohexanone did not exert any effect on activity against MDA-MB231 cell line. Significant reduction in activity was observed in compounds **4b** (IC$_{50}$ = 24.08 ± 0.02 µM) and **4c** (IC$_{50}$ = 20.62 ± 2.16 µM) having non-substituted phenyl rings containing dibenzylidenecyclohexanone moiety attached to 6-chloro and 5-flouro isatin ring, respectively. Compounds **4d–g**, **4k**, **4m**, and **4n** appeared inactive against the breast cancer cell line (MDA-MB231). All results are summarized in Table 1.

2.3. Molecular Docking Study

It has been reported that most of the human cancer cells overexpressed p-53 protein [4,11,36,37]. Therefore, docking studies were performed to rationalize the plausible mechanism of inhibition of p53-MDM2 protein–protein interactions.

A tumor suppressor protein p53 plays a pivotal role in preventing tumor progression and development. Cellular stress in response to DNA damage and hypoxia triggers the stimulation of p53. Up-regulated p53 stimulates the transcription of many important genes involved in apoptosis, senescence, DNA repair, and apoptosis. Consequently, suppression of p53 may be a requisite step in tumor formation. Murine double minute 2 (MDM2) is a central negative regulator of p53. Due to the vital role of MDM2 in inhibiting the tumor suppressor function of p53, blockade of protein–protein interaction of MDM2-p53 is an attractive anticancer therapeutic target. Furthermore, it has been extensively reported that spirooxindole analogs potentially inhibit the activity of MDM2 [19,38–40]. Thus, in this study, molecular docking studies of the potential anticancer di-spirooxindole analogs were carried out using MDM2 crystal structure to explore the observed anticancer activity. The docking studies suggested that **4a**, **4b**, **4i**, and **4l** accommodated well in the binding site of MDM2 with a binding affinity of −7.20, −7.37, −7.83, and −7.90 kcal/mol, respectively (Figure 3).

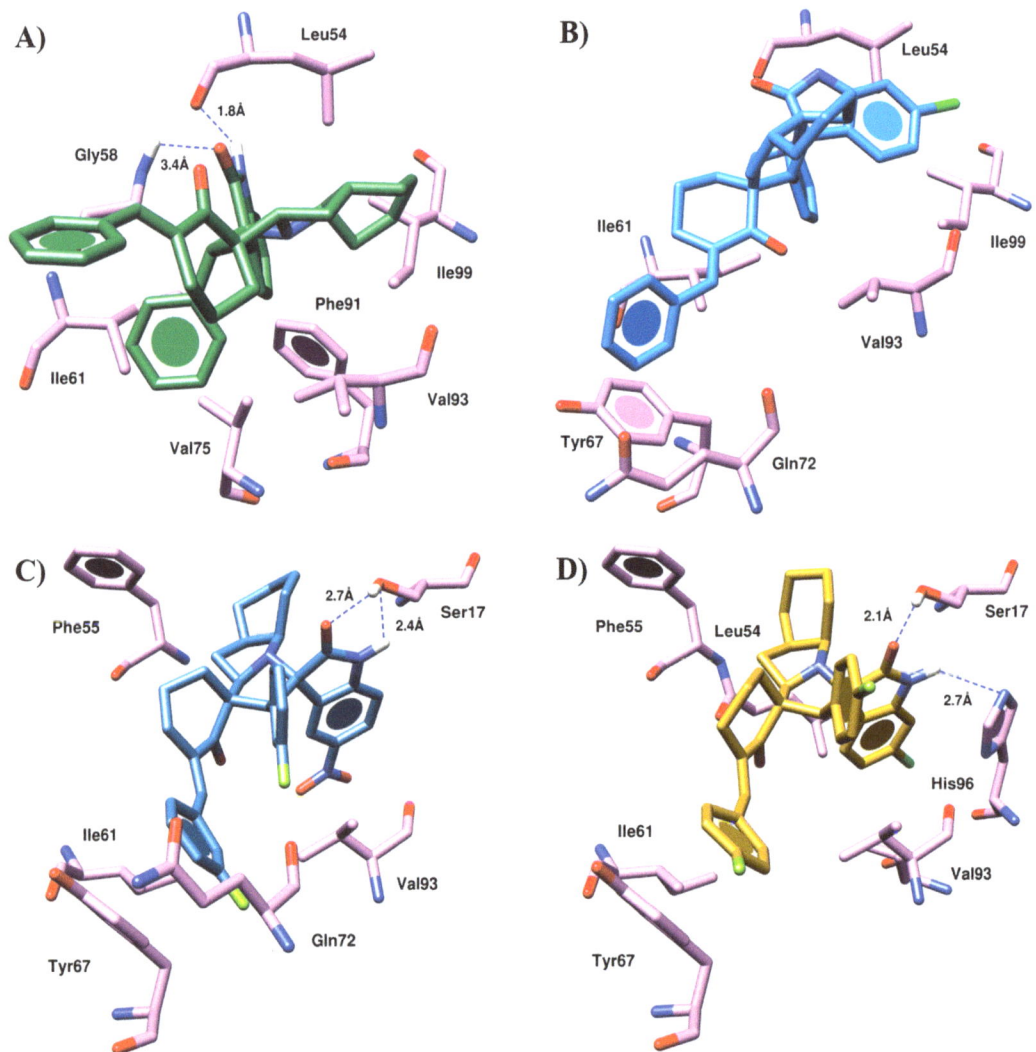

Figure 3. Docked pose of compounds (**A**) 4a, (**B**) 4b, (**C**) 4i, and (**D**) 4l in the binding site of MDM2.

Compound **4a** showed a slightly different binding mode in comparison to **4b**, **4i**, and **4l**. The unsubstituted oxindole ring of **4a** interacts with the side chain of Leu54 and Gly58 while the substituted oxindole ring of **4b**, **4i**, and **4l** is buried deeply in the binding cavity of MDM2 by interacting with Val93, His96, and Ile99. Substitution on the oxindole ring may account for the different binding mode of the di-spirooxindole analogs within the binding cavity of MDM2. Similarly, compound **4a** confers two hydrogen bond contacts with the carboxyl group of Leu54 and Gly58. Six-membered aromatic rings in the **4a** mediate π-π and π-alkyl interactions with the binding site residues of MDM2, including Leu54, Ile61, Val75, Phe91, Val93, and Ile99, which projected **4a** firmly in the binding pocket. The compound **4b** resides comfortably in the binding site extending hydrophobic interactions with Leu54, Ile61, Tyr67, Gln72, Val93, and Ile99, while no hydrogen bond was observed. The docked pose of compound **4i** suggested a number of significant hydrophobic interactions with binding site residues. Fluorinated phenyl rings stacked between Ile61, Tyr67, and Val93 produced hydrophobic effects. Similarly, Phe55 was also observed to mediate hydrophobic interactions. In addition, **4i** confers two hydrogen bonds with the side chain hydroxyl group of Ser17 and a halogen bond with Gln72, whereas fluorinated phenyl rings of compound **4l** establish hydrophobic interactions with Leu57, Phe55, Ile61, Tyr67, Val93, and Ile99. Moreover, two hydrogen bonds were observed with the side chain hydroxyl group and imidazol ring of Ser17 and His96, respectively.

3. Materials and Methods

3.1. General Procedure for the Synthesis of Di-spirooxindoles (4a–n) (GP1)

Substituted (2E,6E)-2,6-dibenzylidenecyclohexanone (**1a–f**) (0.25 mmol), isatin derivatives (**3a–f**) (0.25 mmol) (2S)-octahydro-1H-indole-2-carboxylic acid (**2**) (63 mg, 0.37 mmol) were dissolved in methanol (20 mL) and refluxed for 1–1.5 h. Finally, the products were isolated by flash column chromatography using 100–200 mesh silica gel and 10–20% ethyl acetate/n-hexane as an eluent to afford pure spirooxindoles (**4a-n**). Note for optical rotation measurement: sample prepared in 10 mL, then concentration calculated in g/100 mL. A 100 mm polarimeter tube was used. Instrument used: A.KRÜSS Optronic P8000-PT digital polarimeter (A.KRÜSS Optronic GmbH Alsterdorfer Straße 276–278 22297 Hamburg, Germany).

3.1.1. (1. S,1′S,3′S,4a′S,8a′S,9a′R)-3-((E)-Benzylidene)-1′-phenyl-4a′,5′,6′,7′,8′,8a′,9′,9a′-octahydro-1′H-dispiro[cyclohexane-1,2′-pyrrolo[1,2-a]indole-3′,3″-indoline]-2,2″-dione (**4a**)

2,6-Di((E)-benzylidene)cyclohexan-1-one (**1a**) (69 mg, 0.25 mmol), (2S)-octahydro-1H-indole-2-carboxylic acid (**2**) (64 mg, 0.37 mmol) and isatin (**3a**) (37 mg, 0.25 mmol) were reacted according to GP1 for 1 h and yielded white solid spirooxindole (**4a**) (104 mg, 76%); m.p.: 70–71 °C; ^{1}H-NMR (500 MHz, CDCl$_3$): δ (ppm) = 7.90 (s, 1H, NH), 7.57 (d, J = 7.4 Hz, 1H, Ar-**H**), 7.38 (d, J = 8.0 Hz, 3H, Ar-**H**), 7.25–7.21 (m, 5H, Ar-**H**), 7.14 (t, J = 7.7 Hz, 1H, Ar-**H**), 7.06 (d, J = 6.3 Hz, 1H, Ar-**H**), 7.04 (d, J = 6.3 Hz, 2H, Ar-**H**), 6.96 (d, J = 7.6 Hz, 1H, Ar-**H**), 6.64 (d, J = 7.7 Hz, 1H, Ar-**H**), 4.98 (d, J = 10.3 Hz, 1H, C**H**), 4.58 (m, 1H, NC**H**), 3.39 (q, J = 4.3 Hz, 1H, NC**H**), 2.89–2.81 (m, 1H, C**H**$_2$), 2.36–2.30 (m, 1H, C**H**$_2$), 2.25–2.18 (m, 1H, C**H**$_2$), 2.02–1.97 (m, 3H, C**H**$_2$), 1.70–1.66 (m, 1H, C**H**$_2$), 1.65–1.60 (m, 3H, C**H**$_2$), 1.54–1.52 (m, 2H, C**H**$_2$), 1.02–0.96 (m, 3H, C**H**$_2$); ^{13}C-NMR (126 MHz, CDCl$_3$): δ (ppm) = 202.1 (**C**O), 180.2 (**C**O), 141.3, 138.6, 137.8, 135.8, 134.8, 130.1, 129.7, 129.1, 128.5, 128.3, 128.2, 128.1, 127.1, 126.8, 121.4, 109.7, 79.7, 69.5, 64.3, 57.9, 52.3, 42.6, 36.3, 28.5, 28.4, 27.9, 26.6, 24.8, 21.7, 20.4; IR (KBr, cm^{-1}) $ν_{max}$ = 3057, 2928, 2854, 1711, 1683, 1617, 1600, 1521, 1492, 1471, 1447, 1365, 1321, 1289, 1199, 1154, 1030, 961, 753, 697; (Anal. Calcd. for C$_{36}$H$_{36}$N$_2$O$_2$: C, 81.79; H, 6.86; N, 5.30; Found: C, 81.88; H, 6.94; N, 5.21); LC/MS (ESI, m/z): found 529.3 [M+H]$^+$; exact mass 528.3 for C$_{36}$H$_{36}$N$_2$O$_2$. $[α]_D^{25}$ = −20.72° (c 0.10, MeOH).

3.1.2. (1. S,1′S,3′S,4a′S,8a′S,9a′R)-3-((E)-Benzylidene)-6

-chloro-1′-phenyl-4a′,5′,6′,7′,8′,8a′,9′,9a′-octahydro-1′H-dispiro[cyclohexane-1,2′-pyrrolo[1,2-a]indole-3′,3″-indoline]-2,2″-dione (**4b**)

2,6-Di((*E*)-benzylidene)cyclohexan-1-one (**1a**) (69 mg, 0.25 mmol), (2*S*)-octahydro-1*H*-indole-2-carboxylic acid (**2**) (64 mg, 0.37 mmol) and 6-chloroisatin (**3b**) (45 mg, 0.25 mmol) were reacted according to GP1 for 1 h and yielded white solid spirooxindole (**4b**) (98 mg, 70%); m.p.: 77–78 °C; ^{1}H-NMR (500 MHz, CDCl$_3$): δ (ppm) = 8.14 (s, 1H, N**H**), 7.46 (d, *J* = 8.2 Hz, 1H, Ar-**H**), 7.34 (d, *J* = 8.3 Hz, 3H, Ar-**H**), 7.25–7.21 (m, 6H, Ar-**H**), 7.06 (d, *J* = 8.0 Hz, 2H, Ar-**H**), 6.93 (d, *J* = 8.0 Hz, 1H, Ar-**H**), 6.70 (s, 1H, Ar-**H**), 4.94 (d, *J* = 10.3 Hz, 1H, C**H**), 4.58–4.53 (m, 1H, NC**H**), 3.37 (q, *J* = 4.0 Hz, 1H, NC**H**), 2.79–2.73 (m, 1H, C**H**$_2$), 2.34–2.28 (m, 1H, C**H**$_2$), 2.25–2.18 (m, 1H, C**H**$_2$), 2.01–1.94 (m, 2H, C**H**$_2$), 1.70–1.64 (d, *J* = 6.1 Hz, 2H, C**H**$_2$), 1.64–1.58 (m, 3H, C**H**$_2$), 1.53–1.48 (m, 2H, C**H**$_2$), 1.28–1.22 (m, 2H, C**H**$_2$), 1.07–0.97 (m, 3H, C**H**$_2$); ^{13}C-NMR (126 MHz, CDCl$_3$): δ (ppm) = 202.0 (**C**O), 180.0 (**C**O), 142.6, 138.4, 137.5, 135.7, 135.4, 134.8, 130.8, 130.2, 129.7, 128.5, 128.3, 128.1, 127.9, 126.9, 121.4, 110.3, 79.3, 69.8, 64.2, 57.9, 52.6, 42.6, 36.2, 28.6, 28.4, 28.1, 26.8, 24.8, 21.6, 20.4; IR (KBr, cm^{-1}) ν$_{max}$ = 3058, 2928, 2853, 1716, 1685, 1619, 1608, 1525, 1491, 1470, 1448, 1363, 1317, 1275, 1199, 1153, 1032, 965, 758, 696; (Anal. Calcd. for C$_{36}$H$_{35}$ClN$_2$O$_2$: C, 76.78; H, 6.26; N, 4.97; Found: C, 76.71; H, 6.35; N, 5.07); LC/MS (ESI, *m*/*z*): found 563.1 [M($_{35}$Cl)+H]$^+$; 565.1 [M($_{37}$Cl)+H]$^+$; exact mass 562.1 for C$_{36}$H$_{35}$ClN$_2$O$_2$. [α]$_D^{25}$ = −17.54° (c 0.19, MeOH).

3.1.3. (1. *S*,1′*S*,3′*S*,4a′*S*,8a′*S*,9a′*R*)-3-((*E*)-Benzylidene)-5″-fluoro-1′-phenyl-4a′,5′,6′,7′,8′,8a′,9′,9a′-octahydro-1′H-dispiro[cyclohexane-1,2′-pyrrolo[1,2-a]indole-3′,3″-indoline]-2,2″-dione (**4c**)

2,6-Di((*E*)-benzylidene)cyclohexan-1-one (**1a**) (69 mg, 0.25 mmol), (2*S*)-octahydro-1*H*-indole-2-carboxylic acid (**2**) (64 mg, 0.37 mmol) and 5-fluoroisatin (**3c**) (41 mg, 0.25 mmol) were reacted according to GP1 for 1h and yielded white solid spirooxindole (**4c**) (104 mg, 76%); m.p.: 70–71 °C; ^{1}H-NMR (500 MHz, CDCl$_3$): δ (ppm) = 8.56 (s, 1H, N**H**), 7.37–7.34 (m, 3H, Ar-**H**), 7.24–7.22 (m, 6H, Ar-**H**), 7.09–7.05 (m, 3H, Ar-**H**), 6.86 (td, *J* = 8.8, 2.7 Hz, 1H, Ar-**H**), 6.65 (dd, *J* = 8.5, 4.3 Hz, 1H, Ar-**H**), 4.98 (d, *J* = 10.4 Hz, 1H, C**H**), 4.60–4.56 (m, 1H, NC**H**), 3.42–3.37 (m, 1H, NC**H**), 2.79–2.73 (m, 1H, C**H**$_2$), 2.39–2.20 (m, 4H, C**H**$_2$), 2.07–1.94 (m, 3H, C**H**$_2$), 1.73–1.57 (m, 6H, C**H**$_2$), 1.08–0.99 (m, 3H, C**H**$_2$); ^{13}C-NMR (126 MHz, CDCl$_3$): δ (ppm) = 201.8 (**C**O), 180.7 (**C**O), 159.4, 157.5, 138.4, 137.4, 137.4, 136.5, 135.7, 135.2, 130.7, 130.5, 130.2, 130.1, 129.7, 128.4, 128.3, 128.14, 128.14, 126.9, 115.6, 115.4, 114.7, 114.5, 110.3, 110.3, 79.9, 69.8, 64.2, 57.9, 52.7, 42.5, 36.12, 28.5, 28.3, 28.1, 26.7, 24.7, 21.6, 20.4; IR (KBr, cm^{-1}) ν$_{max}$ = 3054, 2929, 2852, 1715, 1680, 1614, 1605, 1527, 1495, 1476, 1444, 1368, 1321, 1284, 1196, 1151, 1007, 962, 755, 693; (Anal. Calcd. for C$_{36}$H$_{35}$FN$_2$O$_2$: C, 79.09; H, 6.45; N, 5.12; Found: C, 79.21; H, 6.58; N, 5.07); LC/MS (ESI, *m*/*z*): found 547.3 [M+H]$^+$; exact mass 546.3 for C$_{36}$H$_{35}$FN$_2$O$_2$. [α]$_D^{25}$ = −39.87° (c 0.10, MeOH).

3.1.4. (1. *S*,1′*S*,3′*S*,4a′*S*,8a′*S*,9a′*R*)-3-((*E*)-Benzylidene)-5″-nitro-1′-phenyl-4a′,5′,6′,7′,8′,8a′,9′,9a′-octahydro-1′H-dispiro[cyclohexane-1,2′-pyrrolo[1,2-a]indole-3′,3″-indoline]-2,2″-dione (**4d**)

2,6-Di((*E*)-benzylidene)cyclohexan-1-one (**1a**) (69 mg, 0.25 mmol), (2*S*)-octahydro-1*H*-indole-2-carboxylic acid (**2**) (64 mg, 0.37 mmol) and 5-nitroisatin (**3d**) (48 mg, 0.25 mmol) were reacted according to GP1 for 1 h and yielded white solid spirooxindole (**4d**) (98 mg, 68%); m.p.: 111–122 °C; ^{1}H-NMR (500 MHz, CDCl$_3$): δ (ppm) = 8.47 (s, 1H, N**H**), 7.50–7.44 (m, 3H, Ar-**H**), 7.35–7.32 (m, 2H, Ar-**H**), 7.31–7.26 (m, 1H, Ar-**H**), 7.24–7.21 (m, 2H, Ar-**H**), 7.19–7.17 (m, 1H, Ar-**H**), 7.13 (d, *J* = 8.2 Hz, 1H, Ar-**H**), 7.12–7.09 (m, 2H, Ar-**H**), 7.02–6.99 (m, 1H, Ar-**H**), 6.74 (q, *J* = 1.7 Hz, 1H, Ar-**H**), 4.91 (d, *J* = 10.2 Hz, 1H, C**H**), 4.53–4.46 (m, 1H, NC**H**), 3.34 (q, *J* = 3.9 Hz, 1H, NC**H**), 2.92 -2.87 (m, 1H, C**H**$_2$), 2.82–2.73 (m, 1H, C**H**$_2$), 2.39–2.29 (m, 2H, C**H**$_2$), 2.19–2.14 (m, 1H, C**H**$_2$), 2.08–2.00 (m, 3H, C**H**$_2$), 1.96–1.92 (m, 1H, C**H**$_2$), 1.71–1.59 (m, 5H, C**H**$_2$), 1.08–1.01 (m, 3H, C**H**$_2$); ^{13}C-NMR (126 MHz, CDCl$_3$): δ (ppm) = 201.8 (**C**O), 180.1 (**C**O), 142.5, 139.9, 139.5, 137.6, 135.1, 133.7, 132.7, 132.5, 131.4, 130.2, 129.7, 128.6, 127.9, 122.5, 121.6, 110.5, 79.4, 69.6, 64.2, 58.0, 52.1, 42.5, 36.1, 28.6, 28.3, 28.0, 26.8, 24.6, 21.5, 20.9; IR (KBr, cm^{-1}) ν$_{max}$ = 3262, 2926, 2853, 1715, 1681, 1612, 1592,

1558, 1484, 1473, 1447, 1365, 1317, 1260, 1200, 1155, 1102, 1073, 995, 961, 914, 846, 784, 683; (Anal. Calcd. for $C_{36}H_{35}N_3O_4$: C, 75.37; H, 6.15; N, 7.32; Found: C, 75.24; H, 6.01; N, 7.23); LC/MS (ESI, m/z): found 574.3 [M+H]$^+$; exact mass 573.26 for $C_{36}H_{35}N_3O_4$. $[\alpha]_D^{25}$ = −15.78° (c 0.13, MeOH).

3.1.5. (1. S,1′S,3′S,4a′S,8a′S,9a′R)-3-((E)-Benzylidene)-5″-methoxy-1′-phenyl-4a′,5′,6′,7′,8′,8a′,9′,9a′-octahydro-1′H-dispiro[cyclohexane-1,2′-pyrrolo[1,2-a]indole-3′,3″-indoline]-2,2″-dione (**4e**)

2,6-Di((E)-benzylidene)cyclohexan-1-one (**1a**) (69 mg, 0.25 mmol), (2S)-octahydro-1H-indole-2-carboxylic acid (**2**) (64 mg, 0.37 mmol) and 5-methoxyisatin (**3e**) (44 mg, 0.25 mmol) were reacted according to GP1 for 1 h and yielded white solid spirooxindole (**4e**) (91 mg, 65%); m.p.: 111–122 °C; ^{1}H-NMR (500 MHz, CDCl$_3$): δ (ppm) = 7.36 (t, J = 6.9 Hz, 4H, Ar-**H**), 7.23 (d, J = 5.7 Hz, 2H, Ar-**H**), 7.20 (d, J = 2.7 Hz, 1H, Ar-**H**), 7.13 (s, 1H, Ar-**H**), 7.10 (d, J = 6.7 Hz, 2H, Ar-**H**), 7.07 (d, J = 6.4 Hz, 2H, Ar-**H**), 6.70 (dd, J = 8.4, 2.6 Hz, 1H, Ar-**H**), 6.52 (d, J = 8.4 Hz, 1H, Ar-**H**), 4.96 (d, J = 10.4 Hz, 1H, C**H**), 4.59–4.55 (m, 1H, NC**H**), 3.79 (s, 3H, C**H**$_3$), 3.41 (d, J = 4.5 Hz, 1H, NC**H**), 2.86–2.80 (m, 1H, C**H**$_2$), 2.38–2.29 (m, 2H, C**H**$_2$), 2.27–2.15 (m, 2H, C**H**$_2$), 2.09–1.96 (m, 5H, C**H**$_2$), 1.75–1.64 (m, 3H, C**H**$_2$), 1.08–0.98 (m, 4H, C**H**$_2$); ^{13}C-NMR (126 MHz, CDCl$_3$): δ (ppm) = 201.9 (**C**O), 181.1 (**C**O), 155.0, 138.7, 137.7, 137.1, 134.8, 131.6, 130.8, 130.5, 130.1, 129.8, 128.5, 128.3, 128.1, 126.8, 114.1, 109.7, 79.9, 69.6, 64.3, 57.9, 56.1 (O**C**H$_3$), 52.54, 42.55, 36.21, 28.53, 28.39, 27.94, 26.50, 24.79, 21.68, 20.44; IR (KBr, cm^{-1}) ν_{max} = 3267, 2928, 2854, 1718, 1685, 1610, 1597, 1554, 1483, 1471, 1449, 1363, 1317, 1265, 1202, 1154, 1105, 1077, 993, 965, 912, 844, 787, 686; (Anal. Calcd. for $C_{37}H_{38}N_2O_3$: C, 79.54; H, 6.86; N, 5.01; Found: C, 79.68; H, 6.74; N, 5.11); LC/MS (ESI, m/z): found 559.3 [M+H]$^+$; exact mass 558.28 for $C_{37}H_{38}N_2O_3$. $[\alpha]_D^{25}$ = −14.21° (c 0.06, MeOH).

3.1.6. (1. S,1′S,3′S,4a′S,8a′S,9a′R)-3-((E)-4-Bromobenzylidene)-1′-(4-bromophenyl)-6″-chloro-4a′,5′,6′,7′,8′,8a′,9′,9a′-octahydro-1′H-dispiro[cyclohexane-1,2′-pyrrolo[1,2-a]indole-3′,3″-indoline]-2,2″-dione (**4f**)

2,6-Bis((E)-4-bromobenzylidene)cyclohexan-1-one (**1b**) (108 mg, 0.25 mmol), (2S)-octahydro-1H-indole-2-carboxylic acid (**2**) (64 mg, 0.37 mmol) and 6-chloroisatin (**3b**) (45 mg, 0.25 mmol) were reacted according to GP1 for 1h and yielded white solid spirooxindole (**4f**) (124 mg, 69%); m.p: 97–98 °C; ^{1}H-NMR (400 MHz, CDCl$_3$): δ (ppm) = 8.55 (s, 1H, N**H**), 7.48 (d, J = 8.0 Hz, 1H, Ar-**H**), 7.40–7.34 (m, 4H, Ar-**H**), 7.24–7.22 (m, 2H, Ar-**H**), 7.20–7.17 (m, 1H, Ar-**H**), 6.97 (dd, J = 8.1, 1.9 Hz, 1H, Ar-**H**), 6.93 (d, J = 8.5 Hz, Ar-**H**), 6.73 (d, J = 1.8 Hz, 1H, Ar-**H**), 4.89 (d, J = 10.4 Hz, 1H, C**H**), 4.49 (td, J = 10.0, 5.8 Hz, 1H, NC**H**), 3.35 (q, J = 3.9 Hz, 1H, NC**H**), 2.80–2.70 (m, 1H, C**H**$_2$), 2.36–2.26 (m, 1H, C**H**$_2$), 2.19–2.10 (m, 1H, C**H**$_2$), 2.04–1.90 (m, 3H, C**H**$_2$), 1.67–1.58 (m, 3H, C**H**$_2$), 1.52–1.43 (m, 1H, C**H**$_2$), 1.42–1.31 (m, 3H, C**H**$_2$), 1.19–1.09 (m, 2H, C**H**$_2$), 1.05–0.95 (m, 3H, C**H**$_2$); ^{13}C-NMR (101 MHz, CDCl$_3$): δ (ppm) = 202.03 (Hex-**C**O), 180.02 (**C**O), 142.54, 138.77, 136.57, 134.97, 134.38, 134.03, 131.67, 131.60, 131.39, 131.26, 128.30, 127.90, 122.87, 121.56, 120.96, 110.49, 79.58, 69.30, 64.29, 58.08, 51.44, 42.51, 36.17, 28.47, 28.32, 28.02, 26.63, 24.67, 21.59, 20.31; IR (KBr, cm^{-1}) ν_{max} = 3242, 2927, 2853, 1716, 1684, 1612, 1487, 1446, 1316, 1260, 1153, 1073, 1010, 851, 720, 691; (Anal. Calcd. for $C_{36}H_{33}Br_2ClN_2O_2$: C, 59.98; H, 4.61; N, 3.89; Found: C, 60.12; H, 4.73; N, 3.93); LC/MS (ESI, m/z): found 719.1 [M($_{35}$Cl)+H]$^+$; 721.1 [M($_{37}$Cl)+H]$^+$, 723.1 [M($_{37}$Cl+$_{81}$Br)+H]$^+$, exact mass 718.06 for $C_{36}H_{33}Br_2ClN_2O_2$. $[\alpha]_D^{25}$ = −24.26° (c 0.11, MeOH).

3.1.7. (1. S,1′S,3′S,4a′S,8a′S,9a′R)-3-((E)-4-bromobenzylidene)-1′-(4-bromophenyl)-5″-nitro-4a′,5′,6′,7′,8′,8a′,9′,9a′-octahydro-1′H-dispiro[cyclohexane-1,2′-pyrrolo[1,2-a]indole-3′,3″-indoline]-2,2″-dione (**4g**)

2,6-*Bis*((E)-4-bromobenzylidene)cyclohexan-1-one (**1b**) (108 mg, 0.25 mmol), (2S)-octahydro-1H-indole-2-carboxylic acid (**2**) (64 mg, 0.37 mmol) and 5-nitroisatin (**3d**) (48 mg,

0.25 mmol) were reacted according to GP1 for 1 h and yielded white solid spirooxindole (**4g**) (123 mg, 67%); m.p.: 125–126 °C; ^{1}H-NMR (500 MHz, CDCl$_3$): δ (ppm) = 8.47 (d, *J* = 2.4 Hz, 1H, Ar-**H**), 8.14 (dd, *J* = 8.6, 2.4 Hz, 1H, Ar-**H**), 8.01 (s, 1H, N**H**), 7.47 (d, *J* = 7.2 Hz, 1H, Ar-**H**), 7.41 (t, *J* = 7.6 Hz, 1H, Ar-**H**), 7.37 (d, *J* = 7.4 Hz, 1H, Ar-**H**), 7.34–7.31 (m, 3H, Ar-**H**), 7.07 (dd, *J* = 7.7, 1.9 Hz, 2H, Ar-**H**), 6.80 (dt, *J* = 8.6, 1.4 Hz, 1H, Ar-**H**), 4.90 (d, *J* = 10.5 Hz, 1H, C**H**), 4.67–4.61 (m, 1H, NC**H**), 3.38 (q, *J* = 3.8 Hz, 1H, NC**H**), 2.97–2.92 (m, 1H, C**H**$_2$), 2.85–2.78 (m, 1H, C**H**$_2$), 2.43–2.28 (m, 3H, C**H**$_2$), 2.18–2.10 (m, 2H, C**H**$_2$), 1.99–1.92 (m, 2H, C**H**$_2$), 1.73–1.61 (m, 5H, C**H**$_2$), 1.11–0.99 (m, 3H, C**H**$_2$); ^{13}C-NMR (126 MHz, CDCl$_3$): δ (ppm) = 201.8 (**C**O), 179.5 (**C**O), 147. 1, 143.4, 138.1, 137.1, 136.1, 135.4, 130.8, 130.5, 130.2, 129.6, 128.8, 128.5, 128.3, 126.2, 122.6, 109.3, 79.1, 70.6, 64.2, 57.8, 53.8, 42.6, 35.9, 28.7, 28.6, 28.2, 27.2, 24.6, 21.4, 20.2; IR (KBr, cm^{-1}) ν$_{max}$ = 2927, 2854, 1740, 1668, 1619, 1606, 1523, 1507, 1446, 1336, 1272, 1164, 1082, 1028, 965, 909, 842, 773, 747, 732, 696; (Anal. Calcd. for C$_{36}$H$_{33}$Br$_2$N$_3$O$_4$: C, 59.11; H, 4.55; N, 5.74; Found: C, 59.24; H, 4.43; N, 5.81); LC/MS (ESI, *m*/*z*): found 730.1 [M($_{79}$Br)+H]$^+$; 732.1 [M($_{81}$Br)+H]$^+$, exact mass 729.08 for C$_{36}$H$_{33}$Br$_2$N$_3$O$_4$. $[α]_D^{25}$ = −12.64° (c 0.12, MeOH).

3.1.8. (1. S,1′S,3′S,4a′S,8a′S,9a′R)-6″-Chloro-3-((E)-3-fluorobenzylidene)-1′-(3-fluorophenyl)-4a′,5′,6′,7′,8′,8a′,9′,9a′-octahydro-1′H-dispiro[cyclohexane-1,2′-pyrrolo[1,2-a]indole-3′,3″-indoline]-2,2″-dione (**4h**)

2,6-*Bis*((*E*)-3-fluorobenzylidene)cyclohexan-1-one (**1d**) (78 mg, 0.25 mmol), (2*S*)-octahydro-1*H*-indole-2-carboxylic acid **2** (64 mg, 0.37 mmol) and 6-chloroisatin (**3b**) (45 mg, 0.25 mmol) were reacted according to GP1 for 1 h and yielded white solid spirooxindole (**4h**) (109 mg, 73%); m.p.: 83–84 °C; ^{1}H-NMR (500 MHz, CDCl$_3$): δ (ppm) = 8.82 (s, 1H, N**H**), 7.48 (d, *J* = 8.1 Hz, 1H, Ar-**H**), 7.25–7.18 (m, 3H, Ar-**H**), 7.13 (d, *J* = 8.1 Hz, 1H, Ar-**H**), 7.12–7.08 (m, 1H, Ar-**H**), 6.97 (dd, *J* = 8.1, 1.9 Hz, 1H, Ar-**H**), 6.94–6.88 (m, 3H, Ar-**H**), 6.81–6.77 (m, 1H, Ar-**H**), 6.74 (d, *J* = 1.9 Hz, 1H, Ar-**H**), 4.96 (d, *J* = 10.3 Hz, 1H, C**H**), 4.51 (td, *J* = 10.0, 5.8 Hz, 1H, NC**H**), 3.36 (q, *J* = 3.7 Hz, 1H, NC**H**), 2.79–2.73 (m, 1H, C**H**$_2$), 2.37–2.30 (m, 1H, C**H**$_2$), 2.22–2.15 (m, 1H, C**H**$_2$), 2.09–2.05 (m, 2H, C**H**$_2$), 2.01–1.94 (m, 1H, C**H**$_2$), 1.73 -1.67 (m, 1H, C**H**$_2$), 1.66–1.60 (m, 2H, C**H**$_2$), 1.59–1.55(m, 1H, C**H**$_2$), 1.45–1.32 (m, 4H, C**H**$_2$), 1.07–0.97 (m, 3H, C**H**$_2$); ^{13}C-NMR (126 MHz, CDCl$_3$): δ (ppm) = 202.0 (**C**O), 180.4 (**C**O), 163.7, 163.5, 161.7, 161.6, 142.6, 140.3, 140.3, 139.4, 137.8, 137.8, 135.1, 134.0, 129.9, 129.8, 129.6, 129.5, 128.2, 127.9, 126.1, 126.1, 125.6, 121.6, 116.6, 116.5, 116.4, 116.3, 115.5, 113.9, 113.7, 110.6, 79.7, 69.5, 64.4, 58.1, 51.6, 42.5, 36.2, 28.5, 28.3, 28.1, 26.8, 24.7, 21.5, 20.3; IR (KBr, cm^{-1}) ν$_{max}$ = 2929, 2854, 1714, 1681, 1612, 1584, 1366, 1317, 1276, 1236, 1201, 1151, 1074, 976, 906, 787, 732, 686; (Anal. Calcd. for C$_{36}$H$_{33}$ClF$_2$N$_2$O$_2$: C, 72.17; H, 5.55; N, 4.68; Found: C, 71.96; H, 5.63; N, 4.59); LC/MS (ESI, *m*/*z*): found 599.2 [M($_{35}$Cl)+H]$^+$; 601.2 [M($_{37}$Cl)+H]$^+$, exact mass 598.22 for C$_{36}$H$_{33}$ClF$_2$N$_2$O$_2$. $[α]_D^{25}$ = −44.98° (c 0.11, MeOH).

3.1.9. (1. S,1′S,3′S,4a′S,8a′S,9a′R)-3-((E)-3-Fluorobenzylidene)-1′-(3-fluorophenyl)-5″-nitro-4a′,5′,6′,7′,8′,8a′,9′,9a′-octahydro-1′H-dispiro[cyclohexane-1,2′-pyrrolo[1,2-a]indole-3′,3″-indoline]-2,2″-dione (**4i**)

2,6-*Bis*((*E*)-3-fluorobenzylidene)cyclohexan-1-one (**1d**) (78 mg, 0.25 mmol), (2*S*)-octahydro-1*H*-indole-2-carboxylic acid (**2**) (64 mg, 0.37 mmol) and 5-nitroisatin (**3d**) (48 mg, 0.25 mmol) were reacted according to GP1 for 1h and yielded white solid spirooxindole (**4i**) (100 mg, 66%); m.p.: 107–108 °C; ^{1}H-NMR (500 MHz, CDCl$_3$): δ (ppm) = 8.91 (s, 1H, N**H**), 8.46 (d, *J* = 2.2 Hz, 1H, Ar-**H**), 8.15 (dd, *J* = 8.6, 2.4 Hz, 1H, Ar-**H**), 7.23–7.19 (m, 2H, Ar-**H**), 7.12–7.00 (m, 3H, Ar-**H**), 6.99–6.90 (m, 2H, Ar-**H**), 6.90–6.83 (m, 2H, Ar-**H**), 6.81–6.77 (m, 1H, Ar-**H**), 4.90 (d, *J* = 10.53, 1H, C**H**), 4.60–4.55 (m, 1H, NC**H**), 3.36 (q, *J* = 4.1 Hz, 1H, NC**H**), 2.83–2.77 (m, 1H, C**H**$_2$), 2.39–2.33 (m, 2H, C**H**$_2$), 2.31–2.26 (m, 1H, C**H**$_2$), 2.06–2.00 (m, 1H, C**H**$_2$), 1.96–1.91 (m, 1H, C**H**$_2$), 1.74–1.59 (m, 6H, C**H**$_2$), 1.57–1.50 (m, 3H, C**H**$_2$), 1.10–1.00 (m, 3H, C**H**$_2$); ^{13}C-NMR (126 MHz, CDCl$_3$): δ (ppm) = 201.7 (**C**O), 180.3 (**C**O), 163.7, 163.6, 161.8, 161.6, 147.2, 142.9, 139.4, 139.1, 137.4, 134.7, 131.0, 130.0, 130.0, 129.8, 126.3, 125.9, 125.4, 122.6, 116.7, 116.6, 116.5, 116.4, 115.9, 115.7, 114.3, 114.2, 114.1, 109.7, 79.4, 70.2, 64.3, 58.1, 52.9,

42.5, 35.9, 28.6, 28.3, 28.2, 27.2, 24.5, 21.2, 20.2; IR (KBr, cm^{-1}) ν_{max} = 2924, 2854, 1734, 1719, 1610, 1584, 1525, 1507, 1483, 1448, 1337, 1278, 1244, 1224, 1168, 1151, 968, 906, 840, 788, 684; (Anal. Calcd. for $C_{36}H_{33}F_2N_3O_4$: C, 70.92; H, 5.46; N, 6.89; Found: C, 71.08; H, 5.37; N, 6.74); LC/MS (ESI, m/z): found 510 [M+H]$^+$; exact mass 609.24 for $C_{36}H_{33}F_2N_3O_4$. $[\alpha]_D^{25}$ = +20.79° (c 0.13, MeOH).

3.1.10. (1. S,1′S,3′S,4a′S,8a′S,9a′R)-3-((E)-3-Fluorobenzylidene)-1′-(3-fluorophenyl)-5″-methoxy-4a′,5′,6′,7′,8′,8a′,9′,9a′-octahydro-1′H-dispiro[cyclohexane-1,2′-pyrrolo[1,2-a]indole-3′,3″-indoline]-2,2″-dione (**4j**)

2,6-*Bis*((E)-3-fluorobenzylidene)cyclohexan-1-one (**1d**) (78 mg, 0.25 mmol), (2S)-octahydro-1H-indole-2-carboxylic acid (**2**) (64 mg, 0.37 mmol) and 5-methoxyisatin (**3e**) (44 mg, 0.25 mmol) were reacted according to GP1 for 1 h and yielded white solid spirooxindole (**4j**) (106 mg, 71%); m.p.: 92–93 °C; ^{1}H-NMR (500 MHz, CDCl$_3$): δ (ppm) = 8.12 (s, 1H, N**H**), 7.24–7.18 (m, 4H, Ar-**H**), 7.18–7.12 (m, 2H, Ar-**H**), 7.01 (d, J = 10.7 Hz, 2H, Ar-**H**), 6.88 (d, J = 7.0 Hz, 2H, Ar-**H**), 6.71 (dd, J = 8.4, 2.6 Hz, 1H, Ar-**H**), 6.58 (d, J = 8.4 Hz, 1H, Ar-**H**), 4.97 (d, J = 10.3 Hz, 1H, C**H**), 4.50 (dt, J = 10.0, 5.0 Hz, 1H, NC**H**), 3.79 (s, 3H, C**H$_3$**), 3.38 (q, J = 3.8 Hz, 1H, NC**H**), 2.82 (ddd, J = 14.3, 9.7, 4.3 Hz, 1H, C**H$_2$**), 2.38–2.30 (m, 2H, C**H$_2$**), 2.04 (ddt, J = 12.0, 6.7, 3.9 Hz, 3H, C**H$_2$**), 1.99–1.93 (m, 1H, C**H$_2$**), 1.71–1.56 (m, 6H, C**H$_2$**), 1.17–1.13 (m, 4H, C**H$_2$**); ^{13}C-NMR (126 MHz, CDCl$_3$): δ (ppm) = 201.9 (CO), 180.19 (CO), 163.7, 163.5, 161.7, 161.5, 155.1, 139.9, 139.6, 138.1, 138.0, 135.0, 134.8, 133.3, 131.8, 129.8, 129.7, 129.5, 129.4, 128.6, 126.0, 125.6, 116.6, 116.5, 116.5, 116.4, 115.3, 115.1, 114.3, 114.2, 113.9, 113.8, 113.7, 113.6, 110.1, 80.3, 70.0, 64.4, 58.1, 56.11 (OCH$_3$), 51.60, 42.49, 36.21, 28.46, 28.33, 27.94, 26.45, 24.70, 21.56, 20.40; IR (KBr, cm^{-1}) ν_{max} = 2926, 2855, 1736, 1717, 1612, 1581, 1524, 1509, 1485, 1444, 1332, 1274, 1242, 1224, 1165, 1154, 962, 904, 847, 784; (Anal. Calcd. for $C_{37}H_{36}F_2N_2O_3$: C, 74.73; H, 6.10; N, 4.71; Found: C, 74.64; H, 6.25; N, 4.82); LC/MS (ESI, m/z): found 595.2 [M+H]$^+$; exact mass 594.27 for $C_{37}H_{36}F_2N_2O_3$. $[\alpha]_D^{25}$ = −7.51° (c 0.10, MeOH).

3.1.11. (1. S,1′S,3′S,4a′S,8a′S,9a′R)-3-((E)-3-Bromobenzylidene)-1′-(3-bromophenyl)-6″-chloro-4a′,5′,6′,7′,8′,8a′,9′,9a′-octahydro-1′H-dispiro[cyclohexane-1,2′-pyrrolo[1,2-a]indole-3′,3″-indoline]-2,2″-dione (**4k**)

2,6-*Bis*((E)-3-bromobenzylidene)cyclohexan-1-one (**1c**) (108 mg, 0.25 mmol), (2S)-octahydro-1H-indole-2-carboxylic acid (**2**) (64 mg, 0.37 mmol) and 6-chloroisatin (**3b**) (45 mg, 0.25 mmol) were reacted according to GP1 for 1 h and yielded white solid spirooxindole (**4k**) (133 mg, 74%); m.p.: 115–116 °C; ^{1}H-NMR (500 MHz, CDCl$_3$): δ (ppm) = 8.42 (s, 1H, N**H**), 7.48 (d, J = 4.9 Hz, 1H, Ar-**H**), 7.46 (d, J = 3.9 Hz, 1H, Ar-**H**), 7.34 (d, J = 7.9 Hz, 2H, Ar-**H**), 7.23 (s, 1H, Ar-**H**), 7.18 (s, 1H), 7.12 (q, J = 7.9 Hz, 3H, Ar-**H**), 7.00 (d, J = 8.6 Hz, 1H, Ar-**H**), 6.97 (d, J = 8.2 Hz, 1H, Ar-**H**), 6.75 (d, J = 2.3 Hz, 1H, Ar-**H**), 4.91 (d, J = 10.3 Hz, 1H, C**H**), 4.54–4.47 (m, 1H, NC**H**), 3.35 (q, J = 4.0 Hz, 1H, NC**H**), 2.80–2.73 (m, 1H, C**H$_2$**), 2.41–2.29 (m, 2H, C**H$_2$**), 2.19–2.13 (m, 1H, C**H$_2$**), 2.07–2.01 (m, 2H, C**H$_2$**), 1.70–1.60 (m, 4H, C**H$_2$**), 1.58–1.53 (m, 2H, C**H$_2$**), 1.53–1.47 (m, 2H, C**H$_2$**), 1.09–0.98 (m, 3H, C**H$_2$**); ^{13}C-NMR (126 MHz, CDCl$_3$): δ (ppm) = 201.8 (CO), 180.1 (CO), 142.5, 139.9, 139.5, 137.6, 135.1, 133.8, 132.8, 132.7, 132.5, 131.4, 130.2, 129.9, 129.8, 128.6, 128.5, 128.1, 127.9, 122.5, 121.7, 110.5, 79.4, 69.6, 64.2, 58.0, 52.1, 42.5, 36.1, 28.5, 28.3, 28.0, 26.8, 24.6, 21.5, 20.4; IR (KBr, cm^{-1}) ν_{max} = 2926, 2853, 1715, 1682, 1612, 1591, 1558, 1473, 1446, 1316, 1272, 1200, 1155, 1073, 995, 961, 930, 856, 784, 730, 682; (Anal. Calcd. for $C_{36}H_{33}Br_2ClN_2O_2$: C, 59.98; H, 4.61; N, 3.89; Found: C, 60.86; H, 4.53; N, 3.87); LC/MS (ESI, m/z): found 719.1 [M($_{35}$Cl)+H]$^+$; 721.1 [M($_{37}$Cl)+H]$^+$, 723.1 [M($_{37}$Cl+$_{81}$Br)+H]$^+$, exact mass 718.06 for $C_{36}H_{33}Br_2ClN_2O_2$. $[\alpha]_D^{25}$ = −15.68° (c 0.10, MeOH).

3.1.12. (1. S,1′S,3′S,4a′S,8a′S,9a′R)-6″-Chloro-3-((E)-4-fluorobenzylidene)-1′-(4-fluorophenyl)-4a′,5′,6′,7′,8′,8a′,9′,9a′-octahydro-1′H-dispiro[cyclohexane-1,2′-pyrrolo[1,2-a]indole-3′,3″-indoline]-2,2″-dione (4l)

2,6-Bis((E)-4-fluorobenzylidene)cyclohexan-1-one (1e) (78 mg, 0.25 mmol), (2S)-octahydro-1H-indole-2-carboxylic acid (2) (64 mg, 0.37 mmol) and 6-chloroisatin (3b) (45 mg, 0.25 mmol) were reacted according to GP1 for 1 h and yielded white solid spirooxindole (4l) (112 mg, 75%); m.p.: 96–97 °C; ^{1}H-NMR (500 MHz, CDCl$_3$): δ (ppm) = 7.88 (s, 1H, NH), 7.47 (d, J = 8.0 Hz, 1H, Ar-H), 7.35–7.30 (m, 2H, Ar-H), 7.20 (s, 1H, Ar-H), 7.07 (td, J = 5.7, 2.5 Hz, 2H, Ar-H), 6.99–6.91 (m, 5H, Ar-H), 6.65 (d, J = 2.0 Hz, 1H, Ar-H), 4.89 (d, J = 10.3 Hz, 1H, CH), 4.52–4.47 (m, 1H, NCH), 3.35 (q, J = 4.4 Hz, 1H, NCH), 2.93–2.87 (m, 1H, CH$_2$), 2.79–2.72 (m, 1H CH$_2$), 2.36–2.30 (m, 1H CH$_2$), 2.20–2.14 (m, 1H CH$_2$), 2.07–1.98 (m, 3H CH$_2$), 1.97–1.92 (m, 1H CH$_2$), 1.69–1.58 (m, 6H CH$_2$), 1.07–0.97 (m, 3H CH$_2$); ^{13}C-NMR (126 MHz, CDCl$_3$): δ (ppm) = 201.9 (CO), 179.7 (CO), 162.1, 162.0, 159.1, 159.1, 142.3, 137.9, 136.1, 134.9, 134.2, 132.1, 133.1, 132.4, 132.1, 132.0, 131.7, 131.1, 128.4, 128.0, 121.6, 115.7, 115.5, 115.1, 115.0, 110.2, 79.4, 69.5, 64.5, 58.0, 51.6, 42.5, 36.1, 28.5, 28.4, 28.0, 26.6, 24.7, 21.6, 20.4; IR (KBr, cm^{-1}) ν$_{max}$ = 2928, 2853, 1715, 1684, 1611, 1584, 1367, 1312, 1273, 1234, 1207, 1151, 1072, 974, 907, 781, 734, 682; (Anal. Calcd. for C$_{36}$H$_{33}$ClF$_2$N$_2$O$_2$: C, 72.17; H, 5.55; N, 4.68; Found: C, 72.05; H, 5.63; N, 4.49); LC/MS (ESI, m/z): found 599.2 [M($_{35}$Cl)+H]$^+$; 601.2 [M($_{37}$Cl)+H]$^+$, exact mass 598.22 for C$_{36}$H$_{33}$ClF$_2$N$_2$O$_2$. $[α]_D^{25}$ = −39.81° (c 0.10, MeOH).

3.1.13. (1. S,1′S,3′S,4a′S,8a′S,9a′R)-6″-Chloro-3-((E)-4-(trifluoromethyl)benzylidene)-1′-(4-(trifluoromethyl)phenyl)-4a′,5′,6′,7′,8′,8a′,9′,9a′-octahydro-1′H-dispiro[cyclohexane-1,2′-pyrrolo[1,2-a]indole-3′,3″-indoline]-2,2″-dione (4m)

2,6-Bis((E)-4-(trifluoromethyl)benzylidene)cyclohexan-1-one (1f) (103 mg, 0.25 mmol), (2S)-octahydro-1H-indole-2-carboxylic acid (2) (64 mg, 0.37 mmol) and 6-chloroisatin (3b) (45 mg, 0.25 mmol) were reacted according to GP1 for 1 h and yielded white solid spirooxindole (4m) (108 mg, 62%); m.p.: 78–79 °C; ^{1}H-NMR (500 MHz, CDCl$_3$): δ (ppm) = 8.49 (S, 1H, NH), 7.67–7.61 (m, 1H, Ar-H), 7.55 (d, J = 7.3 Hz, 3H, Ar-H), 7.45–7.27 (m, 4H, Ar-H), 7.16 (d, J = 8.0 Hz, 2H, Ar-H), 6.99 (t, J = 6.9 Hz, 1H, Ar-H), 6.78 (q, J = 3.4, 2.9 Hz, 1H, Ar-H), 5.02 (d, J = 10.4 Hz, 1H, CH), 4.64–4.54 (m, 1H, NCH), 3.36 (q, J = 3.9 Hz, 1H, NCH), 2.87–2.74 (m, 1H, CH$_2$), 2.38–2.28 (m, 1H, CH$_2$), 2.22–2.14 (m, 1H, CH$_2$), 2.13–2.00 (m, 2H, CH$_2$), 1.99–1.92 (m, 1H, CH$_2$), 1.74–1.57 (m, 4H, CH$_2$), 1.55–1.47 (m, 2H, CH$_2$), 1.45–1.36 (m, 2H, CH$_2$), 1.06–0.90 (m, 3H, CH$_2$); ^{13}C-NMR (126 MHz, CDCl$_3$): δ (ppm) = 201.88 (CO), 179.9 (CO), 142.5, 141.8, 140.3, 135.8, 135.2, 133.5, 131.0, 130.6, 130.5, 130.2, 130.1, 129.8, 128.2, 128.1, 125.3 (CF$_3$), 125.1 (CF$_3$), 121.8, 110.5, 79.7, 69.4, 64.3, 58.2, 51.8, 42.5, 36.2, 28.5, 28.3, 27.9, 26.7, 24.6, 21.5, 20.3; IR (KBr, cm^{-1}) ν$_{max}$ = 2927, 2856, 1712, 1683, 1615, 1587, 1364, 1316, 1274, 1232, 1205, 1155, 1078, 977, 908, 789, 735, 684; (Anal. Calcd. for C$_{38}$H$_{33}$ClF$_6$N$_2$O$_2$: C, 65.28; H, 4.76; N, 4.01; Found: C, 65.33; H, 4.62; N, 4.13); LC/MS (ESI, m/z): found 699.2 [M($_{35}$Cl)+H]$^+$; 701.2 [M($_{37}$Cl)+H]$^+$, exact mass 698.21 for C$_{38}$H$_{33}$ClF$_6$N$_2$O$_2$. $[α]_D^{25}$ = −34.59° (c 0.15, MeOH).

3.1.14. (1. S,1′S,3′S,4a′S,8a′S,9a′R)-5″-Methyl-3-((E)-4-(trifluoromethyl)benzylidene)-1′-(4-(trifluorom-thyl)phenyl)-4a′,5′,6′,7′,8′,8a′,9′,9a′-octahydro-1′H-dispiro[cyclohexane-1,2′-pyrrolo[1,2-a]indole-3′,3″-indoline]-2,2″-dione (4n)

2,6-Bis((E)-4-(trifluoromethyl)benzylidene)cyclohexan-1-one (1f) (103 mg, 0.25 mmol), (2S)-octahydro-1H-indole-2-carboxylic acid (2) (64 mg, 0.37 mmol) and 5-methylisatin (3f) (40 mg, 0.25 mmol) were reacted according to GP1 for 1 h and yielded white solid spirooxindole (4n) (102 mg, 60%); m.p.: 73–74 °C; ^{1}H-NMR (500 MHz, CDCl$_3$): δ (ppm) = 8.42 (s, 1H, NH), 7.62 (d, J = 8.1 Hz, 1H, Ar-H), 7.57 (d, J = 2.6 Hz, 1H, Ar-H), 7.48 (d, J = 8.1 Hz, 2H, Ar-H), 7.43 (s, 1H, Ar-H), 7.40 (d, J = 8.0 Hz, 1H, Ar-H), 7.35 (d, J = 9.1 Hz, 1H, Ar-H), 7.29 (d, J = 12.5 Hz, 1H, Ar-H), 7.24 (d, J = 8.1 Hz, 1H, Ar-H), 7.14 (d, J = 8.1 Hz, 2H, Ar-H), 6.61 (d, J = 8.1 Hz, 1H, Ar-H), 5.07 (d, J = 10.4 Hz, 1H, CH), 4.62–4.56 (m, 1H, NCH),

3.37–3.33 (m, 1H, NC**H**), 2.96–2.86 (m, 1H, C**H**$_2$), 2.35 (s, 3H, C**H**$_3$), 1.99–1.93 (m, 1H, C**H**$_2$), 1.89–1.85 (m, 1H, C**H**$_2$), 1.73–1.68 (m, 1H, C**H**$_2$), 1.62–1.54 (m, 4H, C**H**$_2$), 1.50–1.39 (m, 3H, C**H**$_2$), 1.16–1.07 (m, 2H, C**H**$_2$), 1.03–0.91 (m, 3H, C**H**$_2$), 0.89–0.83 (m, 1H, C**H**$_2$); ^{13}C-NMR (126 MHz, CDCl$_3$): δ (ppm) = 202.0 (**C**O), 180.2 (**C**O), 142.2, 140.6, 139.3, 138.8, 134.6, 132.7, 131.9, 131.0, 130.7, 130.5, 130.2, 130.1, 129.8, 129.7, 128.1, 125.2 (**C**F$_3$), 125.0 (**C**F$_3$), 109.4, 80.1, 69.1, 64.3, 58.3, 42.4, 36.2, 28.5, 28.3, 27.7, 26.4, 24.6, 21.6, 21.4 (**C**H$_3$), 20.3; IR (KBr, cm^{-1}) ν$_{max}$ = 2926, 2852, 1714, 1687, 1615, 1582, 1363, 1315, 1272, 1234, 1207, 1157, 1075, 979, 904, 785, 737, 685; (Anal. Calcd. for C$_{39}$H$_{36}$F$_6$N$_2$O$_2$: C, 69.02; H, 5.35; N, 4.13; Found: C, 69.25; H, 5.17; N, 4.01); LC/MS (ESI, m/z): found 679.3 [M+H]$^+$; exact mass 678.27 for C$_{39}$H$_{36}$F$_6$N$_2$O$_2$. $[α]_D^{25}$ = −12.18° (c 0.14, MeOH).

3.2. The Biological Activity Assay Protocols

Cytotoxicity against BJ human fibroblast cells and cytotoxicity against PC3, HeLa, MCF-7, and MDA-MB231 cancer cell lines were evaluated by following the procedure as described in the literature [41–47] (Supplementary Materials).

3.3. Molecular Docking Methodology

To rationalize the observed anticancer activity, molecular docking studies of the potential compounds were carried out using MDM2 crystal structure. The selected di-spirooxindole analogs (**4a, 4b, 4i**, and **4l**) were sketched in MOE v.2019 by using Builder module and subsequently subjected to geometry correction and protonation followed by minimization using MMFF94x force field. The 3D structure of MDM2 in complex with a benzodiazepine inhibitor (PDB ID 1T4E) was retrieved from ProteinData Bank [34]. Since there were no conserved water molecules in the utilized pdb, all water molecules were deleted and the structure was corrected and protonated using GB/VI as the electrostatics function with a dielectric value of 80 (for solvent). Consequently, the protein structure was minimized to remove the bad clashes using the Amber99 force field. A grid of 6 Å was generated centered on the co-crystalized ligands and the selected compounds. The triangular method was used as a placement method with an induce fit protocol. The resulting poses of the ligands were scored by London dG scoring function and the top ranked poses were visually analyzed. All the graphics were rendered using MOE software.

4. Conclusions

In conclusion, a new series of hybrid di-spirooxindole analogs, engrafted with substituted oxindole and cyclohexanone moieties, were synthesized successfully by a one-pot multicomponent reaction. The anticancer assay showed promising results, which makes these di-spirooxindole analogs suitable for further research. Synthesized di-spirooxindole analog **4b** (IC$_{50}$ = 3.7 ± 1.0 µM) appeared to be a more potent candidate against PC3 cell line, whereas, di-spirooxindole analogs **4a** (IC$_{50}$ = 7.1 ± 0.2 µM) and **4l** (IC$_{50}$ = 7.2 ± 0.5 µM) possessed promising anticancer activity against cervical cancer HeLa cell line and triple negative breast cancer MDA-MB231 cell line. Compound **4i** (IC$_{50}$ = 7.63 ± 0.08 µM) appeared to be more active among these di-spirooxindole analogs. The docking studies suggested that **4a, 4b, 4i**, and **4l** accommodated well in the binding site of MDM2. However, further mechanistic studies via in vivo animal models are required to validate the results of these in vitro assays.

Supplementary Materials: The following are available online, 1D-NMR and 2D-NMR chemical shift data for compounds **4a–n** and the biological activity assays protocols are provided in SI.

Author Contributions: Conceptualization, A.B. and M.I.C.; methodology, M.S.I., M.A., A.M.A.-M., S.A. and A.S.A.; validation, M.S.I., M.A., A.M.A.-M., S.A. and A.S.A.; formal analysis, M.S.I., M.A., A.M.A.-M., S.A. and A.S.A.; investigation, M.S.I., M.A., A.M.A.-M., S.A. and A.S.A.; Biological activity assays, S.Y. and M.I.C.; resources, A.B.; data curation, M.S.I., M.A., A.M.A.-M., S.A. and A.S.A.; writing—original draft preparation, A.B. and S.Y.; writing—review and editing, M.I.C.; visualization, A.B. and M.I.C.; project administration, M.A.; funding acquisition, A.B. All authors have read and agreed to the published version of the manuscript.

Funding: King Abdulaziz City for Science and Technology, Kingdom of Saudi Arabia, Award Number (14-BIO128-02).

Institutional Review Board Statement: Not applicable.

Informed Consent Statement: Not applicable.

Data Availability Statement: The data presented in this study are available in Supplementary Materials.

Acknowledgments: This project was funded by the National Plan for Science, Technology, and Innovation (MAARIFAH), King Abdulaziz City for Science and Technology, Kingdom of Saudi Arabia, Award Number (14-BIO128-02). The authors would like to thank Zaheer Ul-Haq (Panjwani Center for Molecular Medicine and Drug Research, Karachi, Pakistan) for molecular docking investigation.

Conflicts of Interest: The authors declare no conflict of interest.

Sample Availability: Samples of the compounds **4a–n** are available from the authors.

References

1. Ferlay, J.; Colombet, M.; Soerjomataram, I.; Mathers, C.; Parkin, D.M.; Piñeros, M.; Znaor, A.; Bray, F. Estimating the global cancer incidence and mortality in 2018: GLOBOCAN sources and methods. *Int. J. Cancer* **2019**, *144*, 1941–1953. [CrossRef] [PubMed]
2. Jin, Y.Z.; Wei, X.; Shi, J.Y. Therapeutic potential of spirooxindoles as agents for various diseases. *Pract. J. Clin. Med.* **2018**, *15*, 255–260.
3. Li, G.; Lou, H.X. Strategies to diversify natural products for drug discovery. *Med. Res. Rev.* **2018**, *38*, 1255–1294. [CrossRef] [PubMed]
4. Aziz, Y.M.A.; Lotfy, G.; Said, M.M.; El-Ashry, E.-S.H.; El Tamany, E.-S.H.; Soliman, S.M.; Abu-Serie, M.M.; Teleb, M.; Yousuf, S.; Domingo, L.R.; et al. Design, synthesis, chemical and biochemical insights on to novel hybrid spirooxindoles-based p53-MDM2 inhibitors with potential Bcl2 signaling attenuation. *Front. Chem.-Supramol. Chem* **2021**, *915*, in press. [CrossRef]
5. Omer, A.M.; Ahmed, M.S.; El-Subruiti, G.M.; Khalifa, R.E.; Eltaweil, A.S. pH-Sensitive alginate/carboxymethyl chitosan/aminated chitosan microcapsules for efficient encapsulation and delivery of diclofenac sodium. *Pharmaceutics* **2021**, *13*, 338. [CrossRef]
6. Hosny, M.; Fawzy, M.; Abdelfatah, A.M.; Fawzy, E.E.; Eltaweil, A.S. Comparative study on the potentialities of two halophytic species in the green synthesis of gold nanoparticles and their anticancer, antioxidant and catalytic efficiencies. *Adv. Powder Technol.* **2021**, *32*, 3220–3233. [CrossRef]
7. Omer, A.M.; Tamer, T.M.; Khalifa, R.E.; Eltaweil, A.S.; Agwa, M.M.; Sabra, S.; Abd-Elmonem, M.S.; Mohy-Eldin, M.S.; Ziora, Z.M. Formulation and antibacterial activity evaluation of quaternized aminochitosan membrane for wound dressing applications. *Polymers* **2021**, *13*, 2428. [CrossRef] [PubMed]
8. Kaur, M.; Singh, M.; Chadha, N.; Silakari, O. Oxindole: A chemical prism carrying plethora of therapeutic benefits. *Eur. J. Med. Chem.* **2016**, *123*, 858–894. [CrossRef]
9. Tantawy, M.A.; Nafie, M.S.; Elmegeed, G.A.; Ali, I.A. Auspicious role of the steroidal heterocyclic derivatives as a platform for anti-cancer drugs. *Bioorg. Chem.* **2017**, *73*, 128–146. [CrossRef]
10. Panda, S.S.; Jones, R.A.; Bachawala, P.; Mohapatra, P.P. Spirooxindoles as potential pharmacophores. *Mini.-Rev. Med. Chem.* **2017**, *17*, 1515–1536. [CrossRef]
11. Lotfy, G.A.; Aziz, Y.M.A.; Said, M.M.; El Ashry, E.S.H.; El Tamany, E.S.H.; Abu-Serie, M.M.; Teleb, M.; Dömling, A.; Barakat, A. Molecular hybridization design and synthesis of novel spirooxindole-based MDM2 inhibitors endowed with BCL2 signaling attenuation; a step towards the next generation p53 activators. *Bioorg. Chem.* **2021**, 105427, in press. [CrossRef]
12. Mei, G.J.; Shi, F. Catalytic asymmetric synthesis of spirooxindoles: Recent developments. *Chem. Commun.* **2018**, *54*, 6607–6621. [CrossRef]
13. Monteiro, Â.; Gonçalves, L.M.; Santos, M.M. Synthesis of novel spiropyrazoline oxindoles and evaluation of cytotoxicity in cancer cell lines. *Eur. J. Med. Chem.* **2014**, *79*, 266–272. [CrossRef] [PubMed]
14. Yang, J.; Liu, X.W.; Wang, D.D.; Tian, M.Y.; Han, S.N.; Feng, T.T.; Liu, X.L.; Mei, R.Q.; Zhou, Y. Diversity-oriented one-pot multicomponent synthesis of spirooxindole derivatives and their biological evaluation for anticancer activities. *Tetrahedron* **2016**, *72*, 8523–8536. [CrossRef]

15. Barakat, A.; Islam, M.S.; Al Majid, A.M.; Ghawas, H.M.; El-Senduny, F.F.; Badria, F.A.; Elshaier, Y.A.M.M.; Ghabbour, H.A. Substituted spirooxindole derivatives as potent anticancer agents through inhibition of phosphodiesterase 1. *RSC Adv.* **2018**, *8*, 14335. [CrossRef]
16. Lotfy, G.; Said, M.M.; El Sayed, H.; El Sayed, H.; Al-Dhfyan, A.; Aziz, Y.M.A.; Barakat, A. Synthesis of new spirooxindole-pyrrolothiazoles derivatives: Anti-cancer activity and molecular docking. *Bioorg. Med. Chem.* **2017**, *25*, 1514–1523. [CrossRef] [PubMed]
17. Lotfy, G.; El Sayed, H.; Said, M.M.; Aziz, Y.M.A.; Al-Dhfyan, A.; Al-Majid, A.M.; Barakat, A. Regio- and stereoselective synthesis of novel spiro-oxindole via 1,3-dipolar cycloaddition reaction. Anti-cancer and molecular docking studies. *J. Photochem. Photobiol. B* **2018**, *180*, 98–108. [CrossRef]
18. Tumskiy, R.S.; Burygin, G.L.; Anis'kov, A.A.; Klochkova, I.N. Synthesis of novel spirooxindole-pyrrolidines and evaluation of their cytotoxic activity. *Pharmacol. Rep.* **2019**, *71*, 357–360. [CrossRef]
19. Barakat, A.; Islam, M.S.; Ghawas, H.M.; Al-Majid, A.M.; El-Senduny, F.F.; Badria, F.A.; Elshaier, Y.A.; Ghabbour, H.A. Design and synthesis of new substituted spirooxindoles as potential inhibitors of the MDM2–p53 interaction. *Bioorg. Chem.* **2019**, *86*, 598–608. [CrossRef] [PubMed]
20. Altowyan, M.S.; Atef, S.; Al-Agamy, M.H.; Soliman, S.M.; Ali, M.; Shaik, M.R.; Choudhary, M.I.; Ghabbour, H.A.; Barakat, A. Synthesis and characterization of a spiroindolone pyrothiazole analog via X-ray, biological, and computational studies. *J. Mol. Struct.* **2019**, *1186*, 384–392. [CrossRef]
21. Al-Majid, A.M.; Ghawas, H.M.; Islam, M.S.; Soliman, S.M.; El-Senduny, F.F.; Badria, F.A.; Ali, M.; Shaik, M.R.; Ghabbour, H.A.; Barakat, A. Synthesis of spiroindolone analogue via three components reaction of olefin with isatin and sarcosine: Anti-proliferative activity and computational studies. *J. Mol. Struct.* **2020**, *1204*, 127500. [CrossRef]
22. Islam, M.S.; Ghawas, H.M.; El-Senduny, F.F.; Al-Majid, A.M.; Elshaier, Y.A.; Badria, F.A.; Barakat, A. Synthesis of new thiazolo-pyrrolidine-(spirooxindole) tethered to 3-acylindole as anticancer agents. *Bioorg. Chem.* **2019**, *82*, 423–430. [CrossRef]
23. Lotfy, G.; Aziz, Y.M.A.; Said, M.M.; El Ashry, E.S.H.; El Tamany, E.S.H.; Barakat, A.; Ghabbour, H.A.; Yousuf, S.; Ul-Haq, Z.; Choudhary, M.I. Synthesis of oxindole analogues, biological activity and in silico investigation. *ChemistrySelect* **2019**, *4*, 10510–10516. [CrossRef]
24. Al-Majid, A.M.; Soliman, S.M.; Haukka, M.; Ali, M.; Islam, M.S.; Shaik, M.R.; Barakat, A. Design, construction, and characterization of a new Regioisomer and diastereomer material based on the spirooxindole scaffold incorporating a sulphone function. *Symmetry* **2020**, *12*, 1337. [CrossRef]
25. Chen, S.; Xiao, L.; Chen, Z.Y. Synthesis and antitumor activities of novel pyrimidine-fused spiropyrrolidine oxindoles. *Chin. J. Synth. Chem.* **2017**, *25*, 14–17.
26. Arumugam, N.; Almansour, A.I.; Kumar, R.S.; Periasamy, V.S.; Athinarayanan, J.; Alshatwi, A.A.; Govindasami, P.; Altaf, M.; Menéndez, J.C. Regio- and diastereoselective synthesis of anticancer spirooxindoles derived from tryptophan and histidine via three-component 1,3-dipolar cycloadditions in an ionic liquid. *Tetrahedron* **2018**, *74*, 5358–5366. [CrossRef]
27. Mali, P.R.; Shirsat, P.K.; Khomane, N.; Nayak, L.; Nanubolu, J.B.; Meshram, H.M. 1,3-dipolar cycloaddition reactions for the synthesis of novel oxindole derivatives and their cytotoxic properties. *ACS Comb. Sci.* **2017**, *19*, 633–639. [CrossRef]
28. Huang, Y.; Huang, Y.X.; Sun, J.; Yan, C.G. A [3+2] cycloaddition reaction for the synthesis of spiro[indoline-3,3'-pyrrolidines] and evaluation of cytotoxicity towards cancer cells. *New J. Chem.* **2019**, *43*, 8903–8910. [CrossRef]
29. Shyamsivappan, S.; Vivek, R.; Saravanan, A.; Arasakumar, T.; Subashini, G.; Suresh, T.; Shankar, R.; Mohan, P.S. Synthesis and X-ray study of dispiro 8-nitroquinolone analogues and their cytotoxic properties against human cervical cancer HeLa cells. *Medchemcomm* **2019**, *10*, 439–449. [CrossRef] [PubMed]
30. Ríos-Gutiérrez, M.; Domingo, L.R. Unravelling the Mysteries of the [3+2] Cycloaddition Reactions. *Eur. J. Org. Chem.* **2019**, 267–282. [CrossRef]
31. Domingo, L.R.; Chamorro, E.; Pérez, P. Understanding the high reactivity of the azomethine ylides in [3+2] cycloaddition reactions. *Lett. Org. Chem.* **2010**, *7*, 432–439. [CrossRef]
32. Domingo, L.R.; Kula, K.; Ríos-Gutiérrez, M. Unveiling the reactivity of cyclic azomethine ylides in [3+2] cycloaddition reactions within the molecular electron density theory. *Eur. J. Org. Chem.* **2020**, *2020*, 5938–5948. [CrossRef]
33. Parr, R.G.; Yang, W. *Density-Functional Theory of Atoms and Molecules*; Oxford University Press: New York, NY, USA, 1989.
34. Domingo, L.R.; Chamorro, E.; Pérez, P. Understanding the reactivity of captodative ethylenes in polar cycloaddition reactions. A theoretical study. *J. Org. Chem.* **2008**, *73*, 4615–4624. [CrossRef] [PubMed]
35. Domingo, L.R.; Ríos-Gutiérrez, M.; Pérez, P. A molecular electron density theory study of the role of the copper metalation of azomethine ylides in [3+2] cycloaddition reactions. *J. Org. Chem.* **2018**, *83*, 10959–10973. [CrossRef] [PubMed]
36. May, E.; Jenkins, J.R.; May, P. Endogenous HeLa p53 proteins are easily detected in HeLa cells transfected with mouse deletion mutant p53 gene. *Oncogene* **1991**, *6*, 1363–1365.
37. Hui, L.; Zheng, Y.; Yan, Y.; Bargonetti, J.; Foster, D.A. Mutant p53 in MDA-MB-231 breast cancer cells is stabilized by elevated phospholipase D activity and contributes to survival signals generated by phospholipase D. *Oncogene* **2006**, *25*, 7305–7310. [CrossRef]
38. Zhao, Y.; Liu, L.; Sun, W.; Lu, J.; McEachern, D.; Li, X.; Yu, S.; Bernard, D.; Ochsenbein, P.; Ferey, V.; et al. Diastereomeric spirooxindoles as highly potent and efficacious MDM2 inhibitors. *J. Am. Chem. Soc.* **2013**, *135*, 7223–7234. [CrossRef] [PubMed]

39. Yang, M.C.; Peng, C.; Huang, H.; Yang, L.; He, X.H.; Huang, W.; Cui, H.L.; He, G.; Han, B. Organocatalytic asymmetric synthesis of spiro-oxindole piperidine derivatives that reduce cancer cell proliferation by inhibiting MDM2–p53 interaction. *Org. Lett.* **2017**, *19*, 6752–6755. [CrossRef] [PubMed]
40. Xie, X.; Xiong, S.S.; Li, X.; Huang, H.; Wu, F.B.; Shen, P.F.; Peng, C.; He, G.; Han, B. Design and organocatalytic synthesis of spirooxindole–cyclopentene–isoxazole hybrids as novel MDM2–p53 inhibitors. *Org. Chem. Front.* **2021**, *8*, 1836–1843. [CrossRef]
41. Foye, W.O.; Lemke, T.L.; Williams, D.A. *Principles of Medicinal Chemistry*, 4th ed.; Williams and Wilkins: Philadelphia, PA, USA, 2002; p. 822.
42. Mannerström, M.; Toimela, T.; Sarkanen, J.-R.; Heinonen, T. Human BJ Fibroblasts is an Alternative to Mouse BALB/c 3T3 Cells inIn VitroNeutral Red Uptake Assay. *Basic Clin. Pharmacol. Toxicol.* **2017**, *121*, 109–115. [CrossRef]
43. Price, P.; McMillan1, T.J. Use of the tetrazolium assay in measuring the response of human tumor cells to ionizing radiation. *Cancer Res.* **1990**, *50*, 1392–1396. Available online: https://cancerres.aacrjournals.org/content/canres/50/5/1392.full.pdf (accessed on 1 June 2020). [PubMed]
44. Scudiero, D.A.; Shoemaker, R.H.; Paull, K.D.; Monks, A.; Tierney, S.; Nofziger, T.H.; Currens, M.J.; Seniff, D.; Boyd, M.R. Evaluation of a soluble tetrazolium/formazan assay for cell growth and drug sensitivity in culture using human and other tumor cell lines. *Cancer Res.* **1988**, *48*, 4827–4833. [PubMed]
45. Mosmann, T. Rapid colorimetric assay for cellular growth and survival: Application to proliferation and cytotoxicity assays. *J. Immunol. Methods* **1983**, *65*, 55–63. [CrossRef]
46. Grasberger, B.L.; Lu, T.; Schubert, C.; Parks, D.J.; Carver, T.E.; Koblish, H.K.; Cummings, M.D.; LaFrance, L.V.; Milkiewicz, K.L.; Calvo, R.R.; et al. Discovery and cocrystal structure of benzodiazepinedione HDM2 antagonists that activate p53 in cells. *J. Med. Chem.* **2005**, *48*, 909–912. [CrossRef] [PubMed]
47. Barakat, A.; Islam, M.S.; Ali, M.; Al-Majid, A.M.; Alshahrani, S.; Alamary, A.S.; Yousuf, S.; Choudhary, M.I. Regio- and Stereoselective Synthesis of a New Series of Spirooxindole Pyrrolidine Grafted Thiochromene Scaffolds as Potential Anticancer Agents. *Symmetry* **2021**, *13*, 1426. [CrossRef]

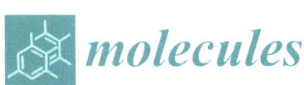

Review

Phytochemistry, Ethnopharmacological Uses, Biological Activities, and Therapeutic Applications of *Cassia obtusifolia* L.: A Comprehensive Review

Md Yousof Ali [1], Seongkyu Park [2] and Munseog Chang [2,3,*]

[1] Department of Physiology and Pharmacology, Hotchkiss Brain Institute and Alberta Children's Hospital Research Institute, Cumming School of Medicine, University of Calgary, Calgary, AB T2N 4N1, Canada; mdyousof.ali@ucalgary.ca

[2] Department of Prescriptionology, College of Korean Medicine, Kyung Hee University, 26, Kyunghee dae-ro, Dongdaemun-gu, Seoul 02447, Korea; comskp@khu.ac.kr

[3] Qgenetics, Seoul Bio Corporation Center, 504, 23 Kyunghee Dae-ro, Dongdaemun-gu, Seoul 02447, Korea

* Correspondence: mschang@khu.ac.kr; Tel.: +82-2-961-9443

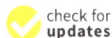

Abstract: *Cassia obtusifolia* L., of the Leguminosae family, is used as a diuretic, laxative, tonic, purgative, and natural remedy for treating headache, dizziness, constipation, tophobia, and lacrimation and for improving eyesight. It is commonly used in tea in Korea. Various anthraquinone derivatives make up its main chemical constituents: emodin, chrysophanol, physcion, obtusifolin, obtusin, au rantio-obtusin, chryso-obtusin, alaternin, questin, aloe-emodin, gluco-aurantio-obtusin, gluco-obtusifolin, naphthopyrone glycosides, toralactone-9-β-gentiobioside, toralactone gentiobioside, and cassiaside. *C. obtusifolia* L. possesses a wide range of pharmacological properties (e.g., antidiabetic, antimicrobial, anti-inflammatory, hepatoprotective, and neuroprotective properties) and may be used to treat Alzheimer's disease, Parkinson's disease, and cancer. In addition, *C. obtusifolia* L. contributes to histamine release and antiplatelet aggregation. This review summarizes the botanical, phytochemical, and pharmacological features of *C. obtusifolia* and its therapeutic uses.

Citation: Ali, M.Y.; Park, S.; Chang, M. Phytochemistry, Ethnopharmacological Uses, Biological Activities, and Therapeutic Applications of *Cassia obtusifolia* L.: A Comprehensive Review. *Molecules* **2021**, *26*, 6252. https://doi.org/10.3390/molecules26206252

Keywords: anthraquinones; antidiabetic; antimicrobial; *Cassia obtusifolia* L.; hepatoprotection; neuro protection

Academic Editors: Imtiaz Khan and Sumera Zaib

Received: 23 September 2021
Accepted: 13 October 2021
Published: 15 October 2021

Publisher's Note: MDPI stays neutral with regard to jurisdictional claims in published maps and institutional affiliations.

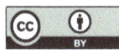

Copyright: © 2021 by the authors. Licensee MDPI, Basel, Switzerland. This article is an open access article distributed under the terms and conditions of the Creative Commons Attribution (CC BY) license (https://creativecommons.org/licenses/by/4.0/).

1. Introduction

Cassia (family Caesalpiniaceae) is a large tropical genus with ~600 species of herbs, shrubs, and trees. *Cassia obtusifolia* (sicklepod) Linn., a member of the genus Cassia (Leguminosae), is a well-known traditional Chinese medicinal plant. It belongs to the medically and economically important family Leguminosae (syn. Fabaceae; subfamily Caesalpinioideae). *C. obtusifolia* L. is found mainly in China, Korea, India, and the western tropical regions. It is an annual semi-shrubby herb that ranges in height from ~0.5 to 2 m. It has two or three pairs of round-tipped leaflets with one to three flowers on a short axillary peduncle with pedicels up to 2 cm; the yellow petals (0.8–1.5 cm) wilt by midday. The pods are linear (up to 20 cm in length), curve gently downward, and contain numerous shiny, dark brown seeds (~0.5 cm in length). The seeds of *C. obtusifolia* L. are rhomboidal or slightly flat, with linear concave ramps on each side. *Cassia tora* L. is considered synonymous with *C. obtusifolia* L., but differs in its botanical and morphological characteristics [1,2]. The main distinguishing morphological feature between the two is the seed coat, which is marked with an obliquely symmetrical dented line on each side of the rib (*C. obtusifolia* L.) or has broad bands on both sides of the rib (*C. tora* L.).

Cassia species are of medicinal interest because of their therapeutic value in traditional medicine. The dry seeds are processed as a crude drug for clinical use or as a dietary supplement. The cultured plants are important sources of Semen Cassiae-derived commercial products in the market. *C. obtusifolia* L. seeds are a well-known medicinal plant in East Asia and are consumed as food to clear liver heat, sharpen vision, lubricate the intestines, and promote bowel movement [3]. In Korea, dried and roasted Cassia seeds are frequently used in brewing tea. In traditional oriental and Chinese (Juemingzi in Chinese) medicine, *C. obtusifolia* L. has been used to treat lacrimation, headaches, dizziness, and constipation [3,4]. *C. obtusifolia* L. has several pharmacological properties, including antiplatelet aggregation, antidiabetic, antimicrobial, anti-inflammatory, hepatoprotective, and neuroprotective activities, and may be used to treat Alzheimer's disease, Parkinson's disease, and cancer [5–12]. It also contributes to histamine release and antiplatelet aggregation. The whole plant, as well as its roots, flowers, leaves, seeds, and pods, possesses medicinal properties. A summary of the ethnomedicinal uses of different parts of the plant is provided in Table 1. This review herein summarizes progress regarding the chemical analysis of *C. obtusifolia* L., primarily focusing on the development of the phytochemistry, botanical aspects, ethnopharmacological, and pharmacological effects of *C. obtusifolia* L. *C. obtusifolia* L. species are rich sources of different types of anthraquinones and naphthopyrone derivatives that exhibit a number of biological activities and may potentially impact human health. Unfortunately, *C. obtusifolia* L. has not been developed as a pharmaceutical agent. The main objective of this review is to present a summary of the studies published to date on this promising plant, with a solid platform to design and conduct clinical studies. This paper reviews the phytochemical and pharmacological activities of *C. obtusifolia* L. and discusses its potential uses as a human food source and/or a pharmacological agent.

Table 1. Ethnomedicinal importance of *Cassia obtusifolia*.

Sr. No.	Plant Part Used	Ethnomedicinal Use
1	Whole plant	In traditional Oriental medicine, the whole plant of *C. obtusifolia* has been used for treatment of Laxative, eye infections, diarrhea, urinary tract infections, gingivitis, fever, and cough remedy [13].
2	Roots	Root is considered bitter, tonic, stomachic and is antidote against snake bite. Other uses are in treatment of fungal diseases, worm infection, abdominal tumors, bronchitis, and asthma. The roots of *C. obtusifolia* are also usually crushed, mixed with lime juice, and applied to ringworms [14].
3	Seeds	The seeds of *C. obtusifolia* are used to treat dizziness and to benefit the eyes by anchoring and nourishing the liver. The dried and roasted seeds are also used as brew a tea. Seeds of *C. obtusifolia* were also used for the treatment of headache, ophthalmic diseases, constipation, hypertension, and hyperlipidemia. In Korea, the hot extract of seeds is taken orally for protection of liver [10,15].
4	Leaves	*C. obtusifolia* leaves and pods have been widely used as purgatives and laxatives. In Indian traditional ayurveda system, the leaves and Pods are used as digestible, laxative, diuretic, stomachic, antipyretic, improves the appetite, biliousness, blood diseases, burning sensation, leprosy, bronchitis, piles, and leucorrhoea [16,17].
5	Stem bark	In Indian traditional ayurveda system, Stem bark extract is used for various skin ailments, rheumatic diseases, and as laxative [18].
6	Pods and fruits	Pods are used in dysentery, in eye diseases and pains in the joints. The unripe fruits are also cooked and eaten [14].

2. Phytochemistry

Several classes of bioactive metabolites have been identified from *C. obtusifolia* L., including anthraquinones, terpenoids, flavonoids, and lipids [1,10,19]. The main plant chemicals include anthraquinone, emodin, chrysophanol, physcion, obtusifolin, obtusin, aurantio-obtusin, chryso-obtusin, alaternin, questin, aloe-emodin, gluco-aurantio-obtusin, gluco-obtusifolin, chrysophanol-2-*O*-tetraglucoside, chrysophanol-2-*O*-triglucosides, and chryso-obtusin-2-glucoside [2,5–12,19]. Other components include naphthopyrone glycosides, toralactone-9-β-gentiobioside, toralactone gentiobioside, cassiaside, rubrofusarin-6-*O*-gentiobiosideol, rubrofusarin-6-β-gentiobioside, cassiaside C, cassiaside B2, cassiaside

C2, xanthones (1,8-dihydroxy-3-methoxy-6-methylxanthone, isogentisin, 1,7-dihydroxy-3-methylxanthone, euxanthone, 1,3,6-trihydroxy-8-methylxanthone), triterpenoids (lupeol, betulinic acid, α-amyrin, sterols, polyketide, steroids, fatty esters), and toralactone [1,17]. The chemical structures of the main compounds are presented in Figure 1. Research on *C. obtusifolia* L. reveals that the nature and number of phytochemicals vary according to climate. Researchers have found that the whole *C. obtusifolia* L. plant (seeds, twigs, leaves, and roots) is rich in free and bound anthraquinones, although the quantities differ markedly. In general, anthraquinone content is higher in seeds and less abundant in other components. The following section discusses the phytochemical contents of the various plant parts.

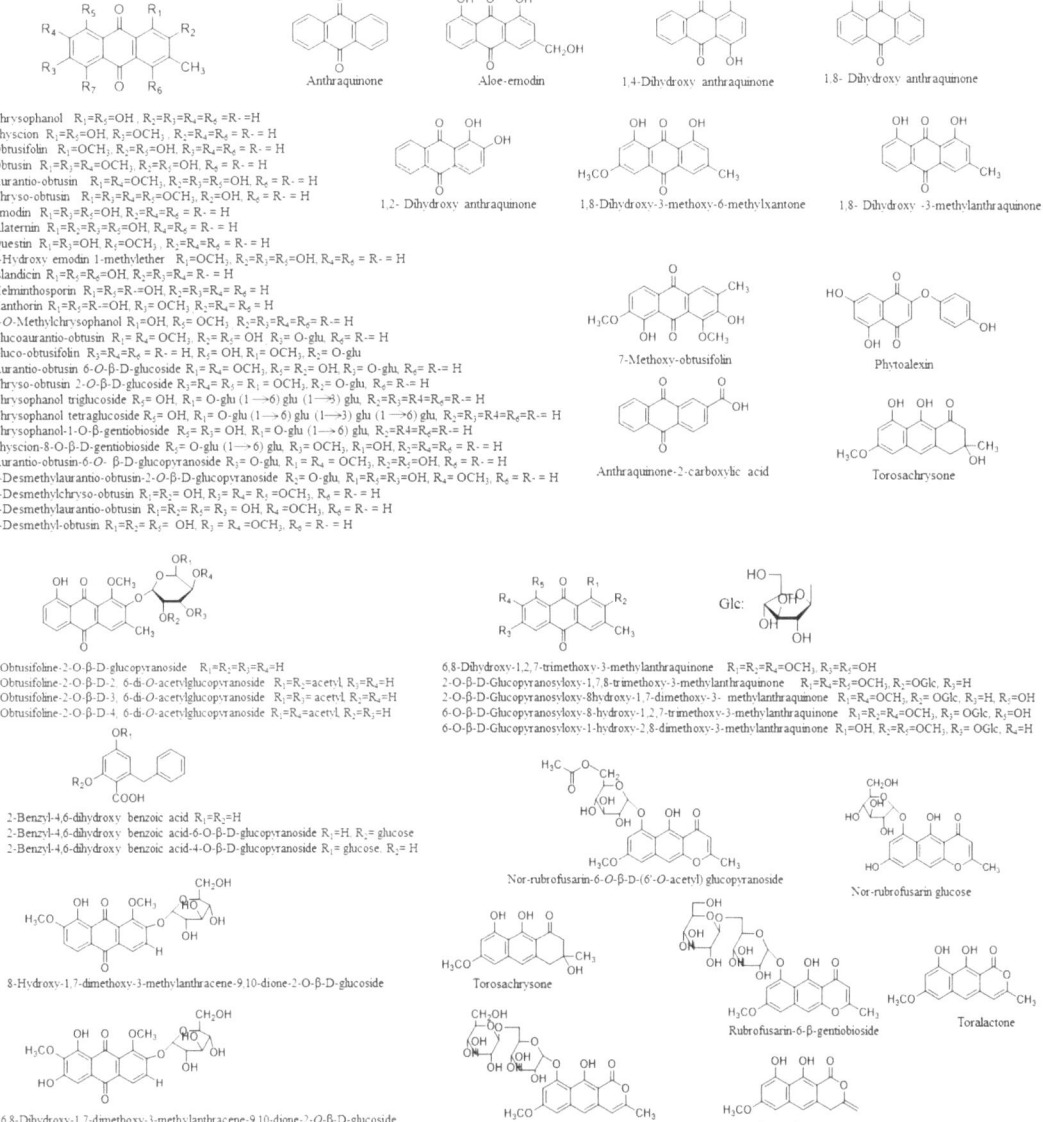

Figure 1. *Cont.*

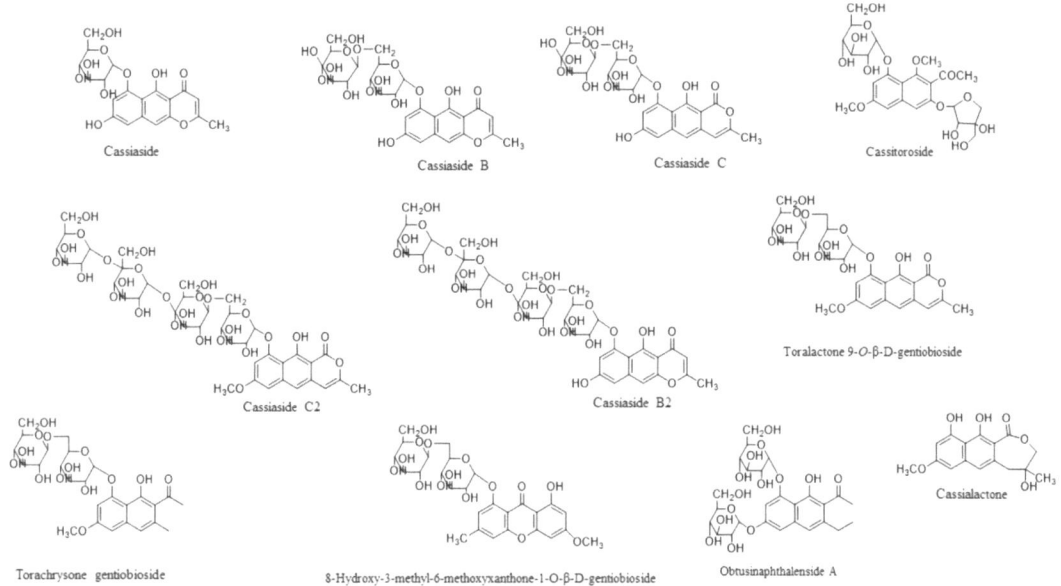

Figure 1. Chemical structures of the main compounds present in *Cassia obtusifolia* L.

2.1. The Whole Plant

Analysis of the whole *C. obtusifolia* L. plant indicates the presence of various anthraquinones and naphthopyrones: aloe-emodin, emodin, 1,2-dihydroxyanthraquinone, obtusin, chryso-obtusin, aurantio-obtusin, gluco-obtusifolin, gluco-aurantio-obtusin, gluco-chryso-obtusin, 1-desmethylaurantio-obtusin-2-*O*-β-D-glucopyranoside, 1-desmethyl-obtusin, aurantio-obtusin-6-*O*-β-D-glucopyranoside, 1-desmethylaurantio-obtusin, alaternin-1-*O*-β-D-glucopyranoside, chryso-obtusin-2-*O*-β-D-glucopyranoside, physicon-8-*O*-β-D-glucoside, obtusifolin, *O*-methyl-chrysophanol, emodin-1-*O*-β-gentio-bioside, chrysophanol-1-*O*-β-gentiobioside, chrysophanol-1-*O*-β-D-glucopyranosyl-(13)-β-D-glucopyranosyl-(1→6)-β-D-glucopyranoside, physcion-8-*O*-β-glucoside, 1,3-dihydroxy-8-methylanthraquinone, torosachrysone, 1-methylaurantio-obtusin-2-*O*-β-D-glucopyranoside, 1-desmethylchryso-obtusin, chrysophanic, acid, physcion, chrysophanol-10,10′-bianthrone, physcion-8-*O*-β-gentiobioside, and questin [20].

2.2. Seeds

Cassia obtusifolia seeds are composed of 1–2% anthraquinones, 5–7% fats, 14–19% protein, and 66–99% carbohydrates [21]. In addition to proteins and fats, the seeds also contain a gum of commercial interest [22]. As much as 41% of the seed is extractable [23]. Several anthraquinone compounds and glycosides have been isolated from the methanol extract of the seeds; examples include anthraquinone, chrysophanol, physcion, emodin, obtusifolin, obtusin, questin, chryso-obtusin, gluco-obtusifolin, aloe-emodin, alaternin, aurantio-obtusin, gluco-aurantio obtusin, chrysophanol tetraglucoside, 2-hydroxyemodin-1 methylether, chryso-obtusin-2-glucoside, chrysophanol triglucoside, 1,2-dihydroxyanthraquinone, 1,4-dihydroxyanthraquinone, 1,8-dihydroxyanthraquinone, 1,8-dihydroxy-3-methylanthraquinone, naphthopyrone glycoside, toralactone gentiobioside, cassiaside, and the naphthalene glycoside cassitoroside [7,10]. Torosachrysone and naphthalenic lactones, isotoralactone, cassialactone, three benzyl-β-resorcylates (2-benzyl-4,6-dihydroxy benzoic acid, 2-benzyl-4,6-dihydroxy benzoic acid-6-*O*-β-D-glucopyranoside, and 2-benzyl-4,6-dihydroxy benzoic acid-4-*O*-β-D-glucopyranoside), a new sodium salt of anthraquinone (sodium emodin-1-*O*-β-gentiobioside), chrysophanol-1-*O*-β-D-glucopyran osyl-(1–3)-β-D-glucopyranosyl-(1–6)-β-D-glucopyranoside, rubrofusarin-6-O-β-D-gentiobioside, obtusifolin-2-O-β-D-glucopyranoside, aurantio-obtusin-6-O-β-D-glucopyranoside, physcion-8-O-β-D-glucopyranoside,1-hydroxyl-2-acetyl-3,8-dimethoxy-6-O-β-D-apiofuranosyl-(1–2)-β-D-glucosylnaphthalene, toralactone-9-O-β-D-gentiobioside, and rubrofusarin-6-O-β-D-apiofuranosyl-(1–6)-O-β-D-glucopyranoside have also been isolated from C. obtusifolia L. seeds [24–26]. In addition, three acetylated anthraquinone glycosides (obtusifoline-2-O-β-D-2,6-di-O-acetylglucopyranoside, obtusifoline-2-O-β-D-3,6-di-O-acetylglucopyranoside, and obtusifoline-2-O-β-D-4,6-di-O-acetylglucopyranoside) have been isolated from the ethanolic extract of the seeds [27]. Recently, Pang et al. [28,29] have isolated four new compounds from the seeds of C. obtusifolia obtusifolin-2-O-β-D-(6′-O-α, β-unsaturated butyryl)-glucopyranoside, epi-9-dehydroxyeurotinone-β-D-glucopyranoside, obtusinaphthalenside A, and obtusinaphthalenside B. Feng et al. [30] also purified various monosaccharides, and polysaccharides from the water extract of C. obtusifolia L.

2.3. Leaves

The leaves of C. obtusifolia L. contain anthraquinones, xanthones, polyketide, steroids, triterpenoids, and fatty esters [17]. The methanol extract of the leaves contains aloe emodin, emodin, 1,8-dihydroxy-3-methoxy-6-methylxantone, euxanthone, chrysophanol, physcion, 1,2,8-trihydroxy-6,7-dimethoxyanthraquinone,1,7-dihydroxy-3-methoxyxanthone,1,5-dihydroxy-3-methoxy-7-methylanthraquinone,3,7-dihydroxy-1-methoxyxanthone,1-O-methyl chrysophanol, 8-O-methylchrysophanol, 1,3,6-trihydroxy-8-methylxanthone, 1-hydroxy-7-methoxy-3-methylanthraquinone, and obtusifolin. The ethyl acetate extract contains (4R*,5S*,6E,8Z)-ethyl-4-([E]-but-1-enyl)-5-hydroxypentdeca-6,8-dienoate, (24S)-24-ethylch olesta-5,22(E),25-trien-3β-ol, (−)-acetoxy-9,10-dimethyl-1,5-octacosanolide, friedelin, stigmasterol, lupeol, and (E)-eicos-14-enoic acid [17]. A single phytoalexin was isolated and purified from 12- to 14-day-old leaves [31].

2.4. Roots

The hairy roots of C. obtusifolia L. contain betulinic acid, sitosterol, stigmasterol, anthraquinones, chrysophanol, physcion, 1-hydroxy-7-methoxy-3-methylanthraquinone, 8-O-methylchrysophanol, 1-O-methylchrysophanol, 1,2,8-trihydroxy-6,7-dimethoxyanthraquinone, emodin, iso-landicin, helminthosporin, obtusifolin, aloe-emodin, and xanthorin [20,32].

3. Bioactivity

Numerous researchers have investigated the pharmacological activities of various C. obtusifolia L. extracts. Table 2 summarizes the pharmacological features that have been observed. They include: antidiabetic, anti-inflammatory, antimicrobial, antioxidant, hepatoprotective, neuroprotective, immune-modulatory, anti-Parkinson's disease, anti-Alzheimer's disease, and larvicidal properties. The anthraquinones and naphthopyrones isolated from C. obtusifolia L. are structurally diverse and exhibit multiple pharmacological properties, which suggests that these compounds contribute to its therapeutic effects (Table 3). C. obtusifolia L. and its major constituents display a vast number of biological activities (Figure 2). Natural products are highly promising sources for antioxidant and anti-inflammatory agents. A wide range of bioactive constituents of plants have antioxidant and anti-inflammatory activities. Based on various assay methods and activity indices, antioxidant or anti-inflammatory activities and nutraceutical and therapeutic effects of traditional Chinese medicines as well as the mechanisms underlying such activities and effects have been investigated. The generation of free radicals can result in damage to the cellular machinery. The seeds of C. obtusifolia L. are widely used in Chinese folk medicine and have been demonstrated to exhibit significant antioxidant and anti-inflammatory. Over the past century, natural products, especially anthraquinone compounds, have become valuable products for achieving chemical diversity in the molecules used for inflammation relief. In addition, COE has traditionally been used in Korea to treat eye inflammation, photophobia, and lacrimation.

Table 2. Pharmacological activities of *Cassia obtusifolia* extracts.

Pharmacological Activity	Part of Plant	Type of Extract	In Vivo/In Vitro	Model	Administration (In Vivo)	Dose Range	Active Concentration	Reference
Neuroprotective Activity	Seeds	85% EtOH ext.	In vivo	Ameliorate scopolamine or 2VO-induced memory impairments by inhibiting AChE	Oral	25–100 mg/kg	50 mg/kg	[8]
	Seeds	85% EtOH ext.	In vivo	Neuroprotection by inhibition of pro-inflammatory genes iNOX, and COX-2, and increased neurotrophic factor expression of pCREB and BDNF	Oral	10, 50 mg/kg	50 mg/kg	[33]
	Seeds	85% EtOH ext.	In vitro	Reduced Aβ toxicity and maintenance of Ca^{2+} dysregulation and excitotoxicity, mitochondrial dysfunction in primary hippocampal cultures	-	0.1–10 μg/mL	1, 10 μg/mL	[11]
	Seeds	EtOH ex.	In vivo	protected the dopaminergic cells against 6-OHDA- and MPP+-induced neurotoxicities in primary mesencephalic cultures and in a mouse model in PD	Intraperitoneal injection	0.1–10 μg/mL for DA, 50 mg/kg mouse	0.1, 1 μg/mL 50 mg/kg	[34]
	Seeds	EtOH ext.	In vitro	Inhibited cell loss against 6-OHDA-induced DA neural toxicity by an anti-oxidant and anti-mitochondrial-mediated apoptosis mechanism in PC12 cells.	-	0.1–10 μg/mL 1000 μg/mL for DPPH, ABTS	1 μg/mL ROS, 10 μg/mL GSH, 75% Casp-3, 92%-DPPH, 85% ABTS	[35]
	Seeds	MeOH ext. EtOAc fr. CH_2Cl_2 fr. BuOH fr.	In vitro	Inhibitory activity against MAO-A, and MAO-B	-	0.25–120 μg/mL	EtOAc fr. exhibited greatest inhibitory IC_{50} = 20, and 56 μg/mL activity against MAO-A, and MAO-B	[36]
	Seeds	MeOH ext. EtOAc fr. CH_2Cl_2 fr. BuOH fr. H_2O fr.	In vitro	Inhibitory activity against AChE, BChE, BACE1	-	0.4–120 μg/mL	IC_{50} = 9.45~29 μg/mL for AChE, IC_{50} = 7.58~49 μg/mL for BChE, IC_{50} = 26~96 μg/mL for BACE1	[10]
	Seeds	85% EtOH ext.	In vivo	Ameliorate Aβ-induced LTP impairment in the acute hippocampal slices and regulates GSK-3β, Akt signaling pathways through the inhibition of iNOS, COX expression	-	1 and 10 μg/mL	10 μg/mL	[35]

Table 2. Cont.

Pharmacological Activity	Part of Plant	Type of Extract	In Vivo/In Vitro	Model	Administration (In Vivo)	Dose Range	Active Concentration	Reference
Hepatoprotective Activity	Seeds	MeOH ext.	In vitro	Protection against tacrine-induced hepatotoxicity in HepG2 cells	-	300 µg/mL	300 µg/mL	[36]
	Seeds	70% EtOH ext. EtOAc, CH_2Cl_2, BuOH, H_2O fr.	In vitro	Protective effect against t-BHP-induced hepatotoxicity in HepG2 cells	-	10–100 µg/mL	EtOAc fr. showed most potent hepatoprotective activity (30 µg/mL)	[12]
	Seeds	EtOH ext.	In vivo	Hepatoprotective effects against CCl_4-induced liver injury in mice	Intraperitoneal injection	0.5, 1, 2 g/kg	Reduced ALT and AST, Ca^{2+}, MDA, and increased GSH, SOD, GR, GPx, GST, CYP2E1 (2 g/kg)	[15]
	seeds	EtOAc fr. CH_2Cl_2 fr. BuOH fr. H_2O fr.	In vitro	Protective effect against t-BHP-induced hepatotoxicity in HepG2 cells	-	12.5–50 µg/mL	EtOAc fr. showed most potent hepatoprotective activity (50 µg/mL)	[37]
	Seeds	70% EtOH ext.	In vivo	(a) Significantly decreased the levels of AST, ALT, TG, TC, TNF-α, IL-6, IL-8 and MDA; (b) Increased the levels of SOD and GSH; (c) Significantly increased the mRNA expression levels of LDL-R	Oral	0.5–2 g/kg	(a) Dose-dependently decreased biomarkers at 0.5–2 g/kg; (b) Dose-dependently decreased at 0.5–2 g/kg; (c) Significantly increased the levels of LDL-R at 2 g/kg	[38]
Anti-diabetic Activity	Seeds	MeOH ext. EtOAc fr. CH_2Cl_2 fr. BuOH fr. H_2O fr.	In vitro	Inhibitory activity against PTP1B and α-glucosidase	-	0.4–400 µg/mL for PTP1B, 0.16–400 µg/mL for α-glucosidase	MeOH ext. (IC_{50} = 14 µg/mL) and EtOAc fr. (IC_{50} = 74 µg/mL) exhibited greatest inhibitory activity against PTP1B and α-glucosidase	[9]
	Seeds	EtOH ext.	In vitro	Inhibitory activity against α-glucosidase	-	1000 µg/mL	20% inhibition of α-glucosidase (1000 µg/mL)	[39]

Table 2. Cont.

Pharmacological Activity	Part of Plant	Type of Extract	In Vivo/In Vitro	Model	Administration (In Vivo)	Dose Range	Active Concentration	Reference
	Roasted seeds	Hot H$_2$O ext.	In vivo	Protection against dextran sulfate sodium (DSS)-induced colitis through the inhibition of (IL)-6, COX-2, NF-κB	Oral	1 g/kg	Significantly reduced clinical signs and the levels of inflammatory mediators (at concentration 1 g/kg)	[40]
Anti-inflammatory, Antioxidant, and Immune-modulatory Activities	Seeds	H$_2$O soluble polysaccharide fr.	In vitro	Increased immune-modulatory activity by promoting phagocytosis and stimulating the production of NO and cytokines TNF- and IL-6 on macrophage cell line RAW264.7	-	62.5–500 μg/mL	Stimulates NO, TNF- and IL-6 expression (250 μg/mL) and promotes phagocytic activity (500 μg/mL)	[41]
	Seeds	MeOH ext.	In vitro	DPPH, Fe [II], superoxide radicals scavenging activity and inhibit β-carotene degradation	-	1 mg/mL	Inhibition 65.79% DPPH, 50.78% superoxide radical, 49.92% inhibit β-carotene degradation, 1292 mM Fe [II] inhibited (at 1 mg/mL)	[14]
	Seeds	MeOH ext. Hexane fr. EtOAc fr. CH$_2$Cl$_2$ fr. BuOH fr. H$_2$O fr.	In vitro	Bifidobacterium adolescentis, B. bifidum, B. longum, B. breve, Clostridium perfringens, Escherichia coli, Lactobacillus casei	-	5 mg discs^{-1}	CH$_2$Cl$_2$ fr, MeOH ext. and Hexane fr. exhibited the greatest antibacterial activity	[7]
Antimicrobial Activity	Leaf	Pet ether ext. EtOH ext. Chloroform ext.	In vitro	Aspergilus fumigatus, Staphylococcus aureus, Enterococcus faecalis, E. coli, Klebsiella sp., Candia albicans	-	0.6–1 mg/mL	Pet ether, chloroform ext. active against C. albicans (MIC 0.3524, and 0.4239 mg/mL), ethanol E. faecalis (MIC 0.2738 mg/mL)	[18]
	stem	Pet ether ext. EtOH ext. Chloroform ext.	In vitro	Aspergilus fumigatus, Staphylococcus aureus, Enterococcus faecalis, E. coli, Klebsiella sp., Candia albicans	-	0.6–1 mg/mL	Ethanol, pet ether, chloroform ext. was more active against E. faecalis (MIC 0.298, 0.254, and 0.589 mg/mL, respectively)	[18]

Table 2. Cont.

Pharmacological Activity	Part of Plant	Type of Extract	In Vivo/In Vitro	Model	Administration (In Vivo)	Dose Range	Active Concentration	Reference
	Whole plant	MeOH ext.	In vitro	E. coli, P. aeruginosa, Enterobacter aerogenes Providencia stuartii, K.pneumoniae, Enterobacter cloacae, S. aureus	-	256 µg/mL	inhibition of S. aureus, E. coli, P. aeruginosa, E. aerogenes, K. pneumoniae (MIC ranges of 64–289 µg/mL	[42]
	Seeds	MeOH ext.	In vitro	Larvicidal activity against Aedes aegypti and Culex pipiens pallens	-	10–300 ppm	40 ppm	[43]
	Seeds	Chloroform fr.	In vitro	Larvicidal activity against A. aegypti, Aedes togoi, and Cx. pipiens	-	25 mg/L	100% Mortality (at concentration 25 mg/L)	[44]
Larvicidal Activity	Leaf	EtOH ext.	In vitro	Larvicidal activity against Anopheles stephensi	-	25–125 mg/L	LC_{50} = 52.2 mg/L, LC_{90} = 108.7 mg/L (at concentration 25 mg/L)	[45]
	Leaf	EtOH ext.	In vitro	Anti-oviposition activity against Anopheles stephensi	-	100–400 mg/L	92.5% for 400 mg/L, 87.2% for 300 mg/L, 83.0% for 200 mg/L	[45]

Table 3. Major Phytochemicals in Cassia obtusifolia and their pharmacological activities.

Compounds	Biological Activity	In Vivo/In Vitro	Model	Administration (In Vivo)	Dose Range	Active Concentration	Reference
Anthraquinones							
	Anti-Alzheimer's activity	In vitro	(a) Acetylcholinesterase inhibitory activity (b) Butyrylcholinesterase inhibitory activity (c) β-secretase inhibitory activity	-	0–100 µg/mL	(a) IC_{50} = 9.17 µg/mL (b) IC_{50} = 157 µg/mL (c) IC_{50} = 4.48 µg/mL	[10]
	Antimicrobial activity	In vitro	Antibacterial activity against (a) Staphylococcus aureus 209P (b) Escherichia coli NIHJ	-	0–1 mg/mL	MIC (a) 4.5 µg/mL (b) 25 µg/mL	[46]
Emodin	Antidiabetic activity	In vitro	(a) PTP 1B inhibitory activity (b) α-glucosidase inhibitory activity (c) Stimulation of glucose uptake in HepG2 cells	-	(a) 0–100 µg/mL (b) 0–400 µg/mL (c) 3.12–12.5 µM	(a) IC_{50} = 3.51 µg/mL (b) IC_{50} = 1.02 µg/mL (c) glucose uptake	[9]
	Platelet anti-aggregatory activity	In vitro	(a) Adenosine 5′-diphosphate inhibitory activity (b) Arachidonic-acid inhibitory activity (c) Collagen inhibitory activity	-	0–1 mg/mL	1 mg/mL	[47]

Table 3. Cont.

Compounds	Biological Activity	In Vivo/In Vitro	Model	Administration (In Vivo)	Dose Range	Active Concentration	Reference
	Larvicidal activity	In vitro	Larvicidal activity against (a) *Culex pipiens pallens* (b), *Aedes aegypti* (c) *Aedes togoi*	-	1–20 mg/L	(a) LC_{50} = 1.4 mg/L (b) LC_{50} = 1.9 mg/L (c) LC_{50} = 2.2 mg/L	[44]
	Hepatoprotective activity	In vitro	Protection against *t*-BHP-induced hepatotoxicity in HepG2 cells	-	25 µM	protect cells damage	[37]
	Parkinson's disease activity	In vitro	(a) MAO-A inhibitory activity (b) MAO-B inhibitory activity	-	25 µM	(a) IC_{50} = 23 µM (b) IC_{50} = 54 µM	[19]
	Neuroprotective activity	In vivo	Prevented nitrotyrosine and lipid peroxidation, as well as BCCAO induced-iNOS expression and significantly reduced microglial activation	Orally	1, 10 mg/kg	10 mg/kg	[48]
	Antidiabetic activity	In vitro	(a) PTP 1B inhibitory activity (b) α-glucosidase inhibitory activity (c) Stimulation of glucose uptake in HepG2 cells	-	(a) 0–100 µg/mL (b) 0–400 µg/mL (c) 12.5–50 µM	(a) IC_{50} = 1.22 µg/mL (b) IC_{50} = 0.99 µg/mL (c) glucose uptake	[9]
Alaternin	Anti-Alzheimer's activity	In vitro	(a) Acetylcholinesterase inhibitory activity (b) Butyrylcholinesterase inhibitory activity (c) β-secretase inhibitory activity	-	0–100 µg/mL	(a) IC_{50} = 6.29 µg/mL (b) IC_{50} = 113 µg/mL (c) IC_{50} = 0.94 µg/mL	[10]
	Hepatoprotective activity	In vitro	Protection against *t*-BHP-induced hepatotoxicity in HepG2 cells	-	50, 100 µM	(a) protect cells damage (b) increased GSH level and reduce ROS level	[37]
	Parkinson's disease activity	In vitro	(a) MAO-A inhibitory activity (b) MAO-B inhibitory activity	-	10 µM	(a) IC_{50} = 5.35 µM (b) IC_{50} = 4.55 µM	[19]
	Neuroprotective activity	In vivo	Significantly reversed scopolamine-induced cognitive impairments in the passive avoidance test, improved escape latencies, swimming times in the target quadrant, and crossing numbers in the zone in Morris water maze test	Orally	0.25–2 mg/kg	0.5 mg/kg	[49]
Obtusifolin	Hyperlipidemia and antioxidant activity	In vivo	Reduced body weight, TC, TG, LDL-C and increased HDL-C levels, as well as increased SOD and NO, and reduced MDA levels in hyperlipidemic rats.	Orally	5 and 20 mg/kg	20 mg/kg	[50]
	Neuropathic and anti-inflammatory activity	In vivo	Inhibition of TNF-α, IL-1β, IL-6 and NF-kB up-regulation in the spinal cord in mice and rat models	Intraperitoneal injection	0.25–2 mg/kg	1 and 2 mg/kg	[51]

Table 3. Cont.

Compounds	Biological Activity	In Vivo/In Vitro	Model	Administration (In Vivo)	Dose Range	Active Concentration	Reference
	Anti-Alzheimer's activity	In vitro	(a) Acetylcholinesterase inhibitory activity (b) Butyrylcholinesterase inhibitory activity (c) β-secretase inhibitory activity	-	0–100 µg/mL	(a) IC_{50} = 18.5 µg/mL (b) IC_{50} = 284 µg/mL (c) IC_{50} = 64.8 µg/mL	[10]
	Antidiabetic activity	In vitro	(a) PTP 1B inhibitory activity (b) α-glucosidase inhibitory activity	-	(a) 0–100 µg/mL (b) 0–400 µg/mL	(a) IC_{50} = 35.2 µg/mL (b) IC_{50} = 142 µg/mL	[9]
	Hepatoprotective activity	In vitro	Protection against tacrine-induced hepatotoxicity in HepG2 cells	-	160 µM	Protection ratio value 41.2% at 160 µM	[36]
	Parkinson's disease activity	In vitro	(a) MAO-A inhibitory activity; (b) MAO-B inhibitory activity	-	100 µM	(a) IC_{50} = 31 µM (b) $IC_{50} \geq$ 400 µM	[19]
	Neuropathic and anti-inflammatory activity	In vivo	Inhibition of TNF-α, IL-1β, IL-6 and NF-kB up-regulation in the spinal cord in mice and rat models	Intraperitoneal injection	0.25–2 mg/kg	1 and 2 mg/kg	[51]
	Anti-Alzheimer's activity	In vitro	(a) Acetylcholinesterase inhibitory activity (b) Butyrylcholinesterase inhibitory activity (c) β-secretase inhibitory activity	-	0–400 µg/mL	(a) IC_{50} = 37.2 µg/mL (b) IC_{50} = 172 µg/mL (c) IC_{50} = 41.1 µg/mL	[10]
Gluco-obtusifolin	Neuroprotective activity	In vivo	Significantly reversed scopolamine-induced cognitive impairments in the passive avoidance test, improved escape latencies, swimming times in the target quadrant, and crossing numbers in the zone in the Morris water maze test	Orally	0.25–2 mg/kg	0.5 mg/kg	[49]
	Antidiabetic activity	In vitro	(a) PTP 1B inhibitory activity (b) α-glucosidase inhibitory activity	-	(a) 0–100 µg/mL (b) 0–400 µg/mL	(a) IC_{50} = 53.35 µg/mL (b) IC_{50} = 23.77 µg/mL	[9]
	Platelet anti-aggregatory activity	In vitro	(a) Adenosine 5'-diphosphate inhibitory activity (b) Arachidonic-acid inhibitory activity (c) Collagen inhibitory activity	-	0–1 mg/mL	(a) IC_{50} = 0.25 µg/mL (b) IC_{50} = 0.05 µg/mL (c) IC_{50} = 0.1 µg/mL	[5]
	Parkinson's disease activity	In vitro	(a) MAO-A inhibitory activity (b) MAO-B inhibitory activity	-	500 µM	(a) $IC_{50} \geq$ 400 µM (b) $IC_{50} \geq$ 400 µM	[19]
	Hepatoprotective activity	In vitro	Protection against tacrine-induced hepatotoxicity in HepG2 cells	-	160 µM	Protection ratio value 55.3% at 160 µM	[36]
Aurantio-obtusin	Anti-Alzheimer's activity	In vitro	(a) Acetylcholinesterase inhibitory activity (b) Butyrylcholinesterase inhibitory activity (c) β-secretase inhibitory activity	-	0–100 µg/mL	(a) IC_{50} = 92.1 µg/mL (b) IC_{50} = 314 µg/mL (c) IC_{50} = 67.9 µg/mL	[10]
	Platelet anti-aggregatory activity	In vitro	(a) Adenosine 5'-diphosphate inhibitory activity (b) Arachidonic-acid inhibitory activity (c) Collagen inhibitory activity	-	0–1 mg/mL	1 mg/mL	[48]

Table 3. Cont.

Compounds	Biological Activity	In Vivo/In Vitro	Model	Administration (In Vivo)	Dose Range	Active Concentration	Reference
	Antidiabetic activity	In vitro	(a) PTP 1B inhibitory activity (b) α-glucosidase inhibitory activity	-	(a) 0–100 µg/mL (b) 0–400 µg/mL	(a) IC_{50} = 27.19 µg/mL (b) IC_{50} = 41.20 µg/mL	[9]
	Anti-cancer activity	In vitro	Cytotoxicity against (a) HCT-116, (b) A549, (c) SGC7901 and (d) LO2 cell lines	-	0.4–50 µg/mL	(a) IC_{50} = 18.9 µg/mL (b) IC_{50} = 20.1 µg/mL (c) IC_{50} = 22.0 µg/mL (d) IC_{50} = 23.1 µg/mL	[52]
	Prevention of bone disease	In vitro	Stimulates osteoblast migration, differentiation, and mineralization in a dose-dependent manner in MC3T3-E1 osteoblast cells	-	0.1–100 µM	10 µM	[53]
	Anti-inflammatory activity	In vitro	(a) Significantly decreased the production of NO, PGE2, and inhibited the iNOS, COX-2, TNF-α and IL-6. (b) Reduced the LPS-induced activation of nuclear factor-κB in RAW264.7 cells.	-	6.12–100 µM	6.12–100 µM	[54]
	Parkinson's disease activity	In vitro	(a) MAO-A inhibitory activity (b) MAO-B inhibitory activity	-	200 µM	(a) IC_{50} = 27.23 µM (b) IC_{50} = 174.40 µM	[19]
Obtusin	Antidiabetic activity	In vitro	(a) PTP 1B inhibitory activity (b) α-glucosidase inhibitory activity	-	(a) 0–100 µg/mL (b) 0–400 µg/mL	(a) IC_{50} = 6.44 µg/mL (b) IC_{50} = 20.92 µg/mL	[9]
	Anti-Alzheimer's activity	In vitro	(a) Acetylcholinesterase inhibitory activity (b) Butyrylcholinesterase inhibitory activity (c) β-secretase inhibitory activity	-	0–100 µg/mL	(a) IC_{50} = 82 µg/mL (b) IC_{50} = 287 µg/mL (c) IC_{50} = 61.9 µg/mL	[10]
	Anti-cancer activity	In vitro	Cytotoxicity against (a) HCT-116, (b) A549, and (c) SGC7901 cell lines	-	0.4–50 µg/mL	(a) IC_{50} = 13.1 µg/mL (b) IC_{50} = 29.2 µg/mL (c) IC_{50} = 15.2 µg/mL	[52]
	Parkinson's disease activity	In vitro	(a) MAO-A inhibitory activity (b) MAO-B inhibitory activity	-	400 µM	(a) IC_{50} = 11.12 µM (b) $IC_{50} \geq$ 400 µM	[19]
Chryso-obtusin	Anti-cancer activity	In vitro	Cytotoxicity against (a) HCT-116, (b) A549, (c) SGC7901 and (d) LO2 cell lines	-	0.4–50 µg/mL	(a) IC_{50} = 10.5 µg/mL (b) IC_{50} = 14.6 µg/mL (c) IC_{50} = 12.0 µg/mL (d) IC_{50} = 15.8 µg/mL	[52]
	Anti-Alzheimer's activity	In vitro	(a) Acetylcholinesterase inhibitory activity (b) Butyrylcholinesterase inhibitory activity (c) β-secretase inhibitory activity	-	0–100 µg/mL	(a) IC_{50} = 68.6 µg/mL (b) IC_{50} = 287 µg/mL (c) IC_{50} = 49.9 µg/mL	[10]

Table 3. Cont.

Compounds	Biological Activity	In Vivo/In Vitro	Model	Administration (In Vivo)	Dose Range	Active Concentration	Reference
	Antidiabetic activity	In vitro	(a) PTP 1B inhibitory activity (b) α-glucosidase inhibitory activity	-	(a) 0–100 μg/mL (b) 0–400 μg/mL	(a) IC$_{50}$ = 14.88 μg/mL (b) IC$_{50}$ = 36.1 μg/mL	[9]
	Platelet anti-aggregatory activity	In vitro	(a) Adenosine 5′-diphosphate inhibitory activity (b) Arachidonic-acid inhibitory activity (c) Collagen inhibitory activity	-	0–1 mg/mL	1 mg/mL	[47]
	Parkinson's disease activity	In vitro	(a) MAO-A inhibitory activity (b) MAO-B inhibitory activity	-	400 μM	(a) IC$_{50}$ = 327.67 μM (b) IC$_{50}$ ≥ 400 μM	[19]
	Antimicrobial activity	In vitro	Antibacterial activity against (a) *Staphylococcus aureus* 209P and (b) *Escherichia coli* NIHJ	-	0–100 μg/mL	MIC (a) 25 μg/mL (b) 50 μg/mL	[48]
Questin	Anti-Alzheimer's activity	In vitro	(a) Acetylcholinesterase inhibitory activity (b) Butyrylcholinesterase inhibitory activity (c) β-secretase inhibitory activity	-	0–100 μg/mL	(a) IC$_{50}$ = 34.0 μg/mL (b) IC$_{50}$ = 138 μg/mL (c) IC$_{50}$ = 32.8 μg/mL	[10]
	Antidiabetic activity	In vitro	(a) PTP 1B inhibitory activity (b) α-glucosidase inhibitory activity	-	(a) 0–100 μg/mL (b) 0–400 μg/mL	(a) IC$_{50}$ = 5.69 μg/mL (b) IC$_{50}$ = 136.1 μg/mL	[9]
	Parkinson's disease activity	In vitro	(a) MAO-A inhibitory activity (b) MAO-B inhibitory activity	-	20 μM	(a) IC$_{50}$ = 0.17 μM (b) IC$_{50}$ = 10.58 μM	[19]
	Platelet anti-aggregatory activity	In vitro	(a) Adenosine 5′-diphosphate inhibitory activity (b) Arachidonic-acid inhibitory activity (c) Collagen inhibitory activity	-	0–1 mg/mL	(a) IC$_{50}$ = 0.25 μg/mL (b) IC$_{50}$ = 0.05 μg/mL (c) IC$_{50}$ = 0.1 μg/mL	[5]
Gluco-aurantio-obtusin	Anti-Alzheimer's activity	In vitro	(a) Acetylcholinesterase inhibitory activity (b) β-secretase inhibitory activity	-	0–100 μg/mL	(a) IC$_{50}$ = 109 μg/mL (b) IC$_{50}$ = 50.9 μg/mL	[10]
	Antidiabetic activity	In vitro	(a) PTP 1B inhibitory activity (b) α-glucosidase inhibitory activity	-	(a) 0–100 μg/mL (b) 0–400 μg/mL	(a) IC$_{50}$ = 31.3 μg/mL (b) IC$_{50}$ = 142.1 μg/mL	[9]
	Hepatoprotective activity	In vitro	Hepatoprotective efficacy against *t*-BHP-induced cell death in HepG2 cells	-	20 μM	Protection ratio value 49.7% at 20 μM	[12]
	Parkinson's disease activity	In vitro	(a) MAO-A inhibitory activity (b) MAO-B inhibitory activity	-	400 μM	(a) IC$_{50}$ = 39.55 μM (b) IC$_{50}$ = 180.76 μM	[19]

Table 3. Cont.

Compounds	Biological Activity	In Vivo/In Vitro	Model	Administration (In Vivo)	Dose Range	Active Concentration	Reference
Chrysophanol; Aloe-emodin; Physcion;	Antidiabetic activity	In vitro	(a) PTP 1B inhibitory activity (b) α-glucosidase inhibitory activity	-	(a) 0–100 μg/mL (b) 0–400 μg/mL	(a) IC_{50} = 5–103 μg/mL (b) IC_{50} = 5–228 μg/mL	[9]
Chrysophanol tri, Tetraglucoside; 2-hydroxyemodin-1methylether;	Anti-Alzheimer's activity	In vitro	(a) Acetylcholinesterase inhibitory activity (b) Butyrylcholinesterase inhibitory activity (c) β-secretase inhibitory activity	-	0–400 μg/mL	(a) IC_{50} = 14–71 μg/mL (b) IC_{50} ≥ 100 μg/mL (c) IC_{50} = 13–59 μg/mL	[10]
Chryso-obtusin-2-O-β-D-glucoside	Parkinson's disease activity	In vitro	(a) MAO-A inhibitory activity (b) MAO-B inhibitory activity	-	400 μM	(a) IC_{50} = 2.47–400 μM (b) IC_{50} ≥ 400 μM	[19]
Dihydroxyan thraquinone	Bacterial growth promoting and inhibiting activity	In vitro	(a) Growth promoting activity against *Bifidobacterium bifidum* (b) Growth inhibiting activity against *Clostridium perfringens* and *Escherichia coli*	-	(a) 0.05–0.5 mg/d (b) 0.1–5 mg/d	(a) GIR > 2.0 at 0.5 mg/disk (b) Inhibitory zone diameter > 30 mm	[7]
Naphthopyrone							
	Anti-Alzheimer's activity	In vitro	(a) Acetylcholinesterase inhibitory activity (b) Butyrylcholinesterase inhibitory activity (c) β-secretase inhibitory activity	-	0–100 μg/mL	(a) IC_{50} = 18.1 μg/mL (b) IC_{50} = 177 μg/mL (c) IC_{50} = 1.85 μg/mL	[10]
	Antidiabetic activity	In vitro	(a) PTP 1B inhibitory activity (b) α-glucosidase inhibitory activity	-	(a) 0–100 μg/mL (b) 0–400 μg/mL	(a) IC_{50} = 48.55 μg/mL (b) IC_{50} = 129.2 μg/mL	[9]
Cassiaside	Hepatoprotective activity	In vitro	Hepatoprotective efficacy against *t*-BHP-induced cell death in HepG2 cells	-	25 μM	(a) protect cells damage (b) increased GSH level and reduce ROS level	[37]
	Parkinson's disease activity	In vitro	(a) MAO-A inhibitory activity (b) MAO-B inhibitory activity	-	400 μM	(a) IC_{50} = 11.26 μM (b) IC_{50} ≥ 400 μM	[19]
Isotoralactone; Toralactone	Antimicrobial activity	In vitro	Antibacterial activity against (a) *Staphylococcus aureus* 209P and (b) *Escherichia coli* NIHJ	-	0–100 μg/mL	MIC (a) 2–3 μg/Ml (b) 5.5–12 μg/mL	[46]
Cassiaside B2, Cassiaside C2	Antiallergic activity	In vitro	Inhibition of histamine release in rat peritoneal mast cells	-	100 μM	Cassiaside B2 inhibit 17.2%; Cassiaside C2 Inhibit 53.9%	[6]

Table 3. *Cont.*

Compounds	Biological Activity	In Vivo/In Vitro	Model	Administration (In Vivo)	Dose Range	Active Concentration	Reference
	Antidiabetic activity	In vitro	(a) PTP 1B inhibitory activity (b) α-glucosidase inhibitory activity	-	(a) 0–100 μg/mL (b) 0–400 μg/mL	(a) IC_{50} = 81.1 μg/mL (b) IC_{50} = 37.60 μg/mL	[9]
Toralactone Gentiobioside	Anti-Alzheimer's activity	In vitro	(a) Acetylcholinesterase inhibitory activity (b) Butyrylcholinesterase inhibitory activity (c) β-secretase inhibitory activity	-	0–100 μg/mL	(a) IC_{50} = 91.3 μg/mL (b) IC_{50} = 117 μg/mL (c) IC_{50} = 69.0 μg/mL	[10]
	Hepatoprotective activity	In vitro	Hepatoprotective efficacy against *t*-BHP-induced cell death in HepG2 cells	-	20 μM	Increased in Nrf2/ARE-luciferase activity, and upregulated NQO1, GLC, HO-1 levels	[12]
rubrofusarin, Rubrofusarin 6-*O*-β-D-glucopyranoside, Rubrofusarin 6-*O*-β-D-gentiobioside, Nor-rubrofusarin 6-*O*-β-D-glucoside	Anti-Alzheimer's activity	In vitro	(a) Acetylcholinesterase inhibitory activity (b) β-secretase inhibitory activity	-	(a) 0–100 μM (b) 0–750 μM	(a) 15.95–148 μM (b) 14.0–190 μM	[55]

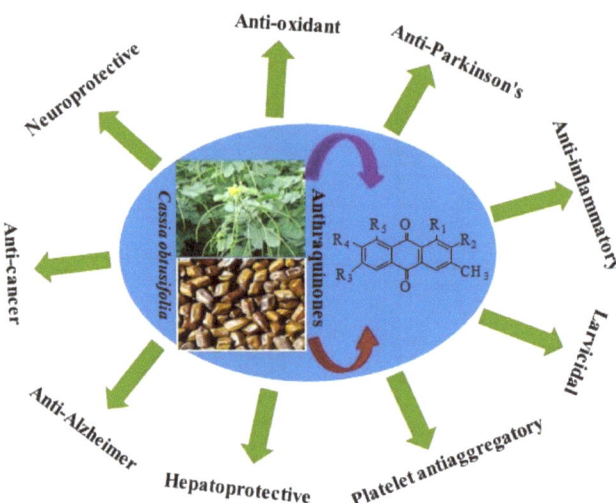

Figure 2. Different biological activities displayed by *Cassia obtusifolia*.

3.1. Neuroprotective Activity

Various studies have demonstrated the direct neuroprotective activities of the *C. obtusifolia* L. seed extract (COE) and its major constituents (anthraquinones). More detailed studies are required to clarify the compositional features and neuroprotective activities of the anthraquinones. The ethanolic COE (25, 50, or 100 mg/kg) ameliorates scopolamine or bilateral common carotid artery occlusion (2VO)-induced memory impairment by inhibiting acetylcholinesterase [8]. COE (10 or 50 mg/kg/day) reduced memory impairment and neuronal damage caused by 2VO in a mouse model of transient global ischemia; it was suggested that the neuroprotective effects of COE are attributable to its anti-inflammatory properties resulting in decreased expression of inducible nitric oxide synthase (iNOX) and cyclooxygenase-2 (COX-2) and increased expression of the neurotrophic factors pCREB and BDNF [33]. Alaternin, the active compound in *C. obtusifolia* L., exhibits neuroprotective activity after transient cerebral hypoperfusion induced by bilateral common carotid artery occlusion. Administration of alaternin (10 mg/kg) prevented or reduced nitrotyrosine and lipid peroxidation, bilateral common carotid artery occlusion (BCCAO)-induced iNOS expression, and microglial activation [48]. Drever et al. [11] reported that ethanolic COE is neuroprotective against NMDA-induced calcium dysregulation and 3-nitropropionic acid-induced cell death in mouse hippocampal cultures. Recently, Paudel et al. [56] also reported that four major compounds (cassiaside, rubrofusarin gentiobioside, aurantio-obtusin, and 2-hydroxyemodin 1-methylether) exhibited neuroprotective effects; among them, aurantio-obtusin showed promising neuroprotective effects via targeting various G-protein-coupled receptors and transient brain ischemia/reperfusion injury C57BL/6 mice model.

3.1.1. Anti-Alzheimer's Disease Activity

The effects of the ethanolic extract of COE in Aβ-induced anti-Alzheimer's disease (anti-AD) models have been reported. The mechanism of COE ameliorated Aβ-induced LTP impairment in acute hippocampal slices and prevented Aβ-induced GSK-3β activation [35]. Moreover, COE prevented microglial activation as well as iNOS and COX activation induced by Aβ in the hippocampus, and in vivo studies have indicated that COE ameliorated Aβ-induced object recognition memory impairment [35]. Two anthraquinones from *C. obtusifolia* L., obtusifolin and gluco-obtusifolin, improved scopolamine-induced learning and memory impairment in mice based on the passive avoidance and Morris water maze tests [49]. Obtusifolin (0.25, 0.5, and 2 mg/kg) and gluco-obtusifolin (1, 2, and 4 mg/kg) significantly reversed scopolamine-induced cognitive impairment on the passive avoidance test; obtusifolin (0.5 mg/kg) and gluco-obtusifolin (2 mg/kg) improved escape latencies, swimming times in the target quadrant, and crossing numbers in the zone where the platform previously existed on the Morris water maze test [49]. The anti-AD properties of COE may be attributed to its constituents, such as anthraquinones and naphthopyrone glycosides. The methanolic seed extract and its solvent-soluble fractions from *C. obtusifolia* L. were tested for their acetylcholinesterase (AChE) and butyrylcholinesterase (BChE) inhibitory activities using Elman's method. Ethyl acetate and butanol fractions significantly inhibited AChE activity at a final concentration of 100 µg/mL, with IC_{50} values of 9.45 ± 0.44 and 9.87 ± 0.70 µg/mL, respectively. Butanol (IC_{50} = 7.58 ± 0.51 µg/mL) and ethyl acetate (IC_{50} = 16.09 ± 0.16 µg/mL) fractions exhibited potent inhibitory activity against BChE. Furthermore, butanol fraction (IC_{50} = 26.19 ± 0.72 µg/mL) significantly inhibited the β-secretase (BACE1) activity [10]. In addition, several anthraquinones (emodin, chrysophanol, physcion, obtusifolin, alaternin, questin, aloe-emodin) that displayed strong anti-AD activity by inhibiting AChE, BChE, and BACE1 enzymes were isolated from this plant [10]. Recently, Shrestha et al. [55] observed anti-AD effects of naphthopyrone and its glycosides including rubrofusarin, rubrofusarin 6-O-β-D-glucopyranoside, rubrofusarin 6-O-β-D-gentiobioside, nor-rubrofusarin 6-O-β-D-glucoside, isorubrofusarin 10-O-β-D-gentiobioside, and rubrofusarin 6-O-β-D-triglucoside by inhibiting AChE, BChE, and BACE1 enzymes. The use of AChE, BChE, and BACE1 inhibitors has been a promising treatment strategy for AD; therefore, *C. obtusifolia* may be an effective agent for treating AD.

3.1.2. Prevention and Treatment of Parkinson's Disease

A neuroprotective effect of COE was observed in both in vitro and in vivo models of Parkinson's disease [34]. In PC12 cells, COE reduced cell damage induced by 100 µM 6-hydroxydopamine and inhibited the overproduction of reactive oxygen species, glutathione depletion, mitochondrial membrane depolarization, and caspase-3 activation at 0.1 to 10 µg/mL. In addition, COE displayed radical scavenging effects in DPPH and ABTS assays, which suggests that COE may be useful for treating Parkinson's disease [34].

3.2. Hepatoprotective Activity

Few studies have demonstrated the hepatoprotective activities of COE [15]. Further studies are required to establish the hepatoprotective mechanisms of major COE anthraquinones. The protective effects of ethanolic COE against the cytotoxicity induced by CCl_4 liver in mice were evaluated by assessing aminotransferase activities, histopathological changes, hepatic and mitochondrial antioxidant indices, and cytochrome P450 2E1(CYP2E1) activity. Administration of COE (0.5, 1, 2 g/kg) markedly reduced ALT and AST release, Ca^{2+}-induced mitochondria membrane permeability transition, and CYP2E1 activity. In addition, COE significantly reduced hepatic and mitochondrial malondialdehyde levels, increased hepatic and mitochondrial glutathione levels, and restored superoxide dismutase, glutathione reductase, and glutathione S-transferase activities [15]. Meng et al. [38] reported the hepatoprotective effects of ethanolic COE on non-alcoholic fatty liver disease (NAFLD). Administration of COE (0.5, 1, 2 g/kg) markedly reduced the levels of AST, ALT, TG, TC, TNF-a, IL-6, IL-8, and MDA. COE treatments also increased the levels of SOD, GSH, and the expression of LDL-R mRNA [38]. Seo et al. [12] observed hepatoprotective effects of ethanolic COE and its components (e.g., toralactone glycoside) in *t*-BHP-induced cell death in HepG2 cells. *Cassia* anthraquinones, aurantio-obtusin, and obtusifolin also protected against tacrine-induced cytotoxicity in HepG2 cells [36]. Recently, Ali et al. [37] investigated the hepatoprotective effects of different soluble fractions of methanolic derived COE and its active components in *t*-BHP-induced oxidative stress in HepG2 cells. The possible mechanism was that alaternin, aloe emodin, and cassiaside potently scavenge ROS in *t*-BHP-induced HepG2 cells and the decrease in ROS generation parallels the up-regulation of glutathione (GSH). Very recently, Paudel et al. [57] investigated the hepatoprotective activity of an anthraquinone (1-desmethylaurantio-obtusin 2-O-β-D-glucopyranoside) and two naphthopyrone glycosides (rubrofusarin 6-O-β-D-apiofuranosyl-(1→6)-O-β-D-glucopyranoside and rubrofusarin 6-O-β-gentiobioside) isolated from the butanol fraction of COE in the t-BHP-induced oxidative stress in HepG2 cells through up-regulated HO-1 via the nuclear factor erythroid-2-related factor 2 (Nrf2) activation and modulation of the JNK/ERK/MAPK signaling pathway.

3.3. Anti-Inflammatory and Antioxidant Activity

COE has traditionally been used in Korea to treat eye inflammation, photophobia, and lacrimation. Pretreatment with the aqueous extract of *C. obtusifolia* L. inhibited interleukin (IL)-6 and cyclooxygenase-2 (COX-2) and reduced the activation of transcription nuclear factor-kB p65 in colon tissues treated with dextran sulfate sodium [40]. Two major anthraquinones from *C. obtusifolia*, obtusifolin and gluco-obtusifolin, reduced neuropathic and inflammatory pain [40]. Pro-inflammatory cytokines (e.g., TNF-α, IL-1β, IL-6) and activation of NF-kB have been strongly implicated in the initiation and development of inflammatory and neuropathic pain, and the administration of obtusifolin and gluco-obtusifolin (1 and 2 mg/kg) significantly inhibited this upregulation. This finding suggests that obtusifolin and gluco-obtusifolin inhibited the overexpression of spinal TNF-α, IL-1β, IL-6, and NF-κB p65 associated with inflammatory and neuropathic pain, which involves the regulation of neuroinflammatory processes and the neuroimmune system [51]. In another study, water-extracted polysaccharides (CP) from the whole seeds of *C. obtusifolia* L. and its two subfractions CP-30 and CP-40 were obtained. CP, CP-30, and CP-40 possessed immunomodulation activity by promoting phagocytosis and stimulating the production of nitric oxide (NO) and cytokines TNF-α and IL-6 [41]. Methanolic COE was investigated for antioxidant and health-relevant functionality. The extract exhibited 1292 mM Fe[II] per 1 mg/mL extract of antioxidant power, 49.92% inhibition of β-carotene degradation, 65.79% of scavenging activity against DPPH, and 50.78% of superoxide radicals (at a concentration 1 mg/mL). These antioxidant properties may be attributed to the total free phenolic content of the raw seeds, which was 13.33 ± 1.73 g catechin equivalent/100 g extract [14]. Recently, Kwon et al. [58] investigated the anti-inflammatory activity of major anthraquinone derivatives; among them, aurantio-obtusin inhibited iNOS expression without affecting iNOS enzyme activity and down-regulation mechanisms included interruption of the JNK/IKK/NF-κB activation and proinflammatory cytokine production from the lung-related cells. Additionally, aurantio-obtusin also dose-dependently (10 and 100 mg/kg) inhibited the inflammatory responses in a mouse model of airway inflammation, LPS-induced acute lung injury. Very recently, Hou et al. [54] reported anti-inflammatory activity by decreasing the production of NO, PGE2, and inhibiting iNOS, COX-2, TNF-α, and IL-6. Additionally, there was a reduction in the LPS-induced activation of nuclear factor-κB in RAW264.7 cells [54].

3.4. Antimicrobial Activity

Because many bacterial and fungal strains are resistant to a wide variety of antibiotics, medicinal plants have been studied for their potential antimicrobial properties. COE was active against several different microbes (*Bifidobacterium adolescentis*, *B. bifidum*, *B. longum*, *B. breve*, *Clostridium perfringens*, *Escherichia coli*, *Lactobacillus casei*). Isolated 1,2-dihydroxyanthraquinone strongly inhibited the growth of *C. perfringens* and *E. coli* and promoted the growth of *B. bifidum* [7]. The *C. obtusifolia* L. leaf extract in petroleum ether and chloroform showed sensitivity against *E. faecalis* (minimal inhibitory concentration [MIC] 0.2725 mg/mL), whereas ethanol extracts showed sensitivity against *A. fumigatus* (MIC 0.3116 mg/mL). Similarly, stem extracts of *C. obtusifolia* L. in petroleum ether showed sensitivity against *E. faecalis* (MIC 0.407 mg/mL), ethanol extracts showed sensitivity against *E. faecalis* (MIC 0.3009 mg/mL), and chloroform extracts showed sensitivity against *E. faecalis* MIC 0.4946 mg/mL [18]. The whole plant extract of *C. obtusifolia* significantly inhibited the growth of *Staphyloccocus aureus* MRSA8 (MIC 64 µg/mL), *E. coli* AG100 (MIC 256 µg/mL), *Pseudomonas aeruginosa* PA01 (MIC 256 µg/mL), *Enterobacter aerogenes* EA289

(MIC 289 µg/mL), and *Klebsiella pneumoniae* KP55 MIC 256 µg/mL [42]. Phytoalexin 2-(phydroxyphenoxy)-5,7-dihydroxychromone isolated from *C. obtusifolia* L. exhibited strong antifungal activity [31]. The *C. obtusifolia* L. root extract and its constituents exhibited strong antibacterial activity. Emodin, 2,5-dimethoxybenzoquione, questin, isotoralactone, and toralactone exhibited strong antibacterial activity against *S. aureus* 209P (MICs 4.5, 19, 25, and 3 µg/mL, respectively) and *E. coli* NIHJ MICs 25, 50, 50, 12, and 5.5 µg/mL, respectively [46].

3.5. Antidiabetic Activity

Two key enzymes, protein tyrosine phosphatase 1B (PTP1B) and α-glucosidase, are effective in treating diabetes mellitus. The effects of methanolic COE revealed inhibitory activities against PTP1B and α-glucosidase. Out of 15 anthraquinones from the extract, compounds with alaternin, physcion, chrysophanol, emodin, obtusin, questin, chryso-obtusin, aurantio-obtusin, 2-hydroxyemodin-1 methylether, gluco-obtusifolin, gluco-aurantio obtusin, and naphthalene glycoside aloe-emodin exhibited the highest inhibitory activities against PTP1B and α-glucosidase in vitro [9]. The effects of alaternin and emodin on the stimulation of glucose uptake by insulin-resistant human HepG2 cells were examined at concentrations ranging from 12.5 to 50 µM and 3.12 to 12.5 µM, respectively. In another study, five new anthraquinones were isolated from ethanol seed extracts of *C. obtusifolia* L. and evaluated for their antidiabetic activities through the inhibition of α-glucosidase in vitro [39]. Obtusifolin isolated from *C. obtusifolia* L. may have an antihyperlipidemic effect; an intraperitoneal obtusifolin injection reduced blood lipid levels in streptozotocin-induced diabetic rats [59]. Results from another study indicated that oral administration of obtusifolin significantly reversed the changes induced by hyperlipidemia in body weight, total cholesterol, triglycerides, low-density lipoprotein cholesterol, and high-density lipoprotein cholesterol; increased serum superoxide dismutase, and nitric oxide, and reduced malondialdehyde [50].

Recently, two new naphthalenic lactone glycosides(3S)-9,10-dihydroxy-7-methoxy-3-methyl-1-oxo-3,4-dihydro-1H-benzo[g]isochromene-3-carboxylic acid 9-O-β-D-glucopyranoside and (3R)-cassialactone 9-O-β-D-glucopyranoside were isolated from seeds of *C. obtusifolia* L. that showed significant inhibitory activities against the formation of advanced glycation end-products (AGEs) with IC_{50} values of 11.63 and 23.40 µM, respectively [60].

3.6. Antiplatelet Aggregation Inhibitory Activity

Ethanolic COE and three major anthraquinones (aurantio-obtusin, chryso-obtusin, and emodin) demonstrated inhibitory activity against ADP (adenosine 5′-diphosphate), arachidonic acid (AA), or collagen-induced platelet aggregation [47]. Methanolic COE and different solvent soluble fractions, including normal butanol (n-BuOH) and dicloromethane (CH_2Cl_2), exhibited antiplatelet aggregation activities. Furthermore, 17 anthraquinones, including gluco-obtusifolin, gluco-aurantio-obtusin, obtusifolin, and gluco-chryso-obtusin, were identified as active antiplatelet aggregation components [5].

3.7. Anticancer Activity

Polysaccharide COB1B1S2 and its sulfated derivative COB1B1S2-Sul were isolated from an alkaline COE. Human hepatocellular carcinoma cell lines Bel7402, SMMC7721, and Huh7, as well as HT-29 and Caco-2, were used to evaluate the anticancer effects of COB1B1S2 and COB1B1S2-Sul [61]. COB1B1S2 had a weak inhibitory effect on Bel7402, Huh7, HT-29, as well as Caco-2 cells. By contrast, COB1B1S2-Sul significantly inhibited the growth of all cell lines, particularly Bel7402 cells at 250 µg/mL; the inhibition ratio was 61.7% [62]. Three acetylated benzyl-beta-resorcylate glycosides (2-benzyl-4,6-dihydroxy benzoic acid-6-O-[2,6-O-diacetyl]-D-glucopyranoside, 2-benzyl-4,6-dihydroxy benzoic acid-6-O-[3,6-O-diacetyl]-D-glucopyranoside, and 2-benzyl-4,6-dihydroxy benzoic acid-6-O-[4,6-O-diacetyl]-D-glucopyranoside) were isolated from seeds of *C. obtusifolia* and exhibited significant cytotoxicity against a human hepatoblastoma cell line, with IC_{50} values of 4.6, 5.0, and 4.3 µg/mL, respectively [62]. In addition, 12 compounds were isolated from seeds of *obtusifolia* and their anticancer activities evaluated in multiple cancer cell lines [52]. 8-Hydroxy-1,7-dimethoxy-3-methylanthracene-9,10-dione-2-O-β-D-glucoside was active against HCT-116, A549, HepG2, SGC7901, and LO2 cell lines, with IC_{50} values of 4.5, 7.6, 22.8, 20.7, and 18.1 µg/mL, respectively. 6,8-Dihydroxy-1,7-dimethoxy-3-methylanthracene-9,10-dione-2-O-β-D-glucoside was only weakly active against HCT-116 (IC_{50}, 43.0 µg/mL). 1-Desmethylobtusin had moderate cytotoxicity against HCT-116, A549, and SGC7901 cell lines, with IC_{50} values of 5.1, 10, and 25.4 µg/mL, respectively. Chryso-obtusin showed significant cytotoxic activity against HCT-116, A549, SGC7901, and LO2 cell lines, with IC_{50} values of 10.5 to 15.8 µg/mL. Obtusin was moderately active against HCT-116, A549, and SGC7901 cell lines, with IC_{50} values of 13.1, 29.2, and 15.2 µg/mL, respectively. Aurantio-obtusin was moderately active against HCT-116, A549, SGC7901, and LO2 cell lines, with IC_{50} values of 18.9 to 22.0 µg/mL. Chryso-obtusin-2-O-β-D-glucopyranoside was selectively cytotoxic against HCT-116, A549, HepG2, SGC7901, and LO2 cell lines, with IC_{50} values of 5.8 to 14.6 µg/mL. Finally, aurantio-obtusin-6-O-β-D-glucopyranoside was weakly cytotoxic against HCT-116 and SGC7901, with IC_{50} values of 31.1 and 23.3 µg/mL, respectively [52].

3.8. Larvicidal Activity

The larvicidal activity of methanol COE against early fourth-stage larvae of *Aedes aegypti* and *Culex pipiens pallens* was investigated [43]. At 200 ppm, extracts of *C. obtusifolia* L. caused more than 90% mortality in larvae of *Ae. aegypti* and *Cx. pipiens pallens*. At 40 ppm, extracts of *C. obtusifolia* L. caused 51.4% and 68.5% mortality in fourth-stage larvae of *Ae. aegypti* and *Cx. pipiens pallens*, respectively. Larvicidal activity of *C. obtusifolia* extract at 20 ppm was significantly reduced [43]. In another study, COE obtained in different fractions showed mosquito larvicidal activity against fourth instar larvae of *A. aegypti*, *Aedes togoi*, and *Cx. pipiens pallens* [44]. However, the chloroform fraction of *C. obtusifolia* extracts exhibited a strong larvicidal activity of 100% mortality (at a concentration 25 mg/L), and the isolated active compound emodin showed strong larvicidal activity, with LC_{50} values of 1.4, 1.9, and 2.2 mg/L against *C. pipiens pallens*, *A. aegypti*, and *A. togoi*, respectively [44]. The ethanolic leaf extract of *C. obtusifolia* L. was also investigated for larvicidal and oviposition deterrence effects against late third instar larvae of *Anopheles stephensi* [45]. Extracts from the leaf displayed significant larvicidal activity, with LC_{50} and LC_{90} values of 52.2 and 108.7 mg/L, respectively (at concentrations of 25 mg/L). In addition, the oviposition study indicated that different concentrations of leaf extract greatly reduced the number of eggs deposited by gravid *A. stephensi*. At concentrations of 100, 200, 300, and 400 mg/L, the maximum percentages of effective repellency against oviposition were 75.5%, 83.0%, 87.2%, and 92.5%, respectively [45].

3.9. Other Activities

The methanol extract of *C. obtusifolia* L. and its isolated naphthopyrones cassiaside B2 and cassiaside C2 inhibited histamine release from rat peritoneal exudate mast cells induced by antigen–antibody reaction [6]. The anti-angiogenic activity of two polysaccharides, COB1B1S2 and COB1B1S2-Sul, from *C. obtusifolia* L. seeds was evaluated by tube formation of HMEC-1 cells on Matrigel. COB1B1S2 at 50 or 100 µg/mL did not impair tube formation, but COB1B1S2-Sul at 50 or 100 µg/mL significantly disrupted tube formation; even at 50 µg/mL, COB1B1S2-Sul could potentially completely inhibit tube formation in HMEC-1 cells [61]. Water-soluble polysaccharides (WSPs) from *C. obtusifolia* L. (pectic polysaccharides and hemicellulose) were identified. These WSPs reduced pancreatic α-amylase activity by 20.5% and 28.9% (at concentrations of 20 and 80 mg/mL, respectively), reduced pancreatic lipase activity by about 18.9% (at a concentration of 80 mg/mL), and increased protease activity 5- to 7-fold (at concentrations of 20 and 80 mg/mL, respectively). These WSPs were also able to bind bile acids and reduce the amount of cholesterol available for absorption [63]. The simultaneous determination and pharmacokinetic study of seven anthraquinones (chrysophanol, emodin, aloe-emodin, rhein, physcion, obtusifolin, and aurantio-obtusin) in rat plasma after oral administration of *C. obtusifolia* L. extract was investigated and may help to explain the bioactivity and clinical applications of *C. obtusifolia* L. [64]. The effects of COE and its anthraquinones on muscle mitochondrial function were evaluated in vivo in rats and in vitro using mitochondrial energy metabolism models. The organic extract of *C. obtusifolia* L. and emodin significantly inhibited NADH: cytochrome c oxidoreductase activity of bovine heart mitochondrial particles and NADH: coenzyme Q oxidoreductase activity of porcine heart mitochondrial NADH dehydrogenase and exhibited protective effects of coenzyme Q against enzyme inhibition by anthraquinones [65]. Inhibition of trypsin activity by *C. obtusifolia* L. seeds was investigated [66]. A Kunitz-type trypsin inhibitor showed strong resistance against the midgut trypsin-like protease of *Pieris rapae*. In addition, a trypsin inhibitor gene (*CoTI1*) was isolated from *C. obtusifolia* L. and exhibited dominant inhibitory activities against trypsin and trypsin-like proteases from *Helicoverpa armigera*, *Spodoptera exigua*, and *Spodoptera litura* [67]. Moreover, Dong et al. [68], has been also reported that Cassia semen (*C. obtusifolia* and *C. tora*) and its major constituents possesses a wide spectrum of pharmacological properties.

4. Conclusions and Perspectives

As presented in this review, pharmacological studies on *C. obtusifolia* L. and its putative active compounds, especially anthraquinones and naphthopyrone, support that several biological activities of *C. obtusifolia* can potentially impact human health. Anthraquinones and naphthopyrone can be effectively isolated and purified from *C. obtusifolia* seeds, leaves, root and its whole plant with various extraction analytical methods, mainly separation-based methods using TLC, HPLC, high-speed counter-current chromatography (HSCCC), and column chromatography (silica gel, reverse-phase, and Sephadex). The semi-shrubby herb *C. obtusifolia* L., which belongs to the family Leguminosae, has gained popularity because of its medicinal and historical importance. It has been widely used in traditional medicine to treat headaches, dizziness, dysentery, and eye disease. In addition, *C. obtusifolia* L. is important to the food industry and possesses a wide spectrum of pharmacological properties (e.g., anti-allergic, antidiabetic, anti-inflammatory, antimicrobial, antioxidant, hepatoprotective, neuroprotective, anti-Alzheimer's disease, antiplatelet aggregation, and larvicidal activities) that are associated with its diverse chemical constituents (e.g., anthraquinones, naphthopyrone, terpenoid, flavonoid, polysaccharides, and lipids). The number of modern studies on bioactive compounds is increasing in biomedicine, suggesting that these compounds might have great medical significance in the future. Although the bioactivities of seed extracts or compounds isolated from *C. obtusifolia* L. have been substantiated using in vitro and in vivo studies, the mechanisms of action remain unknown. Thus, there are still opportunities and challenges for research of seed extracts or compounds. Therefore, additional studies are required before *C. obtusifolia* L. and its components can be considered for further clinical use. In conclusion, *C. obtusifolia* L. is an edible medicinal plant that is important to the food industry and has a wide range of potential pharmacological uses. This review presents a summary of studies published to date on this promising plant.

Author Contributions: Conceptualization, M.Y.A.; data curation, M.Y.A.; writing—original draft preparation, M.Y.A.; review and editing, M.Y.A., S.P. and M.C. All authors have read and agreed to the published version of the manuscript.

Funding: This research did not receive any specific grant from funding.

Institutional Review Board Statement: Not applicable.

Informed Consent Statement: Not applicable.

Conflicts of Interest: All authors agree to the authorship and submission of the manuscript for peer review.

References

1. Sob, S.V.T.; Wabo, H.K.; Tchinda, A.T.; Tane, P.; Ngadjui, B.T.; Ye, Y. Anthraquinones, sterols, triterpenoids and xanthones from Cassia obtusifolia. *Biochem. Syst. Ecol.* **2010**, *38*, 342–345. [CrossRef]
2. Tang, L.; Wu, H.; Zhou, X.; Xu, Y.; Zhou, G.; Wang, T.; Kou, Z.; Wang, Z. Discrimination of Semen cassiae from two re-lated species based on the multivariate analysis of high-performance liquid chromatography fingerprints. *J. Sep. Sci.* **2015**, *38*, 2431–2438. [CrossRef] [PubMed]
3. Yanjun, H.; Yuli, S.; Yuqing, Z. The advancement of the studies on the seeds of Cassia obtusifolia. *Chin. Tradit. Herbal. Drugs.* **2001**, *32*, 858–859.
4. Li, Y.T.; Wang, Z.J.; Fu, M.H.; Yan, H.; Wei, H.W.; Lu, Q.H. A new anthraquinone glycoside from seeds of Cassia obtusifolia. *Chin. Chem. Lett.* **2008**, *19*, 1083–1085.
5. Yun-Choi, H.S.; Kim, J.H.; Takido, M. Potential Inhibitors of Platelet Aggregation from Plant Sources, V. Anthraquinones from Seeds of Cassia obtusifolia and Related Compounds. *J. Nat. Prod.* **1990**, *53*, 630–633. [CrossRef]
6. Kitanaka, S.; Nakayama, T.; Shibano, T.; Ohkoshi, E.; Takido, M. Antiallergic Agent from Natural Sources. Structures and Inhibitory Effect of Histamine Release of Naphthopyrone Glycosides from Seeds of Cassia obtusifolia L. *Chem. Pharm. Bull.* **1998**, *46*, 1650–1652. [CrossRef]
7. Sung, B.K.; Kim, M.K.; Lee, W.H.; Lee, D.H.; Lee, H.S. Growth responses of Cassia obtusifolia toward human intestinal bac-teria. *Fitoterapia* **2004**, *75*, 505–509. [CrossRef]
8. Kim, D.H.; Yoon, B.H.; Kim, Y.-W.; Lee, S.; Shin, B.Y.; Jung, J.W.; Kim, H.J.; Lee, Y.S.; Choi, J.S.; Kim, S.Y.; et al. The seed extract of Cassia obtusifolia ameliorates learning and memory impairments induced by scopolamine or transient cerebral hypoperfusion in mice. *J. Pharmacol. Sci.* **2007**, *105*, 82–93. [CrossRef]
9. Jung, H.A.; Ali, M.Y.; Choi, J.S. Promising Inhibitory Effects of Anthraquinones, Naphthopyrone, and Naphthalene Glycosides, from Cassia obtusifolia on α-Glucosidase and Human Protein Tyrosine Phosphatases 1B. *Molecules* **2017**, *22*, 28. [CrossRef]
10. Jung, H.A.; Ali, M.Y.; Jung, H.J.; Jeong, H.O.; Chung, H.Y.; Choi, J.S. Inhibitory activities of major anthraquinones and other constituents from Cassia obtusifolia against β-secretase and cholinesterases. *J. Ethnopharmacol.* **2016**, *191*, 152–160. [CrossRef]
11. Drever, B.D.; Anderson, W.G.; Riedel, G.; Kim, D.H.; Ryu, J.H.; Choi, D.-Y.; Platt, B. The seed extract of Cassia obtusifolia offers neuroprotection to mouse hippocampal cultures. *J. Pharmacol. Sci.* **2008**, *107*, 380–392. [CrossRef] [PubMed]
12. Seo, Y.; Song, J.-S.; Kim, Y.-M.; Jang, Y.P. Toralactone glycoside in Cassia obtusifolia mediates hepatoprotection via an Nrf2-dependent anti-oxidative mechanism. *Food Res. Int.* **2017**, *97*, 340–346. [CrossRef] [PubMed]
13. Doughari, J.H.; El-mahmood, A.M.; Tyoyina, I. Antimicrobial activity of leaf extracts of Senna obtusifolia (L.). *Afr. J. Pharm. Pharmacol.* **2008**, *2*, 7–13.
14. Vadivel, V.; Kunyanga, C.N.; Biesalski, H.K. Antioxidant Potential and Type II Diabetes-Related Enzyme Inhibition of Cassia obtusifolia L.: Effect of Indigenous Processing Methods. *Food Bioprocess Technol.* **2012**, *5*, 2687–2696. [CrossRef]
15. Xie, Q.; Guo, F.F.; Zhou, W. Protective effects of cassia seed ethanol extract against carbon tetrachloride-induced liver in-jury in mice. *Acta Biochem. Pol.* **2012**, *59*, 265–270.
16. Kirtikar, K.R.; Basu, B.D. *Indian Medicinal Plant*; Lalit Mohan Basu Press: Allahabad, India, 2006.
17. Sob, S.V.T.; Wabo, H.K.; Tane, P.; Ngadjui, B.T.; Ma, D. A xanthone and a polyketide derivative from the leaves of Cassia obtusifolia (Leguminosae). *Tetrahedron* **2008**, *64*, 7999–8002. [CrossRef]
18. Deshpande, S.R.; Naik, B.S. Evaluation of in vitro antimicrobial activity of extracts from Cassia obtusifolia L. and Senna so-phera (L.) Roxb against pathogenic organisms. *J. Appl. Pharm. Sci.* **2016**, *6*, 83–85. [CrossRef]
19. Paudel, P.; Seong, S.H.; Shrestha, S.; Jung, H.A.; Choi, J.S. In vitro and in silico human monoamine oxidase inhibitory po-tential of anthraquinones, naphthopyrones, and naphthalenic lactones from Cassia obtusifolia Linn seeds. *ACS Omega* **2019**, *4*, 16139–16152. [CrossRef]
20. Dave, H.; Ledwani, L. A review on anthraquinones isolated from Cassia species and their applications. *Indian, J. Nat. Prod. Resour.* **2012**, *3*, 291–319.
21. Harry-O'Kuru, R.E.; Mohamed, A. Processing scale-up of sciklepod (Senna obtusifolia L.) seed. *J. Agri. Food Chem.* **2009**, *57*, 2726–2731. [CrossRef] [PubMed]
22. Wu, Y.V.; Abbott, T.P. Gum and protein enrichment from sciklepod (Cassia obtusifolia) seed by fine grinding and sieving. *Ind. Crops. Prod.* **2005**, *21*, 387–390. [CrossRef]
23. Abbott, T.P.; Vaughu, S.F.; Dowd, P.F.; Mojtahedi, H.; Wilson, R.F. Potential uses ofsciklepod (Cassia obtusifolia). *Ind. Crops. Prod.* **1998**, *8*, 77–82. [CrossRef]
24. Kitanaka, S.; Takido, M. Studies on the constituents of the seeds of Cassia obtusifolia: The structures of two new lactones, isotoralactone and cassialactone. *Phytochemistry* **1981**, *20*, 1951–1953. [CrossRef]
25. Wu, X.-H.; Ruan, J.-L.; Cheng, C.-R.; Wu, Z.-Y.; Guan, S.-H.; Tao, S.-J.; Xu, P.-P.; Guo, D.-A. Benzyl-β-resorcylates from Cassia obtusifolia. *Fitoter.* **2010**, *81*, 617–620. [CrossRef]
26. Zhang, C.; Wang, R.; Liu, B.; Tu, G. Structure elucidation of a sodium salified anthraquinone from the seeds of Cassia obtusifolia by NMR technique assisted with acid-alkali titration. *Magn. Reson. Chem.* **2011**, *49*, 529–532. [CrossRef]
27. Wu, X.-H.; Cai, J.-J.; Ruan, J.-L.; Lou, J.-S.; Duan, H.-Q.; Zhang, J.; Cheng, C.-R.; Guo, D.-A.; Wu, Z.-Y.; Zhang, Y.-W. Acetylated anthraquinone glycosides from Cassia obtusifolia. *J. Asian Nat. Prod. Res.* **2011**, *13*, 486–491. [CrossRef]

28. Pang, X.; Li, N.-N.; Yu, H.-S.; Kang, L.-P.; Yu, H.-Y.; Song, X.-B.; Fan, G.-W.; Han, L.-F. Two new naphthalene glycosides from the seeds of Cassia obtusifolia. *J. Asian Nat. Prod. Res.* **2018**, *21*, 970–976. [CrossRef] [PubMed]
29. Pang, X.; Wang, L.M.; Zhang, Y.C.; Kang, L.P.; Yu, H.S.; Fan, G.W.; Han, L.F. New anthraquinone and eurotinone ana-logue from the seeds of Senna obtusifolia and their inhibitory effects on human organic anion transporters 1 and 3. *Nat. Prod. Res.* **2018**, *4*, 1–8.
30. Feng, L.; Yin, J.Y.; Nie, S.P.; Wan, Y.Q.; Xiea, M.Y. Enzymatic purification and structure characterization of glucuronoxy-lan from water extract of Cassia obtusifolia seeds. *Int. J. Biol. Macromol.* **2018**, *107*, 1438–1446. [CrossRef] [PubMed]
31. Sharon, A.; Ghirlando, R.; Gressel, J. Isolation, Purification, and Identification of 2-(p-Hydroxyphenoxy)-5,7-Dihydroxychromone: A Fungal-Induced Phytoalexin from Cassia obtusifolia. *Plant Physiol.* **1992**, *98*, 303–308. [CrossRef]
32. Guo, H.; Chang, Z.; Yang, R.; Guo, D.; Zheng, J. Anthraquinones from hairy root cultures of Cassia obtusifolia. *Phytochemistry* **1998**, *49*, 1623–1625. [CrossRef]
33. Kim, D.H.; Kim, S.; Jung, W.Y.; Park, S.J.; Park, D.H.; Kim, J.M.; Cheong, J.H.; Ryu, J.H. The neuroprotective effects of the seeds of Cassia obtusifolia on transient cerebral global ischemia in mice. *Food Chem. Toxicol.* **2009**, *47*, 1473–1479. [CrossRef] [PubMed]
34. Ju, M.S.; Kim, H.G.; Choi, J.G.; Ryu, J.H.; Hur, J.; Kim, Y.J.; Oh, M.S. Cassiae semen, a seed of Cassia obtusifolia, has neuroprotective effects in Parkinson's disease models. *Food Chem. Toxicol.* **2010**, *48*, 2037–2044. [CrossRef] [PubMed]
35. Yi, J.H.; Park, H.J.; Lee, S.; Jung, J.W.; Kim, B.C.; Lee, Y.C.; Ryu, J.H.; Kim, D.H. Cassia obtusifolia seed ameliorates amyloid β-induced synaptic dysfunction through anti-inflammatory and Akt/GSK-3β pathways. *J. Ethnopharmacol.* **2016**, *178*, 50–57. [CrossRef] [PubMed]
36. Byun, E.; Jeong, G.S.; An, R.B.; Li, B.; Lee, D.S.; Ko, E.K.; Yoon, K.H.; Kim, Y.C. Hepatoprotective compounds of Cassiae Semen on tacrine-induced cytotoxicity in HepG2 cells. *Korean, J. Pharmacogn.* **2007**, *38*, 400–402.
37. Ali, M.Y.; Jannat, S.; Jung, H.A.; Min, B.-S.; Paudel, P.; Choi, J.S. Hepatoprotective effect of Cassia obtusifolia seed extract and constituents against oxidative damage induced by tert-butyl hydroperoxide in human hepatic HepG2 cells. *J. Food Biochem.* **2018**, *42*, e12439. [CrossRef]
38. Meng, Y.; Liu, Y.; Fang, N.; Guo, Y. Hepatoprotective effects of Cassia semen ethanol extract on non-alcoholic fatty liver disease in experimental rat. *Pharm. Biol.* **2019**, *57*, 98–104. [CrossRef]
39. Xu, Y.-L.; Tang, L.-Y.; Zhou, X.-D.; Zhou, G.-H.; Wang, Z.-J. Five new anthraquinones from the seed of Cassia obtusifolia. *Arch. Pharmacal Res.* **2014**, *38*, 1054–1058. [CrossRef] [PubMed]
40. Kim, S.-J.; Kim, K.-W.; Kim, D.-S.; Kim, M.-C.; Jeon, Y.-D.; Kim, S.-G.; Jung, H.-J.; Jang, H.-J.; Lee, B.-C.; Chung, W.-S.; et al. The Protective Effect of Cassia obtusifolia on DSS-Induced Colitis. *Am. J. Chin. Med.* **2011**, *39*, 565–577. [CrossRef] [PubMed]
41. Feng, L.; Yin, J.; Nie, S.; Wan, Y.; Xie, M. Fractionation, physicochemical property and immunological activity of poly-saccharides from Cassia obtusifolia. *Int. J. Biol. Macromol.* **2016**, *91*, 946–953. [CrossRef] [PubMed]
42. Voukeng, I.K.; Beng, V.P.; Kuete, V. Antibacterial activity of six medicinal Cameroonian plants against Gram-positive and Gram-negative multidrug resistant phenotypes. *BMC Complement. Altern. Med.* **2016**, *16*, 388. [CrossRef] [PubMed]
43. Jang, Y.-S.; Baek, B.-R.; Yang, Y.-C.; Kim, M.-K.; Lee, H.-S. Larvicidal activity of leguminous seeds and grains against Aedes aegypti and Culex pipiens pallens. *J. Am. Mosq. Control. Assoc.* **2002**, *18*, 210–213.
44. Yang, Y.C.; Lim, M.Y.; Lee, H.S. Emodin isolated from Cassia obtusifolia (Leguminosae) seed shows larvicidal activity against three mosquito species. *J. Agri. Food. Chem.* **2003**, *51*, 7629–7631. [CrossRef] [PubMed]
45. Rajkumar, S.; Jebanesan, A. Larvicidal and oviposition activity of Cassia obtusifolia Linn (Family: Leguminosae) leaf ex-tract against malarial vector, Anopheles stephensi Liston (Diptera: Culicidae). *Parasitol. Res.* **2009**, *104*, 337–340. [CrossRef] [PubMed]
46. Kitanaka, S.; Takido, M. Studies on the constituents in the roots of Cassia obtusifolia L. and the antimicrobial activities of aonstituents of the roots and the seeds. *Yakugaku Zasshi* **1986**, *106*, 302–306. [CrossRef]
47. Yun-Choi, H.S.; Lee, J.R.; Kim, J.H.; Kim, Y.H.; Kim, T.H. Potential inhibitors oplatelet aggregation from plant sources, IV. Anthraquinones from seeds of Cassia obtusifolia and related compounds. *Korean. J. Pharmacogn.* **1987**, *18*, 203–206.
48. Shin, B.Y.; Kim, D.H.; Hyun, S.K.; Jung, H.A.; Kim, J.M.; Park, S.J.; Kim, S.Y.; Cheong, J.H.; Choi, J.S.; Ryu, J.H. Alater-nin attenuates delayed neuronal cell death induced by transient cerebral hypoperfusion in mice. *Food Chem. Toxicol.* **2010**, *48*, 1528–1536. [CrossRef] [PubMed]
49. Kim, N.H.; Hyun, S.K.; Yoon, B.H.; Seo, J.-H.; Lee, K.-T.; Cheong, J.H.; Jung, S.Y.; Jin, C.; Choi, J.S.; Ryu, J.H. Gluco-obtusifolin and its aglycon, obtusifolin, attenuate scopolamine-induced memory impairment. *J. Pharmacol. Sci.* **2009**, *111*, 110–116. [CrossRef] [PubMed]
50. Zhuang, S.-Y.; Wu, M.-L.; Wei, P.-J.; Cao, Z.-P.; Xiao, P.; Li, C.-H. Changes in Plasma Lipid Levels and Antioxidant Activities in Rats after Supplementation of Obtusifolin. *Planta Medica* **2016**, *82*, 539–543. [CrossRef]
51. He, Z.-W.; Wei, W.; Li, S.-P.; Ling, Q.; Liao, K.-J.; Wang, X. Anti-allodynic effects of obtusifolin and gluco-obtusifolin against inflammatory and neuropathic pain: Possible mechanism for neuroinflammation. *Biol. Pharm. Bull.* **2014**, *37*, 1606. [CrossRef]
52. Shi, B.-J.; Zhang, W.-D.; Jiang, H.-F.; Zhu, Y.-Y.; Chen, L.; Zha, X.-M.; Lu, Y.-Y. A new anthraquinone from seed of Cassia obtusifolia. *Nat. Prod. Res.* **2016**, *30*, 35–41. [CrossRef]
53. Vishnuprasad, C.N.; Tsuchiya, T.; Kanegasaki, S.; Kim, J.H.; Han, S.S. Aurantio-Obtusin stimulates chemotactic migra-tion and differentiation of MC3T3-E1 osteoblast cells. *Planta Med.* **2014**, *80*, 544–549.
54. Hou, J.; Gu, Y.; Zhao, S.; Huo, M.; Wang, S.; Zhang, Y.; Qiao, Y.; Li, X. Anti-Inflammatory Effects of Aurantio-Obtusin from Seed of Cassia obtusifolia L. through Modulation of the NF-κB Pathway. *Molecules* **2018**, *23*, 3093. [CrossRef] [PubMed]

55. Shrestha, S.; Seong, S.H.; Paudel, P.; Jung, A.H.; Choi, J.S. Structure related inhibition of enzyme systems in cholinester-ases and BACE1 in vitro by naturally occurring naphthopyrone and its glycosides isolated from Cassia obtusifolia. *Molecules* **2018**, *23*, 69. [CrossRef] [PubMed]
56. Paudel, P.; Kim, D.; Jeon, J.; Park, S.; Seong, S.; Jung, H.; Choi, J. Neuroprotective Effect of Aurantio-Obtusin, a Putative Vasopressin V_{1A} Receptor Antagonist, on Transient Forebrain Ischemia Mice Model. *Int. J. Mol. Sci.* **2021**, *22*, 3335. [CrossRef]
57. Paudel, P.; Jung, H.A.; Choi, J.S. Anthraquinone and naphthopyrone glycosides from Cassia obtusifolia seeds mediate hepatoprotection via Nrf2-mediated HO-1 activation and MAPK modulation. *Arch. Pharm. Res.* **2018**, *41*, 677–689. [CrossRef] [PubMed]
58. Kwon, K.S.; Lee, J.H.; So, K.S.; Park, B.K.; Lim, H.; Choi, J.S.; Kim, H.P. Aurantio-obtusin, an anthraquinone from cassiae semen, ameliorates lung inflammatory responses. *Phytother. Res.* **2018**, *32*, 1537–1545. [CrossRef] [PubMed]
59. Tang, Y.; Zhong, Z. Obtusifolin Treatment Improves Hyperlipidemia and Hyperglycemia: Possible Mechanism Involving Oxidative Stress. *Cell Biophys.* **2014**, *70*, 1751–1757. [CrossRef] [PubMed]
60. Shrestha, S.; Paudel, P.; Seong, S.H.; Min, B.S.; Seo, E.K.; Jung, H.A.; Choi, J.S. Two new naphthalenic lactone glyco-sides from Cassia obtusifolia L. seeds. *Arch. Pharm. Res.* **2018**, *41*, 737–742. [CrossRef] [PubMed]
61. Cong, Q.; Shang, M.; Dong, Q.; Liao, W.; Xiao, F.; Ding, K. Structure and activities of a novel heteroxylan from Cassia ob-tusifolia seeds and its sulfated derivative. *Carbohydr. Res.* **2014**, *393*, 43–50. [CrossRef] [PubMed]
62. Wu, X.; Ruan, J.; Yang, V.C.; Wu, Z.; Lou, J.; Duan, H.; Zhang, Y.J.; Zhang, A.; Guo, D. Three new acetylated ben-zyl-beta-resorcylate glycosides from Cassia obtusifolia. *Fitoterapia* **2012**, *83*, 166–169. [CrossRef] [PubMed]
63. Huang, Y.-L.; Chow, C.-J.; Tsai, Y.-H. Composition, characteristics, and in-vitro physiological effects of the water-soluble polysaccharides from Cassia seed. *Food Chem.* **2012**, *134*, 1967–1972. [CrossRef]
64. Yang, C.; Wang, S.; Guo, X.; Sun, J.; Liu, L.; Wu, L. Simultaneous determination of seven anthraquinones in rat plasma by ultra-high-performance liquid chromatography–tandem mass spectrometry and pharmacokinetic study after oral admin-istration of semen cassiae extract. *J. Ethnopharmacol.* **2015**, *169*, 305–313. [CrossRef] [PubMed]
65. Lewis, D.C.; Shibamoto, T. Effects of Cassia obtusifolia (sicklepod) extracts and anthraquinones on muscle mitochondrial function. *Toxicon* **1989**, *27*, 519–529. [CrossRef]
66. Liao, H.; Ren, W.; Kang, Z.; Jiang, J.-H.; Zhao, X.-J.; Du, L.-F. A trypsin inhibitor from Cassia obtusifolia seeds: Isolation, characterization and activity against Pieris rapae. *Biotechnol. Lett.* **2007**, *29*, 653–658. [CrossRef]
67. Liu, Z.; Zhu, Q.; Li, J.; Zhang, G.; Jiamahate, A.; Zhou, J.; Liao, H. Isolation, structure modeling and function characteri-zation of a trypsin inhibitor from Cassia obtusifolia. *Biotechnol. Lett.* **2015**, *37*, 863–869. [CrossRef]
68. Dong, X.; Fu, J.; Yin, X.; Yang, C.; Zhang, X.; Wang, W.; Du, X.; Wang, Q.; Ni, J. Cassiae semen: A review of its phyto-chemistry and pharmacology. *Mol. Med. Rep.* **2017**, *16*, 2331–2346. [CrossRef] [PubMed]

MDPI AG
Grosspeteranlage 5
4052 Basel
Switzerland
Tel.: +41 61 683 77 34

Molecules Editorial Office
E-mail: molecules@mdpi.com
www.mdpi.com/journal/molecules

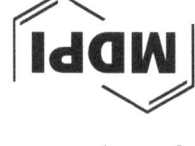

Disclaimer/Publisher's Note: The title and front matter of this reprint are at the discretion of the Guest Editors. The publisher is not responsible for their content or any associated concerns. The statements, opinions and data contained in all individual articles are solely those of the individual Editors and contributors and not of MDPI. MDPI disclaims responsibility for any injury to people or property resulting from any ideas, methods, instructions or products referred to in the content.

www.ingramcontent.com/pod-product-compliance
Lightning Source LLC
LaVergne TN
LVHW072312090526
838202LV00019B/2270